Cesarean Delivery

Cesarean Delivery

Editors

Jeffrey P. Phelan, MD
Associate Professor
Department of Obstetrics and Gynecology
University of Southern California School of Medicine
Los Angeles

Steven L. Clark, MD
Director, Maternal–Fetal Medicine
Utah Valley Regional Perinatal Center
Provo

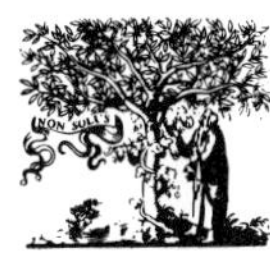

Elsevier
New York • Amsterdam • London

Elsevier Science Publishing Co., Inc.
52 Vanderbilt Avenue, New York, New York 10017

Distributors outside the United States and Canada:
Elsevier Science Publishers B.V.
P.O. Box 211, 1000 AE Amsterdam, the Netherlands

Library of Congress Cataloging-in-Publication Data

Cesarean delivery / editors, Jeffrey P. Phelan, Steven L. Clark.
p. cm.
Includes index.
ISBN 0-444-01304-0
1. Cesarean section. 2. Cesarean section—Complications and sequelae.
I. Phelan, Jeffrey P. II. Clark, Steven L.
[DNLM: 1. Cesarean Section. WQ 430 C4213]
RG761.C457 1988
618.8'6–dc19
DNLM/DLC
for Library of Congress

88-7154
CIP

Current printing (last digit):
10 9 8 7 6 5 4 3 2 1

Manufactured in the United States of America

This textbook is dedicated to
our wives, Marilyn and Kersten,
and their cesarean births

Kelly
Shane
Shannon
Jed
Benjamin
Erika
Christopher

Contents

Foreword

During the past 40 years, the practice of obstetrics has undergone remarkable changes. The introduction of new therapies, such as antibiotics and blood transfusions, has made pregnancy safer for women than driving a car. The safety of surgical procedures has also improved dramatically. With mothers' health almost guaranteed, the next obstetric emphasis was to improve the outcome for infants. New technologies and advances, such as electronic fetal monitoring, ultrasound, and amniocentesis, have made evaluation of the fetus safe, practical, and reliable. During these same years, a concern developed about overpopulation; this was addressed with the development of new contraceptive and sterilization methods. These methods allowed couples to control the size of their families; the result has been a parental expectation of a small family with all children being healthy.

The explosive inflation of medical–legal decisions against health care providers when damaged or dead infants resulted from a pregnancy further modified the practice of obstetrics towards defensive, regionalized, and nontraumatic approaches. The overall change in delivery techniques has been the near disappearance of operative deliveries such as version and extraction of second twins, vaginal breech deliveries, and difficult midforcep rotations. The replacement procedure has been the cesarean. It is anticipated that during the 1990s infants will be delivered either easily and spontaneously via the vagina or by cesarean. Currently, cesarean delivery is used in approximately 25% of all deliveries. The four conditions of fetal distress—failure to progress in labor, prior cesarean birth, and breech presentation—make up 85% of the current indications.

Despite these remarkable changes in the practice of obstetrics, there is no comprehensive textbook on cesarean delivery. This volume by Drs. Phelan and Clark fills that void with a comprehensive, current, and in-depth review of all aspects of the topic. Important chapters written by recognized experts in perinatal medicine include discussions of current indications for the procedure, operative techniques, and common and unusual complications. Other important topics are included such as prophylactic antibiotic usage and vaginal delivery after a prior cesarean. This book is recommended to all who practice obstetrics; it is clearly a benchmark for the specialty as it moves into the 21st century, when the only operative delivery with which residents will have significant experience will be cesarean delivery.

William N. Spellacy, MD

Professor and Chairman
Department of Obstetrics and Gynecology
University of Illinois College of Medicine
Chicago

Preface

Cesarean delivery is a complex issue. Unlike other specialists, obstetricians are unique in that they must simultaneously manage the care of two and sometimes more individuals. When deciding whether or not vaginal delivery is prudent, the attending physician must balance the effects the route of delivery might have not only on the pregnant woman, but also her fetus. The balancing is not limited to the events that surround the birth, but includes the downstream consequences associated with each route of delivery. Once the balancing is done, cesarean delivery may be indicated for the patient, her fetus, or both. This is reflected in the fact that there are at least 25 separate indications for a cesarean delivery. To add to the complexity—especially in the United States today—is the constant threat of medical malpractice litigation. In many respects, the 200% rise in cesarean births may be due to these influences.

We hope that this text will provide a perspective that addresses these complexities in a logical and clinically oriented way. The text is, therefore, a comprehensive compilation of current information regarding all aspects of cesarean delivery. The book is designed to progress along a path from indications for cesarean delivery to anesthetic and surgical techniques associated with cesarean birth to postoperative complications. The book then shifts its focus to concentrate on ways to reduce the cesarean delivery rate by exploring options such as external cephalic version and vaginal birth after cesarean and concludes with pertinent ethical and legal considerations of cesarean birth. By choosing this approach, we hope to provide practicing clinicians and residents in training with both a reference book and a common-sense, practical guide to the clinical management of patients who may require a cesarean. To ensure clinical relevance we invited contributors actively involved in clinical care as well as cesarean research.

We are grateful to Jane Licht, senior editor, Elsevier Science Publishing Co., for her support and constant encouragement during the preparation of this text. Additionally, we are extremely grateful for the secretarial assistance of Fiona Sung, Rosie Curtis, and Cheryl Lake. We are also deeply indebted to Myoung Ock Ahn, MD, for her editorial and graphic support evident throughout this text.

Jeffrey P. Phelan, MD
Steven L. Clark, MD

Contributors

Richard Anane, MD
Department of Obstetrics and Gynecology, Komfo Anokye Teaching Hospital, Kumasi, Ghana

Garland D. Anderson, MD
Professor and Director, Maternal–Fetal Medicine, Department of Obstetrics and Gynecology, University of Tennessee, School of the Health Sciences, Memphis

David L. Barclay, MD
Clinical Professor, Department of Obstetrics and Gynecology, University of Arkansas, Little Rock

Harbinder S. Brar, MD
Assistant Professor, Maternal–Fetal Medicine, Department of Obstetrics and Gynecology, University of Southern California School of Medicine, Los Angeles

Robert C. Cefalo, MD, PhD
Professor and Director, Maternal–Fetal Medicine, Department of Obstetrics and Gynecology, University of North Carolina, Chapel Hill

Frank A. Chervenak, MD
Associate Professor, Director of Obstetric Ultrasound and Ethics, New York Hospital–Cornell Medical Center, New York

Judith L. Chervenak, MD
Maternal–Fetal Medicine, Department of Obstetrics and Gynecology, New Jersey College of Medicine and Dentistry, Newark

Steven L. Clark, MD
Director, Maternal–Fetal Medicine, Utah Valley Regional Perinatal Center, Provo

Charles Drescher, MD
Department of Obstetrics and Gynecology, University of Michigan Medical School, Ann Arbor

Patrick Duff, MD
Director, Division of Maternal–Fetal Medicine, Madigan Army Medical Center, Tacoma, Washington

Gary S. Eglinton, MD
Assistant Professor and Director, Maternal–Fetal Medicine, Uniformed Services, University of the Health Sciences, F. Edward Hebert School of Medicine, Bethesda, Maryland

Thomas E. Elkins, MD MAR
Associate Professor, Chief of Gynecology, Department of Obstetrics and Gynecology, University of Michigan Medical School, Ann Arbor

Stanley A. Gall, MD
Professor and Vice Chairman, Department of Obstetrics and Gynecology, University of Illinois College of Medicine, Chicago

Stanley A. Gall, Jr, MD
Department of Surgery, Duke University Medical Center, Durham, North Carolina

Donald G. Gallup, MD
Associate Professor, Section of Gynecologic Oncology, Department of Obstetrics and Gynecology, Medical College of Georgia, Augusta

Larry C. Gilstrap III, MD
Associate Professor and Director, Maternal–Fetal Medicine, Department of Obstetrics and Gynecology, University of Texas Health Science Center, Dallas

Steven H. Golde, MD
Director of Perinatal Services, St. Joseph's Hospital, Burbank, California

Gary D.V. Hankins, MD
Chairman and Program Director, Department of Obstetrics and Gynecology, Wilford Hall United States Air Force Medical Center, Lackland Air Force Base, Texas

Janet Horenstein, MD
Assistant Professor, Department of Obstetrics and Gynecology, University of Southern California School of Medicine, Los Angeles

Vern L. Katz, MD
Assistant Professor, Department of Obstetrics and Gynecology, University of North Carolina, Chapel Hill

William L. Koontz, MD
Assistant Director, Maternal–Fetal Medicine, Department of Obstetrics and Gynecology, Charlotte Memorial Hospital, Charlotte, North Carolina

J.O. Martey, MD
Professor and Chairman, Department of Obstetrics and Gynecology, Komfo Amokye Teaching Hospital, Kumasi, Ghana

Stephen D. Minton, MD
Director, Utah Valley Regional Perinatal Center, Provo

Thomas R. Moore, MD
Director, Perinatal Medicine, Department of Obstetrics and Gynecology, Naval Regional Medical Center, San Diego

Richard H. Paul, MD
Professor and Director, Maternal–Fetal Medicine, Department of Obstetrics and Gynecology, University of Southern California School of Medicine, Los Angeles

Richard P. Perkins, MD
Professor, Department of Obstetrics and Gynecology and Pediatrics, University of Nevada School of Medicine, Las Vegas

Jeffrey P. Phelan, MD
Associate Professor, Department of Obstetrics and Gynecology, University of Southern California School of Medicine, Los Angeles

Richard P. Porreco, MD
Associate Clinical Professor, Department of Obstetrics and Gynecology, University of Colorado Health Sciences Center; Director, St. Luke's/Children's Perinatal Program, Denver

Susan E. Rutherford, MD
Head of Perinatal Services, Department of Obstetrics and Gynecology, Naval Regional Medical Center, Portsmouth, Virginia

David A. Sacks, MD
Director, Divison of Maternal–Fetal Medicine, Department of Obstetrics and Gynecology, Kaiser Foundation Hospital, Bellflower, California

Carl V. Smith, MD
Director, Labor and Delivery Service, Division of Maternal–Fetal Medicine, Department of Obstetrics and Gynecology, Naval Hospital, Bethesda, Maryland

O. Eduardo Talledo, MD
Professor, Director, Section of Gynecologic Oncology, Department of Obstetrics and Gynecology, Medical College of Georgia, Augusta

L. Magnus R. Westgren, MD
Associate Professor, Department of Obstetrics and Gynecology, Karolinska Institute, Danderyd Hospital, Danderyd, Sweden

Chapter 1

History and Evolution of Cesarean Delivery

Vern L. Katz, MD, and
Robert C. Cefalo, MD, PhD

Cesarean delivery has its origins in prehistoric times. Though anecdotal reports of operations on living women are sprinkled throughout written history during the Middle Ages and Renaissance, only in the late 18th and early 19th centuries was the cesarean seriously considered for living women. Until the last century, cesarean delivery was performed only as a last resort, when vaginal delivery seemed impossible, or postmortem. Most physicians condemned the procedure because of its devastating associated mortality due to hemorrhage and sepsis. In the late 19th century, with the emergence of aseptic techniques and with the acceptance of the revolutionary idea of suturing the uterus, mortality from the operation began to decline. In the 100 years from 1886 to 1986, mortality from cesarean birth has decreased from nearly 100% to less than 1 in 1,000 operations. One recent series reported over 10,000 cesarean deliveries without a maternal death. As mortality has declined, the incidence and indications for cesareans have risen until, in 1985, a physician asked in *The New England Journal of Medicine*, "If an informed patient opts for prophylactic cesarean section at term, can it be denied?"[1]

This chapter outlines and highlights the evolution of cesarean delivery from ancient, oral, and mythological tradition through the current literature. Though most myths about the operation have been lost over time, some have remained and affect our day-to-day approach to this procedure. The evolution of cesarean delivery has, more often than not, reflected the scientific and social environments of the time, from the Church edicts of the Middle Ages requiring postmortem sections on all women who died in childbirth to the recent rise in the incidence of the operation, which many authorities feel reflects the medicolegal pressures of our time.

THE MYTHOLOGY AND FOLKLORE OF ABDOMINAL DELIVERIES

The birth of an infant through an opening in the mother's abdomen has been known since before the period of written history. Stories and legends from cultures throughout the world describe such miraculous births. These myths are exaggerations of reality derived from human experience. Most of the early references are related to the birth of heroes and gods, demonstrating their superhuman origins. Often, but not always, the deliveries were performed as the mother was dying or was already dead. Thompson's *Motif Index of Folk Literature* references legends about abdominal deliveries to English, Egyptian, Persian, Hindu, Malagasy, Haitian, Greek, North American Indian, Oceanic, Patagonian, Central American, and Finnish cultures.[2]

Indo-European mythology is especially marked by references to abdominal birth. Greek mythology describes two notable postmortem sections. Dionysus, the Greek god of wine (in Latin, Bacchus) was delivered prematurely from his dying mother, Semele. Semele was set on fire when Zeus, Dionysus' father, in a fit of jealousy, threw a lightning bolt at her. Hermes, the obstetrician, transplanted Dionysus into the thigh of Zeus. (The thigh in ancient cultures was often used synonymously with the testicle.) Dionysus later emerged full-grown and was named in Latin "Bacchus-Dithrambicus," Dionysus of two gateways. This reference from Ovid's *Metamorphosis* may be the earliest known reference to embryo transfer. Asclepius, the first physician, whose staff was the caduceus, was delivered by his father, Apollo, from the dead nymph Koronis. Rustan, the Persian equivalent of Hercules, was delivered as a 10-lb, 10-oz baby through an incision; his mother did well. Brahma and Buddha were also said to be born through their mother's flanks. All were born by deliberate operations in which the mother survived.[3]

An argument for the prehistoric origins of cesarean delivery can be found in the accounts of explorers and primitive tribes. In 1887, Dr. Robert Felkin witnessed an African shaman in what is now Uganda performing a cesarean delivery on a living woman who survived. The tribal doctor used banana wine as a disinfectant and anesthetic. He did not suture the uterus, but did pin and suture the abdominal wall.[4]

The Talmud, a codification of Jewish law, written in the first few centuries AD, contains several discussions of abdominal delivery. Maimonides, in referring to the Talmud, explained in his commentaries that the operation was performed on living women: "a woman who cannot bear a child in the natural way, shall be opened in the side, and in this way delivered of her offspring."[5,15] The birthrights of twins delivered by section and postpartum purification rites of women having cesarean births are also considered.

The Fah-Nameh, completed in 999 AD by Firdausi, is a textbook of

Persian medicine. It describes a cesarean: "Bring thou a blue steel dagger, . . . bemuse the lady first with wine to ease her pain and fear . . . take the lion from his lair by piercing her waist while all unconscious. Then imbuing her side in blood, stitch up the gash."

Written references to postmortem cesarean section occur several hundred years prior to Christ. Numa Pompilus in 715 BC decreed the "Lex Regis de Inferendo Mortis," which stated that when a pregnant woman died, she should be delivered as quickly as possible to try to save the child. Pliny the Elder referred to the birth of Scipio Africanus, the Roman general who defeated Hannibal, by postmortem section.[6] Over the next millennium, several important persons were said to be born by postmortem cesarean: Gorgias of Sicily, Robert II of Scotland, Andrea Doria the Genovese admiral, Pope Gregory XIV, and Bishop Paulus of Spain.[7]

Shakespeare in the play *Macbeth* refers to a postmortem section. Macbeth, fearing no "man of woman born," is told in the last scene by his adversary, MacDuff, "I was from my mother's womb untimely ripped" (untimely because she died).[8]

ORIGINS OF THE TERM "CESAREAN SECTION"

The origin of the term "cesarean section" has been a disputed issue for the past 200 years. The first written reference to it was by Rousset in 1581 in his treatise on cesarean birth, "Trainte, Nouveau Day L'hysterotomotokie ou L'Enfantement Cesarien." Jacques Guillimeau called such deliveries "sections" in 1598, and thereafter the two terms were joined so that the operation became known as a "cesarean section."[6] Because an interest in Greek and Roman tradition was revived during the Renaissance, the birth of Caesar became a popular motif for painters and writers. One explanation of the origin of the term is that it was named for Julius Caesar. However, Julius Caesar was most likely not delivered abdominally, as was commonly thought during the Renaissance and Enlightenment. We must presume that most sections were fatal to the mother, and Julius Caesar's mother was corresponding with him during his campaigns in northern Europe 30 years later.

Another theory of the derivation of the term refers to the Roman law known as the "Lex Regis," mentioned above, mandating postmortem sections. This law was later referred to as the "Lex Cesare" when the Roman kings became known as the "Roman Caesars."

A third explanation is that "cesarean" refers to the term "to cut," which in Latin is "cadere." In ancient Rome, children born by abdominal delivery were referred to as "caesones." The term "cesarean section" is therefore a tautology.[6] This term has survived into modern times. However, in 1981, the consensus report of the National Institute of Child Health Development of the National Institutes of Health recommended adoption of the term "cesarean birth."

CESAREAN DELIVERY FROM THE MIDDLE AGES THROUGH THE MID-1800S

Postmortem cesarean deliveries were described in midwifery textbooks as early as the 14th century. The *Chirurgia*, written in 1363 by Guy de Cauliac, describes "*de extractione foetus*" as a postmortem procedure.[5] The operation, though, was not suggested or known to be practiced on a living woman until the 16th century. Allegedly, the first successful operation was performed by a Swiss sow gelder, Jacob Nufer, on his wife in the year 1500. She survived, bearing more children and dying of noniatrogenic causes at the age of 77.[3] In 1540 Christopher Bane of Italy performed a cesarean delivery on a woman who survived, but the infant was stillborn.[9] The first authenticated cesarean delivery was performed in 1610 by Jeremiah Trautmann of Saxony. The woman died 25 days after the procedure. In none of these three cases were sutures used on the uterus.[10]

Two important obstetric works appeared in the sixteenth century advocating cesarean delivery on living women in cases where the woman would not otherwise be able to deliver. Francois Rousset, the physician of the Duke of Saxony, advocated the use of cesarean section. He recommended the extraction of the child through a left lateral incision in the abdomen and a median vertical incision in the uterus. Rousset described 15 successful operations, though he had not performed or witnessed any of them. The reason for the use of a left paramedial abdominal incision was to avoid injuring the liver. Rousset recommended against the use of uterine sutures, which he stated caused peritonitis. It is noteworthy that Rousset advocated cesarean delivery because the most renowned physician of the time, Ambrose Pare, spoke out against its use on the living woman.[5,11]

Scipione Mercurio in 1596 published the first Italian guide to obstetrics, *La Comare o Riciglitrice*. This book was reprinted 40 times over the next 200 years.[12] It contains several illustrations describing cesarean delivery. Mercurio suggested that the operation be used for women with contracted pelvises. He also recommended against the use of uterine sutures. Despite Mercurio's and Rousset's works, the operation was performed only rarely on living women over the next 200 years. From 1500 to 1769, only 76 cases with maternal recovery were reported in the European literature.[13]

During this time, cesarean deliveries were not attempted unless the woman had been in labor for a very long time and was unable to deliver vaginally. Maternal mortality from both hemorrhage and infection was overwhelming. The emotions associated with the almost inevitable subsequent maternal death were so great that debates arose regarding the appropriateness and ethics of the operation. These debates were more bitter than anything else in the medical literature to that time. Jean Louis

Baudelocque, an advocate of cesarean delivery in 1790, was called an assassin and a murderer by Jean Francois Sacombe. Sacombe was the leader of an anticesarean society that had been formed in France. Baudelocque accused Sacombe of slander, and Sacombe was found guilty. He was forced to flee France for his life.[3,14] In England in 1754, Pugh declared that advocates of cesarean operations were "sporting with lives." In the Hull–Simmons debates in England in the 1790s, Simmons said that the operation "can never be justified during the patient's life."[15,16] Between 1750 and 1800, only 24 sections were reported in France. During the last quarter of the 18th century, many physicians in Europe, notably France, turned to symphysotomy and improved methods of craniotomy rather than perform cesarean deliveries. By 1865, the mortality rate from cesareans in the British Isles was 85%. In Paris over 90% of cesarean deliveries performed in the 17th and 18th centuries were fatal. During the 100-year period ending in 1880, no woman survived a cesarean delivery in Vienna.[6,17]

From the Middle Ages through the mid-19th century, postmortem cesarean deliveries were performed routinely. The Catholic Church mandated removal of the baby from the body of a pregnant woman who died for the purposes of baptism. Rarely was a liveborn infant reportedly salvaged. Church edicts proclaimed that postmortem sections should be performed by all physicians attending a birth where the mother died. These edicts were issued in Cologne in 1280, in Langres in 1404, and in Sens in 1514.[9] Such official edicts were continued by state governments throughout the 19th century in the spirit of the ancient Roman Lex Regis, in the slight hope of preserving the infant. Venice in 1608, Frankfurt in 1786, and Bavaria in 1816 were three of the many European states that enacted laws mandating cesarean delivery on women who died in childbirth.[18]

THE MODERN DEVELOPMENT OF THE CESAREAN

The modern cesarean operation was developed between the late 19th century and the first three decades of the 20th century. During this period, three developments accounted for the reduction in maternal mortality from cesarean delivery from close to 100% to 2%. These three developments were the adoption of the use of uterine sutures to arrest hemorrhage, the adoption of aseptic technique, and changes in operative technique from the classical to lower-segment operations. The basis for aseptic technique was established during the mid-19th century by Lister, Pasteur, and Semmelweiss. With the adoption of asepsis during this period, important improvements were made in mortality rates. Infection was controlled not only by more attention to aseptic technique but also by the development of lower-segment incisions on the uterus in attempts to limit the spread of contaminated fluid into the peritoneal cavity. Physicians began to emphasize and perform cesarean deliveries prior to the onset of labor when the pelvis was contracted, noting that the longer a woman was in labor, the greater the mortality of the operation.

In 19th-century Europe, the only suture materials used were permanent. Any sutures placed were left long and brought out through the abdominal incision, to be removed postoperatively. Surgeons of the time felt that such material was the cause of peritonitis. Since Rousset's time, the bleeding uterus was thought to contract enough on its own to stop hemorrhage. Sutures, it was thought, would only tear the uterus as it involuted. Ramsbotham, in the English textbook of 1847, *Principles and Practice of Obstetric Medicine and Surgery*, stated, "On the uterine cavity being evacuated, the organ will contract more or less perfectly. Hemorrhage will thus be prevented; . . . and there will be no need of sutures to bring the edges of the uterine womb together."[19]

Jean Lebas in Paris in 1769 was the first surgeon to actually place sutures in the uterus to control hemorrhage. He used three individual silk strands. However, until Max Sanger published on the subject in 1886, the predominant thinking in Europe was that suturing was definitely unnecessary and also dangerous. It was the Americans, on the "frontier of civilization," who began in isolated cases to suture the uterus. Frank Polin of Springfield, Kentucky, was the first of several American surgeons to use silver wire in 1852.[3] Eastman summarized the contribution of these obstetricians in the development of uterine sutures. He discussed 16 cases between 1867 and 1880 where sutures were used by American surgeons. When linen and silk sutures were used, they were left long, brought out through the lower portion of the abdominal womb, and removed 4–6 days postpartum. When silver wire was used, the suture was cut short and buried.[20] American surgeons advocated the use of sutures not only to control hemorrhage interoperatively, but also to inhibit the escape of potentially infecting lochia into the peritoneum. Harris, summarizing the American experience through 1877, discussed 100 cesarean operations, with a maternal mortality of 56%. In his summary he recommended, "To arrest uterine hemorrhage and prevent its return, suture the uterus with silver wire."[21]

In 1882, Max Sanger of Leipzig, an assistant to Crede, published "Der Kaiserschnitt bei Uterusfibromen nebst vergleichender Methodik der Sectio Caesarea und der Porro-Operation." This 200-page work explained the principles and techniques of cesarean section, with careful attention to a 2-step uterine closure with meticulous hemostasis: "The exact closure of the entire uterine womb by a 2-level suture, the lower tier of which is to comprise the whole uterine wall without passing through the cavity of the organ, while the superficial tier placed between the deeper stitches merely unites the surfaces of the serous edge, both tiers to be so close and so numerous as to assure an absolutely perfect reunion of the uterine womb, its covering with peritoneum. . . . The uterus after the suture must be like an uninjured organ." Sanger's landmark publication on cesarean section included a tabulation and review of the American cases.[22]

Sanger's methods included aseptic preparatory steps, such as disinfection of the abdominal wall with a thorough cleansing, and a midline abdominal incision. The uterus was opened and the baby delivered with the uterus inside the abdominal cavity. After delivery of the placenta, it was lifted out for suturing. Sanger advocated incising the uterus in a medial, vertical line, avoiding the lower uterine segment. After the baby was delivered, he recommended either placing an elastic ligature around the lower uterine segment or performing manual compression of the lower uterine segment to prevent bleeding while the uterus was cleansed and sutured. He performed a manual detachment of the placenta and then a disinfection of the uterine cavity with iodoform. He then utilized the two layers of sutures as described above. He recommended silver wire for suture of the deep layer; usually 8–10 were sufficient for the deep stitches. The superficial serosal sutures of fine silk, 10–30 in number, were cut short. If silver wire was not available, deep sutures could be made with strong aseptic silk. (These were also cut short.) Sanger then recommended washing the sutured uterus with an iodine solution and powdering the suture in with an iodoform solution. The uterus was to be replaced in the abdomen only after all bleeding was stopped. He did not recommend draining the abdominal womb, but did use an iodoform dusting of the incision after it was closed. He recommended the use of ergotin if postpartum hemorrhage was a problem.[22,23]

Sanger's work was revolutionary in its emphasis on uterine suture and the fact that the suture could be buried. He disavowed the growing tendency toward the cesarean hysterectomy (discussed below). Sanger felt that his procedure would eliminate the dangers of hemorrhage and sepsis that the cesarean hysterectomy had been developed to combat. Sanger was not the first to use uterine suture. The importance of his work is that he brought the use of uterine suture to the obstetric community's attention, and thus is known as the father of the modern cesarean delivery.

The adoption of Sanger's work led to an explosion in the number and success of cases of cesarean delivery and a silencing of the opposition to the operation on living women. In 1887, Crede reported 57 cases with a 77% survival. Zweifel chronicled 278 cases in Germany from 1889 to 1899 with a 93.3% maternal survival.[24] In the first edition of Williams' *Obstetrics* in 1904, cesarean delivery was presented as a standard technique in the practice of obstetrics.[25] Medical historians have come to feel that the publication of Sanger's work advocating uterine sutures for hemostasis was the turning point in the history of cesarean delivery.

Attempts to prevent mortality from sepsis led to changes in the technique of the operation. In the early 19th century, DeWees wrote that all that was necessary for "cleansing" was that the abdomen be lavaged with warm water mixed with laurel and henbane to remove foreign material and that pressure be kept on the abdominal walls so that the intestines would not seep out during the operation.[26] By 1879, with the work of Lister and Pasteur accepted into the mainstream of medicine, Harris recommended "antiseptic treatment."[22] Sanger reaffirmed in 1880 that "I, as well as surgery in general, have extensively utilized the blessings of antisepsis." Williams wrote in 1904: "This marvelous diminution in the mortality [from cesareans] is due to several factors. Primarily, of course, it must be attributed to the ever-increasing perfection of aseptic techniques."[27] Throughout the 19th century, physicians, no matter how unsophisticated regarding the etiologies of infection, were aware that the mortality from the operation was directly proportional to the amount of time the patient was in labor. Physicians writing on the subject emphasized the importance of operating very early in labor and even electively. In 1904 Williams stated: "The prospects for recovery decrease in almost geometric ratio for every hour elapsing . . . [after the onset of labor]."[28]

In conjunction with better asepsis, surgeons of the 19th and early 20th centuries felt that if the uterine incision could be separated from the peritoneal cavity, the mortality due to infection would be reduced. The extraperitoneal cesarean, the lower uterine segment incision, and the cesarean hysterectomy are three important modifications that began as attempts to limit peritoneal contamination.

The extraperitoneal approach of cesarean delivery was suggested during the first decade of the 19th century by both Bell in England and Baudelocque, though neither of them performed the operation on living patients.[6] In 1820, von Ritgen also suggested the operation, performing it in 1821 and calling the operation a "gastro-elytrotomy."[29] He made a perimedian incision in the abdominal wall and approached the uterus laterally. The vagina and the lower cervix were incised vertically to deliver the baby. Unfortunately his patient died. In 1824 DeWees, in his textbook of obstetrics, published a letter from an anatomist, W.E. Horner, regarding an extraperitoneal approach, that described a midline abdominal incision, displacing the bladder medially from its peritoneal covering.[13] Although this operation was discussed several times over the next 45 years, it was not until 1870 that it was attempted again by Thomas in New York. The patient did not survive. Skene successfully performed the operation on a patient whose diagonal conjugate measured 2.75 in. the following year. The mother did well, as did her 10-lb baby.[30,31] Several successful extraperitoneal sections were performed over the next 10 years, with a less than 50% mortality.[32] In 1907, Frank in Cologne reported 13 cases with no deaths, with an extraperitoneal approach and a transverse lower uterine segment incision. In the next 8 years, Latzko and Sellheim published modifications of Frank's technique.[31,32] In 1912 Kronig argued that the good results of Frank's extraperitoneal sections were primarily due to the location of the incision in the lower uterine segment.[33] There less blood loss, less peritoneal contamination, and better wound healing. He suggested suturing together the visceral and serosal peritoneums before incising the uterus to decrease peritoneal contamination.[34] In the United States in the 1930s, Waters and Norton refined the extraperitoneal section to its present form.[35,36] Most of such operations currently performed use their approaches, although with the advent of antibiotics, the incidence of the extraperitoneal approach has sharply declined.

The surgical technique of incising the uterus in the lower uterine or "cervical" segment was developed initially to decrease pelvic contamination. As it became more popular, several advantages over the classical section were appreciated. The lower uterine segment incision was suggested as early as 1786 by the English obstetrician Johnson and reintroduced by Freidrich Ossiander in 1818.[3] However, Kehrer in 1882 was the first obstetrician to perform the low transverse incision.[3,32] Fritz Frank in 1907 advocated its use with extraperitoneal sections.[37] As mentioned above, Kronig helped to popularize Frank's lower uterine incision in 1912, and used a modification of uniting the peritoneal flaps. In 1919 Beck published a report of 107 cases with a 3.8% mortality using a lower segment vertical incision with careful reperitonealization after the uterus was closed.[38] The two most important advocates of the lower uterine segment incision in this century were Kerr and DeLee. Kerr, writing in 1926, felt that not only was there less infection, postoperative ileus, and bleeding with the lower segment approach, but also less uterine rupture and fewer adhesions. Speaking before the 51st meeting of the American Gynecologic Society, he argued against the "unsatisfactory nature of the uterine scar after the ordinary longitudinal incision."[39] DeLee, in the sixth edition of his very popular textbook, stated in 1933 that the classical fundal cesarean delivery was "rapidly passing into discard."[17]

Perhaps the most interesting modification suggested to avert peritoneal contamination was the "Portes" operation described in the 1920s. In this approach, the uterus was brought out of the abdomen and the abdominal incision was closed and sutured before the uterus was incised. The baby was then delivered, and the uterus was sewn up and left to involute for 4 weeks extra-abdominally. After a month the uterus and adnexa were replaced in the abdomen in a separate operation. The Portes operation was reserved for situations where "frank infection is present. . . . Infection in a dead child, . . . when any manner [of delivery] through the birth canal might rupture the uterus, [or in the] presence of a pelvic indication for abdominal delivery with fetal putrefaction."[40]

The technique of cesarean hysterectomy, like that of extraperitoneal and lower segment incisions, was initially developed to combat mortality due to infection. The first discussions of a cesarean hysterectomy were presented by Joseph Cavallini of Florence in 1768. He performed the operation on animals, but not on women. Other advocates of the potential benefits of the procedure were Machaelis in 1809, Blundell in 1823, and Feser in 1862.[41] All worked only on animals. In 1869, Horatio Storer in Boston was the first physician to perform the operation on a woman. The uterus was removed supracervically, and the stump was ligated and marsupialized into the abdominal wound for drainage. Three days later the patient died.[42] Eduardo Porro in 1876 performed the first successful cesarean hysterectomy on a living woman. In his procedure the cervical stump was also marsupialized into the abdominal wall. When the report of this procedure was published in Europe, Sanger had not yet published his work emphasizing careful uterine suturing. Porro's procedure was hailed as the answer to problems of both hemorrhage and infection. Three years after this procedure was published, Harris summarized 29 cases worldwide.[43] By 1880, 50 cases had been reported. With the improved mortality of Sanger's technique, enthusiasm for cesarean hysterectomies waned. Porro's procedure became known as the "radical cesarean" and Sanger's became known as the "conservative cesarean." From 1876 to 1900, several surgical improvements were developed in order to decrease bleeding, such as Oppenheimer's recommendation in 1880 to clamp the uterine vessels.[42] In the 1890s, the modification was adopted of replacing the cervical stump in the abdomen after covering it with the posterior peritoneum, thus eliminating the gaping scar left by the marsupialized cervical stump.[42] Although cesarean hysterectomy was never as popular as the more conservative cesarean section, it remained an important alternative in patients with severe infection. Through 1922, in 223 cesarean operations at Johns Hopkins Hospital, there were 64 (29%) cesarean hysterectomies, the maternal mortality of which was 4.7%. This low mortality is remarkable in that cesarean hysterectomy was done primarily for infection at the time of surgery. This could be compared with a 22.8% maternal mortality reported in 1891 by R.T. Harris. In 1943, total cesarean hysterectomy began to replace the subtotal variety. In Davis' address in 1951 to the American Gynecologic Society, he called the complete cesarean hysterectomy "a logical advancement in modern obstetric surgery" over the subtotal hysterectomy. He reported on 140 cesarean hysterectomies from 1947 to 1951, 100 of which were complete.[44] Since that time, it has been the exception to perform a subtotal cesarean hysterectomy.

CESAREAN DELIVERY IN THE 20TH CENTURY

The development of the cesarean in this century has been characterized by (1) adoption of the low transverse uterine incision, to the exclusion of the myriad techniques developed in the previous century; (2) increasing indications and increasing incidence of the operation; and (3) an ongoing debate, only recently resolved, about the acceptability of vaginal delivery after cesarean operation. The first two themes will be discussed in the following section; the last will be discussed in Chapters 31–35. The use of modern anesthetic techniques and of blood banking were important improvements in all fields of surgery. The contribution to improved mortality rates is obvious. Anesthesia for cesareans will be discussed in Chapters 10 and 11. With the advent of modern surgical techniques, the mortality from cesarean operations fell dramatically. The technically more difficult, potentially more hemorrhagic extraperitoneal sections lost favor. The uterine eversion of Portes never caught on, and the desire for future fertility limited the use of cesarean hysterectomy. A cervical or lower uterine approach was popularized early in the century by Beck, Kerr, and DeLee. Debating its advantages throughout the 1920s, Kerr wrote in 1926, "Practically all writers have been forced to the conclusion that in a fair percentage of cases the scar, of the ordinary longitudinal incisions, is not satisfactory."[39] The same year, Beck quoted a study of 1,015 classic operations with a maternal mortality of 5.9% and 187 low cervical sections with a mortality of 4.2%.[45] Williams took a slightly more conservative approach in his textbook in 1930. He stated that the lower cervical operation was "somewhat more difficult than the classical operation; it gives excellent results and is the procedure of choice whenever cesarean section is performed six or more hours after the onset of labor. If, however, the patient shows signs of actual infection, much better maternal results are obtained if the body of the uterus is amputated."[46] He wrote later in the chapter that the extraperitoneal section presents "no advantage over the low cervical operation. I have ceased to make use of it."[47] William Danforth, in his discussion of the classical cesarean versus the low cervical in 1936, stated, "It seems to me that the cervical operation is definitely superior to the classical, not only from the standpoint of mortality but also from the standpoint of morbidity."[48] Verch in 1950 reported on 1,231 cesareans performed in a private hospital in Milwaukee from 1933 to 1947. In the period 1933–1937, 60% were low cervical, compared to 92.5% in the period 1947–1957.[49] Douglas, reporting on the results at the New York Lying-In Hospital over the same period, 1933–1947, stated, "From 1933 to 1937, the classical type and a low flap were used with about equal frequency; since 1937 the low flap has greatly superseded all other techniques."[50]

When the operative mortality and morbidity from cesareans fell, the incidence of cesareans rose. The indications for the operation were quickly expanded. In the 1904 edition of *Obstetrics*, Williams argued that the "relative indications to perform surgery be broadened in appropriate cases, and its upper limit placed at a conjugate vera of 8.5 centimeters."[25] Twenty-five years later, Williams listed 4 pages of indications for cesarean delivery.[51] Indeed, the rapid acceptance and increased practice of the operation by the obstetric community led to acrimonious debate. Goldstone wrote in 1937, "Cesarean section is practiced by some as if it were merely an alternate method to normal delivery."[52] The *New York Obstetric Re-*

port in 1943, taking a more moderate position, stated, "Cesarean section is one of the greatest blessings to womankind. It is its abuse that must be deplored."[53] Maternal mortality due to cesarean operation prior to the time of Porro and Sanger was close to 100%. By 1890 the reported mortality was close to 25%; by 1900 it was approximately 10%.[54] Alfred Beck in 1919 reported on a series from Brooklyn with a 3.8% maternal mortality.[38] By 1940 the "acceptable maternal mortality" was 1%.[55]

The New York Obstetric Society in 1933 presented an important survey to the New York Academy of Sciences on maternal mortality throughout the city. In that review of deliveries from 1929 to 1933, 2.2% of all patients were reportedly delivered by cesarean operation. However, 19.8% of all maternal deaths were secondary to the procedure.[52] This figure may be compared to the 0.2% incidence of cesarean delivery in New York in 1910.[56,57] Of cesarean-related deaths, 48% were due to infection, 21% to shock, 8% to toxemia, 8% to hemorrhage, 2% to other causes, and 13% to nonobstetric causes.[55] The authors found that 4.76% of classic sections were fatal, compared to only 1.26% of low cervical sections. In addition, 82% of maternal deaths due to cesarean operations were considered preventable. The advisory committee of the New York Academy of Sciences concluded: "(1) there was an excessive use of cesarean section; (2) classical operation should be limited to elective use."[58]

Maternal mortality due to cesareans continued to decline throughout the next 2 decades. Temple Hospital from 1931 to 1940 had a 1% mortality due to cesarean delivery.[57] The New York Lying-In Hospital from 1932 to 1948 had a 1% mortality in 230 operations. The 1943–1947 period contained 45% of the operations and had no maternal deaths.[51] Anthony D'Esopo reported on 1,266 cases from 1942 to 1947, with only 1 maternal death due to cesarean delivery.[59] The relative causes of death changed as infection became better controlled. In the period 1937–1950 in the United States, 28% of cesarean deaths were due to anesthesia. Prior to that time, less than 1% were due to this cause.[60]

In the period 1950–1965, maternal mortality due to cesarean operations reached a plateau between 0.2 and 0.3%. Physicians at the New York Lying-In Hospital reported a 0.26% mortality.[61] At the University of Southern California from 1948 to 1974, the mortality associated with cesarean delivery was 0.27%.[62] In Britain in 1964 it was 0.13%; in 1974, 0.07%. In the 17th edition of Williams' *Obstetrics*, published in 1985, the authors state, "Maternal mortality from cesarean section should be less than 1 per 1,000."[63] They cite the experience of the Boston Lying-In Hospital, with over 10,000 cesarean operations and no deaths due to the operation. In the approximately 100 years from the time of Max Sanger's report in 1882, maternal mortality has dropped from nearly 100% to less than 1 per 1,000.

As the mortality due to the operation declined, obstetricians found more and more reasons to operate. The biggest shift in thinking occurred in the 1930s and 1940s when surgery began to be performed for the baby's safety, a concept previously ignored. In the sixth edition of Williams' *Obstetrics*, in the section on indications for cesarean delivery, there is no mention of an indication for fetal reasons.[51] At the New York Lying-In Hospital in the period 1933–1937, only 0.8% of the surgeries were done because of fetal distress.[50] In 1956, 11% of the surgeries were performed for fetal reasons.[61] At the University of Southern California, in the period 1948–1953, 4.5% of sections could be considered to have been performed for the baby's sake. The three groups of fetal indications for surgery include breech and other abnormal presentations, fetal distress, and potentially traumatic vaginal manipulations, specifically by midforceps. This switch from vaginal to abdominal deliveries for breech presentations is a phenomenon of the last 15 years. At the Los Angeles County Hospital, breech deliveries accounted for 2% of cesarean operations in 1949, 4% in 1965, and 22% in 1970.[62]

The second indication that accounts for much of the increased incidence of cesarean delivery in this century is repeat cesarean section. This will be covered in detail in Chapters 8 and 30–34. To summarize briefly here, a committee from the American College of Surgeons studied the problem in 1963 and reported that repeat cesarean delivery accounted for 35% of all sections in the United States. From 40% to 50% of all cesarean deliveries in New York in 1963 were repeats.[64] At Los Angeles County Hospital prior to 1970, with a policy of awaiting labor, repeat cesarean section represented 50% of the operations.[62] Prior to 1930, when mortality from the operation was significant, a repeat procedure was unadvisable. Williams wrote in 1930, "The 'Once a cesarean, always a cesarean' dictum: I do not entirely agree with such teaching." In 1920–1929 at Johns Hopkins, less than 6% of cesareans were performed because they were repeat sections.[65] By the 1940s, when mortality had dropped to less than 1%, the risk of the procedure made repetition of the operation more attractive. Obviously, the more primary cesareans performed, the greater the number of repeat sections. The increase in repeat operations occurred at the same time that low cervical operations replaced the classical cesarean in popularity. Ironically, the advocates of low cervical cesareans lobbied in the literature for its adoption because of the better healing and decreased incidence of rupture of the uterus. DeLee stated in 1933: "Rupture of the uterus and subsequent labor is much rarer than after the classical operation."[66] This inherent contradiction was forgotten for close to 50 years.

Cesarean deliveries accounted for only a tiny fraction of deliveries until the end of the first two decades of the century. In all New York hospitals in 1910, cesarean deliveries accounted for only 2 per 1,000 deliveries. From 1910 to 1930, the cesarean delivery rate rose steadily. By 1927 it represented 2.5 per 100 deliveries. In the Chicago Lying-In Hospital in 1910 the incidence was 6 per 1,000. In 1928 it was 3 per 100. In 1929 in Boston it was 3.4 per 100.[55] Private hospitals throughout the country always accounted for more cesarean deliveries than public hospitals. In 1933–1937, at the Milwaukee Hospital private service, the cesarean delivery rate was 7.4%, though there was less than a 3% overall cesarean rate in that city.[49] From 1941 to 1950 at Columbia University's Sloan Hospital in New York, the overall cesarean rate was 5.8%, 4.5% in the public service and 7.7% in the private service.[57] From 1934 to 1943, the incidence at the Boston Lying-In Hospital was 3.1% in the ward service and 6.7% in the private service.[49] In the obstetric community by 1940, the cesarean rate stood at approximately 2.5%. By 1950 it had risen to 5%. In 1950 Verch wrote, "We consider an incidence of 5% to 5.5% the irreducible minimum to which the operative treatment can be reduced under our present indications for cesarean section."[49] In 1963 R. Gordon Douglas wrote, "For the most part an incidence of approximately 5% is considered optimal."[64] The rise in rate remained gradual from 1950 to 1969. At the Los Angeles County Hospital it was 5.3% in 1965.[62] The cesarean delivery rate in the United States in 1970 was still only 5.5%. In Canada in 1972 it was 7.5%.[67] However, from 1970 to 1980, the rate began to rise again, this time much more sharply. At the Los Angeles County Hospital in 1974, it was 9.1%.[62] In the United States overall in 1970, the rate had risen to 15.2%. In Canada the rate had risen to 13.9% in 1979.[67] At Parkland Hospital in Dallas in 1983, the cesarean delivery rate was 18.3%.[63] The overall cesarean delivery rate in the United States in 1984 was 21.6% and is expected to approach 30% in 1988.

THE EVOLUTION OF POSTMORTEM DELIVERIES

The evolution of postmortem sections since 1500 has paralleled that of cesarean delivery on living women. Throughout the Middle Ages and into the Renaissance, the Catholic Church, for the purpose of baptism, mandated the performance of postmortem sections. Throughout the 17th and 18th centuries, edicts were issued by both the papal and municipal authorities requiring its use.[18] The King of Sicily in 1747 condemned a physician to death for not performing one.[18] However, the fetal salvage rate was minimal. In a series in 1836 in Germany, 107 cases of postmortem section were reported, with no fetal survivors. A London hospital report from the first quarter of the 19th century reported 331 operations with 19 infant survivors. A series from 1837 in France found 49 operations and only seven infants surviving. In 1864 the Berlin Obstetric Society's report listed 147 cases of postmortem section with only three infant survivors.[18] This procedure evoked so much disgust and furor that a strong debate arose in the 1850s echoing the debate about cesarean delivery on the living. Scanzoni in 1861 stated, "The fetus in utero is the same as any other internal organ of the woman. If we recognize the instance of the death of the mother, when all organic expression is gone, and organic laws yield to chemical laws, that instance we must recognize also the death

TABLE 1.1 Postmortem Cesarean Deliveries with Surviving Infants[a]

Cases (min)	No. of Patients	Percent
0–5	42 (normal infants)	70
6–10	7 (normal infants) 1 (mild neurologic sequelae)	13
Subtotal	8	
11–15	6 (normal infants) 1 (severe neurologic sequelae)	12
Subtotal	7	
16–20	1 (severe neurologic sequelae)	1.7
21+	2 (severe neurologic sequelae) 1 (normal infant)	3.3
Subtotal	2	
Total	60	100

[a] Reports of time from death of the mother until delivery (cases from 1900 to 1985).[68]

of the child."[18] The debates over the operation's usefulness lasted into the 20th century. However, all major textbooks continued to advocate the operation, since surviving infants were continually being reported. Since 1879 there have been 269 cases of postmortem sections in the English literature, with 188 infants surviving.[68] Medicolegal authorities in this century have concluded that the operation does not need the consent of a family member and is indicated any time that a viable fetus or the potential for one exists.[68]

The percentages of infants surviving in relation to the time of cesarean delivery after maternal death are presented in Table 1.1. Almost all survivors have been delivered within 5 minutes of maternal death. Several cases of maternal recovery after cardiopulmonary arrest and after cesarean operation have been documented in the literature. DeLee cited the first such case in his textbook in 1933.[66]

This phenomenon is secondary to the removal of obstruction of the vena cava by delivery of the infant, allowing venous return. If a woman has cardiopulmonary arrest, the supine position is often the only position in which cardiopulmonary resuscitation is performed.[68] But in the supine position the gravid uterus inhibits venous return, significantly decreasing cardiac output. Since only delivery of the infant restores the potential for adequate cardiac output with cardiopulmonary resuscitation, and since brain damage may occur within 4–6 minutes, both in the mother and in the baby, we have suggested the 4-minute rule: "Cesarean delivery should be begun within 4 minutes, and the baby delivered within 5 minutes after maternal cardiac arrest."[68] If a woman can recover from cardiopulmonary arrest (if the cause of the arrest is reversible—for example, an anesthetic problem), preforming the surgery within 4 minutes will give the greatest chance for resuscitation and salvage of the mother. Delivery within 5 minutes will also give the greatest chance for infant survival. Care must be taken to continue cardiopulmonary resuscitation during and after the procedure.[68]

REFERENCES

1. Feldman GB, Freiman JA: Prophylactic cesarean section at term? *N Engl J Med* 312:1264, 1985.
2. Thompson S: *Motif Index of Folk Literature*, ed 2. Bloomington, Ind, University Press, 1955, p 732.
3. Speert H: *A Pictorial History of Gynecology and Obstetrics*. Philadelphia, FA Davis Co, 1973, p 297.
4. Speert H: *A Pictorial History of Gynecology and Obstetrics*. Philadelphia, FA Davis Co, 1973, p 309.
5. Ramsbotham FH: *Principles and Practices of Obstetrics Medicine and Surgery*. Philadelphia, Lea and Blanchard, 1847, p 503.
6. Horley JMG: Cesarean section. *Clin Obstet Gynecol* 7:529, 1980.
7. Weber CE: Postmortem cesarean section: Review of the literature case reports. *Am J Obstet Gynecol* 110:158, 1971.
8. Shakespeare W: *Macbeth*, Act V, Scene viii, in Harbage A (ed): *William Shakespeare: The Complete Works*. Baltimore, Penguin Books, 1969, p 1134.
9. Findley P: *Priests of Lucina*. Boston, Little, Brown and Co, 1939, p 375.
10. Findley P: *Priests of Lucina*. Boston, Little, Brown and Co, 1939, p 377.
11. Findley P: *Priests of Lucina*. Boston, Little, Brown and Co, 1939, p 379.
12. Cutter IS, Viets HR: *A Short History of Midwifery*. Philadelphia, WB Saunders Co, 1964, p 220.
13. Dewees WP: *A Compendium System of Midwifery*, ed 6. Philadelphia, Carey, Lea and Blanchard, 1833, p 585.
14. Cutter IS, Viets HR: *A Short History of Midwifery*. Philadelphia, WB Saunders Co, 1964, p 230.
15. Cutter IS, Viets HR: *A Short History of Midwifery*. Philadelphia, WB Saunders Co, 1964, p 205.
16. Thomas H: *Our Obstetric Heritage*. Hamden, Conn, Shoe String Press, Inc, 1960, p 84.
17. DeLee JB: *Principles and Practice of Obstetrics*, ed 6. Philadelphia, WB Saunders Co, 1936, p 1078.
18. Duer EL: Postmortem delivery. *Am J Obstet Gynecol* 12:1, 1879.
19. Ramsbotham FH: *Principles and Practice of Obstetric Medicine and Surgery*. Philadelphia, Lea and Blanchard, 1847, p 230.
20. Eastman NJ: The role of frontier American in the development of cesarean section. *Am J Obstet Gynecol* 24:919, 1932.
21. Harris RP: A study and analysis of 100 cesarean operations performed in the United States during the present century and prior to 1878. *Am J Med Sci* 79:43, 1879.
22. Sanger M: My work in reference to the cesarean operation. *Am J Obstet Dis Women Children* 20:593, 1887.
23. Sanger M: Speaking before the German Gynecology Association 1885. *Am J Obstet Dis Women Child* 19:883, 1886.

24. Speert H: *Obstetric and Gynecologic Milestones.* New York, Macmillan Co, 1958, p 381.
25. Williams JW: *Obstetrics.* New York, D Appleton & Co, 1904, p 402.
26. Dewees WP: *A Compendium System of Midwifery*, ed 6. Philadelphia, Carey, Lea and Blanchard, 1833, p 565.
27. Williams JW: *Obstetrics.* New York, D Appleton & Co, 1904, p 409.
28. Williams JW: *Obstetrics.* New York, D Appleton & Co, 1904, p 404.
29. Speert H: *Obstetrics and Gynecology in America.* Baltimore, Waverly Press, 1980, p 155.
30. Thomas GT: Gastro-elytrotomy, a substitute for the cesarean section. *Am J Obstet Gynecol* 3:125, 1871.
31. Douglas RG, Stromme WB: *Operative Obstetrics*, ed 2. New York, Appleton-Century-Crofts, 1957, p 415.
32. Speert H: *Obstetric and Gynecologic Milestones.* New York, Macmillan Co, 1958, p 599.
33. Quillagan EJ, Zuspan F (eds): *Operative Obstetrics*, ed 4. New York, Appleton-Century-Crofts, 1982, p 600.
34. Titus P: *Management of Obstetric Difficulties*, ed 3. St Louis, CV Mosby Co, 1945, p 699.
35. Waters EG: Supravesical extraperitoneal cesarean section. *Am J Obstet Gynecol* 39:423, 1940.
36. Norton JF: A paravesical extraperitoneal cesarean section technique. *Am J Obstet Gynecol* 51:519, 1946.
37. Frank F: Die suprasymphysare entbindung und ihr verhaltnisszu den anderen operationen bei engen becken. *Archiv fur Gynaekologie* 81:58, 1907.
38. Beck AC: Observations on a series of cesarean sections done at the Long Island College Hospital during the past six years. *Am J Obstet Gynecol* 79:197, 1919.
39. Kerr JM: The technique of cesarean section with special reference to the lower uterine segment incision. *Am J Obstet Gynecol* 12:729, 1926.
40. Phaneuf LE: Cesarean section followed by temporary exteriorization of the uterus. *Surg Gynecol Obstet* 44:788, 1927.
41. Speert H: *Obstetric and Gynecologic Milestones.* New York, Macmillan Co, 1958, p 585.
42. Durfee RB: Evolution of cesarean hysterectomy. *Clin Obstet Gynecol* 12:575, 1969.
43. Harris RP: The results of the first fifty cases of cesarean ovarohysterectomy 1869–1880. *Am J Med Sci* 80:129, 1880.
44. Davis EM: A complete cesarean hysterectomy: A logical advance in modern obstetric surgery. *Am J Obstet Gynecol* 62:838, 1951.
45. Beck AC: Improved technique of the two flap low incision cesarean section. *JAMA* 92:22, 1929.
46. Williams JW: *Obstetrics*, ed 6. New York, Appleton-Century-Crofts, 1930, p 543.
47. Williams JW: *Obstetrics*, ed 6. New York, Appleton-Century-Crofts, 1930, p 546.
48. Danforth WC: Discussion of Falls FH: A critical study of the low cervical and classical cesarean section operations. *Am J Obstet Gynecol* 32:989, 1936.
49. Verch LH: A 15-year survey of cesarean sections. *Am J Obstet Gynecol* 59:108, 1950.
50. Douglas RG, Landesman R: Recent trends in cesarean section. *Am J Obstet Gynecol* 59:96, 1950.
51. Williams JW: *Obstetrics*, ed 6. New York, Appleton-Century-Crofts, 1930, p 533.
52. Goldston I: *Maternal Death and Ways to Prevention.* New York, Commonwealth Fund, 1937, p 57.
53. Goldston I: *Maternal Death and Ways to Prevention.* New York, Commonwealth Fund, 1937, p 56.
54. Morris RC (ed): *Obstetrics.* Philadelphia, WB Saunders Co, 1895, p 917.

55. Goldston I: *Maternal Death and Ways to Prevention.* New York, Commonwealth Fund, 1937, p 132.
56. Goldston I: *Maternal Death and Ways to Prevention.* New York, Commonwealth Fund, 1937, p 127.
57. Titus P, Wilson JR: *The Management of Obstetric Difficulties*, ed 5. St Louis, CV Mosby Co, 1955, p 557.
58. Goldston I: *Maternal Death and Ways to Prevention.* New York, Commonwealth Fund, 1937, p 138.
59. D'Esopa DA: A review of cesarean section at Sloane Hospital for Women 1942–1947. *Am J Obstet Gynecol* 59:77, 1950.
60. Titus P, Wilson JR: *The Management of Obstetric Difficulties*, ed 5. St Louis, CV Mosby Co, 1955, p 558.
61. Douglas RG, Stromme WB: *Operative Obstetrics*, ed 2. New York, Appleton-Century-Crofts, 1965, p 416.
62. Hibbard LT: Changing trends in cesarean section. *Am J Obstet Gynecol* 125:798, 1976.
63. Pritchard JA, MacDonald PC, Gant NF: *Williams' Obstetrics*, ed 17. Norwalk, Conn, Appleton-Century-Crofts, 1985, p 868.
64. Douglas RG, Birnbaum SJ, MacDonald FA: Pregnancy and labor following cesarean section. *Am J Obstet Gynecol* 86:961, 1963.
65. Williams JW: *Obstetrics*, ed 6. New York, Appleton-Century-Crofts, 1930, p 536.
66. DeLee JB: *Principles and Practices of Obstetrics.* Philadelphia, WB Saunders Co, 1933, p 1078.
67. Cesarean childbirth, Report of a consensus developmental conference. National Institutes of Health Pub No. 82-2067. Washington, DC, US Dept of Health and Human Services. October 1981.
68. Katz VL, Dotters DJ, Droegemueller W: Perimortem cesarean delivery. *Obstet Gynecol* 68:571, 1986.

Indications for Cesarean

Chapter 2

Abnormal Labor

William L. Koontz, MD

The leading component of the tremendous increase in the rate of cesarean births over the past several years has been the procedures performed for the diagnosis of abnormal labor, or dystocia.[1] Although the term "dystocia" may be used to describe all cases of difficult labor, it is now commonly used in a more restricted sense. This limited definition excludes cases of breech presentation, which are considered in a separate category. In clinical practice, dystocia is probably most often listed as "failure to progress" or "cephalopelvic disproportion (CPD)." Dystocia is unique among the most common diagnoses contributing to the increased rate of cesarean birth, as it is the only one for which significant controversy exists in terms of both diagnosis and management.

It is difficult to demonstrate that an increased number of cesarean deliveries performed for dystocia has had a beneficial effect on perinatal morbidity or mortality.[1] Some authors have reported a greatly decreased perinatal mortality rate over the past several years while maintaining a stable rate of cesarean birth.[2] Although some investigators have found that increased numbers of cesareans have replaced midforceps deliveries,[3,4] the opposite has been found by others.[5] The NIH Consensus Development Task Force on cesarean childbirth[1] examined data from New York City and concluded that cesarean delivery for dystocia was not associated with greater survival than that which occurs with vaginal delivery. Unfortunately, definitive long-term morbidity data are not available.

Friedman has underscored our lack of understanding of abnormal labor patterns by listing 65 terms in use to describe labor variants.[6] This is further emphasized by the fact that cesarean deliveries are most often done for labors involving normal-sized infants in the vertex presentation.[1] Because of these uncertainties, it is widely held that study of the management of dystocia could result in lower numbers of cesareans for this indication. Indeed, some authors have already reported that better understanding and more aggressive management of labor may safely result in a lower or stabilized rate of cesarean birth.[7,8]

Many cesarean deliveries are performed because of a lack of understanding of disorders of labor and their appropriate management.[8–10] The components of labor have traditionally been called the "three P's": powers, passage, and passenger. Cardozo and Studd[11] have suggested that a fourth "P," poor understanding of labor curves, is a frequent cause of the rise in cesareans. When intensive education and monitoring programs have been instituted,[8,9] a decrease in the rate of cesareans performed for dystocia has resulted. Clearly, more study of this problem is needed in this critical area.[1]

Although some large series involving labor disorders and their treatment were published several years ago,[12,13] their conclusions are difficult to apply to modern obstetrics. Many aspects of intrapartum management, such as the widespread use of electronic fetal monitoring, have changed considerably since these studies were done. O'Brien and Cefalo[14] have discussed the difficulties involved in analyzing these studies and applying them to current practice. Only recently has labor again become a popular subject for study, probably as a result of concern over the increased number of cesarean births done for disorders of labor.

DISORDERS OF EARLY LABOR

An understanding of early labor is essential to the acceptable management of the laboring gravida because this area has the greatest potential for resulting in unnecessary cesareans. The latent phase is defined by Friedman[6] as the portion of labor that occurs between the onset of regular uterine contractions and the sharp increase in the rate of cervical dilatation that heralds the onset of the active phase. There is, however, much disagreement concerning this concept. Hendricks feels that what is commonly known as "latent phase labor" is simply the late stage of prelabor cervical preparation. Cardozo and Studd[11] accept the concept of the latent phase but define it as the time (if any) between admission in labor and the time when the cervix becomes 3 cm dilated. Crawford[15] simply denies the existence of the latent phase. This debate is concerned primarily with semantics, as all would agree that there is an early stage of labor during which cervical dilatation takes place very slowly.

Individualized therapy, usually consisting of either therapeutic rest or oxytocin infusion, should be employed when prolongation of the latent phase occurs. Koontz and Bishop[16] have stated that therapy should be based on the patient's physical and mental status, parity, and cervical status, without adhering to Friedman's strictly statistical criteria. Regardless of the treatment chosen, cesarean delivery for failure to progress in the latent phase does not appear reasonable.

Although it may seem obvious, one of the inherent problems of labor management is accuracy in making the diagnosis of labor. Recent investigators[7,17] have emphasized that aggressive management, with oxytocin administration in this phase of labor, often leads to cesarean delivery. This is underscored by the fact that elective inductions are associated with increased rates of intervention.[18–20] Data on the contribution of elective induction to the cesarean birth rate are difficult to obtain, because the diagnosis in this situation is often listed as failure to progress or CPD. However, Smith and associates[21] found that the cesarean birth rate was doubled when nulliparous patients were electively induced.

When labor is induced for valid indications, there are insufficient data as to what constitutes an adequate trial of induction. There is certainly a phase of induced labor that is comparable to the latent phase in spontaneous labor. During this period, any change in the cervix takes place very slowly. However, little data are currently available to characterize this phase of induced labor.[16] One of the most common situations in which labor induction is undertaken is premature rupture of the membranes (PROM). Immediate induction for PROM in the presence of a mature fetus has been the rule in the past. Recently, however, it has been shown that short-term expectant management up to 24 hr, even with a mature fetus, can safely decrease the rate of cesarean delivery associated with this complication without increasing maternal or neonatal infectious morbidity.[22]

PREDICTION OF DIFFICULT LABOR

It would be ideal if difficult labor could be predicted accurately and avoided. In practice, however, this has been extremely difficult. Sokol and associates[23] evaluated approximately 100 pregnancy risk factors and found that the need for primary cesarean birth could not be predicted prior to the onset of labor in the great majority of patients. Risk factors detectable in the antenatal period were significantly associated with increased primary cesarean birth rates in only 11% of their cases.

Although fetal macrosomia often results in cesarean delivery, it occurs in only a very small percentage of pregnancies.[24] As a result, macrosomia does not contribute significantly to the current rate of cesarean births. The great majority of infants delivered abdominally because of CPD are normal-sized babies delivered from a normal-sized maternal pelvis. Bottoms and associates[10] have pointed out that it is highly unlikely that the incidence of true CPD has doubled in the last 10 years, although this is exactly what has happened to the incidence of the diagnosis. This emphasizes that, in the great majority of cases, abnormal labor is a functional, rather than an anatomic, diagnosis.

Although some authors have recommended more liberal use of abdominal delivery for fetal macrosomia, the antenatal diagnosis of this condition remains very difficult. Parks and Ziel[24] found that macrosomia (defined in their study as fetal weight greater than 4,500 g) was diagnosed antenatally only 20% of the time. Strikingly, fetal weight was underestimated by more than 3 lb in more than 6% of the macrosomic group. Recently some success has been reported in the use of ultrasound to predict difficult labor and delivery related to macrosomia.[25]

IDENTIFICATION OF ABNORMAL ACTIVE PHASE LABOR

Normal labor can be diagnosed only in retrospect. If a healthy infant is born within a reasonable length of time, without major intervention and without significant injury to the mother or the fetus, normal labor has occurred. Identification of abnormal labor is somewhat more complicated. O'Brien and Cefalo[14] have discussed in detail the two major classifications of labor abnormalities. Briefly, the cervicographic method involves evaluation of labor by serially determining the status of the cervix and station of the presenting part. These data are then recorded in graphic form, and the curve thus obtained is compared to "normal" curves derived from studies of large populations.[6,26–28] Although these curves do have differences, they are very similar during the active phase, when most significant labor abnormalities occur. Bowes[29] recently superimposed these curves and found that their active phase portions were virtually identical.

The second major school of labor evaluation analyzes labor through measurement of contraction frequency, intensity, and duration.[30,31] In this system, labor disorders are classified in terms of whether uterine contractions are hypertonic or hypotonic, and therapy is chosen accordingly.

The cervicographic method of evaluation has become favored in the United States for two main reasons. First, the data required are easily obtained, whereas an intrauterine pressure catheter is required in the latter method. Second, normal labor is defined by normal progress, and this is precisely what is measured with the cervicographic method. The best way of following progress in labor is to use the cervicographic method primarily. The nanometric methods are then reserved for further evaluation of abnormalities of the cervicographically derived labor curve.

Friedman[6] describes three major disorders of active labor that are recognizable with graphic analysis of cervical dilatation (Table 2.1). These are primary dysfunctional labor (protracted active phase), secondary arrest of cervical dilatation, and combined disorders. Primary dysfunctional labor is statistically defined as active phase cervical dilatation that progresses at a rate below 1.2 cm/hr in nulliparas and 1.5 cm/hr in multiparas. Secondary arrest of cervical dilatation is defined as cessation of progress in cervical dilatation for at least 2 hours in the active phase. Combined disorders involve arrest of labor superimposed on a labor that was already progressing abnormally slowly. In the second stage, protracted descent is diagnosed if the presenting part descends at a rate of less than 1.0 cm/hr

TABLE 2.1 Major Disorders of Labor

Active phase	
Primary dysfunctional labor (protracted active phase)	Nullipara <1.2 cm/hr Multipara <1.5 cm/hr
Secondary arrest of cervical dilatation	No cervical change for 2 hr
Combination	Protraction and secondary arrest
Second stage	
Protracted descent	Nullipara <1.0 cm/hr Multipara <2.0 cm/hr
Arrest of descent	No descent for 1 hr

Source: Friedman EA: *Labor: Clinical Evaluation and Management*, ed 2. New York, Appleton-Century-Crofts, 1978.

in nulliparas or less than 2.0 cm/hr in multiparas. Arrest of descent is defined as cessation of descent for 1 hour or more. Although Friedman refers to the above classifications as "diagnoses," it is suggested that they are instead clinical signs calling for further investigation in order to arrive at a diagnosis. Indeed, for each of the classifications, Friedman lists various diagnoses that he feels are most often responsible for the abnormal labor pattern. Thus, it is preferable to view cervicographic labor abnormalities as signals that call for further evaluation, rather than as firm diagnoses on which treatment should be based. Friedman's studies were done at a time when obstetric practice was considerably different from what it is today. For this reason, "Friedman's curve" is primarily of value in alerting the clinician to abnormalities that require a closer look. Friedman's discussions of the causes of abnormal patterns and his recommendations for treatment are often difficult to apply to present-day obstetrics.

EVALUATION OF ABNORMAL ACTIVE PHASE LABOR

Several authors have stressed the importance of confirming the diagnosis of active labor.[7,8,16,17] Although the active phase is defined by the rate of change in cervical dilatation rather than by its actual value, it is unlikely that the active phase has been entered unless the cervix is at least 4 cm dilated. If care is not taken in this regard, inappropriate intervention in the latent phase is likely to result.

There appears to be no strong consensus regarding the frequency and timing of pelvic examinations in the identification and management of abnormal labor. Cardoza and Studd[11] recommend examinations every 3–4 hours, changing to every 2 hours if progress is abnormally slow. O'Driscoll's protocol[7] calls for hourly examinations.

Many authorities consider the understanding of the mechanism of labor and the clinical evaluation of the pelvis a lost art. Increasing emphasis on abdominal delivery for labor abnormalities has resulted in deemphasis of the importance of pelvic types and their influence on the course and outcome of labor. Bowes[29] has nicely summarized the clinical assessment of the pelvis in labor and has stressed that the outcome of this evaluation is of value in predicting or explaining labor abnormalities. Nonetheless, the works of Caldwell et al[32] and Steer[33] on pelvic architecture and labor provide important insights into the condition of the patient with abnormal labor.

X-ray pelvimetry as a technique for the evaluation of abnormal labor has recently come under close scrutiny. A routine part of the evaluation of abnormal labor several years ago, its frequent use has been seriously questioned. Varner and associates[34] studied 101 consecutive x-ray pelvimetry examinations and found no new information regarding pelvic architecture that had any effect on labor management. The new information, which was obtained in seven cases, involved fetal presentation. The authors concluded that this information could be more appropriately obtained via the use of sonography. In a review of the use of x-ray pelvimetry, O'Brien and Cefalo[35] state that although harm to the fetus as a result of the procedure remains controversial, the possible risks of x-ray pelvimetry outweigh the benefits. In addition, many factors other than the bony pelvic architecture contribute to an unsuccessful labor. Thus, the only indications for x-ray pelvimetry in contemporary obstetrics are the breech fetus, in whom vaginal delivery is contemplated (Chapter 3), and possibly selected cases of severe distortion of pelvic architecture. The U.S. Department of Health and Human Services is currently funding a study of the effect of intensive educational efforts on the use of x-ray pelvimetry. The post-education portion of this study has not yet been reported.[36]

Evaluation of the fetus should also be undertaken when it is determined that labor is not progressing normally. If not already in use, electronic fetal monitoring should be initiated. Even in this age of sophisticated fetal monitoring techniques, abnormal labor remains a factor causing increased fetal morbidity. Ott[37] has shown a significant increase in abnormal fetal heart rate patterns associated with abnormal labor. This finding applied even to those fetuses thought to be in good condition at the onset of labor.

An attempt to estimate fetal size should also be made. Clinical evaluation of fetal weight is notoriously inaccurate. Sonographic techniques have been used in an attempt to estimate fetal size more accurately.[38] Although sonographic methods have yielded good results with small premature infants, the standard deviation (106 g per kilogram of fetal weight) becomes larger with advancing gestation. Tamura and co-workers[39] improved the predictive value of these techniques at term by using an equation derived specifically for this use (Table 2.2).

In summary, the results of clinical and sonographic estimation of fetal size suffer from the same limitations as clinical and x-ray pelvimetry. Abnormal results may alert the clinician to the possibility or probability of

TABLE 2.2 Ultrasound-Derived Formulas for Estimating Fetal Weight That Can Be Entered into Programmable Calculators

Warsof[38]	$\log_{10}(\text{birth weight}) = -1.599 + 0.144(\text{BPD}) + 0.032(\text{AC}) - 0.111(\text{BPD}^2 \times \text{AC})/1{,}000$
Tamura[39]	$\log_2(\text{EFW}) = 0.02597\text{AC} + 0.2161\text{BPD} - 0.1999(\text{AC} \times \text{BPD}^2)/1{,}000 + 1.2659$
Shepard[40]	$\log_{10}(\text{birth weight}) = -1.7492 + 0.1666(\text{BPD}) + 0.046(\text{AC}) - 2.646(\text{AC} \times \text{BPD})/1{,}000$

EFW, estimated fetal weight; AC, abdominal circumference; BPD, biparietal diameter.

a subsequent problem, but are not sufficiently accurate to serve as a basis for management, except in very unusual circumstances. One of these circumstances occurs when labor is obstructed secondary to sonographically detectable fetal anomalies. Clark and co-workers[41] have recently described their experience with this situation. They reported 11 cases; in 10 of them, fetal decompression resulted in uneventful vaginal delivery. As the authors have stated, these techniques raise many ethical questions, and the required expertise is not widespread. Thus, the exact role of such techniques remains undefined.

One of the most important aspects of the study of abnormal labor is the evaluation of uterine contractions. Several older studies remain the foundation of our understanding of the physiology of uterine contractions during labor.[42–45] The stimulus for uterine contraction begins in one cornu of the uterus and descends through the myometrium toward the cervix. Contractions are longer and stronger in the fundus, gradually becoming weaker and shorter as they approach the cervix. This "descending gradient" of myometrial activity tends to propel the fetus in the appropriate direction. Although intraamniotic pressure of 15 mm Hg may be sufficient to produce normal progress in labor, contraction intensity of 60 mm Hg often occurs in spontaneous labors. Abdominal palpation or external monitoring may provide accurate information concerning the frequency and duration of uterine contractions, but these techniques may be misleading when used to estimate contraction intensity. Factors such as maternal obesity, polyhydramnios or oligohydramnios, and fetal size and position may result in erroneous conclusions.

The most direct method for the evaluation of the quality of uterine contractions is the recording of intraamniotic pressures via a transcervically placed, fluid-filled catheter connected to a pressure transducer. Two disorders of contractility may be diagnosed: hypotonic and hypertonic uterine dysfunction. In hypotonic dysfunction, the baseline intrauterine pressure (tonus) is normal or low, and infrequent uterine contractions generate low levels of pressure. Hypertonic dysfunction is thought to be the result of incoordinate uterine action, and typically involves contractions that are frequent but of low intensity, along with elevated tonus. Although much has been made of the distinction between hypotonic and hypertonic dysfunction, hypertonic dysfunction is usually associated with early labor in nulliparous patients. Thus, it is often part of the picture of prolonged latent phase labor, rather than of disorders of the active phase. This is undoubtedly one of the reasons that both prolonged latent phase and hypertonic dysfunction are thought to respond well to therapeutic sedation. Intrauterine pressure monitoring requires the presence of ruptured membranes. For this reason, it should generally not be instituted until a firm diagnosis of labor is made.

TREATMENT OF DISORDERS OF ACTIVE PHASE LABOR

Only six methods are currently available for treatment of abnormal active phase labor: (1) observation (watchful waiting), (2) ambulation, (3) maternal sedation or analgesia, (4) amniotomy, (5) stimulation of uterine contractions, and (6) operative delivery.

Supporters of noninterference maintain that the progress of labor is highly variable and that intervention should be undertaken only as a last resort.[46] It has been suggested that the obstetrician's compulsion about forcing labor to conform to an ideal curve results in inappropriate intervention, and that this intervention is primarily responsible for the increased morbidity associated with prolonged labor. Herzfeld[46] states that time in labor is not in itself a factor in poor outcomes. This is contradicted by recent studies that have shown an increased morbidity rate in prolonged labor both with and without intervention.[37] In addition, studies of the so-called active management of labor have demonstrated that aggressive, intervention-oriented protocols may serve to decrease safely the incidence of the ultimate intervention, cesarean birth.[7]

The effect of maternal ambulation on labor has not been extensively studied. Some authors have found that ambulated patients have more rapid, distress-free labors than those patients who labor in bed.[47] Others have found no significant difference.[48] Very little study has been done of the effect of maternal ambulation on disorders of labor. On a very small study of 14 patients, Read and associates[49] found no significant differences between the use of ambulation and oxytocin as therapy for nonprogressive labor.

Maternal sedation and analgesia have been studied primarily as part of the therapy for latent phase disorders. Adequate pain relief may act as therapy for desultory progress in the active phase by decreasing maternal catecholamines and thereby removing their negative effect on uterine contractibility. Although some clinicians believe that analgesia may act as therapy for nonprogressive active phase labor,[15] little data exist in this area.

Amniotomy has long been used as therapy for desultory labor, although solid evidence of beneficial results is lacking.[6] Friedman observes that the widespread use of internal fetal monitoring, which requires amniotomy, has almost made this a moot point.

The most common therapy for failure to progress in the active phase of labor is intravenous infusion of a dilute solution of synthetic oxytocin in order to stimulate uterine contractility. Although oxytocin infusion is widely accepted as the therapy of choice for some abnormalities of labor, there are other areas in which its use is extremely controversial. In addition, there is little agreement on optimal dosage schedules, the importance of the diagnosis of CPD, or criteria for adequacy of a trial of oxytocin augmentation.

Little controversy exists concerning the use of oxytocin in secondary arrest of labor when the fetus is thought to be in good condition, CPD is not thought to be present, and uterine hypocontractility has been demonstrated. Clearly abnormal fetal heart rate patterns are obvious contraindications to the use of oxytocin augmentation. Nonreassuring patterns call for extremely close monitoring of the fetus and discontinuation of oxytocin at the first sign of distress.

Although few would argue for oxytocin infusion in the very few cases of obvious absolute CPD, there is little agreement concerning optimum management when relative CPD is suspected. Some authorities contend that oxytocin stimulation is contraindicated in the presence of suspected CPD.[50,51] However, in recent studies, the importance of pelvic evaluation has been deemphasized and stimulation of labor in all active phase disorders has been advocated.[2,26] These studies reported no deleterious effects on the fetus from a trial of labor in the presence of retrospectively diagnosed CPD when the fetus was carefully monitored. This approach to uterine stimulation is probably the one most commonly used in the United States today. This controversy arises for two reasons: (1) Older studies showed increased fetal morbidity with CPD, but were often done without benefit of fetal monitoring and with delivery techniques that are now seldom employed. (2) CPD is more properly viewed as a functional rather than an anatomic diagnosis. Undoubtedly, many women with perfectly normal intrapartum courses would be diagnosed as having CPD if classic x-ray parameters were singularly applied.

Ideally, documentation of uterine hypocontractility should take place before oxytocin stimulation is instituted. However, where external fetal heart rate monitoring and a careful clinical evaluation document infrequent contractions, further documentation with an intrauterine pressure catheter is not mandatory. Normal contractile activity in the active phase of labor is about 250 Montevideo units (average amplitude $\times$ frequency per 10 min).[52] Stimulation of normal patterns of contractility is unlikely to correct abnormal progress of labor and may result in dangerous hyperstimulation.

Oxytocin stimulation as therapy for primary dysfunctional labor or a protracted active phase is also controversial. Although Friedman's data[6] show a low success rate for oxytocin in this situation, his studies suffer from the limitations previously discussed. Oxytocin has been used by several groups in the presence of primary dysfunctional labor or protracted active phase with good results.[27,53] Bowes[29] has stated that oxytocin used more aggressively has the potential to correct most protraction disorders.

There is currently no controversy regarding the method of intrapartum administration of oxytocin. It should be given intravenously via a constant infusion pump. There is no place for the use of intramuscular, subcutaneous, buccal, or intranasal oxytocin prior to delivery. These routes of administration are not approved for intrapartum use because of unpredictability regarding the amount of drug absorbed.

Standard dosage schedules have recently been questioned as the pharmacokinetics of oxytocin have been more thoroughly studied. Formerly recommended regimens called for increasing (even doubling) the rate of infusion as often as every 15 minutes. Seitchik and associates[54] state that these recommendations are based on confusion between in vivo and in vitro characteristics of oxytocin. They found that 40 minutes is required for a given dose of oxytocin to reach a steady state and the maximum contractile response. The same group had previously demonstrated that increasing the rate of infusion more often than every 30 minutes is associated with a doubled incidence of fetal distress and/or uterine hypercontractility.[55] It has also been demonstrated that dosage regimens based on these findings are very effective.[56]

The proper length of time for an adequate trial of oxytocin stimulation in protraction disorders remains undefined, with most authors recommending a trial of "only a few hours."[51] Friedman found that all patients who were going to respond did so within 7 hours, and that most did within 4 hours.[57] Bowes[29] recommended a trial of 4–6 hours. Hard data concerning what constitutes adequate progress are not available. However, active phase arrest of dilatation for 2 hours after an adequate uterine contraction pattern has been achieved is an indication for cesarean delivery. Because it has been shown that oxytocin was not used at all prior to many cesarean births performed for dystocia,[58] one must suspect that inadequate trials of oxytocin stimulation may be a significant factor in the performance of some unnecessary operative deliveries.

Oxytocin is also used for arrest of descent of the fetal presenting part. Evaluation becomes even more complicated when this occurs because adequacy of the maternal expulsive efforts must also be taken into account. Some authors condemn the practice of having the mother start pushing as soon as complete dilatation has occurred, regardless of the station of the head and whether or not she feels the urge to push. Crawford[15] feels that this is likely to increase the rate of operative intervention because of the maternal exhaustion thus induced. Although it has been shown that arbitrary time limits placed on second-stage labor are not necessary,[59] it is important that some progress be maintained. After a prolonged second stage, midforceps delivery is associated with an increased incidence of shoulder dystocia and birth injury.[60]

NONOBSTETRIC FACTORS

Blumenthal and associates[61] found a large difference between the incidence of dystocia in public and private patients, and concluded that the difference probably resulted from differences in the criteria used for the two groups. However, they were unable to determine whether the difference resulted from excessive intervention in the private group or from less than optimal intervention in the public group.

Phillips and co-workers[62] studied the daily distribution of nonscheduled cesarean deliveries. They felt that if physician convenience was a significant factor in the performance of cesareans, this would show up as an increased number of operations performed on weekends. No significant difference was demonstrated. However, in letters commenting on the above study, both Goodlin[63] and Poma[64] suggested that there are significant trends regarding the time-of-day distribution of abdominal deliveries. Poma speculated that the need for the physician to be present during office hours may be a major influence.

CONCLUSIONS AND RECOMMENDATIONS

The management of abnormal labor should be approached in an organized, logical fashion (Figure 2.1). The NIH Consensus Development Task Force[1] made the following recommendations concerning cesarean delivery for dystocia:

1. In the absence of fetal distress, management of dysfunctional labor may include such measures as patient rest, hydration, ambulation, sedation, and the use of oxytocin prior to consideration of cesarean birth.
2. There is a compelling reason to examine the diagnostic category of dystocia because of its prominent association with the increase in the primary cesarean birth rate and the absence of a survival advantage for cesarean births of infants weighing more than 2,500 g.
3. Included among approaches to the issue of dystocia should be (a) peer review within hospitals; (b) examination of the efficacy of methods for assessing the progress of labor, with specific attention to infant and maternal mortality and morbidity; and (c) research clarifying the factors that affect the progress of labor, including the effects of emotional support, ambulation, rest, sedation, and oxytocin stimulation.

It is hoped that application of these guidelines (Figure 2.1) and the aforementioned principles will result in an appropriate rate of cesarean birth for the problem of abnormal labor.

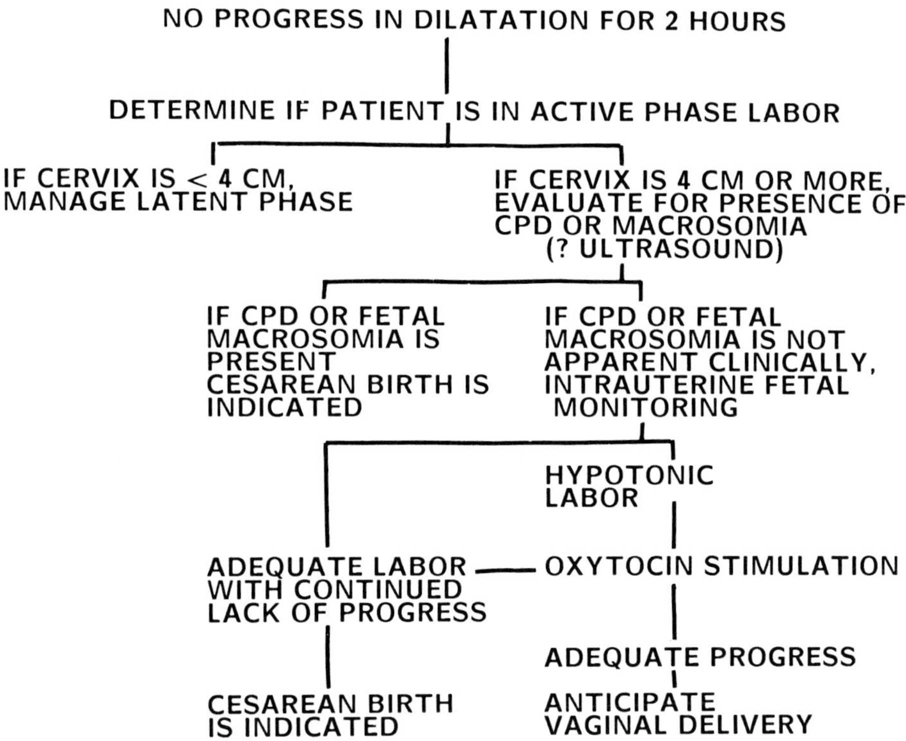

FIGURE 2.1 A management scheme for abnormal active phase labor.

REFERENCES

1. NIH Consensus Development Task Force Statement on Cesarean Childbirth. *Am J Obstet Gynecol* 139:902, 1981.
2. O'Driscoll K, Foley M: Correlation of decrease in perinatal mortality and increase in cesarean section rate. *Obstet Gynecol* 61:1, 1983.
3. Minkoff HL, Schwarz RH: The rising cesarean section rate: Can it safely be reversed? *Obstet Gynecol* 56:135, 1980.
4. Anderson GM, Lomas J: Determinants of the increasing cesarean birth rate. *N Engl J Med* 311:887, 1984.
5. Baskett TF, McMillen RM: Cesarean section: Trends and morbidity. *Can Med Assoc J* 125:723, 1981.
6. Friedman EA: *Labor: Clinical Evaluation and Management*, ed 2. New York, Appleton-Century-Crofts, 1978.
7. O'Driscoll K, Foley M, MacDonald D: Active management of labor as an alternative to cesarean section for dystocia. *Obstet Gynecol* 63:485, 1984.
8. Philipson EH, Rosen MG: Trends in the frequency of cesarean births. *Clin Obstet Gynecol* 28:691, 1985.
9. Gilstrap LC, Hauth JC, Toussaint S: Cesarean section: Changing incidence and indications. *Obstet Gynecol* 63:205, 1984.
10. Bottoms SF, Rosen MG, Sokol RJ: The increase in the cesarean birth rate. *N Engl J Med* 302:559, 1980.
11. Cardozo L, Studd J: Abnormal labour patterns, in Studd J (ed): *The Management of Labour*. Oxford, Blackwell Scientific Publications, 1985.

12. Hellman LM, Kohl SG, Schechter BS: Pitocin—1955. *Am J Obstet Gynecol* 73:507, 1957.
13. Moore DB, D'Esopo DA: The treatment of uterine inertia with dilute intravenous pituitrin. *Am J Obstet Gynecol* 70:1338, 1955.
14. O'Brien W, Cefalo RC: Abnormalities of the active phase: Recognition and treatment. *Clin Obstet Gynecol* 25:115, 1982.
15. Crawford JS: The stages and phases of labour: An outworn nomenclature that invites hazard. *Lancet* 1:271, 1983.
16. Koontz WL, Bishop EH: Management of the latent phase of labor. *Clin Obstet Gynecol* 25:111, 1982.
17. Iams JD, Reiss R: When should labor be interrupted by cesarean delivery? *Clin Obstet Gynecol* 28:745, 1985.
18. Keetel WC: Inducing labor by rupturing membranes. *Postgrad Med* 44:199, 1968.
19. Studd J, Cardozo L: Evaluation of induction of labour, in Studd J (ed): *The Management of Labour.* Oxford, Blackwell Scientific Publications, 1985.
20. Yudkin P, Frumar AM, Anderson ABM, et al: A retrospective study of induction of labour. *Br J Obstet Gynaecol* 86:257, 1979.
21. Smith LP, Nagourney BA, McLean FH, et al: Hazards and benefits of elective induction of labor. *Am J Obstet Gynecol* 148:579, 1984.
22. Berkowitz RL, Hoder L, Freedman RM, et al: Results of a protocol for premature rupture of the membranes. *Obstet Gynecol* 60:271, 1982.
23. Sokol RJ, Rosen MG, Bottoms SF, et al: Risks preceding increased primary cesarean birth rates. *Obstet Gynecol* 59:340, 1982.
24. Parks DG, Ziel HK: Macrosomia—a proposed indication for primary cesarean section. *Obstet Gynecol* 52:407, 1978.
25. Tamura RK, Sabbagha RE, et al: Diabetic macrosomia: Accuracy of third trimester ultrasound. *Obstet Gynecol* 67:828, 1986.
26. Philpott RH, Castle WM: Cervicographs in the management of labour in primigravidae. 1. The alert line for detecting abnormal labour. *J Obstet Gynaecol Br Commonw* 79:592, 1972.
27. Beazley JM, Kurjak A: The influence of a partograph on the active management of labour. *Lancet* 2:348, 1972.
28. Hendricks CH, Brenner WE, Kraus G: Normal cervical dilatation pattern in late pregnancy and labor. *Am J Obstet Gynecol* 106:1065, 1970.
29. Bowes WA: Clinical aspects of normal and abnormal labor, in Creasy RK, Resnick R (eds): *Maternal-Fetal Medicine: Principles and Practice.* Philadelphia, WB Saunders Co, 1984.
30. Caldeyro-Barcia R, Alvarez H: Abnormal uterine action in labor. *J Obstet Gynaecol Br Emp* 59:646, 1952.
31. Jeffcoate TNA, Baker K, Martin RH: Inefficient uterine action. *Surg Gynecol Obstet* 95:257, 1952.
32. Caldwell WE, Moloy HC, D'Esopo DA: Further studies on the mechanism of labor. *Am J Obstet Gynecol* 30:763, 1935.
33. Steer CM (ed): *Moloy's Evaluation of the Pelvis in Obstetrics.* Philadelphia, WB Saunders Co, 1959.
34. Varner MW, Cruikshank DP, Laube DW: X-ray pelvimetry in clinical obstetrics. *Obstet Gynecol* 56:296, 1980.
35. O'Brien W, Cefalo RC: Evaluation of x-ray pelvimetry and abnormal labor. *Clin Obstet Gynecol* 25:157, 1982.
36. Arcarese JS, Morrison JL: The utilization of x-ray pelvimetry in the United States. *Clin Obstet Gynecol* 25:165, 1982.
37. Ott W: Relationship of normal and abnormal late labor patterns to perinatal mortality. *Clin Obstet Gynecol* 25:105, 1982.

38. Warsof SL, Gohari P, Berkowitz RL, et al: The estimation of fetal weight by computer-assisted analysis. *Am J Obstet Gynecol* 128:881, 1977.
39. Tamura RK, Sabbhaga RE, Dooley SL, et al: Real-time ultrasound estimation of weight in fetuses of diabetic gravid women. *Am J Obstet Gynecol* 153:57, 1985.
40. Shepard MJ, Richards VA, Berkowitz RL, et al: An evaluation of two equations in predicting fetal weight by ultrasound. *Am J Obstet Gynecol* 142:47, 1982.
41. Clark SL, DeVore GR, Platt LD: The role of ultrasound in the aggressive management of obstructed labor secondary to fetal malformations. *Am J Obstet Gynecol* 152:1042, 1985.
42. Caldeyro-Barcia R, Alvarez H, Reynolds SRM: A better understanding of uterine contractility through simultaneous recording with an internal and a seven channel external method. *Surg Obstet Gynecol* 91:641, 1950.
43. Reynolds SRM, Heard OO, Bruns P, et al: A multichannel strain-gauge tokodynamometer: An instrument for studying patterns of uterine contractions in pregnant women. *Bull Johns Hopkins Hosp* 82:446, 1948.
44. Larks SD: *Electrohysterography*. Springfield, Ill, Charles C Thomas Co, 1960.
45. Hendricks CH, Quilligan EJ, Tyler AB, et al: Pressure relationships between intervillous space and amniotic fluid in human term pregnancy. *Am J Obstet Gynecol* 77:1028, 1959.
46. Herzfeld J: *Sense and Sensibility in Childbirth: A Guide to Supportive Obstetrical Care*. New York, WW Norton and Co, 1985.
47. Flynn AM, Kelly J, Hollins G, et al: Ambulation in labour. *Br Med J* 2:591, 1978.
48. Williams RM, Thorn MH, Studd JW: A study of the benefits and acceptability of ambulation in spontaneous labour. *Br J Obstet Gynaecol* 87:122, 1980.
49. Read JA, Miller FC, Paul RH: Randomized trial of ambulation versus oxytocin for labor enhancement: A preliminary report. *Am J Obstet Gynecol* 139:669, 1981.
50. Friedman EA: Dysfunctional labor. III. Secondary arrest of dilatation in the nullipara. *Obstet Gynecol* 19:576, 1962.
51. Pritchard JP, MacDonald PC, Gant NF: *Williams Obstetrics*, ed 17. Norwalk, Conn, Appleton-Century-Crofts, 1985.
52. Silverman F, Hutson JM: The clinical and biological significance of the bottom line. *Clin Obstet Gynecol* 29:43, 1986.
53. O'Driscoll K, Meagher D: *Active Management of Labour*. Philadelphia, WB Saunders Co, 1980.
54. Seitchik J, Amico J, Robinson AG, et al: Oxytocin augmentation of dysfunctional labor. IV. Oxytocin pharmacokinetics. *Am J Obstet Gynecol* 150:225, 1984.
55. Seitchik J, Castillo M: Oxytocin augmentation of dysfunctional labor. I. Clinical data. *Am J Obstet Gynecol* 144:899, 1983.
56. Seitchik J, Amico JA, Castillo M: Oxytocin augmentation of dysfunctional labor. V. An alternative oxytocin regimen. *Am J Obstet Gynecol* 151:757, 1985.
57. Friedman EA: Trail of labor: Formulation, application, and retrospective clinical evaluation. *Obstet Gynecol* 10:1, 1957.
58. Evrard JR, Gold EM, Cahill TF: Cesarean section—a contemporary assessment. *J Reprod Med* 24:147, 1980.
59. Cohen WR: Influence of the duration of second stage of labor on perinatal outcome and puerperal morbidity. *Obstet Gynecol* 49:266, 1977.
60. Benedetti TJ, Gabbe SG: Shoulder dystocia—a complication of fetal macrosomia and prolonged second stage of labor with midpelvic delivery. *Obstet Gynecol* 52:526, 1978.
61. Blumenthal NJ, Harris RS, O'Connor MC, et al: Changing caesarean section rates experience at a Sydney obstetric teaching hospital. *Aust NZ J Obstet Gynaecol* 24:246, 1984.

62. Phillips RN, Thornton J, Gleicher N: Physician bias in cesarean sections. *JAMA* 248:1082, 1982.
63. Goodlin R: Physician bias in cesarean section (letter). *JAMA* 249:1005, 1983.
64. Poma PA: Physician bias in cesarean section (letter). *JAMA* 249:1005, 1983.

Chapter 3

Malpresentation
Breech and Transverse Lie

Thomas R. Moore, MD

Of all the contemporary changes in the indications for cesarean delivery, none has changed more dramatically than delivery of the breech fetus. In the last two decades, cesarean delivery of the breech fetus has become routine in many practice settings. Collea noted that the rate of cesarean delivery for breech babies rose from 32% in 1970 at the Los Angeles County-University of Southern California Medical Center to almost 100% by 1979.[1]

Why has there been such a rapid increase in the number of cesareans for breech fetuses? Several factors have contributed. First, the breech delivery carries an increased risk of fetal injury and death. In 1964 Morgan and Kane[2] demonstrated a fivefold increase in perinatal mortality (PNM) when all breech deliveries were compared with vertex deliveries. Subsequent reports by Brenner et al[3] and Kaupilla[4] demonstrated that vaginal delivery of the breech baby frequently produces fetal injury that is avoidable with cesarean delivery and helped spur a trend toward abdominal delivery of the more risky breeches (prematures and footlings).

Second, well-informed patients are increasingly demanding that birth be free from fetal trauma and asphyxia. This has forced many experienced obstetricians to reconsider their former practices involving high-risk vaginal delivery. Finally, as cesarean births have become more frequent, many patients and practitioners have concluded that the maternal risks accompanying cesarean delivery have less long-term impact than the neonatal sequelae following suboptimal breech vaginal birth.

In summary, because breech presentation represents such a small proportion of total deliveries (3%–4%[5]), and because the maternal complications of cesarean delivery are perceived as manageable, many obstetricians have chosen the "safest route" by delivering all breeches abdominally.

Is there, then, any place for vaginal delivery of the breech in contemporary obstetrics?

FETAL AND NEONATAL RISKS OF VAGINAL BREECH DELIVERY

Prematurity

Much of the excess mortality in breech deliveries is associated with prematurity. Prematurity is more common among breech babies (20%–30%[6,7]) than among vertex fetuses (6%–8%). Because birth asphyxia and morbidity occur more frequently during delivery of premature infants in general, it is not surprising that the vaginally delivered premature breech neonate fares less well than the term neonate.[8] Duenholter et al compared the outcomes of premature breech infants delivered either by cesarean section or vaginally and found the PNM rate increased from 2.3% to 15.9% when vaginal delivery was elected.[9] The premature breech fetus tolerates vaginal birth poorly because of its narrower margin for oxygen desaturation and asphyxia and a greater propensity to hypoxic lung injury, intraventricular hemorrhage, and long-bone fracture during difficult delivery. Additionally, because the unmolded fetal head is larger than the fetal trunk until approximately 35–36 weeks,[10] the small breech body frequently prolapses through the cervix prior to full dilatation, trapping the aftercoming head. Except for the "nonviable" fetus of less than 25–26 weeks gestation,[11] vaginal delivery of premature breech infants has been generally abandoned.

Fetal Position: Head Attitude and Cord Prolapse

In 1929 Edmund B. Piper identified three major factors contributing to increased breech PNM when he introduced his breech forceps: umbilical cord prolapse, nuchal arms, and entrapment of the aftercoming head.[12] The incidence of umbilical cord prolapse is increased 5- to 20-fold in the breech presentation, most of which occurs when the breech is nonfrank.[5] Table 3.1 is a tabulation of the relative incidence of cord prolapse with the various arrangements of the fetal legs.[13]

The Nonfrank Breech

Moreover, Table 3.1 suggests that vaginal delivery of the nonfrank breech exposes the fetus to a greater risk of harm.[13,14] Gimovsky and co-workers studied the outcomes of 105 nonfrank breech deliveries randomly assigned to cesarean birth or attempted vaginal delivery. Of these, 35% were randomized to cesarean delivery and 70 candidates were evaluated for attempted vaginal delivery. Of these, 25 (35%) required cesarean delivery because of an inadequate pelvis by x-ray pelvimetry. Fourteen (20%) were

TABLE 3.1 Incidence of Umbilical Cord Prolapse by Breech Type in Patients Delivered Vaginally (N = 208)

Breech Type	Incidence of Cord Prolapse (%)
Frank	1.9
Complete	10.0
Incomplete	28.5
Double footling	8.3
Total of series	4.3

Source: Gimovsky ML, Petrie RH, Todd WD: Neonatal performance of the selected term vaginal breech delivery. *Obstet Gynecol* 56:687, 1980.

delivered operatively for arrested labor or fetal distress, giving a final success rate of 44% (31/70). When babies delivered by cesarean section were compared to those delivered vaginally, the outcomes were not statistically different.

In another series,[13] Gimovsky et al compared breech babies delivered vaginally under a protocol requiring strict predelivery fetal and maternal evaluation with babies delivered without complete predelivery assessment. One-fourth of the series were nonfrank. Vertex vaginal deliveries were used as controls. On final analysis, there was no statistical difference between the *appropriately evaluated* breech deliveries and the vertex vaginal births. However, among the breech infants delivered vaginally without complete fetal/maternal evaluation, 15% had 5-minute Apgar scores of less than 7 and 1 of 78 delivered vaginally died intrapartum. These studies showed that the use of stringent protocols can minimize but not eliminate morbidity during vaginal birth. They also confirmed earlier findings that unless candidates for vaginal delivery are carefully selected, the breech infant is at a greater risk of harm. The cesarean delivery rates for the types of nonfrank breech babies who attempted vaginal delivery are summarized in Table 3.2.

Is a success rate for trial of labor below 50% worth exposing the nonfrank breech fetus to a greater risk of harm? On the basis of the work of Gimovsky and associates (fewer than 40 patients in each protocol arm),

TABLE 3.2 Cesarean Delivery Rates for Nonfrank Breeches, by Type, Who Underwent a Trial of Labor

Nonfrank Breech	Number	Cesarean
Complete	32	14 (43%)
Double footling	21	14 (67%)
Single footling	6	2 (33%)
Incomplete	11	9 (82%)

Source: Gimovsky ML, Wallace RH, Schifrin BS, et al: Randomized management of the nonfrank breech presentation at term: A preliminary report. *Am J Obstet Gynecol* 146:34, 1983.

TABLE 3.3 Cesarean Delivery Rates for Trial of Labor in Selected Frank and Nonfrank Breech Presentation

Breech	Nonfrank (Gimovsky et al[14])	Frank (Collea et al[15])
Number	70	112
Inadequate pelvis	25 (35%)	52 (46%)
Trial of labor	45 (67%)	60 (54%)
Cesarean delivery	14 (31%)	11 (18%)

Source: Gimovsky ML, Wallace RH, Schifrin BS, et al: Randomized management of the nonfrank breech presentation at term: A preliminary report. *Am J Obstet Gynecol* 146:34, 1983; Collea JV, Chien C, Quilligan EJ: The randomized management of term frank breech presentation: A study of 208 cases. *Am J Obstet Gynecol* 137:235, 1980.

comparing morbidity rates is difficult. Nevertheless, it should be noted that the perinatal deaths occurred in the attempted vaginal delivery group; one infant had lethal anomalies but another died following a difficult vaginal delivery under halothane anesthesia requiring 5 minutes for extraction, with Apgar scores of 1, 0, and 0. Thus, despite the overall acceptable results of these recent investigations, most practitioners presently deliver term nonfrank breech infants by cesarean section.

The Frank Breech

The outcomes of frank breech infants delivered vaginally are generally less morbid than those of nonfrank breech infants because of the smaller risk of umbilical cord prolapse (Table 3.1). This led Collea et al[15] (Table 3.3) to compare the outcomes of breech deliveries using a randomized, prospective protocol. The results of this study are summarized in Figure 3.1. Three facts emerge from this study: (1) Of 112 gravidas with frank breech presentations, almost one-half were excluded from trial of labor because

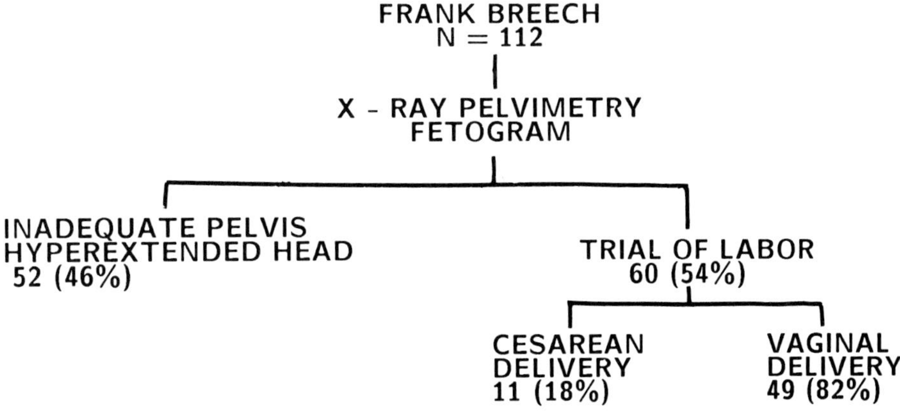

FIGURE 3.1 Flow diagram illustrating the results of the frank breech investigation by Collea and associates.[15]

of an inadequate pelvis by x-ray pelvimetry or a hyperextended fetal head. (2) Of 60 patients permitted to labor, 49 (82%) delivered vaginally. This represented 44% of the original group. (3) When neonates delivered vaginally were compared with those delivered by cesarean section, no statistical difference in morbidity was demonstrated. However, as in the studies of Gimovsky and colleagues, all of the significant fetal morbidity (three occurrences of nuchal arms, resulting in two brachial palsies and a 7.06 umbilical cord pH) occurred in the vaginal delivery group. *No* fetal injury or asphyxia occurred in the group delivered by cesarean section.

Entrapment of the Fetal Head

Entrapment of the fetal head is an obstetric emergency that can occur in association with (1) fetal macrosomia, (2) deflexion of the fetal neck and head, and (3) delivery of the trunk through an incompletely dilated cervix. Macrosomic fetuses face additional hazards regardless of presentation, but breech delivery of the fetus weighing over 4,000 g multiplies the risk of perinatal death by a factor of 10 (Figure 3.2).[16] The problem of macrosomic breech is compounded by the currently inaccurate methods used to judge fetal weight at term. Clinical estimations of fetal size using Leopold's maneuvers are notoriously inaccurate and typically *underestimate* fetal weight by as much as 1,000 g. Ultrasound methodology is accurate to within 10% for fetal weights of less than 2,000 g[17] but is much less reliable above 3,000 g, particularly when the examination is conducted during labor.[18] For these reasons, setting an upper limit to estimated fetal weight of 3,800 g will minimize the chance of head entrapment during delivery.

Hyperextension of the fetal head (Figure 3.3) increases the risk of head entrapment because the occipitomental diameter is the largest of the fetal cephalic dimensions. Ballas and Toaff[19] noted that if the attitude of the fetal head was extended beyond 90°, vaginal delivery was associated with more than a 70% incidence of spinal cord transection. These findings have been confirmed by other studies.[20,21] It is also important to note that these studies found that the "military" head position (head-neck angle = 90°) carried no increased risk during vaginal birth. The diagnosis and degree of hyperextension can be established with either fetography or ultrasonography. If a breech with a hyperextended head is identified, ultrasonography is helpful in searching the neck region for potential causes such as thyroid enlargement or loops of cord[22] (Figure 3.4).

Arrest of the aftercoming head may also occur in premature gestation. Typically, the fetal body (which has a diameter some 20% smaller than that of the fetal head) "prolapses" through the cervix. Entrapment of the premature infant's head above a partially dilated cervix frequently results in fetal injury or death. Therefore, in gestations earlier than 35 weeks,

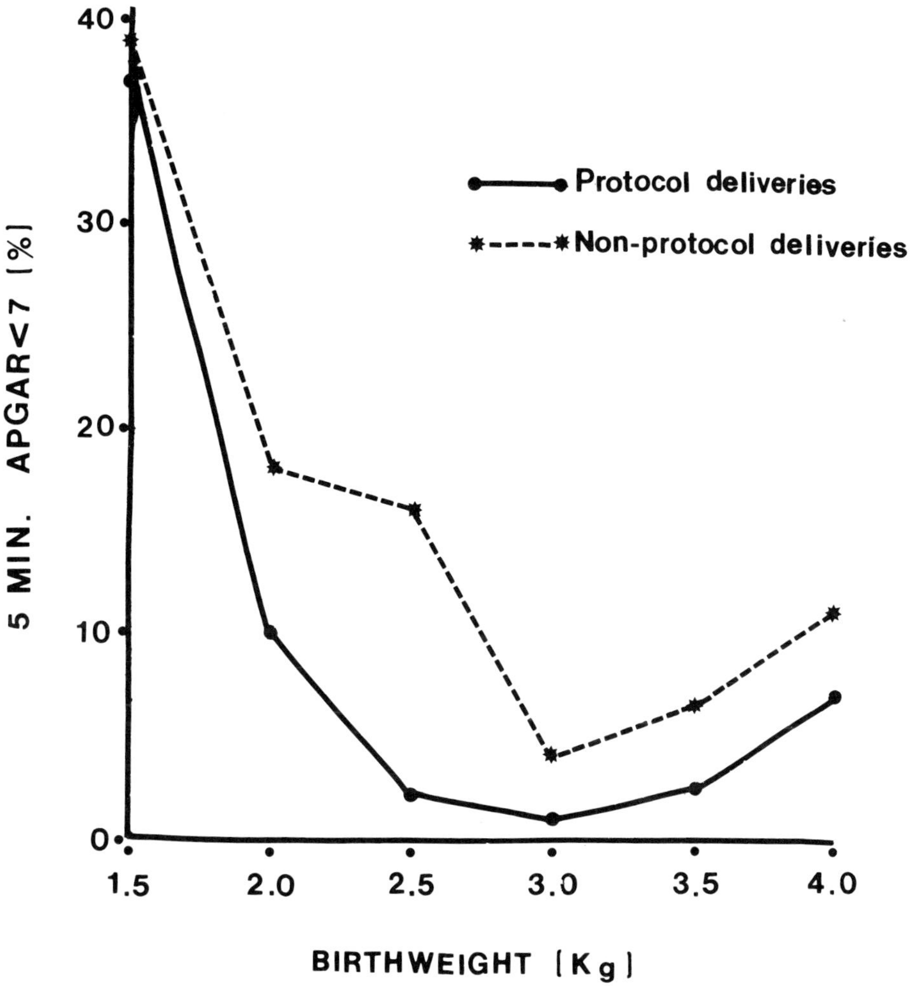

FIGURE 3.2 Percentage of low Apgar deliveries (5-minute Apgar <7) versus birth weight of breech fetus. Open boxes plot nonprotocol births; crosses plot results of deliveries fully evaluated by protocol. (After Gimovsky et al, *Obstet Gynecol* 56:687, 1980.)

regardless of estimated fetal weight, consideration should be given to cesarean delivery rather than a trial of labor.

The studies reviewed thus far consistently underscore the necessity of fully evaluating both the mother and the fetus prior to attempting vaginal delivery.[13–15] Indeed, the patient dilated 8 cm with a rapidly descending breech poses a very dangerous situation if all the steps of fetomaternal assessment cannot be methodically completed. Considering the danger of an undetected extended fetal head alone (Gimovsky and Paul noted this condition in 14% of labor candidates[23]), sufficient time must be available to evaluate the fetal position and maternal pelvic dimensions adequately. How can these assessments be completed accurately and quickly, thus minimizing the risk of harm to the fetus and mother? The

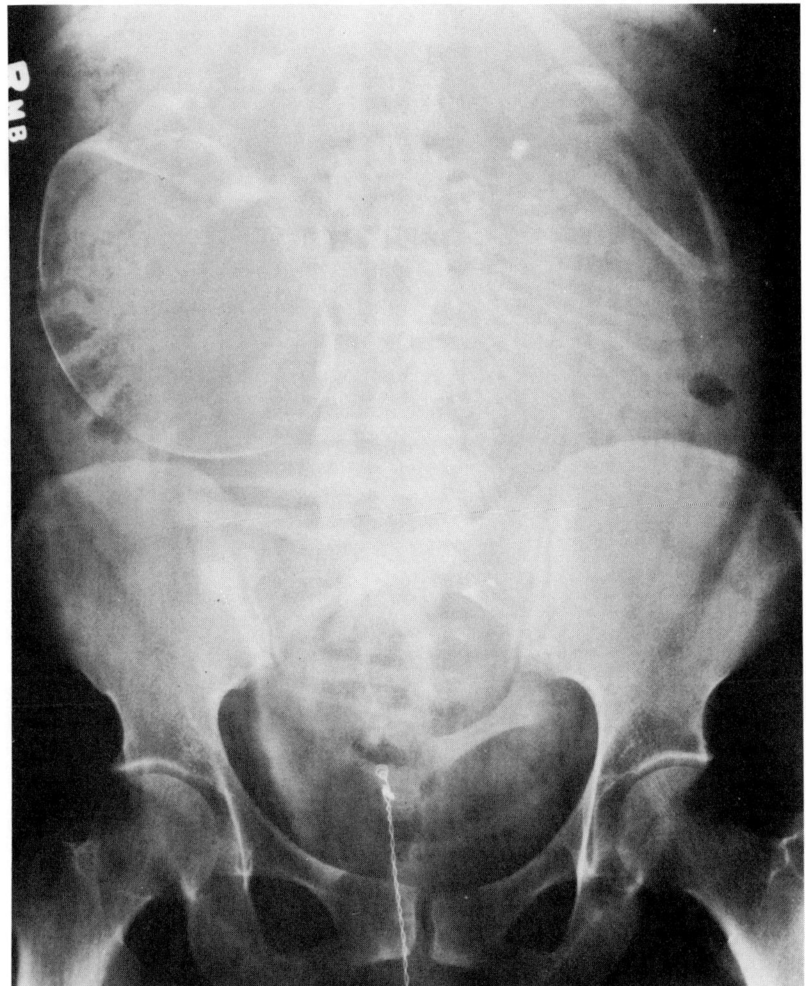

FIGURE 3.3 Fetogram of a breech presentation with a hyperextended head. (From Phelan JP, et al: *J Ultrasound Med* 2:373, 1983. Reprinted with permission from the American Institute of Ultrasound in Medicine.)

following discussion offers a potential approach to the breech presentation.

Step 1: Obtain Informed Consent

Before undertaking the breech workup, it is essential to determine if the patient is amenable to a trial of labor. In some regions of the United States where operative delivery is the de facto standard for the breech infant, many couples will demand cesarean delivery before being counseled. Attempts to dissuade such patients invite loss of patient confidence and arouse suspicion and distrust. Ideally, the issues of risk/benefit alternatives

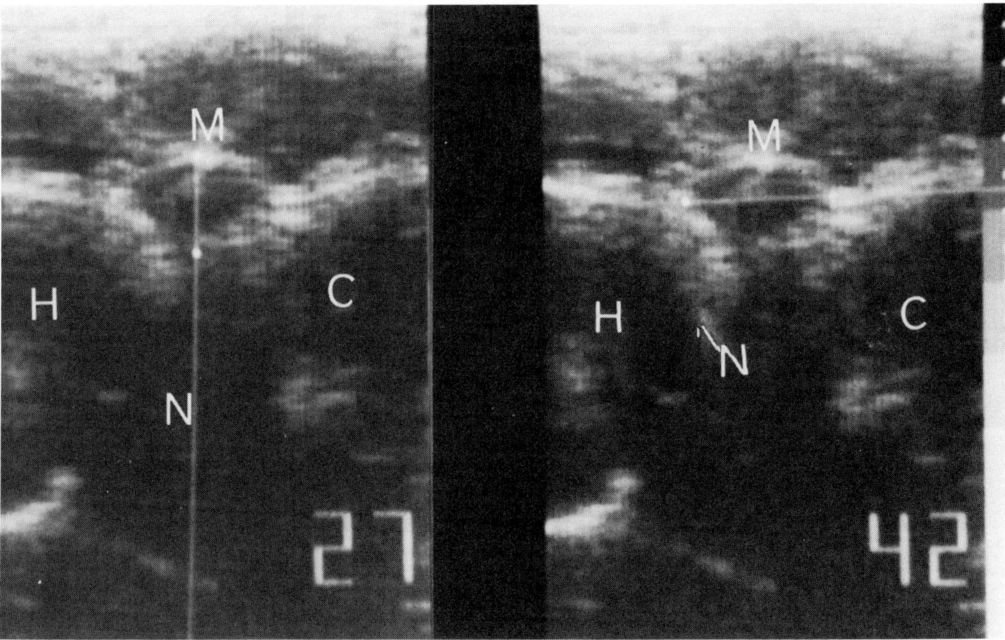

FIGURE 3.4 Ultrasound of fetal neck demonstrating a 2.7 × 4.2 cm mass. (From Phelan JP, et al: *J Ultrasound Med* 2:373, 1983. Reprinted with permission from the American Institute of Ultrasound in Medicine.)

should be routinely addressed during the antepartum period. Included in the alternatives should be the option of external cephalic version (Chapter 36). Nevertheless, because 30% or more of breech presentations are not discovered until the onset of labor, many discussions requiring informed consent will necessarily be conducted during labor.

In counseling the patient, it is essential to ensure that she understands the potential hazards of breech vaginal delivery—both maternal and fetal—compared to those of cesarean delivery. Moreover, the elements of risk assessment should be tailored to fit the patient's specific circumstances. For example, a patient with a term, frank breech should not be given the statistics of Hall and Kohl, indicating that the risk of perinatal death or asphyxia is increased 6- to 10-fold,[24,25] because those data were collected from pregnancies at all gestational ages. More realistic predictions can be made from the study of Collea and co-workers, which demonstrated no statistical benefit of cesarean delivery in properly selected cases.[15] Similarly, the patient who presents at 30 weeks should understand that premature breech infants delivered vaginally encounter a markedly increased risk of injury and death.[26] Finally, all patients should be informed that the risk of maternal morbidity following cesarean delivery may be as high as 30%–50%.[14]

TABLE 3.4 Cesarean Rate during Trial of Labor in the Breech Fetus

Pelvimetry	No. of Patients	Cesarean Section Rate
Adequate	42	17 (40%)
Marginal	26	16 (61%)
Inadequate	18	16 (89%)

Source: Ridley WJ, Jackson P, Stewart JH, et al: Role of antenatal radiology in the management of breech deliveries. *Br J Obstet Gynecol* 89:342, 1982.

Step 2: Exclude the Premature Fetus

With the exception of the extremely premature fetus (Chapter 6) and the fetus with a lethal congenital anomaly, pregnancies of less than 36 weeks gestation should be considered for cesarean delivery rather than a trial of labor. If the obstetrical dates are unknown or unsure, fetal weight estimation guidelines can be employed (see below). For the gravida who, despite counseling, insists upon vaginal delivery, careful and complete documentation of her informed choice should be entered into the medical record.

Step 3: Assess the Type of Breech and the Fetal Head Attitude

The next level of exclusion from trial of labor should focus on identifying the hyperextended head and breech types other than the frank type. Although these can be determined by a skillful ultrasonographer, many clinicians lack bedside sonography and/or experience with this technique. Consequently, the technique usually employed is the fetogram, obtained radiographically as a "flat plate." Fetuses with an angle between the mandible and cervical spine of more than 90° should be excluded from vaginal delivery. Additionally, excluding breech types other than the frank type minimizes the 10%–20% risk of fetal distress from umbilical cord prolapse. However, in some centers with continuous anesthesia availability in the *hospital* and immediate access to an operating room, trial of labor may be considered. This should be attempted only if informed consent is obtained and carefully documented.

Step 4: Perform Pelvimetry

Validation of the adequacy of the diameters of the maternal pelvis is essential to avoid head entrapment and dystocia. Ridley and associates[27] demonstrated a direct relationship between the adequacy of the maternal pelvis on x-ray pelvimetry and the success of trial of labor (Table 3.4). In their series, only 1 in 10 patients with inadequate pelvic dimensions delivered successfully. The minimum acceptable measurements (Table 3.5) do not ensure a successful outcome but rather provide an acceptable margin of safety for the fetus weighing up to 3,800 g.[28,29] The 12-11-10 rule

TABLE 3.5 Critical Pelvic Dimensions on X-Ray Pelvimetry

	Watson-Benson Criteria[28,29]	12-11-10 Rule[30]
Inlet		
Transverse	11.5–12 cm	12 cm
Anteroposterior	10.5–11 cm	11 cm
Midplane (interspinous)		
Transverse	9.5–10 cm	10 cm

(Table 3.5) has also been recommended as the minimum pelvic dimensions because it is easier to remember and provides a greater margin of safety for the fetus.[30] More recently, the use of computed tomography (CT) scanning for pelvimetry has been advocated.[31,32] This technique provides markedly superior image quality and precision of measurement, as well as a significant reduction in the dose of radiation to the fetus. Finally, attempted vaginal delivery of the breech baby is considered reasonable when all three measurements are equal to or exceed these minimums.

Step 5: Estimate Fetal Weight

As documented in Figure 3.2, fetal weights greater than 4,000 g are associated with increased morbidity and death. Similarly, immature fetuses weighing less than 2,000 g are at higher risk.[33] Estimating fetal weight as accurately as possible will avoid inadvertent vaginal delivery of a fetus at the dangerous ends of the spectrum. This can be done either clinically, using a combination of the tape measure and bimanual palpation, or through the use of ultrasonically derived fetal measurements. The disadvantages of the manual method are poor accuracy[34] and misjudgments regarding salvageability. The disadvantage of the sonographic method is the requirement to obtain accurate measurements of the biparietal and abdominal diameters and to consult tables or a programmable calculator. Nevertheless, the formulas of Warsof et al[35] and Shepard et al[36] (Table 3.6) predict fetal weight accurately to within 10% of the actual weight more than 90% of the time.[17] Fetuses whose manually or sonographically estimated weights fall outside the 2,500- to 3,800-g range should be considered for cesarean delivery.

TABLE 3.6 Formulas for Estimating Fetal Weight from Ultrasound-Derived Measurements

Warsof[35]	$\text{Log } 10 \text{ (birth weight)}_2 = -1.599 + 0.144 \text{ (BPD)} + 0.032 \text{ (AC)} - 0.111 \text{ (BPD}^2 \times \text{AC)}/1{,}000$
Shepard[36]	$\text{Log } 10 \text{ (birth weight)} = -1.7492 + 0.166 \text{ (BPD)} + 0.046 \text{ (AC)} - 2.646 \text{ (AC} \times \text{BPD)}/1{,}000$

BPD, biparietal diameter; AC, abdominal circumference.
These formulas can be inserted in programmable calculators.

Step 6: Evaluate the Delivery Team

Once the essential elements of fetal and maternal adequacy have been ensured, it is important to make certain that the delivery unit and obstetrical team are adequately prepared for breech delivery. In order to conduct a vaginal breech delivery, the following conditions should be considered prerequisites:

1. An anesthesia provider (anesthesiologist or qualified nurse anesthetist) is immediately available to the labor suite to assist in delivery. For nonfrank breeches, the anesthesia provider should be physically present or available within 2–4 minutes at all times. For frank breeches, the provider should be present at the beginning of the second stage.
2. A pediatrician should be available throughout labor and present at the delivery to resuscitate the newborn if necessary.
3. The delivery should be conducted in a room capable of supporting cesarean delivery. An individual who can perform as scrub nurse and another individual who can circulate should be in the delivery room during preparation for birth. The cesarean delivery instruments should be in the delivery room, although the sterile packs need not be opened until needed.
4. The obstetrician should be skilled and experienced in the management of complications of breech delivery.

The importance of a skilled delivery team cannot be overemphasized. If any of these elements are missing, the assumptions used in the Collea et al[15] and Gimovsky et al[14] studies, which established the ground rules for safe vaginal breech delivery, will not be satisfied, and the outcomes of these studies will not necessarily be achieved. Medicolegally, conducting vaginal breech delivery without satisfying these requirements exposes the mother and fetus to a greater risk of harm and the physician to a more difficult case to defend.

The importance of an experienced and skilled obstetrician attending the breech delivery deserves further discussion. The delivering physician should be familiar with the management of nuchal arms and head entrapment, as well as with application of the Piper forceps to the aftercoming head. Not all obstetricians, particularly those trained in the past decade, will be skilled in this type of delivery. Moreover, many previously experienced practitioners may be "rusty." Consider the typical experience with vaginal breech delivery that the average practitioner might have in the course of a year in practice (Table 3.7). These calculations for a hypothetical practitioner demonstrate that the opportunity to deliver a breech baby vaginally will occur only once or twice per year if all of the recommended guidelines are followed. One has to ask, is this adequate experience to continue to consider oneself experienced in breech vaginal

TABLE 3.7 A Year's Experience with Breech Delivery in the Average Obstetrical Practice

20 deliveries per month = 240 deliveries per year	
4% of 240 deliveries = 10 breech deliveries per year	
Exclude:	4/10 Premature
	3/10 Inadequate pelvimetry
	1/10 Deflexed fetal head
	2/10 Trial of labor
	1/10 Cesarean section for labor arrest or fetal distress
	1/10 Successful vaginal delivery

delivery? Clearly, this question must be considered carefully by each obstetrician who attempts vaginal breech birth.

INTRAPARTUM MANAGEMENT OF THE BREECH BABY

When to Interrupt Breech Labor with Cesarean Delivery

In general, the usual guidelines for conducting vertex labor should be observed with breech delivery. Dystocia is diagnosed when cervical dilatation proceeds at a rate of less than 1.2 cm/hr in the primipara or less than 1.5 cm/hr in the multipara during the active phase of labor. This should prompt an evaluation of labor forces with an intrauterine pressure catheter. If the contractions are adequate in amplitude and frequency, progress should be monitored closely. If labor progress arrests in the active phase for 2 hours or more despite adequate uterine contractions, cesarean delivery is indicated.

If the contraction pattern is inadequate, using oxytocin to stimulate desultory labor is controversial. The studies of both Gimovsky[14] and Collea[15] and their colleagues utilized oxytocin for protraction disorders, but none of Collea's seven patients who received labor augmentation delivered vaginally.[15] Of nine augmented labors in Gimovsky's series, eight of which were in multipara, only two involved vaginal delivery. One of them involved entrapment of the aftercoming head and fetal asphyxia.[21] If oxytocin is used in protracted labor, care should be taken to ensure that progress is adequate and that the second stage is limited to 2 hours or less.

Technical Aspects of Cesarean Delivery of the Breech Baby

Surgical delivery of the breech baby requires technical skill to avoid the same types of fetal injuries that can occur during vaginal delivery. After opening the peritoneum, the surgeon should assess the adequacy of the abdominal incision for delivery. This is important because the fetal head can be trapped by the maternal abdomen. If this is a possibility, consideration should be given to widening the incision with either a Cherney or Maylard incision, as outlined in Chapter 12. Once the adequacy of the abdominal incision has been established, the orientation of the lower uterine segment must be assessed. At least 10 cm should be available if a transverse incision is to be made. Using the bandage scissors to curve a transverse uterine incision upward may provide some additional room, but if doubt exists, a vertical incision is preferable.

Prior to making the uterine incision, the lie and station of the fetus should be verified by palpation. The fetus initially presenting as a breech may be found unexpectedly in a transverse lie at the time of surgery, especially if it is premature. If this is the case, the fetus can be repolarized by manual version, held in place by an assistant, and delivered via a transverse uterine incision. If version is unsuccessful, and especially if the fetus is in a back-down transverse lie, a vertical incision is recommended to avoid the potentially traumatic manipulations necessary for extraction.

It is possible, despite the best preparations, to encounter nuchal arms or head entrapment after delivering the fetal body at cesarean delivery. The technique for reducing extended arms is similar to that practiced in vaginal delivery. Inadvertent extension of the uterine incision can be minimized by turning the fetus on its side and reducing the posterior arm first. Usually the remaining arm will be delivered easily. If the head becomes trapped by the uterus contracting vigorously around the fetal neck, all efforts should be directed to enlarging the surgical opening and avoiding forcible extraction of the head. Even with the head trapped, the umbilical circulation will provide an adequate oxygen supply during the time required to complete the delivery. Occasionally it is possible to free the head by enlarging the uterine incision laterally with bandage scissors, but a vertical incision into the fundus is always successful and is often a better choice.

INDUCTION OF LABOR VERSUS SCHEDULED CESAREAN DELIVERY FOR THE BREECH PRESENTATION

An especially vexing problem concerns the timing of cesarean delivery for the gravida who is approaching or past her due date with a breech lie. Occasionally, such patients will push for cesarean delivery as early as 37 weeks. In the patient who has refused external cephalic version (Chapter 36) and does not desire a trial of labor, the timing of cesarean delivery should be balanced between the probability of spontaneous conversion to vertex and the risk of cord prolapse. At 37 weeks, the spontaneous conversion rate is approximately 15%–20%.[37] This incidence is considerably less in the primigravida breech.[38] After 40 weeks, the number of breech fetuses spontaneously converting to vertex is negligible.[39] Finally, the risk of umbilical cord prolapse depends on the type of breech (Table

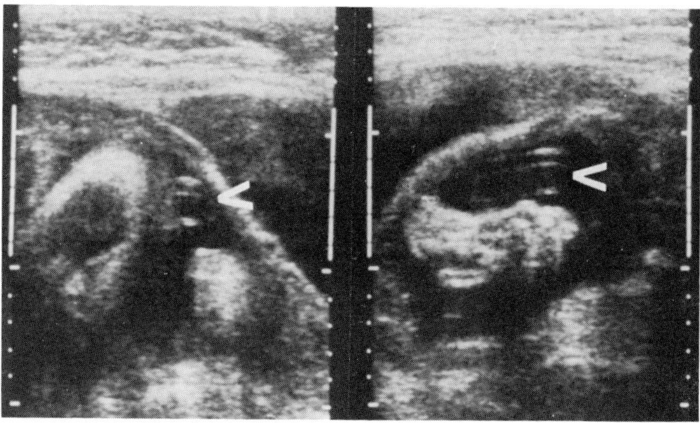

FIGURE 3.5 Ultrasound evaluation of a breech presentation demonstrating a funic presentation at the arrow.

3.1) and increases as the patient approaches her due date.[13] An ultrasound evaluation of the lower uterine segment may help identify a funic presentation (Figure 3.5) and lead to earlier operative intervention. In the absence of a funic presentation, in patients who have elected operative delivery, cesarean delivery should be planned 1 week prior to the due date. Waiting longer is of little value and exposes the fetus to a greater risk of harm. Prior to actually performing the planned cesarean, it is important to verify that the fetus is still in the breech presentation.

For the gravida who wishes to attempt vaginal delivery, it is convenient to determine, prior to labor, the adequacy of the pelvic dimensions and the type of breech. Near the due date, scheduled pelvimetric studies can be done (CT will be easier to perform on a scheduled basis) and patients with inadequate pelvic dimensions should be scheduled for cesarean delivery. The type of breech should be confirmed whenever a breech is suspected clinically. If a nonfrank breech is confirmed, the patient should be informed of the attendant risks, and cesarean delivery, as previously outlined, should be recommended.

Management of the term frank breech patient who qualifies for a trial of labor should be expectant until 42 weeks. Antepartum fetal heart rate testing should be initiated 7 days past the due date and should be done twice weekly. Labor induction with amniotomy or oxytocin can be considered at any time when the Bishop score is favorable (>5) and the frank breech is engaged. However, because of the additive risks of breech presentation and postdatism, many practitioners will quite reasonably perform a cesarean for breech pregnancies that reach 42 weeks.

The Transverse Lie at Term

Optimal management of the transverse lie at term consists of polarization to vertex and vaginal delivery. Version of the transverse fetus can be per-

TABLE 3.8 Etiologic Factors in Transverse Lie

Maternal Factors	Fetal Factors
Multiparity	Prematurity
Uterine anomaly[a]	Hydramnios
Pelvic tumors[a]	Fetal anomalies[a]
Contracted pelvis[a]	Hydrocephaly[a]
	Myotonic dystrophy
	Placenta previa[a]

[a] May not be candidates for version and vaginal delivery.

formed prior to or during labor if the membranes are intact.[40] If version is unsuccessful, contraindicated, or refused by the patient, management of the transverse lie is by cesarean delivery. When determining management plans in these patients, and before committing them to version or cesarean delivery, it is crucial to identify potential complicating factors at the outset.

Incidence, Etiology, and Diagnosis

Transverse lie occurs at a rate of 3–4 per 1,000 births.[41,42] The actual rate of nonaxial lie is higher earlier in gestation (approximately 20 per 1,000 at 32 weeks) because of the continuing trend toward spontaneous polarization as term approaches.[37] Indeed, Edwards and Nicholson documented spontaneous polarization prior to labor in 20% of 254 patients, with transverse lie detected at 38 to 39 weeks.[43] But Phelan et al[44] found an 83% spontaneous conversion rate to a longitudinal lie in patients at 37 weeks or later.

Transverse lie may be associated with a number of abnormal maternal and fetal states (Table 3.8). The transverse lie is best evaluated by a combination of ultrasound and physical examination. Sonographic assessment should include verification of gestational age, determination of placental location (rule out placenta previa), a thorough search for fetal anomalies that would contraindicate vaginal birth (eg, significant hydrocephalus), and a survey of the uterus and adnexae for myomata or ovarian tumors, which may prevent fetal polarization.

If none of these factors are present and the patient is in labor, the cervix should be examined to ensure that there is adequate time for the version attempt. The fetal heart rate tracing should give assurance of fetal well-being. The final preparatory step, especially if the version is being attempted with significant cervical dilatation, should involve anesthesia consultation to ensure the ability to manage cord prolapse or persistent fetal bradycardia promptly.

Management

The actual technique of version of the transverse lie is similar to that employed for breeches (Chapter 36). Because such fetuses tend to revert to a transverse position, antepartum external version should be undertaken when the cervix is favorable for induction of labor. Hydramnios presents a unique problem during version because the fetus tends to return to a nonaxial lie. This can be avoided by first performing the version and then starting contractions with oxytocin while the operator holds the fetal head at the pelvic inlet. Alternatively, one can cautiously rupture the membranes while the head is held engaged subsequent to the version. Occasionally, rupturing of the membranes will precipitate a rapid rush of amnionic fluid, leading to uterine decompression and umbilical cord prolapse, placental abruption, or both. This emergency can be minimized by (1) performing amniotomy in the delivery room, (2) using an 18-gauge spinal needle to puncture the membranes and thus control fluid release, or (3) performing a percutaneous amniocentesis high on the fundus and draining the fluid slowly into a sterile drainage system. If fetal distress supervenes during these maneuvers, the capability for rapid cesarean section should be immediately available.

For the fetus who persists in a transverse lie, operative delivery should be begun without delay, particularly if the cervix is dilated and the umbilical cord or extremities are presenting. The intraoperative precautions mentioned previously for delivery of the breech baby by cesarean section should be observed with the transverse lie as well.

Outcome

Although earlier studies indicated that the transverse lie engenders PNM rates as high as 24%,[45] contemporary practice should limit perinatal death to the fetus with severe congenital anomalies or extreme prematurity.[39]

SUMMARY

The nonvertex fetus presents a situation fraught with maternal, fetal, and malpractice peril. These risks are magnified by the relative infrequency of these presentations. Successful management depends on careful and meticulous predelivery evaluation. Skilled anesthetic support is essential throughout. As a general principle, cesarean section should be the delivery route of choice unless the obstetrician can be satisfied that the dangers of fetal injury and asphyxia are minimal.

The opinions expressed in this chapter are those of the author and not necessarily those of the United States Navy or the Department of Defense.

REFERENCES

1. Collea JV: Reducing mortality from breech presentations. *Contemp ObGyn*, 1985, January: 171.

2. Morgan HS, Kane SH: An analysis of 16,327 breech births. *JAMA* 187:262, 1964.
3. Brenner WE, Bruce RD, Hendricks CH: The characteristics and perils of breech presentation. *Am J Obstet Gynecol* 118:700, 1974.
4. Kaupilla O: The perinatal mortality in breech deliveries and observations on affecting factors: A retrospective study of 2227 cases. *Acta Obstet Gynecol Scand* 39:1, 1975.
5. Pritchard JA, MacDonald PC, Gant NF: *Williams Obstetrics*, ed 17. New York, Appleton-Century-Crofts, 1984.
6. Smith RS, Oldham RR: Breech delivery. *Obstet Gynecol* 36:151, 1970.
7. Moore WT, Steptoe PP: The experience of the Johns Hopkins Hospital with breech presentation. *South Med J* 36:295, 1943.
8. Goldenberg RL, Nelson KG: The premature breech. *Am J Obstet Gynecol* 127:240, 1977.
9. Duenholter JH, Wells CE, Reisch JS, et al: A paired controlled study of vaginal and abdominal delivery of the low birthweight breech fetus. *Obstet Gynecol* 54:310, 1979.
10. Jeanty P, Romero R: The head perimeter-to-abdominal perimeter ratio, in *Obstetrical Ultrasound*. New York, McGraw-Hill Book Co, 1983, pp 168–169.
11. Moore TR, Resnik R: Management of the very low birthweight fetus. *Contemp ObGyn* 1984, June: 174–191.
12. Piper EB, Bachman C: The prevention of fetal injuries in breech delivery. *JAMA* 92:217, 1929.
13. Gimovsky ML, Petrie RH, Todd WD: Neonatal performance of the selected term vaginal breech delivery. *Obstet Gynecol* 56:687, 1980.
14. Gimovsky ML, Wallace RL, Schifrin BS, et al: Randomized management of the nonfrank breech presentation at term: A preliminary report. *Am J Obstet Gynecol* 146:34, 1983.
15. Collea JV, Chien C, Quilligan EJ: The randomized management of term frank breech presentation: A study of 208 cases. *Am J Obstet Gynecol* 137:235, 1980.
16. Moir JC, Meyerscough PR: *Kerr's Operative Obstetrics*. London, Bailliere, Tindall, Cassell, 1971, p 478.
17. Key TC, Dattel B, Resnik R: The ultrasonographic estimation of fetal weight in the very low birthweight infant. *Am J Obstet Gynecol* 145:574, 1983.
18. Yarkoni S, Reece AE, Wan M, et al: Intrapartum fetal weight estimation: A comparison of three formulae. *J Ultrasound Med* 5:707, 1986.
19. Ballas S, Toaff R: Hyperextension of the fetal head in breech presentation: Radiological evaluation and significance. *Br J Obstet Gynecol* 83:201, 1976.
20. Caterini H, Langer A, Sama JC, et al: Fetal risk in hyperextension of the fetal head in breech presentation. *Am J Obstet Gynecol* 119:564, 1976.
21. Daw E: Hyperextension of the head in breech presentation. *Am J Obstet Gynecol* 119:564, 1974.
22. Phelan JP, Bethel M, Devore G, et al: Use of ultrasound in the breech presentation with hyperextension of the fetal head: A case report. *J Ultrasound Med* 2:373, 1983.
23. Gimovsky ML, Paul RH: Singleton breech presentation in labor: Experience in 1980. *Am J Obstet Gynecol* 143:733, 1982.
24. Collea JV: Current management of breech presentation. *Clin Obstet Gynecol* 23:525, 1980.
25. Hall JE, Kohl SG: Breech presentation. *Am J Obstet Gynecol* 72:977, 1956.
26. Goldenberg RL, Nelson KG: The premature breech. *Am J Obstet Gynecol* 127:240, 1977.
27. Ridley WJ, Jackson P, Stewart JH, et al: Role of antenatal radiography in the management of breech deliveries. *Br J Obstet Gynecol* 89:342, 1982.
28. Benson WL, Boyce DC, Vaughn DL: Breech delivery in the primigravida. *Obstet Gynecol* 40:417, 1972.

29. Watson WJ, Benson WL: Vaginal delivery for the selected frank breech infant at term. *Obstet Gynecol* 64:638, 1984.
30. Phelan JP: Management of the breech presentation, in Mishell DR, Brenner PF (eds): *Management of Common Problems in Obstetrics and Gynecology*, ed 2. Oradell, NJ, Medical Economic Books (in press).
31. Gimovsky JL, Petrie WK, Petrie R, et al: X-ray pelvimetry in a breech protocol: A comparison of digital radiography and conventional methods. *Am J Obstet Gynecol* 153:887, 1985.
32. Kopelman JN, Duff P, Karl RT, et al: Computed tomographic pelvimetry in the evaluation of the breech presentation. *Obstet Gynecol* 68:455, 1986.
33. Gimovsky ML, Petrie RH: The intrapartum and neonatal performance of the low-birth-weight vaginal breech delivery. *J Reprod Med* 27:451, 1982.
34. Paul RH, Koh KS, Monfared AH: Obstetric factors influencing outcome in infants weighing from 1001 to 1500 grams. *Am J Obstet Gynecol* 133:503, 1979.
35. Warsof SL, Gohari P, Berkowitz RL: The estimation of fetal weight by computer-assisted analysis. *Am J Obstet Gynecol* 128:881, 1977.
36. Shepard MJ, Richards VA, Berkowitz RL, et al: An evaluation of two equations in predicting fetal weight by ultrasound. *Am J Obstet Gynecol* 142:47, 1982.
37. VanDorsten JP, Schifrin BS, Wallace RL: Randomized control trial of external cephalic version with tocolysis in late pregnancy. *Am J Obstet Gynecol* 141:417, 1981.
38. Westgren M, Edvall H, Nordstrom L, et al: Spontaneous cephalic version of breech presentation in the last trimester. *Br J Obstet Gynecol* 92:19, 1985.
39. Ranney B: The gentle art of external cephalic version. *Am J Obstet Gynecol* 116:239, 1973.
40. Phelan JP, Stine LE, Edwards NB, et al: The role of external version in the intrapartum management of the transverse lie presentation. *Am J Obstet Gynecol* 151:724, 1985.
41. Cruikshank DP, White CA: Obstetric malpresentations—Twenty years' experience. *Am J Obstet Gynecol* 116:1097, 1973.
42. Johnson CE: Transverse presentation of fetus. *JAMA* 187:642, 1964.
43. Edwards RL, Nicholson HO: The management of the unstable lie in late pregnancy. *J Obstet Gynaecol Br Commonw* 76:713, 1969.
44. Phelan JP, Boucher M, Mueller E, et al: The nonlaboring transverse lie: A management dilemma. *J Reprod Med* 31:184, 1986.
45. Yates MJ: Transverse foetal lie in labour. *J Obstet Gynaecol Br Commonw* 71:245, 1964.

Chapter 4

Multiple Gestations

Frank A. Chervenak, MD, and
Judith L. Chervenak, MD

Obstetricians have long recognized that multiple gestations are inherently at high risk for both maternal and fetal complications. The former include pregnancy-induced hypertension, anemia, hyperemesis gravidarum, pyelonephritis, hepatic cholestasis, and antepartum and postpartum hemorrhage. The latter include prematurity, intrauterine growth retardation, malpresentation, congenital anomalies, hydramnios, and cord accidents.[1]

Twins are not an uncommon occurrence, with a reported incidence in the United States of 12 per 1,000 births.[2] Approximately one-third of these are monozygotic, that is, they result from a single fertilized ovum. The incidence of monozygotic twins is thought to be nearly constant throughout the world regardless of maternal age, race, or parity at 4 per 1,000 births. Dizygotic twins, which result from two separate fertilized ova, are much more variable in frequency. The incidence of dizygotic twins is higher in certain families, although the inheritance pattern is not well defined. They are more common in blacks and less common in Asians. They occur more frequently in women of higher age and higher parity, as well as higher weight and height. Lastly, women who receive fertility medications that result in multiple ovulations will, of course, have a higher frequency of dizygotic twins.[2,3] Triplet pregnancies spontaneously occur at the rate of 1 per 10,000 births,[4] and births of higher order are even more rare.

The modern management of multiple gestation is based on its accurate antenatal diagnosis. Until recently, 50% of multiple gestations were not identified until the time of delivery.[5] The widespread use of obstetrical ultrasound has greatly reduced this rate to less than 5%.[6] The presence of multiple gestational sacs with respective fetal poles can define a multiple gestation during the first trimester. During the second and third trimesters, a membrane should be seen separating each fetus. Failure to see this mem-

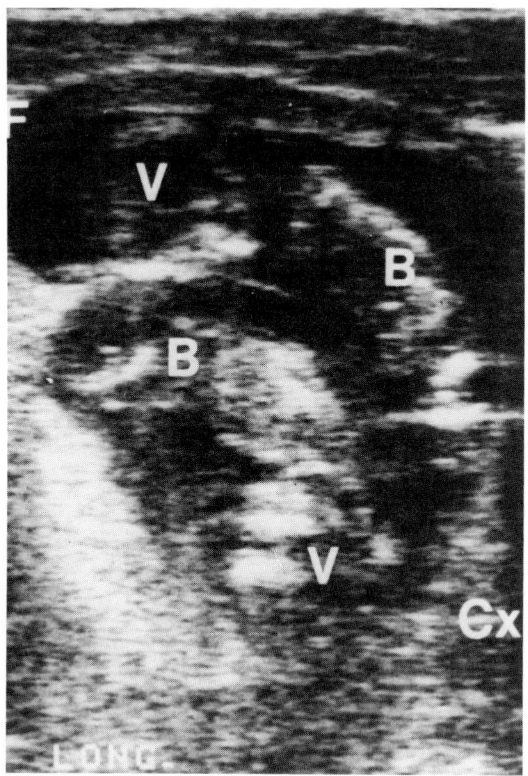

FIGURE 4.1 Longitudinal sonogram demonstrating twin gestation in vertex-breech presentation. F, uterine fundus; Cx, cervix; V, vertex; B, breech.

brane should alert the examiner to the possibility of monoamniotic twins. Ultrasound is also valuable to define the fetal presentations in a multiple gestation (Figure 4.1).

Considerations in the antepartum management of multiple gestations include prevention of prematurity, evaluation of fetal growth, fetal assessment, detection of fetal anomalies, and management of fetal death.

The greatest cause of perinatal morbidity and mortality associated with multiple gestation is premature birth. Prophylactic bed rest, although widely prescribed, is of uncertain therapeutic benefit.[7] The authors do not advocate hospitalized bed rest unless it is warranted for other indications. Prophylactic cerclage placement and prophylactic tocolysis usage have not been found to be clinically efficacious in the prevention of premature birth for multiple gestations.[8] These interventions should be utilized, of course, when there is clinical evidence of an incompetent cervix or premature labor. Any patient with a multiple gestation should be educated about the early signs of premature labor. Home monitoring is a recently described option that may be of value.[9]

Multiple gestations are at substantially increased risk for intrauterine growth retardation. The higher the number of fetuses, the greater the risk because of an excessive demand on the uteroplacental circulation. It is rare for this phenomenon to occur prior to 26 weeks of gestation. Although twin-to-twin transfusion due to placental vascular anastomoses may result in growth retardation of one twin, this phenomenon is responsible for only a small minority of cases of growth retardation among multiple gestations. It is impossible to assess clinically individual fetal growth in multiple gestation with fundal height measurements or other manual determinations. It is therefore the standard of care that every multiple gestation be followed with monthly ultrasound examinations, beginning at about 26 weeks.

Ultrasound examination can then suggest intrauterine growth retardation in one or both twins based on a decrease in estimated fetal weight or other ultrasound parameters.[10] It is important to remember, however, that constitutional differences among the fetuses may occur that are not pathologic.

Because fetuses of multiple gestation are at increased risk for uteroplacental insufficiency, fetal assessment in the third trimester may be valuable.[11] Although there is no consensus concerning the optimal method of fetal assessment, nonstress testing, amniotic fluid assessment, biophysical profiles, and Doppler studies[12] are currently the most widely used methods in this clinical setting.

Among monozygotic twins, there is a generalized increase in fetal anomalies. Two anomalies that are specific to multiple gestations are conjoined twins and the acardiac twin. In the former case, delayed separation of a single zygote is responsible; in the latter, arterial-to-arterial anastomoses permit sustained growth.[10] In those cases in which fetal anomalies are diagnosed prior to 24 weeks gestation, termination of pregnancy may be elected by the parents. Management during the third trimester and during labor is dependent upon the specific anomaly.

It is possible for one embryo of a multiple gestation to die spontaneously during the first trimester. This phenomenon, termed a "vanishing twin," is of uncertain frequency and may be responsible for vaginal bleeding in what may then evolve as a singleton pregnancy or a multiple gestation of lower order.[13] Occasionally, death of a single fetus of a multiple gestation may occur during the second or third trimester. In such cases, maternal coagulopathy due to the retained dead fetus may result. Weekly surveillance of the maternal clotting status is therefore indicated in any case of second- or third-trimester fetal demise.[14]

INTRAPARTUM MANAGEMENT OF MULTIPLE GESTATION

The intrapartum management of multiple gestation has long challenged the obstetrical profession. Currently this controversy primarily involves the role of elective cesarean delivery for certain subsets of twin gestation. Any delivery plan requires consideration of the varied possible presentations for twin A and twin B. Whereas Figure 4.2 illustrates these varied

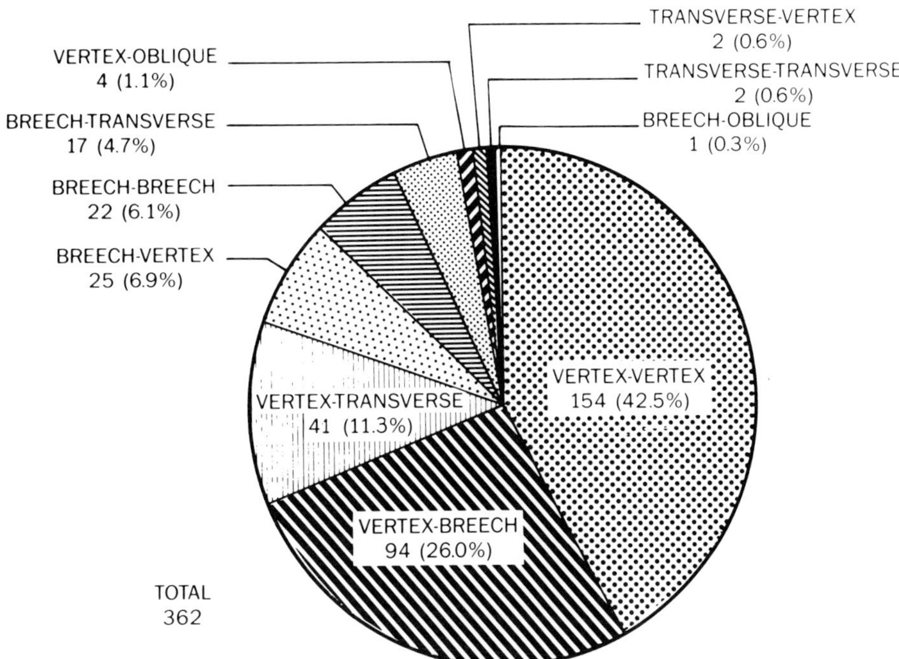

FIGURE 4.2 Diagram showing occurrence of intrapartum presentations for 362 consecutive twin gestations. (From Chervenak FA, Johnson RE, Youcha S, et al: Intrapartum management of twin gestation. *Obstet Gynecol* 65:119, 1985. Reprinted with permission.)

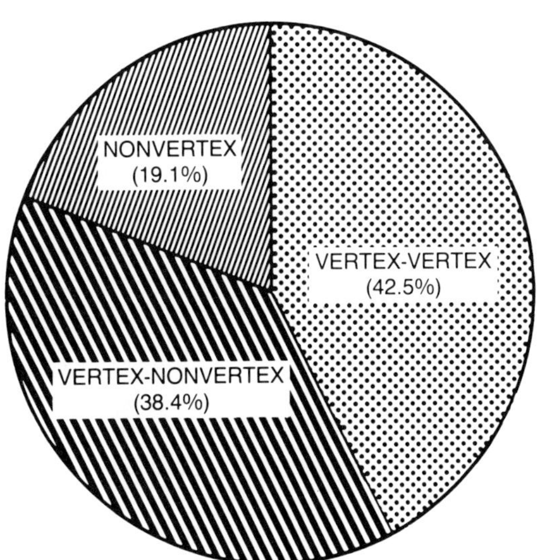

FIGURE 4.3 Diagram showing the occurrence of twin A, vertex with twin B, vertex; twin A, vertex with twin B, nonvertex; and twin A, nonvertex for 362 consecutive twin gestations.

combinations for a population of twins, Figure 4.3 illustrates a clinically more useful classification of twin presentations, with all combinations of twin presentations being classified into three groups: (1) twin A, vertex with twin B, vertex (42.5% of the total twin population); (2) twin A, vertex with twin B, nonvertex (38.4% of the total twin population); and (3) twin A, nonvertex (19.1% of the total twin population).[6] The authors will present an intrapartum management plan for each of these three subsets of twin gestation and discuss controversial areas.

Twin A, Vertex with Twin B, Vertex

There is a broad consensus that attempted vaginal delivery is appropriate for vertex–vertex twins.[1,6,15–21] Although it has been suggested that vertex–vertex twins weighing less than 1,500 g should have a cesarean delivery,[22] there are few data to support this position. Recent series[6,15] have shown that 70%–80% of vertex–vertex twins deliver vaginally.

Previously, it was believed that the time interval between twin deliveries should be no more than 30 minutes; otherwise there would be risk of asphyxia to the second twin from diminished placental circulation.[5,23,24] However, more recently, 5-minute Apgar scores have been shown not to correlate with the time interval between twin deliveries.[6,15,21] After delivery of twin A, there is no urgency to deliver twin B if electronic fetal heart rate monitoring or sonographic visualization of the fetal heart shows no abnormality. In fact, although rare, intervals between deliveries of twins of up to 131 days have been reported.[25–27] This phenomenon may occur either in a bicornuate or a normal uterus. If a prolonged delivery interval is ever considered after delivery of a very premature twin, the membranes of the second twin must be intact, and if the placenta is retained, the umbilical cord of the first twin must be clamped close to the cervix. The authors agree with the recommendation that cervical suture and tocolysis are probably not indicated in this setting.[27]

For all vertex–vertex presentations, if labor has not resumed within 10 minutes of delivery of the first twin, oxytocin augmentation with careful surveillance of the fetal heart may be valuable.[20] Once the vertex is in the pelvic inlet, amniotomy is recommended. There is no current series demonstrating the safety of internal podalic version in cases of fetal distress. If deterioration of the fetal heart rate tracing of twin B occurs before atraumatic vaginal delivery is possible, cesarean delivery should be considered the management of choice. Because of this possibility, the availability of immediate cesarean delivery should be considered the standard of care for all twins.

Lastly, the authors do not believe that the vary rare possibility of spontaneous conversion of a vertex second twin to a nonvertex presentation justifies the routine use of pelvimetry for all cases. If this rare situation occurs, external version under sonographic guidance but not breech delivery of the second twin may be attempted.

Twin A Vertex with Twin B, Nonvertex

The management of twin gestations in vertex-breech or vertex-transverse presentation is especially controversial. Several investigators have advocated cesarean delivery as the proper management when the second twin is in a breech or transverse lie.[15–20] This approach has been justified by reports of an association of increased perinatal mortality[28–30] and depressed Apgar scores[24,30–32] with breech delivery of the second twin. Cetrulo has recently reviewed the experience at St. Margaret's Hospital in Boston, where almost all vertex–nonvertex twins have a cesarean delivery. He found that the usual differential mortality and morbidity for twin B versus twin A was virtually eliminated in his population.[15] The authors believe, however, that routine cesarean is not necessary in order to achieve nontraumatic birth. The options of intrapartum external version and breech delivery of the second twin will now be discussed, and the effects of using these options on neonatal morbidity and mortality of the vaginally delivered second twin in malpresentation will be analyzed.

Intrapartum External Version

Recently, there has been an increase in the popularity of version of the singleton breech. Several investigators have advocated this method,[33–36] whereas others[37,38] believe that the risk of cord accident or placental abruption is substantial. In a prospective randomized study, external cephalic version was found to be a safe and efficacious way of managing breech presentation late in the singleton pregnancy.[39]

There have been several reports of external cephalic version of the second twin.[40–43] Ramney reported successful version with subsequent vaginal delivery in 9 transverse and 2 breech second twins.[40] In a recent series, in 10 of 14 (71%) transverse presentations and 8 of 11 (73%) breech presentations, version was successful and resulted in vertex vaginal delivery (Figure 4.4). The success of the version was not related to gestational age or birth weight. However, when the birth weight of twin B was more than 500 g greater than that of twin A, two version attempts did not result in vaginal vertex deliveries. The success of version was not related to parity. All eight versions attempted under peridural anesthesia were successful, suggesting that relaxation of the abdominal wall musculature may be helpful in successful execution of the version. The 5-minute Apgar score was depressed in only two cases in this entire series (6 and 6). The time interval between delivery of twin A and twin B was not related to a 1- or 5-minute Apgar score, suggesting that the time spent in version did not have a detrimental effect. The maternal morbidity in

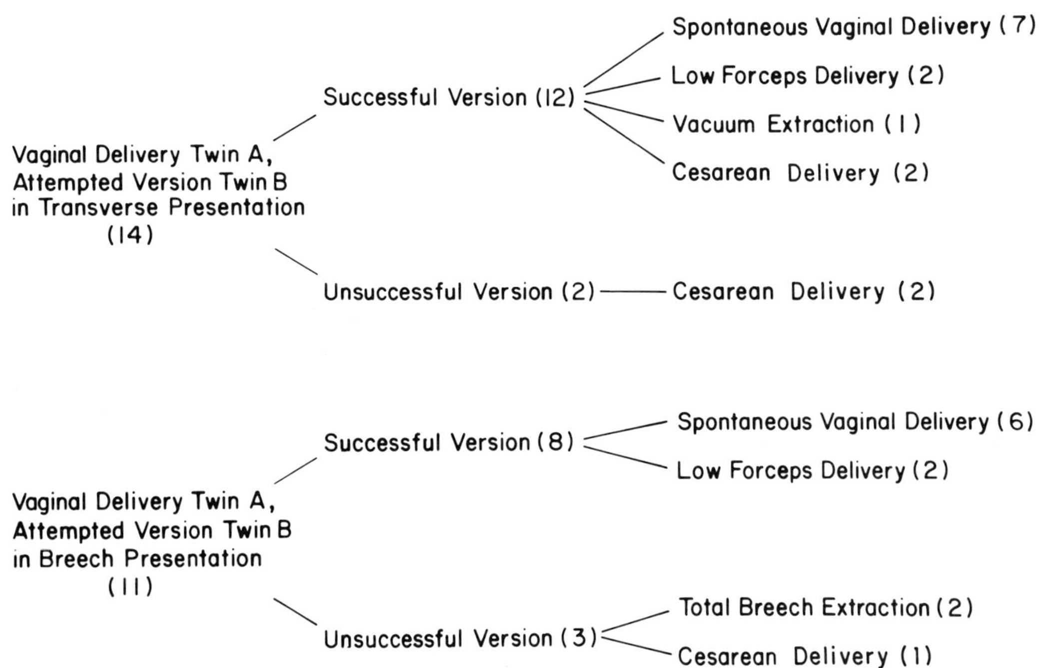

FIGURE 4.4 Mode of delivery after attempted external version of second twins in transverse or breech presentation. (From Chervenak FA, Johnson RE, Berkowitz RL, et al: Intrapartum external version of the second twin. *Obstet Gynecol* 62:160, 1983. Reprinted with permission.)

this series was not excessive; only two cases of endometritis and one case of uterine atony managed by uterine massage and oxytocin administration were present.[43]

The following guidelines for performance of intrapartum external version of the second twin are recommended: (1) Sonographic assessment of the size of both fetuses should be made. If twin B is larger than twin A and a great disparity exists, version with attempted vaginal delivery is best avoided. (2) Epidural anesthesia is advisable before delivery to provide for abdominal wall relaxation. (3) The procedure should be performed only if access to immediate cesarean is possible. (4) A real-time ultrasound machine should be present in the delivery room to determine accurately the fetal presentation after delivery of the first twin. Fetal heart rate should be monitored throughout delivery. Also, gentle pressure with the transducer can guide the infant in vertex presentation into the birth canal (Figure 4.5). (5) If this is not successful, version can be attempted either as a forward or a backward roll. The shortest arc between the vertex and the pelvic inlet should be attempted first. Undue force should always be avoided. (6) If version to vertex presentation is successful, the membrane should be ruptured and oxytocin augmentation may be used. (7) If version is unsuccessful, if the heart tones of twin B show evidence of fetal distress,

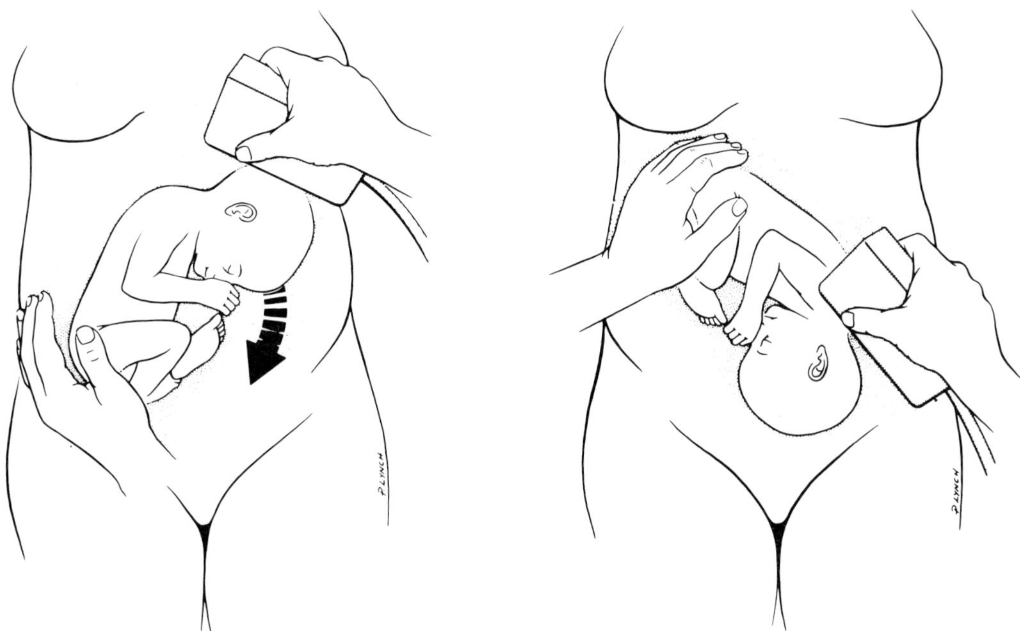

FIGURE 4.5 Method of using an ultrasound transducer to guide the vertex fetus into the pelvis. (From Chervenak FA, Johnson RE, Berkowitz RL, et al: Intrapartum external version of the second twin. *Obstet Gynecol* 62:160, 1983. Reprinted with permission.)

or if twin B fails to descend after version, cesarean delivery or breech extraction is necessary.

Breech Delivery

Acker et al have found no increase in perinatal mortality or depressed 5-minute Apgar scores when the second twin was delivered vaginally as a breech.[44] Our experience is in agreement with this finding. Figure 4.6 illustrates 5-minute Apgar scores of vaginally delivered second twins by birth weight. Above a birth weight of 1,500 g, there were no 5-minute Apgar scores in the low range: three infants (5%) had scores in the midrange and 55 infants (95%) had scores in the high range. One of the three twins with 5-minute Apgar scores in the midrange was not diagnosed until after delivery of the first twin; the second had a monoamniotic placenta, and its cord was intertwined with that of twin A; the third occurred in a 32-week gestation in which the first twin also had a depressed Apgar score.[45] These data suggest that there is not an excessive risk of asphyxia for the vaginally delivered breech second twin.

Examination of our entire twin population, in which 71% of 139 twins in vertex–nonvertex presentation were delivered vaginally, does not

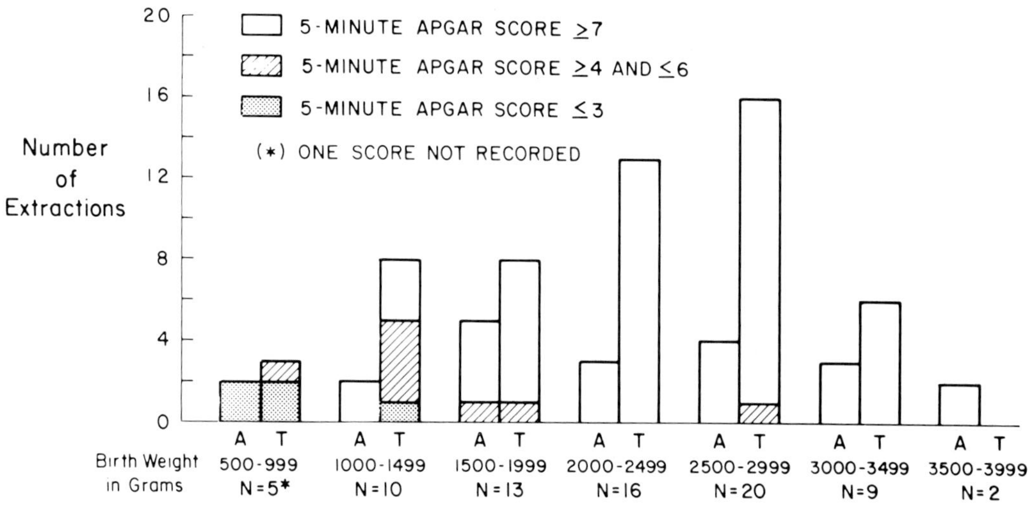

FIGURE 4.6 Five-minute Apgar scores of extracted second twins by birth weight. (From Chervenak FA, Johnson RE, Berkowitz RL, et al: Is routine cesarean section necessary for vertex-breech, vertex–vertex twin gestation? *Am J Obstet Gynecol* 148:1, 1984. Reprinted with permission.)

reveal a high occurrence of birth trauma due to vaginal breech delivery. The four cases of significant birth trauma for our entire twin population are summarized in Table 4.1. The one instance of neonatal death clearly related to birth trauma occurred in a 1,000-g second breech of a breech–breech pair, both of whom were *delivered by cesarean section through a low vertical uterine incision.* The uterus clamped down around the head during breech extraction of the second twin, and extension of the uterine incision was necessary for delivery. Neonatal death occurred at 12 hours.

TABLE 4.1 Significant Birth Trauma for 362 Consecutive Twin Gestations

Birth Trauma	Presentation	Birth Weight (g)	Mode of Delivery
Nenonatal death, 12 hr, perinatal asphyxia	Breech–breech; twin B	1,000	Cesarean section with low vertical uterine incision
Erb's paralysis, paralysis left hemidiaphragm	Vertex–vertex; twin A	2,100	Vertex vaginal delivery (mid forceps, prolonged second stage of labor)
Greenstick fracture right clavicle; nondisplaced fracture, right humerus	Vertex–breech; twin B	3,420	Vaginal delivery; total breech extraction
Large cephalohematoma, resultant anemia and hyperbilirubinemia	Vertex–breech; twin A	2,640	Vertex vaginal delivery (vacuum extraction, prolonged second stage of labor)

Source: Modified from Chervenak FA, Johnson RE, Youcha S, et al: Intrapartum management of twin gestation. *Obstet Gynecol* 65:119, 1985.

The three remaining cases of significant birth trauma occurred during vaginal delivery. One was related to a difficult total breech extraction of a second twin, and the other two were associated with operative vertex deliveries. In all three cases, follow-up examinations revealed no residual deficits in the infants. In addition to the 4 cases of significant birth trauma, there were 2 infants with transient facial nerve palsies and 10 with small, uncomplicated cephalohematomas. Of these, eight occurred in first twins and four occurred in second twins. In this series, there were seven additional cases of neonatal death in which birth weight was ≥1,000 g. Six of these (2, twin A; 4, twin B) were due to complications of prematurity, and one was due to complications resulting from a severe fetomaternal transfusion. The latter occurred in association with bradycardia and placental abruption in the first twin of a vertex-transverse pair delivered by cesarean section. Lastly, there were 20 deaths among neonates with birth weights between 500 and 1,000 g (12, twin A; 8, twin B). All of these were due to complications from prematurity.[6]

For our study population, comparison of the outcome of vaginally delivered second twins in the vertex and nonvertex presentations is enlightening. In Table 4.2, neonatal mortality and morbidity for twin B of vertex–vertex and vertex–nonvertex vaginal deliveries are shown. There were seven nonvertex vaginal deliveries in the 500- to 999-g range; there were no vertex vaginal deliveries in this group. For infants below 1,500 g, the occurrence of 5-minute Apgar scores <7 in twin B was 14.3% for vertex–vertex presentations versus 55.6% for vertex–nonvertex presentations, and the occurrence of neonatal death was 14.3% and 36.8%, respectively. However, in neither comparison was the difference statistically significant ($P > .1$). For infants above 1,500 g, there were no neonatal deaths and no significant differences ($P > .1$) between twin B of vertex–vertex and vertex–nonvertex presentations in any of the measures of outcome.[6] The statistical power of this absence of meaningful difference is weak, however, due to the rarity of adverse outcomes. Therefore, the strong possibility of a type 2 statistical error should be considered, especially in the subgroup of twins weighing <1,500 g where the occurrence of a low 5-minute Apgar score was 14.3% (vertex) versus 55.6% (nonvertex). For nonvertex second twins with a birth weight of >1,500 g, however, the rarity of adverse outcomes both in absolute terms and relative to the vertex second twin is reassuring. It should be emphasized that only one of the four cases of significant birth trauma in this entire series occurred in the second twin of vaginally delivered vertex–nonvertex pairings.[6]

The low incidence of neonatal morbidity and mortality in this series is probably related to the high rate of antepartum and intrapartum diagnosis of twin gestation. Only 4.7% of these twin gestations remained undiagnosed before the delivery of twin B. Antenatal diagnosis is essential for intrapartum monitoring and avoidance of a difficult operative vaginal

TABLE 4.2. Nenonatal Mortality and Morbidity of Twin B in Vertex–Vertex[a] and Vertex–Nonvertex Vaginal Deliveries According to Birth Weight

Birth Weight (g)	Neonatal Death		RDS		IVH		5-Min Apgar Score < 6		Total	
	Vertex–Vertex	Vertex–Nonvertex	Vertex–Vertex	Vertex–Nonvertex	Vertex–Vertex	Vertex–Nonvertex	Vertex–Vertex	Vertex–Nonvertex	Vertex–Vertex	Vertex–Nonvertex
500–999		5/7 (71.4%)		2/7 (28.6%)		1/7 (14.3%)		6/6[b] (100%)	0	7
1,000–1,499	1/7 (14.3%)	2/12 (16.7%)	5/7 (71.4%)	8/12 (75%)	2/7 (28.6%)	4/12 (33.3%)	1/7 (14.3%)	4/12 (33.3%)	7	12
1,500–1,999			6/32 (18.8%)	5/18 (27.8%)	1/32 (3.1%)		3/32 (9.4%)	3/18 (16.7%)	32	18
2,000–2,499			1/31 (3.2%)						31	17
>2,500								1/45 (2.2%)	49	45
500–1,499	1/7 (14.3%)	7/19 (36.8%)	5/7 (71.4%)	10/19 (52.6%)	2/7 (28.6%)	5/19 (26.3%)	1/7 (14.3%)	10/18 (55.6%)	7	19
	($P > 0.1$)		($P > 0.1$)		($P > 0.1$)		($P > 0.1$)			
			7/112 (6.3%)	5/80 (6.3%)	1/112 (.9%)		3/112 (2.7%)	4/80 (5%)	112	80
			($P > 0.1$)				($P > 0.1$)			

RDS, respiratory distress syndrome; IVH, intraventricular hemorrhage.
[a] Six cases not included in which the second twin of vertex–vertex pairings was delivered by internal podalic version.
[b] One 5-min Apgar score not recorded.
Source: Modified from Chervenak FA, Johnson RE, Youcha S, et al: Intrapartum management of twin gestation. *Obstet Gynecol* 65:119, 1985.

delivery when there is fetal distress of twin B. The lack of intrapartum monitoring for twin B and breech delivery in the presence of undetected fetal distress may explain the poorer outcome of vaginally delivered non-vertex twins reported in other series.[5,29–31]

The documented ill effects of vaginal delivery for low-birth-weight (<1,500 g) singleton breech presentations,[46,47] although controversial, should be considered in a plan of intrapartum management for vertex–nonvertex twin gestations. Neither the present series nor those of others has demonstrated any protection against the hazards of breech delivery for the low-birth-weight nonvertex second twin. Because of the lack of data demonstrating its safety, the authors believe that vaginal breech delivery is currently not warranted when the birth weight is <1,500 g. Fortunately, fetal weight can be estimated with fair reliability using antenatal sonography.[48–50] With the methods currently being used, there is approximately a 10% standard deviation in the sonographic estimation of fetal weight, so that 95% of the time estimations are accurate to within 20%. Therefore, use of a cutoff of 2,000 g for estimated fetal weight would be very unlikely to result in an infant with a birth weight of <1,500 g.

Recently, Blickstein et al have reported on the experience of the Kaplan hospital in Rehovot, Israel, of 39 vertex-breech twin pairs delivered vaginally. They found no difference in the outcome between the breech second twin delivered and a control group of vertex second twins delivered vaginally.[51]

The authors' plan for the intrapartum management of vertex–nonvertex twins is summarized in Figure 4.7. The authors admit, however, that a more liberal cesarean delivery policy such as described by Cetrulo[15] is also acceptable. During the intrapartum period, sonographic estimation of fetal weight is done and assessment is made of the standard criteria for vaginal breech delivery (ie, an adequate maternal pelvis,[52] flexed fetal head, and estimated fetal weight less than 3,500 g). If the sonographic estimation of fetal weight is >2,000 g and the criteria for vaginal breech delivery are satisfied, external cephalic version is attempted; if unsuccessful, a breech delivery is performed.

If the sonographic estimation of fetal weight is <2,000 g or the criteria for vaginal breech delivery are not satisfied, external cephalic version is attempted. If this is unsuccessful, a cesarean is performed. Even in those hospitals where breech delivery under any circumstance is not acceptable, routine cesarean may not be necessary for vertex–nonvertex twin gestations, as intrapartum external cephalic version of the second twin may be successful.[43]

It should be emphasized that cesarean delivery is no panacea[53] and does not preclude the possibility of birth injury. The only neonatal death clearly related to intrapartum asphyxia due to birth trauma in our series occurred in a 1,000-g second twin delivered by breech extraction at the

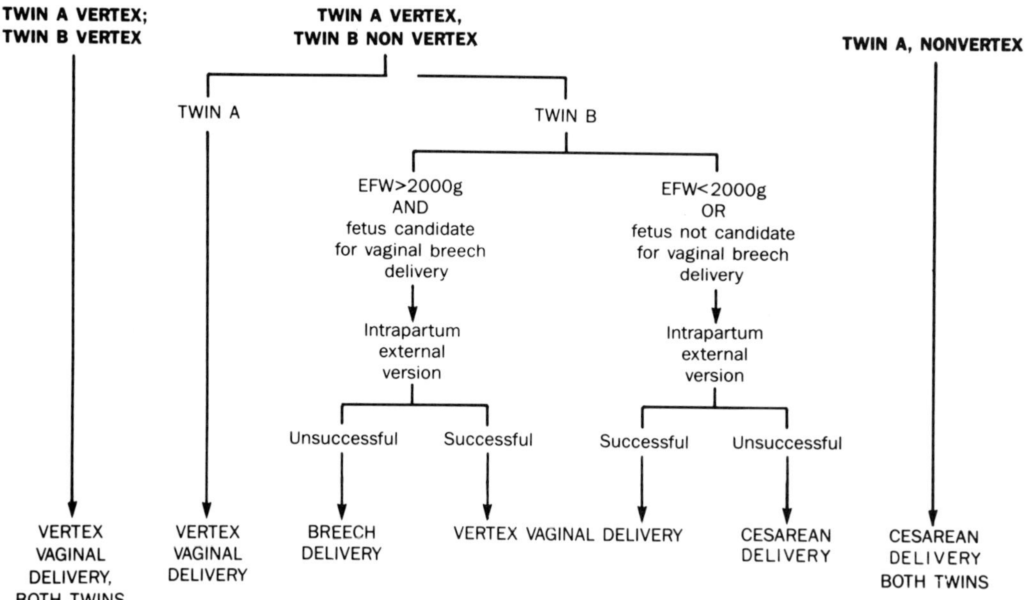

FIGURE 4.7 Protocol for the intrapartum management of twin gestation. (From Chervenak FA, Johnson RE, Youcha S, et al: Intrapartum management of twin gestation. *Obstet Gynecol* 65:119, 1985. Reprinted with permission.)

time of a low vertical cesarean.[6] When cesarean section is performed, an adequate uterine incision is mandatory if birth injury is to be avoided.

Twin A, Nonvertex

Currently, the cesarean seems to be the delivery method of choice when the first twin is nonvertex, as there are no studies to document the safety of vaginal delivery for this group.[54] External cephalic version of a nonvertex first twin would be difficult, if not impossible. Interlocking of fetal heads is a potentially disastrous complication of vaginal breech delivery of the first twin.[55] It is not inconceivable that the second twin might also interfere with breech vaginal delivery of the first twin in more subtle ways, such as by deflexion of the descending vertex. The authors recognize, however, that fears of nonvertex vaginal delivery of the first twin may not be warranted and that vaginal delivery may be proved to be safe in well-defined cases.[1]

SPECIAL CONSIDERATIONS IN THE INTRAPARTUM MANAGEMENT OF MULTIPLE GESTATION

There are special circumstances in which the above plan of management is not appropriate. Monoamniotic twins, which occur in about 1% of twin pregnancies, have such a high risk of cord entanglement and subsequent intrauterine death[56] that elective cesarean after documentation of lung maturity should be performed. Likewise, conjoined twins for whom there is some hope of salvage or for whom dystocia is feared should be delivered by elective cesarean section.[57] Lastly, in the rare instance when three or more fetuses are present, the authors advocate cesarean delivery. Although Loucopoulos and Jewelewicz[58] have suggested that cesarean delivery does not improve the outcome in multifetal pregnancies, the difficulties associated with intrapartum surveillance and atraumatic vaginal delivery warrant that only the most experienced operator[58,59] attempt vaginal delivery.

REFERENCES

1. Hays PM, Smeltzer JS: Multiple gestation. *Clin Obstet Gynecol* 29:264, 1986.
2. Hrubec Z, Robinette D: The study of human twins in medical research. *N Engl J Med* 310;435, 1984.
3. MacGillvray L: Epidemiology of twin pregnancy. *Semin Perinatol* 10:4, 1986.
4. Guttmacher AF: The incidence of multiple births in man and some of the other unipara. *Obstet Gynecol* 2:22, 1953.
5. Faroqui MO, Grossman JH, Shannon RS: A review of twin pregnancy and perinatal mortality. *Obstet Gynecol Surv* 28:144, 1973.
6. Chervenak FA, Johnson RE, Youcha S, et al: Intrapartum management of twin gestation. *Obstet Gynecol* 65:119, 1985.
7. Saunders MC, Dick JS, Brown I, et al: The effects of hospital admissions for bed rest on the duration of twin pregnancy. A randomized trial. *Lancet* 2:793, 1985.
8. Marivate M, Normal RJ: Twins. *Clin Obstet Gynaecol* 9:723, 1982.
9. Katz M, Gill PJ, Newman RB: Detection of preterm labor by ambulatory monitoring of uterine activity: A preliminary report. *Obstet Gynecol* 68:773, 1986.
10. Berkowitz RL: Multiple gestation, in Gabbe SG, Niebyl JR, Simpson JL (eds): *Obstetrics: Normal and Problem Pregnancies.* New York, Churchill Livingstone, 1986, pp 739–767.
11. Devoe LD, Azor H: Simultaneous nonstress fetal heart rate testing in twin pregnancy. *Obstet Gynecol* 58:450, 1981.
12. Farmakides G, Schulman H, Saldana LR, et al: Surveillance of a twin pregnancy with umbilical arterial velocimetry. *Am J Obstet Gynecol* 153:789, 1985.
13. Landy HJ, Keith L, Keith O: The vanishing twin. *Acta Genet Med Gemellol* 31:179, 1982.
14. Dudley DKL, D'Alton ME: Single fetal death in twin gestation. *Semin Perinatol* 10:65, 1986.
15. Cetrulo C: The controversy of mode of delivery in twins: The intrapartum management of twin gestation. *Semin Perinatol* 10:39, 1986.
16. Cetrulo CL, Ingardia CJ, Sbarra AJ: Management of multiple gestation. *Clin Obstet Gynecol* 23:533, 1980.
17. Taylor ES: Editorial. *Obstet Gynecol Surv* 31:535, 1976.
18. Taylor ES: Editorial. *Obstet Gynecol Surv* 38:272, 1983.
19. Keith L, Hughey MJ: Twin gestation, in Gerbie AB, Sciarra JJ (eds): *Gynecology and Obstetrics*, ed 2. New York, Harper and Row Publishers, Inc, 1981, pp 1–10.
20. Pritchard JA, MacDonald PC: *Williams Obstetrics*, ed 16. New York, Appleton-Century-Crofts, 1980, pp 660–661.

21. Rayburn WF, Lavin JP, Miodovnik M, et al: Multiple gestation: Time interval between delivery of the first and second twin. *Obstet Gynecol* 63:502, 1984.
22. Barrett JM, Staggs SM, Van Mooydonk JE, et al: The effect of type of delivery upon neonatal outcome in premature twins. *Am J Obstet Gynecol* 143:360, 1982.
23. Ferguson WF: Perinatal mortality in multiple gestations: A review of perinatal deaths from 1609 multiple gestations. *Obstet Gynecol* 23:861, 1964.
24. Ware HH: The second twin. *Am J Obstet Gynecol* 110:865, 1971.
25. Simpson CW, Olatunbosun OA, Baldwin VJ: Delayed interval delivery in triplet pregnancy: Repeat of a single case and review of the literature. *Obstet Gynecol* 64:8S, 1984.
26. Banchi MT: Triplet pregnancy with second trimester abortion and delivery of twins at 35 weeks gestation. *Obstet Gynecol* 63:728, 1984.
27. Woolfson J, Fay T, Bates A: Twins with 54 days between deliveries. Case report. *Br J Obstet Gynecol* 90:685, 1983.
28. Kauppila A, Jouppila P, Koivisto M, et al: Twin pregnancy: A clinical study of 335 cases. *Acta Obstet Gynecol Scand* 54(suppl):5, 1975.
29. Brown EJ, Dixon HG: Twin pregnancy. *Br J Obstet Gynaecol* 70:251, 1963.
30. Kelsick F, Minkoff H: Management of the breech second twin. *Am J Obstet Gynecol* 144:783, 1982.
31. Ho SK, Wu PYK: Perinatal factors and neonatal morbidity in twin pregnancy. *Am J Obstet Gynecol* 122:979, 1975.
32. Koivisto M, Jouppila P, Kauppila A, et al: Twin pregnancy: Neonatal morbidity and mortality. *Acta Obstet Gynecol Scand* 54(suppl):21, 1975.
33. Stine LE, Phelan JP, Wallace R, et al: Update on external cephalic version performed at term. *Obstet Gynecol* 65:642, 1985.
34. Fall O, Nilsson BA: External cephalic version in breech presentation under tocolysis. *Obstet Gynecol* 53:712, 1979.
35. Ylikorkala O, Hartikainen-Sorri A: Value of external version in fetal malpresentation in combination with use of ultrasound. *Acta Obstet Gynecol Scand* 56:63, 1977.
36. Saling E, Mueller-Holve W: External cephalic version under tocolysis. *J Perinatol Med* 3:115, 1975.
37. Bradley-Watson PJ: The decreasing value of external cephalic version in modern obstetric practice. *Am J Obstet Gynecol* 123:237, 1975.
38. Berg D, Kunze U: Critical remarks on external cephalic version under tocolysis: Report on a case of antepartum fetal death. *J Perinatol Med* 5:32, 1977.
39. Van Dorsten JP, Schifrin BS, Wallace RL: Randomized control trial of external cephalic version with tocolysis in late pregnancy. *Am J Obstet Gynecol* 141:417, 1981.
40. Ranney B: The gentle art of external cephalic version. *Am J Obstet Gynecol* 116:239, 1973.
41. Ganesh V, Apuzzio J, Iffy L: Clinical aspects of multiple gestation, in Iffy L, Kaminetsky HA (eds): *Principles and Practice of Obstetrics and Perinatology*. New York, John Wiley & Sons, Inc, 1981, pp 1183–1192.
42. Camilleri AP: In defense of the second twin. *Br J Obstet Gynaecol* 70:258, 1963.
43. Chervenak FA, Johnson RE, Berkowitz RL, et al: Intrapartum external version of the second twin. *Obstet Gynecol* 62:160, 1983.
44. Acker D, Leiberman M, Holbrook H, et al: Delivery of the second twin. *Obstet Gynecol* 59:710, 1982.
45. Chervenak FA, Johnson RE, Berkowitz RL, et al: Is routine cesarean section necessary for vertex-breech, vertex-transverse twin gestation? *Am J Obstet Gynecol* 148:1, 1984.
46. Kauppila O, Groncoos M, Aro P, et al: Management of low birth weight breech delivery: Should cesarean section be routine? *Obstet Gynecol* 57:289, 1981.

47. Duenmoelter JH, Wells CE, Reisch JS: A paired controlled study of vaginal and abdominal delivery of the low birth weight breech fetus. *Obstet Gynecol* 54:310, 1979.
48. Shepard MJ, Richards VA, Berkowitz RL, et al: An evaluation of the two equations for predicting fetal weight by ultrasound. *Am J Obstet Gynecol* 142:47, 1982.
49. Deter RL, Hadlock FP, Harrist RB, et al: Evaluation of three methods for obtaining fetal weight estimates using dynamic image ultrasound. *J Clin Ultrasound* 9:421, 1981.
50. Hadlock FP, Harrist RB, Carpenter RJ, et al: Sonographic estimation of fetal weight: The value of femur length to head and abdomen. *Measurements Radiol* 150:535, 1984.
51. Blickstein I, Schwartz-Shoham Z, Lancet MD, et al: Vaginal delivery of the second twin in breech presentation. *Obstet Gynecol* 69:774, 1987.
52. Collea JV, Rabin SC, Weghorst GR, et al: The randomized management of term frank breech presentation: Vaginal delivery vs cesarean section. *Am J Obstet Gynecol* 131:186, 1978.
53. Olofsson P, Rydhstrom H: Twin delivery: How should the second twin be delivered? *Am J Obstet Gynecol* 153:479, 1985.
54. Ismajovich B, Confino E, Sherzer A, et al: Optimal delivery of nonvertex twins. *Mt Sinai J Med* 52:106, 1985.
55. Nissen ED: Twins: Collison, impaction, compaction, and interlocking. *Obstet Gynecol* 11:514, 1958.
56. Sutter J, Arab H, Manning FA: Monoamniotic twins: Antenatal diagnosis and management. *Am J Obstet Gynecol* 155:836, 1986.
57. Filler RM: Conjoined twins and their separation. *Semin Perinatol* 10:82, 1986.
58. Loucopoulos A, Jewelewicz R: Management of multifetal pregnancies: Sixteen years experience at the Sloane Hospital for Women. *Am J Obstet Gynecol* 143:902, 1982.
59. Ron-El R, Caspi E, Schreyer P, et al: Triplet and quadruplet pregnancies and management. *Obstet Gynecol* 57:458, 1981.

Chapter 5

Fetal Distress

Carl V. Smith, MD

Continuous electronic fetal monitoring (EFM) remains a universally accepted method by which to assess fetal well-being.[1–3] Its use enables the obstetrician to identify fetal heart rate (FHR) patterns likely to be associated with an increased likelihood of fetal harm. These patterns not infrequently result in cesarean delivery for fetal distress. On most obstetrical units, this fetal distress occurs in 1%–2% of patients.[4,5] This rate has been known to vary among hospitals, patient populations, and individual practitioners. The reasons for these differences are unclear but may be related to differences in FHR pattern recognition and management. The primary goal of the practitioner is to monitor the fetus antepartum and intrapartum accurately and to initiate treatment in an attempt to mitigate the effects of hypoxia on fetal neurologic function.

The discussion that follows includes the rationale for EFM, pattern recognition, and management. Emphasis will be placed on the pathophysiology, methods of assessing fetal acid-base status, and newer methods of assessing fetal well-being.

RATIONALE FOR CONTINUOUS EFM

The ability of EFM to predict a nonacidotic fetus is well recognized. The presence of a normal FHR pattern ensures the virtual absence of acidosis. Less well defined, however, is its ability to predict fetal compromise. It is, therefore, reasonable to view continuous EFM as a method of screening a population for fetal acidosis. Consequently, if the FHR pattern is abnormal, a more definitive assessment of the fetal condition must be undertaken. As with many screening tests, fetal monitoring is best applied to the general population, as it is difficult to predict with reasonable accuracy the at-risk population.[6] This statement is further supported by the work of Westgren et al, who demonstrated no intrapartum deaths, a 0.3% incidence of depressed 5-minute Apgar scores, and, at the same time, a 0.7% incidence of cesarean section for fetal distress.[4] Although this was not a randomized comparison, the data suggest that benefits may be derived from monitoring even the low-risk gravida.

Other authors have presented a similar experience with routine EFM. Ingemarsson et al demonstrated a 7.5% reduction in adverse neurologic sequelae in the fetuses monitored routinely.[7] This was accomplished with an overall cesarean delivery rate for fetal distress of 1%, which remained constant throughout the study period.

A large body of retrospective evidence was presented by Paul and Hon.[8] They observed a twofold reduction in both fetal and perinatal deaths, with implementation of routine FHR monitoring in a high-risk population. Similar findings were reported by Tutera and Newman[9] in routine monitoring of high-risk gravidas in labor.

More current investigations have also demonstrated the benefit of routine EFM.[1,10,11] However, questions regarding sample size, the particular outcome measure, and the effect on cesarean delivery rates remain. It is clear that controlled, randomized investigations with a large number of patients are required to show differences in fetal death rates due to its rare occurrence. It is unlikely that, in the current medicolegal crisis, such an investigation will be initiated in the United States. Of more importance is the less dramatic but equally serious issue of neonatal morbidity. Retrospective investigations have demonstrated a reduced incidence of these events in patients undergoing monitoring. One prospective study suggested that EFM with fetal scalp sampling reduces the incidence of adverse neonatal neurologic sequelae.[10] Chalmers, who pooled the data from the five available randomized trials, demonstrated similar results.[1,10,12–15]

The last, and perhaps most controversial, randomized investigation was reported from the National Maternity Hospital in Dublin.[16] Although no difference in death or fetal distress rates was identified, an increase in the incidence of neonatal seizure activity was observed in those gravidas randomized to the group undergoing intermittent auscultation. Also of critical importance is the 14% incidence of severe neurologic handicap in this group of infants by 1 year of age.

Although controversial, the use of EFM is commonplace, even among low-risk obstetric populations. A detailed analysis of the impact of such a policy is beyond the scope of this chapter. However, at a minimum, the practitioner will encounter abnormal FHR patterns and will deal with these problems by cesarean delivery in at least 1% of his or her patients.

EQUIPMENT CONSIDERATIONS

In order to interpret FHR tracings accurately, a basic understanding of the FHR monitor is highly desirable. This knowledge may prevent unnecessary action for bradycardia that results from the maternal electrocardiographic (ECG) complex and may lead the clinician to suspect FHR rhythm disturbances that can be confused with artifacts. The final FHR tracing reflects two distinct processes. First, input is derived from either the fetal ECG complex or Doppler signals. Second, that signal undergoes some form of processing in order to convert the input into an interpretable tracing. Lastly, and frequently overlooked, is the uterine activity portion of the record. Each of these features will be discussed individually.

DOPPLER CARDIOTOCOMETRY

Fetal monitoring systems are either direct or indirect. The indirect system most frequently relies on the Doppler principle. The transducer emits continuous ultrasound waves. In addition, it measures the change or shift in frequency (Doppler shift) that is generated by movement of the fetal heart. The ventricular septum walls and valves all contribute, but valvular motion probably contributes the most. As all movements under the ultrasound beam can generate noise, monitors possess editing or logic functions to process the signal. These functions consist of filtering high- and low-frequency signals and an editing function to emphasize selectively sounds or signals that are most likely to emanate from the fetal heart.

The newest fetal monitoring systems have built-in autocorrelation functions.[17] This technique selectively enhances the repetitive movement of the fetal heart and separates it from the background noise. In effect, it compares each signal with the previous one; hence, the name "autocorrelation." Although this function produces a "cleaner" FHR tracing, it can, in the patient with a fetal demise, produce an artificial FHR from any periodic movement, such as maternal heart rate and/or respiration.

PHONOCARDIOGRAPHY

In contradistinction to Doppler monitoring, phonocardiography converts actual cardiac sounds into an FHR tracing. Modification with editing and logic functions occurs, as with Doppler techniques.

Neither of the indirect or "external" monitoring techniques provide meaningful information about beat-to-beat FHR variability. In fact, the recorded rate represents an average obtained over several heartbeats. However, by the utilization of autocorrelation techniques, the printed FHR more accurately reflects variability.

Another important feature unique to indirect systems is the presence of a refractory period of a few milliseconds after the first heart sound. Its function is to avoid counting the second heart sound as a separate heartbeat. Consequently, with fetal tachycardias, usually in excess of 180 bpm, the second beat would fall within the refractory period and the monitor would artificially halve the rate. Similarly, with bradycardias, usually below 90 bpm, the monitor may double the rate by counting the second heart sound as a separate second beat.

DIRECT (INTERNAL) FETAL ELECTROCARDIOGRAPHY

This system requires the placement of a stainless steel electrode into the subcutaneous tissue of the fetal presenting part after amniorrhexis. A maternal ground plate, commonly attached to the thigh, completes the connection through the two leads of the spiral electrode. Thus, the input to the monitor consists of a mixed signal containing both maternal and fetal contributions.[18] The monitor contains an automatic gain control amplifier that emphasizes the fetal signal (represented by the R wave of the fetal ECG). This direct system allows a more accurate assessment of FHR variability.

Although halving and doubling of the FHR do not occur with the direct system, transmission of the maternal ECG in cases of fetal demise or misapplication of the electrode are potential sources of error. Auscultation of the FHR with simultaneous palpation of the maternal pulse should eliminate the confusion.

TOCODYNAMOMETRY

Measurement of uterine activity with a strain gauge placed on the maternal abdomen or with placement of an intrauterine pressure catheter (IUPC) is essential to the interpretation of monitor tracings, because the basis for pattern recognition is the relationship between FHR changes and uterine activity. Errors can occur with either system, but the timing of uterine contractions is the least affected and, perhaps, the most important component. Finally, monitoring of resting uterine tonus and absolute intrauterine pressure is possible only with the internal (IUPC) system.

Intrapartum FHR Patterns and Etiologies

Perhaps the most difficult task facing the obstetrician is to determine that the FHR pattern is normal. Although abnormal tracings are frequently associated with normal or, rather, nonacidotic fetuses, the presence of a normal tracing is associated with a universally good outcome.[19–22] Interpretation of an FHR tracing should proceed in a systematic fashion. A detailed discussion of FHR pattern recognition is described by Hon.[23] When approaching a tracing, each of the following should be ascertained: baseline FHR, uterine activity, periodic and non-periodic FHR changes, and variability. Normal values for each of these variables are depicted in Table 5.1.

TABLE 5.1 Normal FHR Parameters

Baseline rate	120–160 bpm
Periodic changes	Absent, accelerations or early (type 1) decelerations are present
Variability	>5 bpm in amplitude

Alterations of Baseline FHR

The most ominous condition associated with a baseline FHR <120 bpm is acute fetal hypoxia. Events such as placental abruption, umbilical cord prolapse, and uterine hypertonus may be etiologic. A rapid search for these conditions is warranted. In their absence, oxygen administration or maternal position change may alleviate the pattern, particularly if it is due to occult umbilical cord compression. Less common causes of bradycardia are congenital bradyarrhythmias such as heart block, maternal β-blocker administration (eg, propanolol), and hypothyroidism. A final diagnostic consideration, especially when bradycardia is noted immediately after applying monitors, is the maternal pulse derived from an external system or the maternal ECG derived from an internal system.

Clearly, not all bradycardias are pathologic. The majority of fetuses with rates ≥100 bpm are clinically and biochemically normal. This is true, however, only when normal FHR variability is noted and no deceleration patterns are present.[21,24–26] Alternatively, in the absence of congenital heart block, most fetuses will not tolerate bradycardias <100 bpm for extended periods of time. As a rule, such a rate represents an obstetric crisis, which generally requires emergency cesarean delivery.

Tachycardia

A baseline FHR of >160 bpm may have several etiologies. The most common include maternal fever, chorioamnionitis and other infections, maternal administration of beta sympathomimetics (eg, ritodrine), hyperthyroidism, fetal cardiac arrhythmias, and, more rarely, fetal acidosis. Like bradycardia, fetal tachycardia is more likely to be pathologic when other FHR abnormalities coexist, especially late or severe variable decelerations.[24–27] Consequently, tachycardia by itself is rarely an indication for intervention.

FHR Variability

Variability of the FHR is often subdivided into short-term or so-called beat-to-beat variability and long-term variability. However, in clinical practice, simultaneous consideration of both types leads to an overall impression of variability. Although precise amplitudes have been discussed

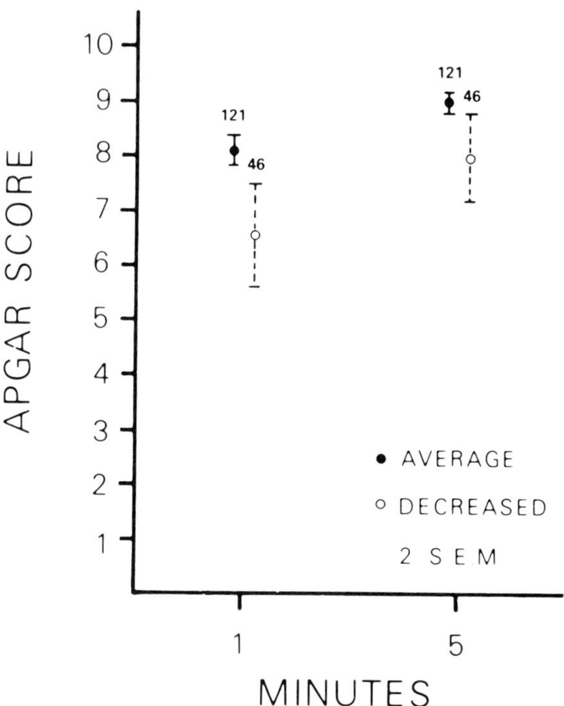

FIGURE 5.1 The presence of average FHR variability immediately prior to delivery is associated with higher mean Apgar scores at 1 and 5 minutes. (From Paul RH, Suidan AK, Yeh S-Y, et al: *Am J Obstet Gynecol* 123:206, 1975. Reproduced with permission from CV Mosby Co, St. Louis.)

in the literature, a clinically useful method is to categorize variability as either average or decreased. Paul and colleagues noted significant reductions in the mean 1- and 5-minute Apgar scores when the two groups were compared[28] (Figure 5.1). More significant is its potential role as an arbiter of abnormal FHR patterns. In the investigation cited above, mild and moderate late decelerations associated with average variability were significantly less likely to be acidotic (pH <7.20)[28] (Figure 5.2).

A variant of long-term variability requires special comment. A sinusoidal pattern, first described with isoimmunized pregnancies, is a regular sine-wave variation of the baseline with a frequency of 3–6 cycles/min.[29] Subsequently, it was reported to be associated with fetal anemia, hypoxemia, and maternal alphaprodine (Nisentil) administration, and was found in the otherwise normal fetus.[30–32] The presence of a sinusoidal pattern should prompt a search for an etiology and perhaps additional assessment of fetal well-being.

Variable Decelerations

Compression of the umbilical cord is held by most to be etiologic in variable decelerations.[33] As their name implies, variable decelerations manifest

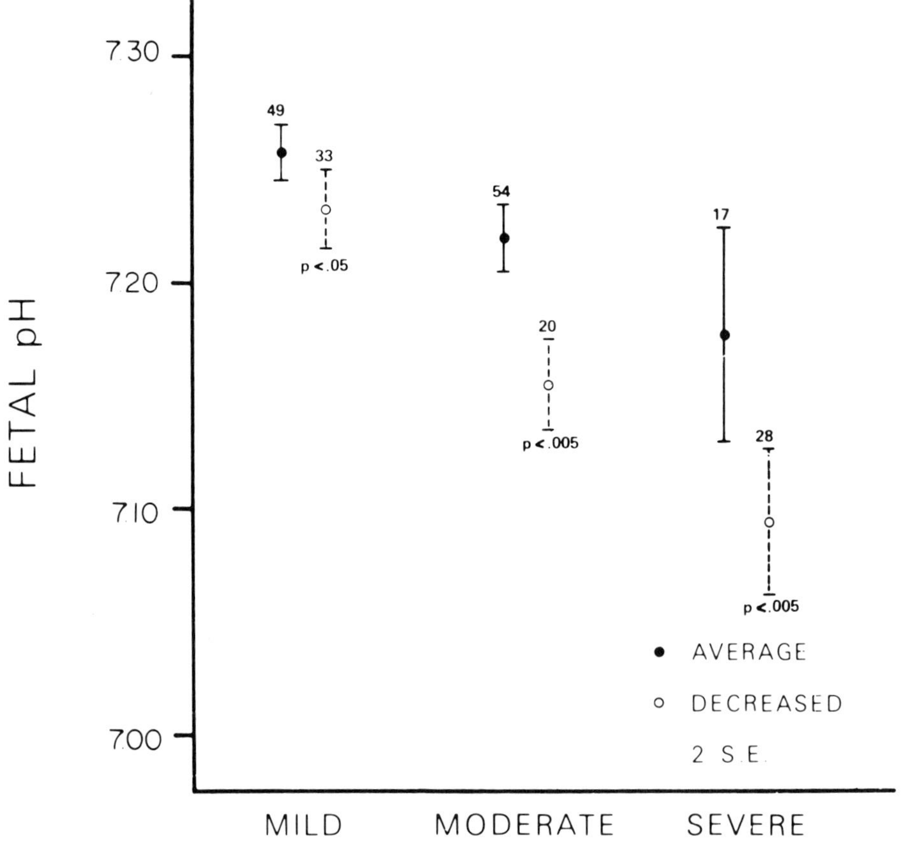

FIGURE 5.2 As the severity of late decelerations increases, the mean fetal pH decreases. In the presence of average rather than absent FHR variability, a higher mean fetal pH was observed for every degree of late deceleration. (From Paul, et al: *Am J Obstet Gynecol* 123:206, 1975. Reproduced with permission from CV Mosby Co, St. Louis.)

no consistent relationship to uterine activity. Similarly, the wave form itself is not uniform in shape. This compression may be secondary to occult umbilical cord prolapse or decreased amniotic fluid volume.[34,35] Variable decelerations occur with increased frequency in patients whose pregnancies are complicated by intrauterine growth retardation (IUGR), postdates, or premature rupture of the membranes.

Variable decelerations have been subclassified into mild, moderate, and severe categories on the basis of their duration and depth.[21] Perhaps a more clinically useful classification is that proposed by Krebs and coworkers.[36] They described atypical variable decelerations that, when present, were associated with a greater likelihood of acidosis (Figure 5.3).

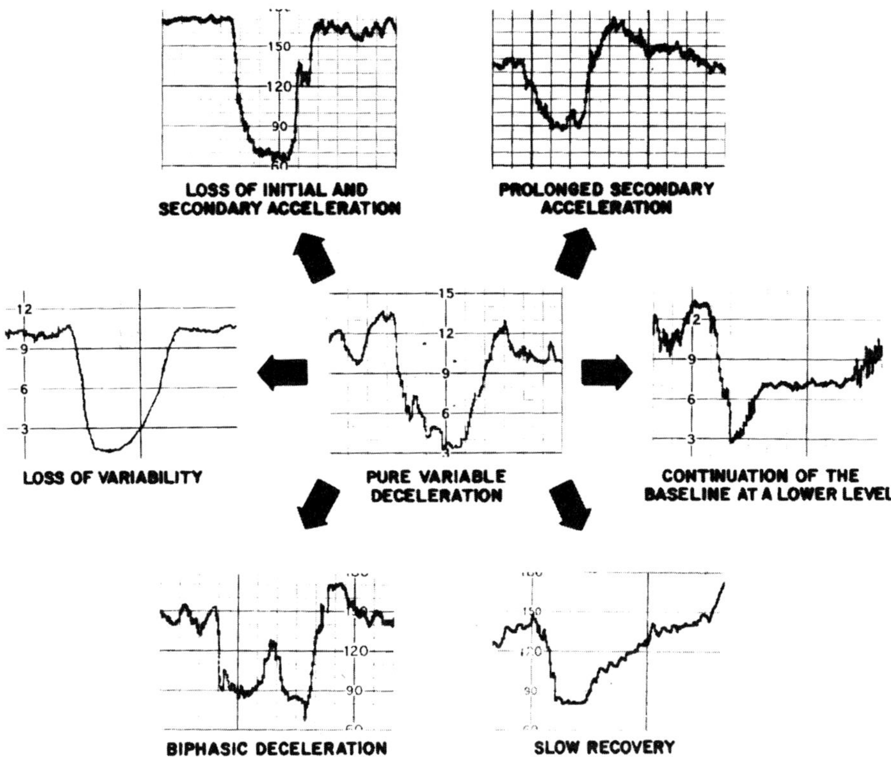

FIGURE 5.3 The potential for an adverse fetal outcome is greater when atypical variable FHR decelerations are encountered during labor. (From Krebs, et al: *Am J Obstet Gynecol* 123:297, 1983. Reproduced with permission from CV Mosby Co, St. Louis.)

These atypical features include (1) loss of initial acceleration, (2) delayed return of the FHR to baseline, (3) loss of secondary acceleration, (4) prolonged acceleration after the deceleration, (5) biphasic deceleration, (6) decreased FHR variability within the deceleration, and (7) continuation of the baseline rate at a level lower than that proceeding the deceleration. The potential for an adverse outcome was noted irrespective of the severity of the decelerating pattern. As an example, the mean fetal scalp pH was 7.19 in patients with atypical variable decelerations. Similarly, depressed 5-minute Apgar scores occurred three times more frequently in the former group. Other investigators have likewise shown a poorer outcome in patients with atypical variable decelerations.[37,38]

Of perhaps more significance is the additive effect of other FHR abnormalities, notably reduced variability. The combination of atypical variable decelerations and reduced variability has resulted in a 22% incidence of depressed 5-minute Apgar scores. Consequently, when these FHR patterns are observed, consideration should be given to additional assessment of fetal well-being.

Late Decelerations

The appearance of repetitive late decelerations may alert the obstetrician to fetal hypoxia or acidosis (Figure 5.4). The incidence of the latter varies from 26% to 83%.[19,25,26] The mechanism for late decelerations is generally accepted to be fetal hypoxia, most commonly resulting from uteroplacental insufficiency (UPI). This condition may be acute or chronic. Patients affected by postdatism or IUGR are notably at risk for UPI. Other conditions such as chronic vascular disease, hypertensive disorders, or diabetes may also place the fetus at risk. Superimposed upon this chronic state are the stresses of labor, which may cause a further reduction in intervillous blood flow.

Alternatively, the acute appearance of UPI and associated late decelerations may be observed with uterine hypertonus, maternal hypotension, and placental abruption.

As with variable decelerations, the assessment of FHR variability is of critical importance when evaluating patients who demonstrate this pattern. As discussed in the section on variability, when diminished variability is present in association with moderate or severe late decelerations, the mean fetal scalp pH was ≤7.15.[28]

Meconium-Stained Amniotic Fluid

A final indicator of fetal stress is the presence of meconium-stained amniotic fluid. The significance of thin meconium is controversial, but it probably does not adversely affect the outcome.[39] However, thick meconium is associated with a higher incidence of fetal acidosis.[39–41] Miller and colleagues reported that meconium by itself was not associated with a higher incidence of acidosis, although they reported an increased frequency of low 5-minute Apgar scores.[39] Krebs et al reported a poorer outcome in the meconium-stained fetus but related it to a higher incidence of abnormal FHR patterns. The combination of meconium passage and an abnormal FHR pattern increases the likelihood of low 1- and 5-minute Apgar scores.[40]

Assessment of Fetal Acid-Base Status

When fetal heart rate patterns, with or without meconium staining, are confusing or cause concern, fetal scalp sampling is frequently the final arbiter of fetal condition. First described by Saling, fetal scalp sampling allows biochemical assessment of fetal well-being.[42] Several investigators have independently verified the validity of this approach. During the first stage of labor, fetal scalp blood pH ranges between 7.20 and 7.35.[43] Values below 7.20 are associated with a higher incidence of depressed 5-minute Apgar scores.[44] A similar correlation can be made between normal outcome and nonacidotic scalp blood pH.

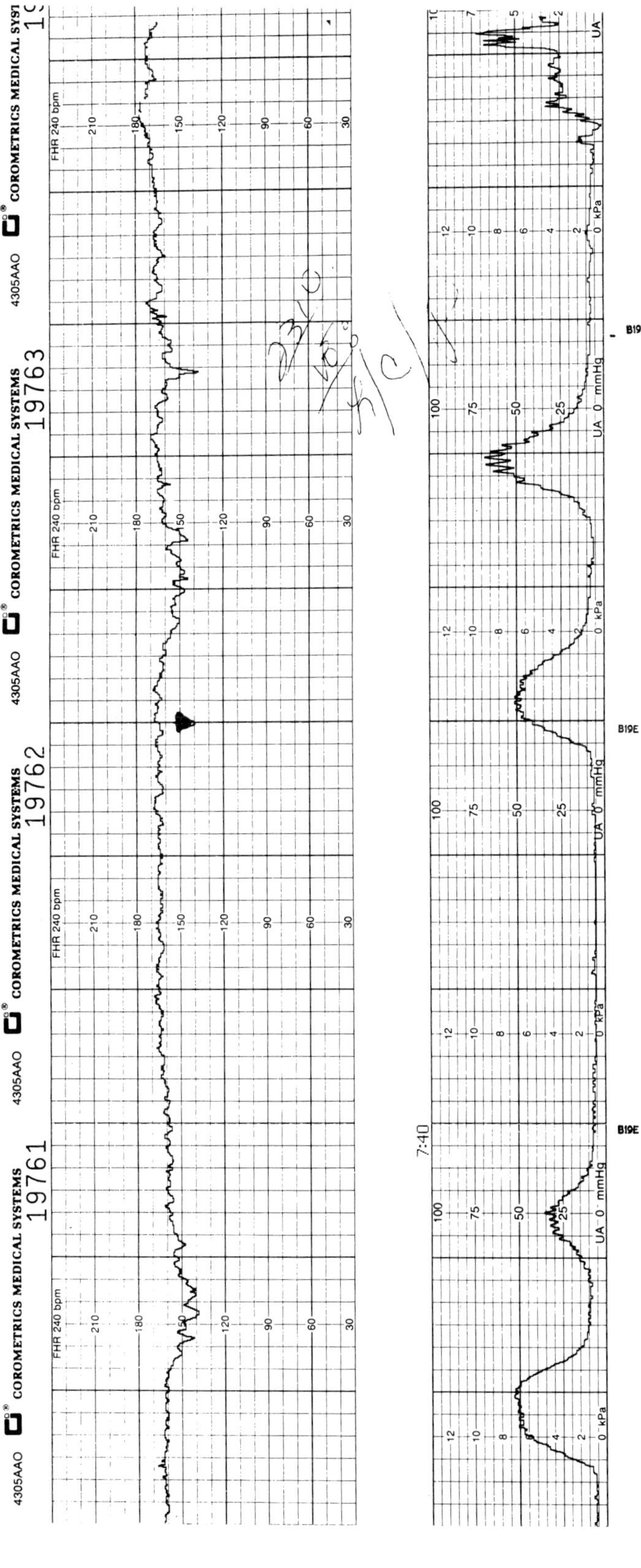

FIGURE 5.4 A FHR tracing with repetitive late decelerations.

TABLE 5.2 Indications for Fetal Acoustic/Scalp Stimulation or Scalp Blood Sampling

Repetitive late decelerations
Absent FHR variability not explainable on the basis of narcotic administration
Repetitive severe variable decelerations
Atypical variable decelerations
Sinusoidal patterns
A combination of FHR patterns that is clinically confusing

Table 5.2 outlines the commonly accepted indications for fetal scalp sampling. The largest group of patients will fall into the last category of confusing patterns.

Of paramount importance is the understanding that fetal pH represents the acid-base status of the fetus at the moment of sampling. It offers little prognostic value unless obtained immediately prior to delivery. Patterns that persist after sampling may warrant periodic assessment of pH if labor is allowed to continue. Similarly, if the FHR tracing suggests deterioration of the fetal condition, an additional assessment of fetal acid-base status or consideration for delivery is warranted.

As with any laboratory test, false-positive and false-negative results may occur. Factors responsible for falsely low readings include maternal hypotension, aortocaval compression, sampling during a uterine contraction, laboratory error, and scalp edema.[45] Similarly, scalp sampling immediately following an episode of bradycardia, severe variable deceleration, uterine hypertonus, or maternal hypotension (particularly in association with conduction anesthesia) may result in a transient fetal respiratory acidosis, rather than an indication of fetal distress. Waiting for 10–15 minutes following correction of these events results in a more accurate picture of the fetal condition.

Values that are falsely reassuring can lead to disastrous outcomes. Perhaps the most easily identifiable source of error is maternal alkalosis. With abnormalities in the FHR, maternal anxiety is likely to lead to hyperventilation and respiratory alkalosis. Simultaneous measurement of maternal venous or arterial pH is recommended at the time of fetal scalp sampling. One should not be reassured by a normal scalp blood pH in the face of an ominous FHR pattern and a maternal pH of 7.45 or greater. On the other hand, it is also unwise to act on a single pH determination that is clinically inconsistent with the FHR pattern.

ALTERNATIVES TO FETAL SCALP SAMPLING

The need for fetal scalp blood sampling varies with the obstetric population and the clinical experience of the practitioner. A survey of 25 university-based perinatal units showed an average use of 3% or less.[5] In a much lower risk population, such as in a private practice, the need for this procedure would probably be less. A number of factors contribute to the lack of widespread utilization of fetal blood sampling. Lack of readily available equipment to perform the microanalysis, its cumbersome nature, and its low incidence of use have led to a disenchantment of some with the technique.[5]

This has led to studies of less invasive methods of fetal assessment. In a retrospective review of FHR tracings, Clark and colleagues noted that an acceleration of 15 bpm for 15 seconds in response to scalp puncture was associated in all cases with a scalp pH greater than 7.20.[46] A later prospective investigation of scalp pressure and/or gentle pinching with an Allis clamp confirmed the relationship.[47] Although a positive or reactive scalp stimulation test correlated with a nonacidotic pH, a lack of response was associated with acidosis only 50% of the time. Thus, it appears that this rapid, noninvasive test may reduce by at least 50% the need for fetal scalp sampling. Another test that offers promise in the assessment of fetal well-being is acoustic stimulation using an artificial larynx (Figure 5.5). Its use in antenatal FHR testing has been shown to increase the number of reactive tests.[48] In a subsequent report, the incidence of reactive tests was increased, testing time was reduced, and reliability of evoked FHR reactivity was comparable to that of nonevoked FHR reactivity.[49] Acoustic stimulation was then applied intrapartum to assess fetal acid-base status in 64 patients with FHR tracings suggestive of an acid-base abnormality.[50] A positive response (Table 5.3), defined as a 15-bpm, 15-second acceleration (Figure 5.6), was associated with the virtual absence of acidosis ($pH \geq 7.25$). If the fetus failed to respond, acidosis was present in about 50%. This technique offers the additional advantage of being noninvasive.

Additional considerations regarding the role of fetal scalp sampling and its alternatives have been presented by Clark and Paul, who showed that with proper FHR interpretation, fetal scalp blood sampling could be abandoned without compromising the clinician's ability to detect fetal distress or significantly increasing the cesarean delivery rate.[5] It appears that acoustic or scalp stimulation may supplant sampling as an arbiter of abnormal FHR patterns.

A final technique that merits limited discussion is the recording of continuous tissue pH.[51] Stamm and associates originally reported the use of a glass electrode for this purpose.[52] However, the correlation between tissue pH and blood pH was suboptimal. Other authors have reported on its use with mixed results.[50,53] A fiberoptic tissue pH sensor with simultaneous recording of the fetal ECG has been more encouraging.[54,55] Practical clinical application of this technique remains unlikely, as the equipment is expensive, the technique cumbersome, and the cost prohibitive.

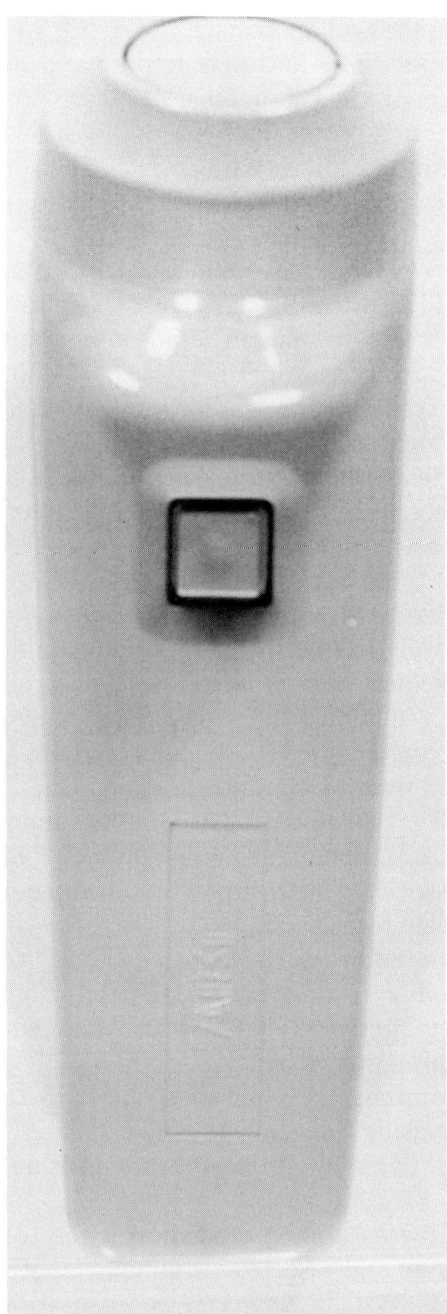

FIGURE 5.5 A model 5C Electronic Artificial Larynx manufactured by Western Electric.

MANAGEMENT SCHEMA FOR ABNORMAL FHR PATTERNS

By understanding the pathophysiologic mechanisms outlined above, rational management approaches may be developed. Table 5.4 lists FHR abnormalities and suggested therapeutic and diagnostic interventions.

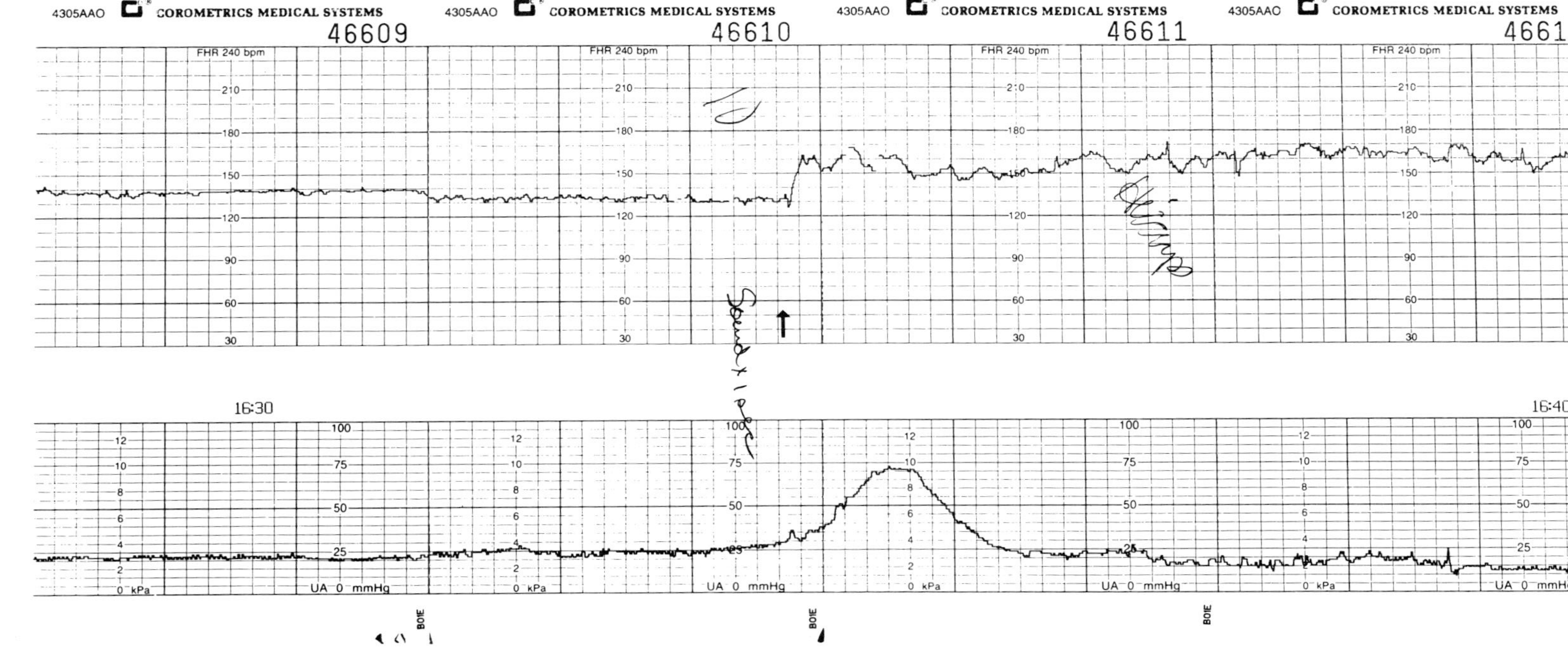

FIGURE 5.6 Fetal response to acoustic stimulation is noted by a FHR acceleration.

TABLE 5.3 Comparison of Fetal pH and Response to Acoustic Stimulation

	Fetal pH	pH
FHR response	<7.25	≥7.25
Reactive	0 (0%)	30 (100%)
Nonreactive	18 (53%)	16 (47%)

Source: Smith CV, Nguygen HV, Phelan JP, et al: Intrapartum assessment of fetal well-being: A comparison of fetal acoustic stimulation with acid-base determinations. *Am J Obstet Gynecol* 155:726, 1986. Reproduced with permission.

In general, mild variable decelerations require no specific therapy other than observation for increasing severity or for atypical features. Severe or atypical variable decelerations, being associated with an increased likelihood of acidosis, are a cause of greater concern. Maternal position change in an attempt to relieve umbilical cord compression is worthwhile. Persistence of the abnormal pattern requires further assessment of fetal status.

Similarly, the therapy of late deceleration is largely empiric. Administration of oxygen, hydration, and positioning the parturient in the left lateral recumbent position in an effort to increase uteroplacental blood flow and avoid aortocaval compression are important steps. As with severe or atypical variable deceleration, persistence demands further fetal evaluation or delivery.

Figure 5.7 presents a flow diagram outlining salient features of therapy and evaluation. If noninvasive strategies have failed to restore a nor-

TABLE 5.4 Management Approach to FHR Abnormalities

Pattern	Etiologies	Treatment
Variable decelerations	Cord compression	
Mild		None
Moderate to severe		Position change
Atypical		Oxygen and assessment of fetal status
Late decelerations	Uteroplacental insufficiency	Position change
	Hypoxia	Oxygen and assessment of fetal status
Tachycardia	Fever	Search for etiology
	Amnionitis	Acid-base assessment
	Acidosis	
	Medication	
	Hyperthyroidism	
Bradycardia	Cord prolapse	Vaginal examination
	Congenital heart block	Oxygen: evaluate cesarean delivery
	Monitor artifact	
	Paracervical block	

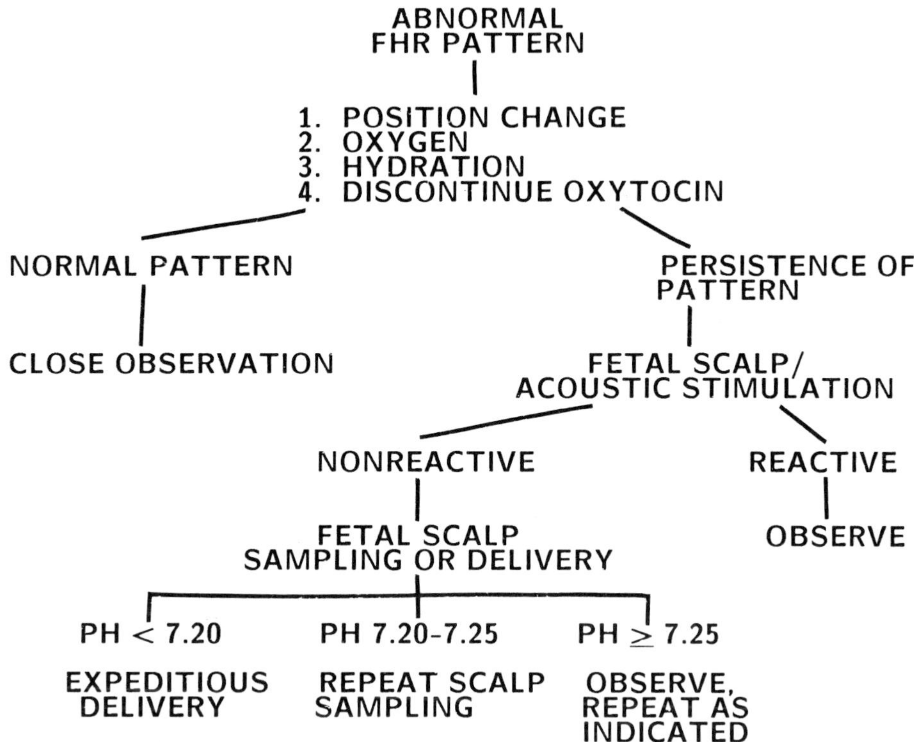

FIGURE 5.7 Evaluation and management schema for abnormal FHR patients.

mal FHR pattern, further assessment of fetal condition should be considered. Fetal scalp or acoustic stimulation offers a less invasive approach than assessing fetal acid-base status. Assessment of capillary pH in fetuses that are unresponsive to either scalp or acoustic stimulation may offer the clinician an alternative to immediate cesarean delivery. However, in light of low utilization rates, technical difficulties, and the possibility of inaccurate FHR tracing interpretation, it also appears reasonable to omit fetal scalp sampling and proceed directly to cesarean delivery under these circumstances.

A final therapeutic alternative is that of intrauterine resuscitation. In a clinical situation such as a markedly abnormal pattern or cord prolapse, when expeditious cesarean delivery is not possible, consideration should be given to the administration of a tocolytic to reduce the added stress of uterine contractions. Katz et al reported on the use of a continuous infusion of ritodrine in the management of umbilical cord prolapse.[56] The prolapse-to-delivery interval was 53 minutes, and none of the 12 newborns so managed had depressed 5-minute Apgar scores. In a limited number of cases, Lipschitz and later Arias also reported on the successful use of β-sympathomimetics in the treatment of fetal distress.[57,58] A later investigation using a 250-μmg intravenous bolus of terbutaline described its usefulness in the abolition of labor.[59,60] It was effective in eliminating uterine contractions within 1–2 minutes of administration and remained effective for a mean duration of 17 minutes in patients in spontaneous labor. In patients with abrupt FHR bradycardia, terbutaline allowed recovery in 28 of 33 patients, 22 of whom delivered nonacidotic babies vaginally. The authors were quick to point out that administration of terbutaline should not replace preparation for emergency abdominal delivery. Likewise, patients who are hemodynamically unstable, those with intrinsic cardiovascular disease, patients with diabetes mellitus, or anyone with other contraindications to β-sympathomimetics should not be treated with these agents.

A final technique that may be of value in the treatment of acute fetal distress is saline amnioinfusion. Miyazaki and Taylor reported its apparent effectiveness in restoring a normal FHR tracing[61] in cases of significant variable deceleration, presumably due to umbilical cord entrapment. In brief, the technique consisted of infusing saline through an intrauterine pressure catheter in patients experiencing repetitive or prolonged decelerations. It was effective in 68% and 86% of the cases, respectively. Although controversial, this technique may offer the clinician and the patient an alternative to cesarean delivery for severe variable decelerations associated with a reduced volume of amniotic fluid due to rupture of the membranes.

The Abnormal Fetus

An important consideration when evaluating a fetus with an abnormal FHR tracing is the possibility of anatomic or chromosomal abnormalities. Whether such tracings are encountered during antepartum fetal heart rate testing (AFHRT) or intrapartum monitoring, the incidence of structural abnormalities is increased when abnormal FHR patterns are present. Biale et al reviewed retrospectively the tracings of 73 fetuses with clinically significant congenital anomalies.[62] Pathologic tracings were found in 55% of the cases. The highest rates of abnormalities were found in fetuses with multiple congenital anomalies (83.3%), central nervous system lesions (72.4%), and chromosomal abnormalities (81.8%). No consistent type of FHR could be associated with a particular type of abnormality. Garite et al, however, identified late decelerations and reduced FHR variability as especially prominent in their series of anomalous fetuses.[63]

Given this association, and if the clinical situation permits, ultrasound examination of the fetus with an abnormal tracing may prove useful. This may be of particular importance in cases of oligohydramnios, hydramnios, or abnormal fetal lie, all of which may be associated with an even greater likelihood of anomalies.

The Role of Antenatal Fetal Surveillance

The objective of prenatal care is to maximize the benefits of in utero existence so that the fetus is in the best possible condition to withstand the stresses of labor. Given a well-compensated fetus at the onset of labor, a normal neonate is likely. Close attention to the basic tenets of prenatal care and liberal use of antenatal FHR testing are methods by which to achieve this goal. The lower incidence of fetal distress in labor associated with a normal nonstress test (NST) or a contraction stress test (CST) supports this premise. Using the NST as the primary method of surveillance, Phelan noted a threefold increase in fetal distress in association with the nonreactive compared to the reactive test.[64] Although a reactive NST does not preclude fetal distress, its presence within 7 days prior to labor makes fetal distress or death less likely.[65] Additional parameters such as perinatal mortality, meconium-stained amniotic fluid, and depressed Apgar scores are also less common in fetuses with normal tests. These data suggest that a normal fetus entering labor will almost always emerge intact. Obvious exceptions include those that suffer from acute events such as cord prolapse, major placental abruptions, and metabolic derangements such as ketoacidosis.

SUMMARY

Fetal distress remains an omnipresent concern of the obstetrician. The presence of a normal FHR tracing ensures its virtual absence. Systematic interpretation of the abnormal tracing, with particular attention to its variability, should allow discrimination between fetal stress patterns and those of distress. In situations where additional clarification is necessary, assessment of fetal condition with evocative tests such as scalp or acoustic stimulation should reduce the requirements for fetal scalp sampling. Appreciation of these principles should allow the obstetrician to make informed decisions regarding the need for cesarean delivery for fetal distress.

The opinions expressed in this chapter are those of the author and not necessarily those of the United States Navy or the Department of Defense.

REFERENCES

1. Wood C, Renou P, Oats J: A controlled trial of fetal heart rate monitoring in a low-risk obstetric population. *Am J Obstet Gynecol* 141:527, 1981.
2. Paul RH, Gauthier RJ, Quilligan EJ: Clinical fetal monitoring: The usage and relationships to trends in cesarean delivery and perinatal mortality. *Acta Obstet Gynaecol Scand* 59:289, 1980.

3. Shenker L, Post RC, Seiler JS: Routine electronic monitoring of fetal heart rate and uterine activity during labor. *Obstet Gynecol* 46:185, 1980.
4. Westgren M, Ingemarsson E, Ingemarsson I, et al: Intrapartum electronic fetal monitoring in low-risk pregnancies. *Obstet Gynecol* 56:301, 1980.
5. Clark SL, Paul RH: Intrapartum fetal surveillance: The role of fetal scalp sampling. *Am J Obstet Gynecol* 153:717, 1985.
6. Hobel C, Hyvarinen MA, Okada DM, et al: Prenatal and intrapartum high risk screening. I. Prediction of the high risk neonate. *Am J Obstet Gynecol* 117:1, 1973.
7. Ingemarsson E, Ingemarsson I, Svenningsen NW: Impact of routine fetal monitoring during labor on fetal outcome with long-term follow-up. *Am J Obstet Gynecol* 141:29, 1981.
8. Paul RH, Hon EH: Clinical fetal monitoring. V. Effect on perinatal outcome. *Am J Obstet Gynecol* 118:529, 1974.
9. Tutera G, Newman RL: Fetal monitoring: Its effect on the perinatal mortality and cesarean section and its complications. *Am J Obstet Gynecol* 122:750, 1975.
10. Renou P, Chang A, Anderson I, et al: Controlled trial of fetal intensive care. *Am J Obstet Gynecol* 126:470, 1976.
11. Neutra RR, Fineberg SE, Greenland S, et al: Effects of fetal monitoring on neonatal death rates. *N Engl J Med* 299:324, 1978.
12. Haverkamp AD, Thompson HE, McFee JG, et al: The evaluation of continuous fetal heart rate monitoring in the high risk pregnancy. *Am J Obstet Gynecol* 125:310, 1976.
13. Haverkamp AD, Orleans M, Langendoerfor S, et al: A controlled trial of the differential effects of intrapartum fetal monitoring. *Am J Obstet Gynecol* 134:399, 1979.
14. Kelso IM, Parsons RJ, Lawrence GF, et al: An assessment of continuous fetal heart rate monitoring in labor. *Am J Obstet Gynecol* 131:526, 1978.
15. Chalmers I: Randomized controlled trials of intrapartum monitoring, in Thalhammer O, Baumgarten KV, Pollak A (eds): *Perinatal Medicine.* Stuttgart, George Thiem, 1979, pp 260–265.
16. MacDonald D, Grant A, Sheridan-Pereira M, et al: The Dublin randomized controlled trial of intrapartum fetal heart rate monitoring. *Am J Obstet Gynecol* 152:524, 1985.
17. Divon MY, Torres FP, Yeh S-Y, et al: Autocorrelation techniques in fetal monitoring. *Am J Obstet Gynecol* 151:2, 1985.
18. Hon EH: Instrumentation of fetal heart rate and fetal electrocardiography. III. Fetal ECG electrodes: Further observations. *Obstet Gynecol* 30:281, 1967.
19. Tejani N, Mann L, Bhakthavathsalan A, et al: Correlation of fetal heart rate–uterine contraction patterns and fetal scalp blood pH. *Obstet Gynecol* 46:392, 1975.
20. Krebs HB, Petres RE, Dunn LJ, et al: Intrapartum fetal heart rate monitoring. I. Classification and prognosis of fetal heart rate patterns. *Am J Obstet Gynecol* 133:762, 1979.
21. Kubli FW, Hon EH, Khazin AF, et al: Observations in heart rate and pH in the human fetus during labor. *Am J Obstet Gynecol* 104:1190, 1969.
22. Schfrin BS, Dame L: Fetal heart rate patterns: Prediction of Apgar score. *JAMA* 219:1322, 1972.
23. Hon EH (ed): *An Atlas of Fetal Heart Rate Patterns.* New Haven, Conn, Hardy Press, 1968.
24. Beard RW, Filshie GM, Knight CA, et al: The significance of the changes in the continuous fetal heart rate in the first stage of labor. *J Obstet Gynaecol Br Commonwealth* 78:865, 1971.
25. Young DC, Gray JN, Luther ER, et al: Fetal scalp blood pH sampling: Its value in an active unit. *Am J Obstet Gynecol* 136:276, 1981.
26. Low JA, Cox MJ, Karchmer EJ, et al: The prediction of intrapartum fetal metabolic acidosis by fetal heart rate monitoring. *Am J Obstet Gynecol* 135:299, 1981.

27. Miller FC: Prediction of acid-base values from intrapartum fetal heart rate data and their correlation with scalp and funic values. *Clin Perinatol* 9:353, 1982.
28. Paul RH, Suidan AK, Yeh S-Y, et al: Clinical fetal monitoring. VII. The evaluation and significance of intrapartum baseline FHR variability. *Am J Obstet Gynecol* 123:206, 1975.
29. Manseau P, Vaquier J, Chavinie J, et al: Le rythme cardiaque foetal "sinusoidal" aspect evocateur de souffrance fortale au coufs de la grossesse. *J Gynecol Obstet Biol Reprod* 1:343, 1972.
30. Young BK, Katz M, Wilson SJ: Sinusoidal fetal heart rate. I. Clinical significance. *Am J Obstet Gynecol* 136:587, 1980.
31. Mondanlou HD, Freeman RK: Sinusoidal fetal heart rate pattern: Its definition and clinical significance. *Am J Obstet Gynecol* 142:1033, 1982.
32. Johnson TRB, Compton AA, Rotmensch J, et al: Significance of the sinusoidal fetal heart rate pattern. *Am J Obstet Gynecol* 139:446, 1981.
33. Gabbe SG, Ettinger RB, Freeman RK, et al: Umbilical cord compression associated with amniotomy: Laboratory observations. *Am J Obstet Gynecol* 126:253, 1976.
34. Phelan JP, Platt LD, Yeh S-Y, et al: The continuing role of the nonstress test in the management of the postdates pregnancy. *Obstet Gynecol* 64:60, 1984.
35. Moberg LG, Garite TJ, Freeman RK: Fetal heart rate patterns and fetal distress in patients with preterm premature rupture of the membranes. *Obstet Gynecol* 64:60, 1984.
36. Krebs H-B, Petres RE, Dunn LH: Intrapartum fetal heart rate monitoring. VII. Atypical variable decelerations. *Am J Obstet Gynecol* 145:297, 1983.
37. James LS, Yeh M-N, Morishima HO, et al: Umbilical vein occlusion and transient acceleration of the fetal heart rate. Experimental observation in subhuman primates. *Am J Obstet Gynecol* 126:276, 1976.
38. Young BK, Katz M, Wilson S: Fetal blood and tissue pH with variable deceleration patterns. *Obstet Gynecol* 56:170, 1980.
39. Miller FC, Sacks DA, Yeh S-Y, et al: Significance of meconium during labor. *Am J Obstet Gynecol* 122:573, 1975.
40. Krebs HB, Petres RE, Dunn LJ, et al: Intrapartum fetal heart rate monitoring. III. Association of meconium with abnormal fetal heart rate patterns. *Am J Obstet Gynecol* 137:936, 1980.
41. Starks GC: Correlation of meconium-stained amniotic fluid, early intrapartum fetal pH and Apgar scores as predictors of perinatal outcome. *Obstet Gynecol* 56:604, 1980.
42. Saling E: Technik der endoskopischen microbluentnahme am feten. *Geburtshilfe Frauenheilkunde* 24:464, 1964.
43. Beard RW, Morris ED, Clayton SG, et al: Foetal capillary pH as an indicator of the condition of the foetus. *J Obstet Gynaecol Br Commonwealth* 74:812, 1967.
44. Saling E, Schneider D: Biochemical supervision of the foetus during labor. *J Obstet Gynaecol Br Commonwealth* 74:799, 1967.
45. Wood C: Fetal scalp sampling: Its place in management. *Semin Perinatol* 2:169, 1978.
46. Clark SL, Gimovsky ML, Miller FC: Fetal heart rate response to scalp blood sampling. *Am J Obstet Gynecol* 144:706, 1982.
47. Clark SL, Gimovsky ML, Miller FC: The scalp stimulation test: A clinical alternative to fetal scalp blood sampling. *Am J Obstet Gynecol* 148:274, 1984.
48. Smith CV, Phelan JP, Broussard PM, et al: Fetal acoustic stimulation testing: A retrospective experience with the fetal acoustic stimulation test. *Am J Obstet Gynecol* 153:567, 1985.
49. Smith CV, Phelan JP, Platt LD, et al: Fetal acoustic stimulation testing (the Fas-Test). II. A randomized clinical comparison with the nonstress test. *Am J Obstet Gynecol* 155:131, 1986.

50. Smith CV, Nguygen HN, Phelan JP, et al: Intrapartum assessment of fetal well-being: A comparison of fetal acoustic stimulation with acid-base determinations. *Am J Obstet Gynecol* 155:726, 1986.
51. Lauersen NN, Miller FC, Paul RH: Continuous intrapartum monitoring of fetal scalp pH. *Am J Obstet Gynecol* 133:441, 1979.
52. Stamm O, Latscha U, Janecek P, et al: Development of a special electrode for continuous subcutaneous pH measurements in the infant scalp. *Am J Obstet Gynecol* 124:193, 1976.
53. Young BK, Noumoff J, Klein AS, et al: Continuous tissue pH in labor. *Obstet Gynecol* 52:533, 1978.
54. Peterson FI, Goldstein SR, Fitzgerald RV: Fiberoptic pH probe for physiological use. *Anal Chem* 5:864, 1980.
55. Chatterjee MS, Hetze F, Kaminetzky HA: Fetal tissue pH continuous intrapartum monitoring. *Int J Gynaecol Obstet* 22:41, 1984.
56. Katz Z, Lancet M, Borenstein R: Management of labor with umbilical cord prolapse. *Am J Obstet Gynecol* 142:239, 1982.
57. Lipschitz J: Use of a B_2-sympathomimetic drug as a temporizing measure in the treatment of acute fetal distress. *Am J Obstet Gynecol* 129:31, 1977.
58. Arias F: Intrauterine resuscitation with terbutaline: A method for the management of acute intrapartum fetal distress. *Am J Obstet Gynecol* 131:39, 1978.
59. Ingemarsson I, Arulkumaran S, Ratnam SS: Single injection of terbutaline in term labor. I. Effect on fetal pH in cases with prolonged bradycardia. *Am J Obstet Gynecol* 153:859, 1985.
60. Ingemarsson I, Arulkumaran S, Ratnam SS: Single injection of terbutaline in term labor. II. Effect on uterine activity. *Am J Obstet Gynecol* 153:865, 1985.
61. Miyazaki F, Taylor NA: Saline amnioinfusion for relief of variable or prolonged decelerations. A preliminary report. *Am J Obstet Gynecol* 146:670, 1983.
62. Biale Y, Brawer-Ostrovsky Y, Insler V: Fetal heart rate tracings in fetuses with congenital anomalies. *J Reprod Med* 30:43, 1985.
63. Garite TJ, Linzey EM, Freeman RK, et al: Fetal heart rate patterns and fetal distress in fetuses with congenital anomalies. *Obstet Gynecol* 53:716, 1979.
64. Phelan JP: The nonstress test: A review of 3000 tests. *Am J Obstet Gynecol* 139:7, 1981.
65. Phelan JP, Cromartie AD, Smith CV: The nonstress test: The false negative test. *Am J Obstet Gynecol* 142:293, 1982.

Chapter 6

Delivery of the Low-Birth-Weight Infant

L. Magnus R. Westgren, MD

The present frequent use of cesarean delivery for certain categories of preterm deliveries represents a major change from the noninterventional management that predominated until recently in most countries. In 1974, Stewart and Reynolds questioned this noninterventional approach and showed a better prognosis for certain very-low-birth-weight infants after abdominal delivery.[1] At the same time, several investigators in the United States and Europe reported an improved long-term outcome for preterm infants following cesarean birth.[2,3] These reports formed the basis for a changing attitude in favor of cesareans for select preterm fetuses. Numerous authors subsequently reported on improved survival, reduction of hypoxia, and less intracranial trauma and intraventricular hemorrhage after cesarean section in some subgroups of low-birth-weight infants. Cesarean delivery has been recommended routinely in cases of preterm malpresentation, and with improvements in neonatal care, many obstetricians will now perform cesareans for fetal indications as early as 25–26 weeks of gestation. However, during the last few years, an increasing number of authors have questioned the value of cesarean section for preterm fetuses.[4–7] This chapter reviews some areas of controversy surrounding cesarean delivery for the preterm infant.

INDICATIONS

In 1987 the proportion of planned, preterm deliveries continues to increase and parallels improved survival rates of preterm infants. Today elective delivery due to fetal and maternal complications represents approximately one-third of all preterm deliveries. Most of these patients are delivered abdominally due to the presence of an unfavorable maternal cervix. In such cases, preterm infants may do better following abdominal delivery, although comparison of elective cesarean delivery to induction with careful fetal monitoring has not been adequately performed. Experience with prostaglandin E_2 for cervical ripening in this group of preterm patients remains limited and requires further investigation.

It has long been recognized that the breech or transverse presentation may involve an increased risk of birth trauma compared to vertex presentations.[8,9] Vaginal breech delivery in the preterm fetus has been associated with a greater likelihood of cord accident and a tendency for the relatively large aftercoming head to be trapped in an incompletely dilated cervix.[10,11] Postmortem examinations suggest noticeably higher rates of birth injury, which are assumed to be directly related to the vaginal delivery process.[10] Moreover, in some cases, preterm breech presentations may suggest fetal compromise per se, because breech presentation is more common in premature fetuses than in normal fetuses that eventually deliver at term. It is also significant that recent studies reveal an increase in respiratory distress syndrome (RDS), low Apgar scores, intracranial hemorrhage, birth trauma, and subsequent neurologic handicaps among very-low-birth-weight breech fetuses regardless of the mode of delivery.[5,12] Effer and associates conclude, "The prematurity itself, with all its accompanying pathophysiology, is so overwhelming that maneuvers involving method of delivery do not alter outcome."[5]

In assessing the risk of vaginal breech delivery for the preterm fetus, only retrospective observational studies are available.[13–27] The limitations of such studies have been extensively discussed.[4,6,28] Despite the limitations inherent in retrospective studies, most obstetricians currently favor cesarean delivery for the preterm breech fetus. In addition, centers with low overall perinatal mortality rates demonstrate that cesarean delivery offers the greatest apparent benefit to the preterm breech fetus (Table 6.1). However, it has not been documented that the policy of liberal cesarean delivery at such institutions can eliminate the difference in long-term outcome between preterm infants born in breech presentation by cesarean and cephalic infants born vaginally. This again suggests that the outcome in the delivery of preterm breech infants is related not only to the technique of delivery but, more importantly, to the essentially different pathophysiology of these low-birth-weight infants.

Twin deliveries represent approximately one-sixth of all preterm deliveries.[29] Several authors have presented evidence to suggest that cesarean delivery is beneficial in preterm twin deliveries in which the presentation is other than vertex–vertex.[30–35] These data appear to be especially valid for infants delivered prior to the 33rd week of gestation. Evidence in support of routine cesearean for vertex–vertex premature twin pregnancies, however, is limited and inconclusive.

To date there is no substantial evidence suggesting that cesarean section is the optimal mode of delivery for the low-birth-weight infant presenting as a vertex. Although this issue has been addressed extensively,

TABLE 6.1 Mortality at Preterm Breech Delivery in Infants Weighing Less Than 1,500 g: Vaginal Delivery versus Cesarean Section

Source	Years of Birth	Mortality		Overall Mortality	Mortality CS/Vaginal
		Vaginal	CS		
Goldenberg and Nelson[43]	1970–1975	49/64 (77%)	13/23 (57%)	(72%)	0.8
Mann and Gallant[16]	Not given	34/44 (77%)	7/15 (47%)	(70%)	0.6
Bowes et al[14]	1970–1977	39/57 (68%)	3/12 (25%)	(61%)	0.4
Woods[17]	1970–1975	10/16 (63%)	1/4 (25%)	(55%)	0.4
Effer et al[5]	1973–1980	15/33 (46%)	26/60 (33%)	(45%)	0.7
Main et al[23]	1977–1981	71/123 (58%)	27/93 (29%)	(45%)	0.5
Westgren et al[6]	1979–1982	20/37 (54%)	37/99 (37%)	(42%)	0.7
Rosen and Chik[26]	1976–1982	22/40 (55%)	10/49 (20%)	(36%)	0.4
Smith et al[18]	1976–1979	31/59 (53%)	17/89 (19%)	(32%)	0.4
Duenholter et al[15]	1972–1977	5/9 (55%)	1/9 (11%)	(33%)	0.2
Sachs et al[22]	1974–1978	1,929/4,455 (43%)	664/3,787 (17%)	(31%)	0.4
Yu et al[24]	1977–1980	20/40 (50%)	2/32 (6%)	(31%)	0.1
Ingemarsson et al[13]	1971–1977	5/13 (38%)	1/11 (9%)	(25%)	0.2

no investigator has conclusively demonstrated any difference in outcome between preterm vertex infants delivered vaginally and via cesarean.[36–38] It must be emphasized, however, that if vaginal delivery is selected, close surveillance of the fetus is mandatory because intrapartum asphyxia is more common in preterm deliveries; in patients with premature rupture of the membranes and preterm delivery, the incidence of birth asphyxia is reported to be three times that of patients delivering with intact membranes.[39] It has been suggested that the high incidence of fetal distress in such cases may, in part, be due to the loss of the cushioning effect of amniotic fluid on the umbilical cord. Recent studies have suggested that in cases of preterm rupture of the membranes with variable decelerations, amnioinfusion may be effective in relieving the pattern of cord compression to achieve successful vaginal delivery.[40,41] Because preterm infants appear to be exquisitely sensitive to the effects of intrauterine asphyxia, a lower threshold for intervention via cesarean delivery may be appropriate for preterm fetuses exhibiting nonreassuring heart rate patterns.[39,42]

Although the advantage of cesarean delivery in the premature breech fetus has been suggested for such fetuses as a group, there is, to date, no evidence that cesarean delivery in the very-low-birth-weight infant improves or contributes to survival or long-term neurologic benefit.[12,43] Thus, in infants delivering prior to 27 weeks gestation, maternal informed consent is vital. After counseling regarding the dismal prognosis for survival, as well as the uncertainty regarding the benefit of cesarean for such fetuses, some mothers may elect nonintervention. It is indeed unfortunate that the medicolegal climate in the United States and the factual ignorance of many so-called expert witnesses often lead to operative intervention in situations where benefit has not been clearly demonstrated.

TABLE 6.2 Maternal Characteristics in Relation to Type of Incision

Factors	Incision		
	Low Transverse (N = 54)	Low Vertical (N = 82)	Classical (N = 38)
Maternal age (M ± 1 SD)	27.9 ± 7.1	27.3 ± 7.0	29. 7 ± 6.5
Maternal weight (kg M ± SD)	63 ± 8.0	60 ± 4.0	68 ± 9.0
Parity			
Nullipara	18 (33%)	26 (32%)	8 (21%)
1 para	36 (67%)	56 (68%)	30 (79%)
Previous CS	6 (11%)	4 (5%)	10 (26%)
Elective	34 (63%)	42 (51%)	19 (50%)
Emergency	20 (37%)	40 (49%)	19 (50%)
Cervical dilatation			
at CS closed	16 (30%)	27 (33%)	13 (34%)
0–5 cm	28 (52%)	43 (52%)	19 (50%)
5 cm	10 (18%)	12 (15%)	6 (16%)
Delivered by:			
Resident (1–2 years)	8 (15%)	13 (16%)	4 (11%)
Sr. resident	43 (79%)	68 (83%)	33 (86%)
Faculty	3 (6%)	1 (1%)	1 (3%)

TECHNIQUE AND COMPLICATIONS

One problem often encountered in performing a cesarean in a preterm fetus is the presence of a poorly developed lower uterine segment. Morrison[44] followed patients prospectively with ultrasound and estimated the width of the normal lower uterine segment to be 0.5 cm at 20 weeks, 1.0 cm at 28 weeks, and 4.0 cm at 34 weeks. In many cases, unless labor has expanded and thinned the lower uterine segment, a transverse incision may be technically difficult to perform. Such inadequate incisions can lead to birth trauma of the fetus or to lateral extensions of the lower uterine segment incision, resulting in broad ligament lacerations and significant maternal morbidity. Such considerations have led many obstetricians to use a low vertical incision at the time of preterm cesarean section.[45] Other authors, however, have expressed doubts about the necessity for a vertical incision in all cases of preterm cesarean delivery.[7] At the Los Angeles County-University of Southern California Women's Hospital, records of 174 patients who were delivered of infants weighing less than 1,500 g between 1983 and 1984 were reviewed. In 31% of the cases, a low transverse incision was performed compared with a low vertical incision in 47% and a classical uterine incision in 22%. Maternal and fetal characteristics did not differ in relation to the type of incision chosen (Table 6.2). This study revealed no differences in the incidence of maternal or fetal complications (Table 6.3). Difficult delivery was noted by the surgeon in one case of low transverse and three cases of low vertical incision.

TABLE 6.3 Maternal and Fetal Complications and Fetal Outcome in Relation to Type of Incision

	Incision		
Complication	Low Transverse	Low Vertical	Classical
Maternal complications			
Required transfusion	4 (7%)	5 (6%)	3 (8%)
Injury to bladder	2 (4%)	1 (1%)	—
Laceration of broad ligament	1 (2%)	—	—
Bleeding from uterine artery	2 (4%)	—	—
Endometritis	4 (7%)	1 (13%)	3 (8%)
Maternal postpartum stay	5.1 ± 2.2	5.2 ± 2.4	5.4 ± 2.0
Fetal complications			
Difficult traumatic delivery	1 (2%)	3 (4%)	—
Skin incision/delivery time	5.9 ± 2.7	6.3 ± 3.2	6.7 ± 4.2
Birth injury[a]	1 (2%)	2 (2%)	1 (3%)
Fetal outcome			
Apgar score <7 at 1 min	45 (79%)	61 (71%)	35 (85%)
<7 at 5 min	6 (11%)	24 (28%)	7 (17%)
Neonatal mortality	5 (9%)	15 (17%)	7 (17%)

[a] Injuries caused by knife or scissors.

Interestingly, all four cases of traumatic cesarean delivery occurred in fetuses presenting as breech or transverse lie with the mother in active labor. In each case, the head or neck was trapped by the contractile part of the uterus at the level of the upper uterine segment or the juncture between the lower and upper uterine segments. Thus, despite the fact that cesarean delivery was carried out including a vertical incision, the preterm breech was not protected from traumatic delivery. In view of the inconclusive nature of the present data, it seems reasonable to decide on the type of incision on an individual basis. Such a decision is best made intraoperatively. Especially in cases of malpresentation, if the lower uterine segment is not of sufficient width to allow an adequate transverse incision, strong consideration should be given to a low vertical or classical incision. The use of β-mimetic agents for uterine relaxation at the time of preterm cesarean has been recommended by some authors.[46] Such a procedure may facilitate the controlled, atraumatic delivery of the tiny infant. Excess intraoperative bleeding in such cases is usually controlled easily by the injection of propranolol following clamping of the cord.

Regardless of the type of incision chosen, intraoperative complications including bladder injury, broad ligament laceration, and uterine artery laceration are more common at the time of preterm cesarean than with term infants.[47] This fact emphasizes the importance of ensuring that these operations are performed by an experienced surgeon with adequate assistance. Clinical experience suggests that the performance of a true low vertical uterine incision (ie, one that does not enter the upper contractile portion of the uterus) is extremely rare. Further investigation is needed to determine the safety of vaginal delivery following a presumed low vertical uterine incision. At the present time, however, the safety of a trial of labor following a vertical uterine incision has not been conclusively demonstrated. Therefore, it seems reasonable to consider the potential for the limitation of future family size, as well as the risk of spontaneous uterine rupture associated with a vertical incision in determining the incision type for the delivery of the low-birth-weight infant.

REFERENCES

1. Stewart A, Reynolds EOR: Improved prognosis for infants of very low birthweight. *Pediatrics* 54:724, 1974.
2. Lubchenco LO, Bard H, Goldman AL, et al: Neonatal intensive care and long-term prognosis. *Dev Med Child Neurol* 16:421, 1974.
3. Davies PA, Tizard JPM: Very low birthweight and subsequent neurological defects (with special reference to spastic diplegia). *Dev Med Child Neurol* 17:3, 1975.
4. Crowley P, Hawkins DF: Premature breech delivery—the cesarean section debate. *J Obstet Gynaecol* 1:2, 1980.
5. Effer SB, Saigal S, Rand C, et al: Effects of delivery method on outcome in the very low birthweight breech infant: Is the improved survival related to cesarean section or other perinatal care maneuvers? *Am J Obstet Gynecol* 145:123, 1983.
6. Westgren M, Sangster G, Paul R: Preterm breech delivery, another retrospective study. *Obstet Gynecol* 66:481, 1985.
7. Janovic R: Incision of the pregnant uterus and delivery of low birthweight infants. *Am J Obstet Gynecol* 152:971, 1985.
8. Galloway WH, Bartholomew RA, Calvin ED, et al: Premature breech presentation. *Am J Obstet Gynecol* 99:975, 1976.
9. Brenner WE, Bruce RD, Hendrics CH: The characteristics and perils of breech presentation. *Am J Obstet Gynecol* 118:700, 1974.
10. Kauppila O: The perinatal mortality in breech deliveries and observations on affecting factors. *Acta Obstet Gynaecol Scand* (suppl) 39:29, 1975.
11. Rovinsky JJ, Miller JA, Kaplan S: Management of breech presentation at term. *Am J Obstet Gynecol* 115:497, 1973.
12. Kauppilla O, Gronros M, Aro P, et al: Management of low birthweight breech delivery: Should cesarean section be routine? *Obstet Gynecol* 57:289, 1981.
13. Ingemarsson I, Westgren M, Svenningsen NW: Long-term follow-up of preterm infants in breech presentation delivered by cesarean section: A prospective study. *Lancet* 2:172, 1978.
14. Bowes WA, Taylor ES, O'Brian M, et al: Breech delivery: Evaluation of the method of delivery on perinatal results and maternal morbidity. *Am J Obstet Gynecol* 135:965, 1979.
15. Duenholter JH, Wells CE, Reisch JS: A paired, controlled study of vaginal and abdominal delivery of the low birthweight breech fetus. *Obstet Gynecol* 54:310, 1979.
16. Mann LJ, Gallant JM: Modern management of the breech delivery. *Am J Obstet Gynecol* 134:611, 1979.
17. Woods JR: Effects of low birthweight breech delivery on neonatal mortality. *Obstet Gynecol* 53:735, 1979.

18. Smith ML, Spencer SA, Hull D: Mode of delivery and survival in babies weighing less than 2000 gr at birth. *Br Med J* 281:1118, 1980.
19. Nisell H, Nistoletti P, Palme C: Preterm breech delivery early and late complications. *Acta Obstet Gynaecol Scand* 60:363, 1981.
20. Cos C, Kendall AC, Hommers M: Changed prognosis of breech-presenting low birthweight infants. *Br J Obstet Gynaecol* 89:881, 1982.
21. Geirsson RT, Namunkangula R, Calder AA: Preterm singleton breech presentation: The impact of traumatic intracranial hemorrhage on neonatal mortality. *J Obstet Gynecol* 2:219, 1982.
22. Sachs BP, McCarthy BJ, Rubin G, et al: Cesarean section: Risks and benefits for the mother and fetus. *JAMA* 250:2157, 1983.
23. Main DM, Main EK, Maurer MM: Cesarean section versus vaginal delivery for the breech fetus weighing less than 1500 grams. *Am J Obstet Gynecol* 146:580, 1983.
24. Yu VYH, Najuh B, Cutting D, et al: Effect of mode of delivery on outcome of very low birthweight infants. *Br J Obstet Gynaecol* 91:633, 1984.
25. van Eyk EA, Huisjes JH: Neonatal mortality and morbidity associated with preterm breech presentation. *Eur J Obstet Gynecol Reprod Biol* 15:17, 1983.
26. Rosen MG, Chik L: The effect of delivery route on outcome in breech presentation. *Am J Obstet Gynecol* 148:909, 1984.
27. Westgren M, Paul R: Delivery of the low birthweight infant by cesarean section. *Clin Obstet Gynecol* 28:752, 1985.
28. Papiernik E: Prediction of the preterm baby. *Clin Obstet Gynecol* 11:315, 1984.
29. Nordenskjold F, Sjoberg NO, Aberg A, et al: Mortality and morbidity in preterm twins. *Dan Med Bull* 26:139, 1979.
30. McCarthy NJ, Sachs BP, Layde PM, et al: The epidemiology of neonatal death in twins. *Am J Obstet Gynecol* 141:252, 1981.
31. Barrett JM, Staffs SM, van Hooylink JE, et al: The effect of type of delivery upon neonatal outcome in premature twins. *Am J Obstet Gynecol* 143:360, 1982.
32. McGilliwray I: Twins and other multiple deliveries. *Clin Obstet Gynaecol* 7:581, 1980.
33. Chervenak FA, Johnson RE, Berkowitz RL, et al: Is routine cesarean section necessary for vertex breech and vertex transverse twin gestations? *Am J Obstet Gynecol* 148:1, 1984.
34. Chervenak FA, Johnson RE, Youcha S, et al: Intrapartum management of twin gestation. *Obstet Gynecol* 65:110, 1985.
35. Wallace RL, Schifrin BS, Paul RH: The delivery route for very low birthweight infants: A preliminary report of a randomized prospective study. *J Reprod Med* 29:736, 1984.
36. Rosen MG, Chik L: The association between cesarean birth and outcome in vertex presentation: Relative importance of birthweight on Dubowitz scores and delivery route. *Am J Obstet Gynecol* 150:775, 1984.
37. Westgren M, Dolfin T, Halperin M, et al: Mode of delivery in the low birthweight fetus: Delivery by cesarean section independent of a fetal lie versus vaginal delivery in vertex presentation. *Acta Obstet Gynaecol Scand* 65:51, 1985.
38. Moberg LJ, Garite T, Freeman R: Fetal heart rate patterns and fetal distress in patients with premature rupture of membranes. *Obstet Gynecol* 64:60, 1984.
39. Westgren M, Holmquist P, Ingemarsson I, et al: Intrapartum fetal acidosis in preterm infants: Fetal monitoring and long-term morbidity. *Obstet Gynecol* 63:355, 1984.
40. Miyazaki FS, Nevarez F: Saline amnioinfusion for relief of repetitive variable decelerations: A prospective randomized study. *Am J Obstet Gynecol* 153:301, 1985.
41. Nageotte MP, Freeman RK, Garite TJ, et al: Prophylactic intrapartum amnioinfusion in patients with preterm premature rupture of membranes. *Am J Obstet Gynecol* 153:557, 1985.

42. Westgren M, Malcus P, Svenningsen N: Intrauterine asphyxia and long-term outcome in preterm infants. *Obstet Gynecol* (in press).
43. Goldenberg RL, Nelson KG: The premature breech. *Am J Obstet Gynecol* 127:240, 1977.
44. Morrison J: The development of the lower uterine segment. *Aust NZ J Med* 12:182, 1972.
45. Haesslein HL, Goodlin RC: Delivery of the tiny newborn. *Am J Obstet Gynecol* 134:192, 1979.
46. Westgren M, Ingemarsson I, Ahlstrom H, et al: Delivery and long-term outcome of very low birthweight infants. *Acta Obstet Gynaecol Scand* 61:25, 1982.
47. Nielson TF, Hokegard KH: Cesarean section and intraoperative surgical complications. *Acta Obstet Gynaecol Scand* 63:103, 1984.

Chapter 7

Abruptio Placenta and Placenta Previa

Garland D. Anderson, MD

Abruptio placenta and placenta previa are serious obstetric complications that occur in the latter half of pregnancy and are frequently manifested by third trimester bleeding. Although the overall incidence of third trimester bleeding is 3%–4% of pregnancies, in approximately half of these cases no specific cause can be identified. However, in the remaining half, placenta previa accounts for 22% and abruptio placenta for 31%.[1] Placenta previa and abruptio placenta are frequent reasons for the delivery of the very-low-birth-weight infant and accounted for 20% of 338 liveborn infants weighing 500–1,000 g at the E.H. Crump Women's Hospital and Perinatal Center during a 5-year period ending December 31, 1984.

ABRUPTIO PLACENTA

Abruptio placenta is defined as a separation of the normally implanted placenta prior to the birth of the fetus. The overall incidence of abruptio placenta varies widely. In the E.H. Crump Women's Hospital and Perinatal Center, the incidence is 1:108 deliveries. The syndrome of abruptio placenta was originally described by Edward Rigby in 1875.[2] Chantreuil[3] reported the association between abruption and the toxemias of pregnancy. Placental abruption is frequently an acute process of increasing severity over a few hours. At other times, abruptio placenta has a variable presentation that may be self-limited without further problems or may become a chronic abruption. In this latter circumstance, the initial episode of abruptio placenta will become quiescent, only to recur subsequently.

The pathophysiology of abruptio placenta is separation of the placenta, initiated by bleeding into the decidua basalis. The bleeding usually begins in the small vessels in the basal layer of the decidua basalis, but it may originate from fetal-placental vessels. This hemorrhage splits the de-

TABLE 7.1 Risk Factors in Abruptio Placenta

Prior history of abruptio placenta
Cigarette smoking
Chronic pregnancy-induced hypertension
Prior history of HELP syndrome
Abdominal trauma
Advanced parity and age

cidua and leaves a thin layer attached to the placenta and myometrium. Once the bleeding starts, a hematoma forms and causes additional separation of the placenta from the uterine wall, with destruction and compression of adjacent placental tissue. The net effect is a reduction in the amount of functional area available to the fetus for exchange of nutrients and respiratory gases. Occasionally blood will extravasate into and through the myometrium to the peritoneal surfaces, resulting in the so-called Couvelaire uterus.

The external manifestation of abruption is vaginal bleeding. This is the result of blood reaching the placenta edge and then dissecting between the decidua and the fetal membranes. Port wine staining of the amniotic fluid, which is almost pathognomonic for abruptio placenta, results from blood passing through the membranes into the amniotic cavity.

ETIOLOGY

Underlying disease of the decidua and uterine blood vessels appears to be a common basis for the diversity of factors associated with abruptio placenta. For instance, disorders associated with abruption range from preeclampsia to the bite of venomous snake (genus *Bothrops*). Table 7.1 lists the factors considered to have an etiologic role in the development of abruptio placenta.

Smoking

Cigarette smoking during pregnancy is associated with a 1.5 times greater risk of abruptio placenta. The Collaborative Perinatal Project of the National Institute of Neurological and Communicative Disorders and Stroke followed the course of 53,518 pregnancies in 12 medical-school-affiliated hospitals in the United States between 1959 and 1966.[4] In that report, the frequency of abruptio placenta was found to be greater in smokers than in nonsmokers. For instance, the incidence was 24.2 per 1,000 in women who smoked during the current pregnancy, 18.7 per 1,000 if they stopped smoking during pregnancy, and 16.9 per 1,000 if they had never smoked. However, the incidence of abruptio placenta increased to 32.0 per 1,000 if the pregnant woman had smoked more than 10 cigarettes per day for more than 6 years.[5] The theoretical basis for abruptio placenta in smoking gravidas is necrosis of the decidua at the margin of the placenta. Under normal circumstances, the central areas of the placenta are perfused better than the periphery. However, during cigarette smoke inhalation, uterine perfusion is decreased for 15 minutes.[6] During this period of diminished perfusion, the decidua and placental edge theoretically are inadequately perfused. As a result, decidual necrosis may develop and result in bleeding.

Trauma

Trauma is the leading cause of death among women 15–33 years of age. Approximately half of these deaths are due to automobile accidents. Of the known causes of abruptio placenta, trauma accounts for 1%.

The most common cause of fetal death in an automobile accident is the death of the mother. If the mother survives the accident, the fetus usually survives. However, in those fetuses who die, the most common cause of death is abruptio placenta. The incidence of abruptio placenta following an accident is variable and depends on the severity of the maternal injury. For instance, Crosby reported a direct relationship between the severity of the motor vehicle accident and the incidence of abruption (minor, 0%; severe, 5.7%). If the pregnant woman herself was severely injured, the rate rose to 29%.[7,8]

In a combined series of 176 women with major injuries, 45 (25.6%) had abruptio placenta.[7] Many of the women had abruption within a few hours of the accident, and all cases occurred within 48 hours of the accident. However, two cases of abruptio placenta have been reported, each occurring 5 days after a serious injury in an automobile accident[9,10]; however, these two cases may have been unrelated to the traumatic event.

Hypertension

Hypertensive disease and abruptio placenta are intimately related. Although the incidence of hypertension among women with abruptio placenta ranges from 11.3% to 64.6%,[11] the 42-month experience at the E.H. Crump Women's Hospital and Perinatal Center ending December 31, 1980, demonstrated hypertension to be a factor in 71 of 265 (26.8%) women with abruptio placenta. Moreover, the perinatal mortality rate was higher among hypertensive women than among normotensive women who developed abruptio placenta. This increase was due to a larger number of fetal deaths, with no significant increase in the number of neonatal deaths. The incidence of abruptio placenta varies widely depending on the specific hypertensive disorder. Women with mild preeclampsia did not have an increased incidence of abruption, whereas those with antepartum eclampsia or hypertension with superimposed preeclampsia had an incidence of approximately 15%[12] (Table 7.2).

TABLE 7.2 Incidence of Abruptio Placenta in Hypertensive Disorder of Pregnancy

Patient Group	No. of Patients	Incidence	
		N	Percent
Normotensive	50,435	472	0.93
Hypertensive disorders	5,923	177	3.00
Mild preeclampsia	4,167	33	0.80
Severe preeclampsia	962	99	10.20
Eclampsia	186	21	11.30
Antepartum eclampsia	134	20	14.90
Chronic hypertension	847	61	7.20
Hypertension only	603	26	4.00
Hypertension + preeclampsia or eclampsia	244	37	15.10

Maternal Age

Abruptio placenta has long been known to occur in older women. Whether this is principally due to advanced age or parity is unclear; however, some investigators have found a direct correlation between abruption and both maternal age and parity. Others have reported that the increase in advanced maternal age is due only to increased parity.[1] In our study group of 265 women with abruptio placenta, both maternal age and parity were positively correlated with the incidence of abruption.[11]

Past History of Abruption

Several studies have reported a high rate of recurrence for abruptio placenta. Our study at the E.H. Crump Women's Hospital and Perinatal Center found recurrent abruptio placenta in 15 of 265 women (9.1%).[11] Of these, 7 women (47%) had chronic hypertension. In multiparous women with chronic hypertension, the incidence of recurrent abruptio placenta was 4.2%. This compares to an incidence in the general obstetric population of 0.93%. After two consecutive abruptions the risk of a third rises to 25% and that about 30% of all future pregnancies fail to produce a healthy child.[12]

Cocaine

Abruptio placenta has been reported within a few hours or minutes after intravenous self-administration of cocaine and within a few hours after intranasal administration (snorting) of cocaine.[13] Cocaine causes tachycardia and immediate but transient hypertension. These physiologic responses are induced secondary to an increase in central stimulation and potentiation of a peripheral response of sympathetically mediated organs by blockade of catecholamine reuptake at adrenergic nerve endings.[14]

Physical Work and Stress

A recent series describing the outcome of pregnancy in female physicians reported a high incidence of placental abruption.[15] Of the 49 deliveries, 27 occurred during residency or fellowship training, 19 during practice, and 5 by physicians who were not working at the time of the delivery; most of them had just completed their residency. Six of the 49 pregnancies (12%) were complicated by either an acute or chronic abruptio placenta. Of the three acute cases of abruptio placenta, two required operative intervention for fetal distress.

Snake Bite

Abruptio placenta has been reported following the bite of the poisonous snake of the genus *Bothrops*.[16] Snakes belonging to this genus are responsible for most of the snake venom poisoning in Brazil. The toxins contained in the venom are potent activators of the coagulation system; this may have led to the abruptio placenta.

DIAGNOSIS

The clinical diagnosis of abruptio placenta requires a high degree of suspicion and a careful history and physical examination. The classical signs and symptoms include abdominal pain, vaginal bleeding, and uterine activity and/or tenderness. The findings of vaginal bleeding, a tightly contracted, "boardlike" uterus, uterine tenderness, and absence of fetal heart tones occur together in only a minority of cases.

Vaginal bleeding occurs in 80%–90% of cases of abruptio placenta. The external bleeding is characteristically dark and nonclotting, but may be serosanguineous when extruded from a retroplacental clot or bright red in cases of sudden abruption.

Abdominal pain can be extremely variable and is absent in approximately 50% of cases upon admission to the hospital. The pain may be severe, intermittent, crampy, or persistent. Abdominal pain frequently indicates extravasation of blood into the myometrium. Associated symptoms may include a feeling of faintness, without evidence of hypovolemia, and nausea and vomiting. Patients with a posterior placental abruption may also present with crampy lower abdominal pain.

More reliable signs of abruptio placenta include uterine tenderness and varying degrees of uterine rigidity. The amount of uterine rigidity is frequently related to the size of the abruption. Associated uterine contractions are characteristically of high frequency and low amplitude, and may be clinically difficult to appreciate. If the baseline uterine tonus is elevated, such contractions may not register on an external tocodynamometer.

TABLE 7.3 Initial Management of Abruptio Placenta

Insert secure large-bore peripheral intravenous line
Obtain laboratory studies
Hematocrit, clot observation test
Fibrinogen, platelet count
Prothrombin time, partial thromboplastin time
Fibrin degradation products
Electrolytes, serum creatinine
Crossmatch 4 units of type-specific packed cells
Determine fetal status
General measures
Oxygen, 8 L/min by nasal cannula
Foley catheter in bladder
Monitor vital signs every 15 minutes

In cases of fetal distress, a large portion of villous exchange area has been lost. In cases where fetal death occurs frequently, over 50% of the placenta will usually have separated from the uterus.

Ultrasonography is of little help in making the diagnosis of abruptio placenta except in cases where there are large retroplacental hematomas and the diagnosis is obvious clinically. Sonographic evidence of abruption includes retroplacental and intraplacental sonolucent areas, separation and rounding of the placental edge, and a placental thickness >5.5 cm.[17,18]

MANAGEMENT OF ABRUPTIO PLACENTA

The proper management of abruptio placenta requires a stepwise approach to minimize the risks to both the mother and the fetus (Table 7.3).

1. A large-bore peripheral intravenous line should be placed and well secured. If there is evidence of maternal hypovolemia, two intravenous lines should be considered. Lactated Ringer's solution or Plasmalyte may be given. Once a coagulopathy has been excluded or has been aggressively treated with component blood therapy, a central line, preferably a pulmonary artery catheter, may be inserted in severe cases if indicated by the patient's condition.
2. Obtain initial laboratory studies and crossmatch for blood. The hematocrit may be initially high if the abruptio is of sudden onset. From 2 to 4 units of type-specific packed red blood cells should be ordered. Fresh frozen plasma can be used to replace coagulation factors if needed. The whole blood clotting time (clot observation test) is useful both initially and serially in determining whether a significant coagulation abnormality is present and whether fresh frozen plasma should be ordered. If fetal distress is present, the woman can safely undergo a cesarean in the presence of a normal whole blood clotting time without waiting for the results of the other coagulation studies. The whole blood clotting time is unaffected by a moderate decrease in coagulation factors, and clotting within 4–8 minutes excludes a clinically significant

coagulopathy. If the blood does not clot in 8 minutes, a significant coagulation disorder is present and cryoprecipitate or fresh frozen plasma should be ordered initially, along with type-specific packed cells. Each unit of cryoprecipitate will raise the serum fibrinogen level by 4–5 mg per 100 mL. Each unit of fresh frozen plasma will raise the serum fibrinogen level approximately 8–10 mg/100 mL. The need for platelet infusions should be guided by a platelet count. Additional coagulation studies may assist in the detection of a subclinical coagulopathy. Baseline renal function tests are useful for the detection of preexisting renal compromise or later detection of renal complications.

3. Determine the fetal status. The fetal heart tones should be auscultated. If possible, both an internal scalp electrode and an internal pressure catheter should be placed. Internal electronic fetal rate monitoring may identify subtle late decelerations that may not be detected by external electronic fetal heart rate monitoring. In addition, internal monitoring allows the assessment of heart rate variability. An internal pressure catheter can identify resting hypertonus (>15 mm Hg), a condition associated with a significant decrease in uterine blood flow, which often accompanies placental abruption.
4. Amniotomy should be performed if expeditious delivery by cesarean section is not planned. This is done principally to allow internal monitoring and perhaps to better quantify the hemorrhage. Although amniotomy is said to reduce extravasation of blood into the myometrium and entry of thromboplastic substance into the maternal circulation, little scientific evidence of this benefit exists.

General Measures

Oxygen (8 L/min) should be given by nasal prongs or mask. In severe cases, a Foley catheter should be inserted in the bladder. The vital signs should be monitored every 15 minutes. A woman with hypertension or preeclampsia may have a blood pressure in the normal range as a result of hypovolemia. Blood loss is usually grossly underestimated in placental abruption. Liberal intravenous fluid therapy should be instituted until blood is available. A urine output of at least 30 mL/hr and a hematocrit of >30% are rational goals of therapy. This may require blood transfusion in excess of the observed blood loss.

Route of Delivery

Vaginal delivery is desirable, especially if the fetus is dead. Cesarean section is indicated if fetal distress is present and if the mother is not experiencing serious disseminated intravascular coagulation (DIC). If the fetal heart rate tracing is normal and the uterus relaxes well between contractions, vaginal delivery may be attempted. However, some authors feel that cesarean section is always the preferred route of delivery with placental abruption when the fetus is alive and considered viable. This is particularly true when abruptio placenta occurs in the preterm fetus.[19] In such circumstances, the risk of fetal distress is high and the risk of sudden, complete separation of the placenta is ever present. With sudden additional placental separation, the fetus may be severely compromised even if delivered within several minutes by emergency cesarean. In one series of abruptio placenta, 75% of fetal deaths occurred more than 90 minutes after admission to the hospital. In addition, 70% of all perinatal mortality occurred in infants who were delivered more than 2 hours after the time of diagnosis.[20] In our series of 265 women, 110 (41.5%) underwent cesarean section. Of the 182 survivors, 25 (13.7%) had a documented abnormality on follow-up in the first year of neonatal life.[11] In any case, all the personnel necessary to perform an emergency cesarean section and resuscitate the infant should be readily available whenever placental abruption is diagnosed or strongly suspected.

In cases of fetal demise, the uterus may be refractory to amniotomy and oxytocin stimulation, especially in primigravid women. These cases are usually associated with hyperfibrinolysis and serum fibrin degradation products of >300 μg/mL.[20] It has been reported that the administration of the antifibrinolytic, antithromboplastic agent Transylol will stimulate uterine contractions in some of these cases.[20] However, this drug is not approved for this use in this country.

Additional serious maternal complications that may be encountered in women with abruptio placenta include hemorrhagic shock, disseminated intravascular coagulation, and acute renal failure.

Hemorrhagic Shock

The risk of hemorrhagic shock is high in severe placental abruption because blood loss is frequently underestimated. In some cases, the uterus may contain upward of 2,500 mL of blood. Additional blood may also be found in the myometrium. Aggressive fluid resuscitation and, in some severe cases, initiation of blood transfusion regardless of initial hematocrit, may reduce this complication. Monitoring of urine output is the best method of assessing effective blood volume. The urine output should be at least 30 mL/hr and the hematocrit kept at >30%.

Acute Renal Failure

Acute renal failure is caused by anoxia due to hemorrhagic shock or microvascular obstruction by fibrin deposition. Almost all cases of acute renal failure are due to reversible acute tubular necrosis. Bilateral cortical necrosis is unlikely to occur unless there is preexisting renal disease or chronic hypertension. The key to prevention of acute renal failure is aggressive blood and fluid replacement to prevent or combat hypovolemic shock.

Disseminated Intravasculation Coagulation (DIC)

DIC in the pregnant woman is defined as a fibrinogen level of <300 mg/100 mL, a platelet count of <100,000/mm,[3] or fibrin degradation products >40 mg/mL, with prolonged partial thromboplastin and prothrombin times. DIC can be present without obvious clinical signs. The key to management is removal of the underlying cause, aggressive blood transfusion, and replacement of clotting factors.

Four units of fresh whole blood or 8–10 units of fresh frozen plasma or 16 units of cryoprecipitate will increase the serum fibrinogen by 100 mg/dL. If the whole blood clotting time is greater than 8 minutes, if oozing from venipuncture sites is observed when the initial blood work is done, or if the fibrinogen is less than 100 mg/dL, we administer 16 units of cryoprecipitate. When DIC is present, serial testing of coagulation should be performed every 2–4 hours.

If the platelet count is <20,000/mm^3 or less than 50,000/mm^3 in a woman who is to have a cesarean section, we give 10 units of platelets. This volume of platelets will increase the platelet count by 80,000–100,000/mm^3. Because potassium is lost from banked blood cells, serum potassium levels may become dangerously elevated. The serum potassium should be checked after the woman receives 4–6 units of packed red cells. In addition, continuous maternal monitoring by electrocardiogram is highly desirable.

PLACENTA PREVIA

Placenta previa is defined as implantation of the placenta in the lower segment of the uterus, with the placenta either overlying or reaching the vicinity of the internal os of the cervix.[21] The placenta previa can be of varying degree; the common terminology is defined in Table 7.4.

In the first quarter of this century, maternal mortality was 10% and perinatal mortality 40%–80% in women with placenta previa.[21] Two major advances led to the decrease in fetal and maternal mortality. In 1927 Bill advocated liberal blood transfusions to counteract the effects of hypovolemia and urged that cesarean section be performed as a method of reducing maternal trauma and hemorrhage.[22] Adoption of this method of treatment for placenta previa reduced maternal mortality to 2% and perinatal mortality to 32%. The second major advance was made in 1945 and 1948 by MacAfee et al,[23] Johnson,[24] and Williams.[25] They demonstrated that in the absence of rectal or vaginal examination, serious bleeding could often be avoided and delivery thus postponed.

TABLE 7.4 Classification of Placenta Previa

United States	Europe	Definition
Lateral placenta previa (low-lying placenta)	Grade I	The placental edge is implanted in the lower uterine segment but does not reach the cervical os
Marginal placenta	Grade II	The placental edge just reaches the internal os
Partial placenta	Grade III	The placenta covers part of the internal cervical os
Total (complete) placenta previa	Grade IV	The placenta completely covers the internal os

Recently, aggressive use of antepartum transfusion in the presence of moderate hemorrhage in lieu of delivery, use of tocolytic agents for inhibition of preterm labor, and elective termination of pregnancy utilizing lecithin/sphingomyelin (L/S) to determine pulmonary maturation have led to further improved maternal and perinatal mortality.

Incidence

The incidence of placenta previa varies widely. Brenner et al reported an incidence of 6 per 1,000 in women beyond 20 weeks gestation. Complete placenta previa was seen in 1.2 per 1,000 patients, and partial placental previa was observed in 4.8 per 1,000 patients.[26] Placenta previa occurred in up to 1 in 20 grand multiparas but in only 1 in 1,500 nulliparas.[27] The overall incidence in the Collaborative Perinatal Project was 1 in 150 births.

In 1,098 women referred for diagnostic ultrasound at 16–18 weeks gestation for genetic indications, placenta previa was diagnosed in 58 (5.3%).[28] Only 5 of the 58 women had placenta previa at delivery. Another study reported the same 5.0% of placenta previa in women having mid-trimester genetic amniocentesis, with 90% "resolving" and never becoming symptomatic.[29] The phenomenon of "placental migration" away from the cervix and lower segment with advancing gestation has not been fully elucidated but appears to involve different rates of growth of the fundus and the lower uterine segment.

Etiology

The two most common factors associated with placenta previa are multiparity and previous cesarean delivery, the latter being associated with a sixfold increase in the incidence of placenta previa.[30,31] Both of these conditions involve damage to the endometrium and may make certain areas of the endometrium unsuitable for implantation in subsequent pregnancies. Furthermore, the risk of subsequent placenta previa appears to increase with an increasing number of previous cesareans.[31]

TABLE 7.5 Incidence of Intrauterine Growth Retardation in Women with Placenta Previa

Type of Placenta Previa	No. of Fetuses	Fetuses with IUGR	Percent of IUGR
Complete	13	6	46.1
Partial	16	4	25.0
Marginal	74	7	9.6
Total	103	17	16.5

Source: Modified from Varma TR: *J Obstet Gynecol Br Commonwealth* 80:313, 1973.

There has also been concern about the role that induced abortion may play in the subsequent development of placenta previa. Although retrospective studies have reported an association between prior abortion and placenta previa,[32,33] other epidemiologic studies have not confirmed this association.[34,35] A recent retrospective cohort study reported a sevenfold increase in subsequent placenta previa in women with induced first trimester abortion compared to women with no such history.[34] However, Grimes and Techman, in a retrospective review of 28,000 pregnancies from Grady Memorial Hospital in Atlanta, found that women with one or more legal abortions did not have an increased risk of symptomatic placenta previa in subsequent pregnancies.[35]

Women with placenta previa have been reported to have a lower incidence of pregnancy-induced hypertension (PIH) than the general population. During an 87-month period ending June 30, 1981, 51 primiparous women were managed at the City Hospital in Nottingham, England, with three (5.9%) developing PIH. During the same time period, there were 9,990 total deliveries of primiparous women, with 1,960 (19.6%) developing PIH.[36] Because maternal levels of human placental lactogen are higher in patients with placenta previa, the authors speculated that improved placental function may protect against the development of PIH. However, these findings remain unconfirmed and are complicated by the fact that over one-third of the women with placenta previa were delivered prior to 37 weeks gestation, possibly before they could develop PIH. There is an increased incidence of intrauterine growth retardation (IUGR) in women with placenta previa. Serial ultrasonography was performed on 103 women with the diagnosis of placenta previa referred to Queen Mary Hospital, London. The overall incidence of IUGR was 16.5%; however, 34.5% of the women who had partial or complete placenta previa had growth-retarded fetuses (Table 7.5).[37] In a similar study, the incidence of IUGR in 297 women with placental previa at Groote Schuur Hospital Maternity Center, Capetown, South Africa, was 17%, compared to an overall incidence of IUGR during this time period of 9.5%.[38] Such studies cast further doubt upon reports of improved placental function in patients with placenta previa.

TABLE 7.6 Mortality by Birth Weight in Women with Placenta Previa

	500–1,000 g	1,001–1,500 g	1,501–2,000 g	2,000–2,500 g	>2,500 g
Birth	20	28	32	62	175
Survivors	4	19	30	59	171
Deaths	16 (80%)	9 (32%)	2 (6%)	3 (5%)	4 (2%)
Fetal	9 (45%)	1 (4%)	1 (3%)	2 (3%)	2 (1%)
Neonatal	7 (35%)	8 (29%)	1 (3%)	1 (2%)	2 (2%)

Source: Cotton DB, Read JA, Paul RH, et al: The conservative aggressive management of placenta previa. *Am J Obstet Gynecol* 137:687, 1980; McShane PM, Heye PS, Epstein MF: Maternal and perinatal morbidity resulting from placenta previa. *Obstet Gynecol* 65:176, 1985.

The incidence of congenital anomalies is also increased in the fetuses of women with placenta previa. Green found an incidence of congenital anomalies of 6.7% in fetuses whose mother had placenta previa compared to an overall incidence of 3.2%.[19] Most series have reported a doubling of the rate of serious congenital malformations in women with placenta previa. Malformations of the cardiovascular system, central nervous system, respiratory tract, and gastrointestinal tract are most common.

Prematurity remains the major factor in the perinatal outcome of pregnancies complicated by placenta previa. In the combined series of Cotton et al[30] and McShane et al,[39] of 317 cases of placenta previa, 48 (15.1%) of the infants had birth weights of ≤1,500 g. This group accounted for 16 of the 34 perinatal deaths (47.0%). Fetal hypoxia secondary to maternal blood loss may also contribute to perinatal morbidity and mortality[40]; there is increased perinatal mortality in all birth-weight groups in women who have placenta previa compared to the control group.[41] A review of the birth certificates of upstate New York for the years 1958–1962 revealed 14,740 women with singleton pregnancies who had placenta previa. Only 15% of the excess perinatal mortality in women with placenta previa could be attributed to those women who delivered fetuses weighing <1,500 g.[40] A more than tenfold perinatal mortality rate occurred in the women who delivered fetuses weighing >2,500 g at ≥ 37 weeks gestation compared to the control group in the same category. In a combined series (Table 7.6) there was a significant decrease in all perinatal mortality in infants weighing ≥1,500 g but no further improvement as birth weight increased.

Diagnosis

Placenta previa is characterized by painless vaginal bleeding. In some women there is no obvious cause for the bleeding, whereas in others bleeding follows pelvic examination, intercourse, or the onset of labor. In the majority of cases, there are no uterine contractions or abdominal pain.

However, in 20% of the cases there is also labor with or without rupture of the membranes.

The mean gestational age at diagnosis is 32.5 weeks, with roughly a third of patients presenting prior to 30 weeks gestation, and a third presenting after 36 weeks of gestation.

Abnormal presentation is common in placenta previa. In 35% of the cases the fetus is either a breech or transverse lie. The rate of malpresentation increases to 50% at less than 36 weeks gestation.[42] When the presentation is vertex, the fetus is often high above the pelvic rim and may be difficult to palpate if the placenta is anterior.

The diagnosis of placenta previa should be made by ultrasonography rather than speculum or pelvic examination, procedures that may precipitate heavy bleeding. Ultrasonography is highly accurate but not infallible. One study published in 1980 reported a false-negative rate of 7.3% in the diagnosis of placenta previa by ultrasonography.[30] The most common reason for failure to diagnose placenta previa is failure to scan the lateral uterine wall and the region of the cervix obscured by the fetal head.[43] With today's instrumentation and experienced sonographers, such errors should be negligible. Today there are few indications for the double setup examination in the diagnosis or management of placenta previa.

Asymptomatic Placenta Previa

Women with diagnosis of placenta previa by ultrasonography in the third trimester should be told to report to the hospital if they have uterine contractions or vaginal bleeding. At 37 weeks, they should have repeat ultrasonography to confirm the continued presence of placenta previa. Amniocentesis should be performed to confirm the presence of fetal lung maturity. if fetal lung maturity is present, delivery should be accomplished by cesarean section.

We favor a low transverse uterine incision in women with posterior placenta previa or when the previa involves the lateral uterine walls. When the placenta is implanted over the anterior lower uterine segment or when the fetus is very immature and the lower uterine segment is undeveloped, we favor a vertical uterine incision. Despite such precautions, an occasional incision will be made that enters the placenta, resulting in profuse bleeding. If the edge of the placenta cannot be identified quickly and the amniotic sac entered, the operation should proceed promptly through the placenta itself. In such circumstances, the cord should be found and clamped (if possible) prior to delivery of the fetus.

Symptomatic Placenta Previa

The treatment of symptomatic placenta previa at or near term is delivery by cesarean section. A woman at ≥36 weeks gestation with symptomatic placenta previa should be delivered by cesarean section if the lung profile is mature.

In cases of bleeding placenta previa remote from term, the patient should be hospitalized. A large-bore intravenous line should be established, a blood count obtained, and the patient crossmatched for blood (4 units of packed red blood cells). Occasionally the patient may be hypovolemic and fluid resuscitation may be required. The fetus should be monitored with external continuous electronic heart rate monitoring. Ultrasonography should be performed to establish the gestational age and to detect associated fetal anomalies.

In the past, patients were categorically delivered after their second episode of hemorrhage that required transfusion, based on the fact that the third episode of bleeding was frequently severe. Today this approach should be modified in the presence of an immature fetus and cesarean section performed only if the patient has massive bleeding or if fetal distress is present. Patients with very immature fetuses in labor may receive tocolytic therapy and repeated transfusion in an effort to gain additional fetal maturity.[30,42] Any patient with significant bleeding should receive continuous fetal monitoring because of the risk of concomitant abruption or fetal distress from blood loss. There is a statistically significant correlation between the degree of maternal hemorrhage and the need for neonatal transfusion, and between neonatal anemia and the amount of intrapartum blood loss.[42]

A prospective randomized trial has recently been reported in a small number of patients at <30 weeks gestation with central placenta previa and at least two bleeding episodes requiring admission to the hospital.[44] Twelve patients had a cerclage placed under general or epidural anesthesia, using a 5-mm Mersilene band. Eleven patients were managed with bed rest in the hospital, tocolysis, and steroids. Patients in both groups were delivered if severe bleeding recurred or if amniocentesis demonstrated a mature lung profile. Pregnancy was prolonged 7.9 weeks in the cerclage group compared to 2.7 weeks in the control group. Five of the 11 fetuses of patients in the control group had significant hyaline membrane disease compared to none of the 12 fetuses of the patients who underwent cerclage. The women in the cerclage group received 42 units of blood compared to 64 units in the control group. Although these results are encouraging, independent confirmation is needed before such therapy can be recommended.

Placenta Accreta

Placenta accreta is an abnormal adherence of the placenta to the uterine wall resulting from defective formation of the decidua, with chorionic villi being in direct contact with the myometrium. In its more severe forms, the chorionic villi penetrate the myometrium (placenta increta) or the entire thickness of the uterine wall, reaching the serosa and sometimes rupturing into the peritoneal cavity (placenta percreta). The incidence of placenta accreta has been reported as 1 in 2,562 deliveries, increasing to 4% in patients with placenta previa.[45] The association of placenta previa with placenta accreta is especially likely in the presence of one or more uterine scars. In such cases, the incidence of placenta accreta may exceed 25%.[31] Although uterine conservation may be possible with focal placenta accreta, when the entire placenta is involved, the treatment is total abdominal hysterectomy.

REFERENCES

1. Golditch IM, Boyce NE: Management of abruptio placenta. *JAMA* 212:288, 1970.
2. Rigby E: *An Essay on the Uterine Haemorrhage Which Precedes the Delivery of the Full Grown Foetus: Illustrated with Cases.* London, Joseph Johnson, 1875.
3. Sexton LI, Hertin AT, Reid DE, et al: Premature separation of the normally implanted placenta. *Am J Obstet Gynecol* 59:13, 1968.
4. Niswander NR, Gordon M: *The Women and Their Pregnancies.* Philadelphia, WB Saunders Co, 1972.
5. Naeye RL: Abruptio placenta and placenta previa: Frequency, perinatal mortality and cigarette smoking. *Obstet Gynecol* 55:701, 1980.
6. Lehtovirta P, Forss M: The acute effect of smoking on intervillous blood flow of the placenta. *Br J Obstet Gynaecol* 85:729, 1978.
7. Crosby W: Trauma during pregnancy: Maternal and fetal injury. *Obstet Gynecol Surv* 29:683, 1974.
8. Crosby W, Costiloe J: Safety of lap-belt restraint for pregnant victims of automobile collisions. *N Engl J Med* 284:632, 1971.
9. Higgins SD, Garite TJ: Late abruptio placenta in trauma patients: Implications for monitoring. *Obstet Gynecol* (suppl)63:10, 1984.
10. Lavin JP, Miodovnik M: Delayed abruption after maternal trauma as a result of an automobile accident. *J Reprod Med* 12:621, 1981.
11. Abdella TN, Sibai BM, Hays JM, et al: Relationship of hypertensive disease to abruptio placenta. *Obstet Gynecol* 634:365, 1984.
12. Hibbard BM, Jeffcoate TNA: Abruptio placentae. *Obstet Gynecol* 27:155, 1966.
13. Acker D, Sachs BP, Tracey KJ: Abruptio placenta associated with cocaine use. *Am J Obstet Gynecol* 146:220, 1983.
14. Ritchie JM, Greene NM: *Local Anesthesia, Pharmacological Basis of Therapeutics,* ed 6. New York, Macmillan Co, 1980, pp 300–320.
15. Schwartz RW: Pregnancy in physicians: Characteristics and complications. *Obstet Gynecol* 66:672, 1985.
16. Zugaib M, deBarros ACSB, Bittar RE, et al: Abruptio placenta following snake bite. *Am J Obstet Gynecol* 151:754, 1985.
17. Blair RG: Abruption of placenta: A review of 189 cases occurring between 1965 and 1969. *J Obstet Gynaecol Br Commonwealth* 80:242, 1973.
18. Jaffe MH, Schoen WC, Silver TM, et al: Sonography of abruptio placentae. *Am J Roentgenol* 133:877, 1979.
19. Green JR: Placental abnormalities: Placenta previa and abruptio placenta, in Creasy RK, Resnick R (eds): *Maternal-Fetal Medicine: Principles and Practice.* Philadelphia, WB Saunders Co, 1984, pp 539–559.
20. Sher G: Trasylol in the management of abruptio placenta with consumption coagulopathy and uterine inertia. *J Reprod Med* 25:113, 1980.

21. Crenshaw C, Jones D, Parker RT: Placenta previa: A survey of twenty years experience with improved perinatal survival by expectant therapy and cesarean delivery. *Obstet Gynecol Surv* 28:461, 1927.
22. Bill AH: Treatment of placenta previa by prophylactic blood transfusion and cesarean section. *Am J Obstet Gynecol* 14:523, 1927.
23. MacAfee CHG, Millar WG, Graham H, et al: Maternal and fetal mortality in placenta previa. *J Obstet Gynaecol Br Commonwealth* 69:203, 1962.
24. Johnson HW: The conservative management of some varieties of placenta previa. *Am J Obstet Gynecol* 50:398, 1945.
25. Williams TJ: The expectant management of placenta previa. *Am J Obstet Gynecol* 55:169, 1948.
26. Brenner WE, Edelman DA, Hendricks CH: Characteristics of patient with placenta previa and results of "expectant management." *Am J Obstet Gynecol* 132:180, 1978.
27. Hibbard LT: Placenta previa, in Sciara JJ (ed): *Gynecology and Obstetrics*, vol 2. New York, Harper and Row, 1981.
28. Rizos N, Doran TA, Miskin M, et al: Natural history of placenta previa ascertained by diagnostic ultrasound. *Am J Obstet Gynecol* 133:287, 1979.
29. Wexler P, Gottesfeld KR: Early diagnosis of placenta previa. *Obstet Gynecol* 54:231, 1979.
30. Cotton DB, Read JA, Paul RH, et al: The conservative aggressive management of placenta previa. *Am J Obstet Gynecol* 137:687, 1980.
31. Clark SL, Koonings PP, Phelan JP: Placenta previa-accreta and previous cesarean section. *Obstet Gynecol* 66:89, 1985.
32. Schoenbaum SC, Monson RR, Stubblefield PG, et al: Outcome of the delivery following an induced or spontaneous abortion. *Am J Obstet Gynecol* 136:19, 1980.
33. Madore C, Hawes WE, Many F, et al: A study on the effects of induced abortion on subsequent pregnancy outcome. *Am J Obstet Gynecol* 139:516, 1981.
34. Barrett JM, Boehm RH, Killam AP: Induced abortion: A risk factor for placenta previa. *Am J Obstet Gynecol* 141:769, 1981.
35. Grimes DA, Techman T: Legal abortion and placenta previa. *Am J Obstet Gynecol* 149:501, 1984.
36. Nicolaides KH, Faratian B, Symonds EM: Effect on low implantation of the placenta on maternal blood pressure and placental function. *Br J Obstet Gynecol* 89:806, 1982.
37. Varma TR: Fetal growth and placental function in patients with placenta previa. *J Obstet Gynaecol Br Commonwealth* 80:311, 1973.
38. Dommisse J: Placenta praevia and intrauterine growth retardation. *South Afr Med J* 89:291, 1985.
39. McShane PM, Heyl PS, Epstein MF: Maternal and perinatal morbidity resulting from placenta previa. *Obstet Gynecol* 65:176, 1985.
40. Nesbitt REL Jr, Yankauer A, Schlesinger ER, et al: Investigation of perinatal mortality rates associated with placenta previa in upstate New York. *N Engl J Med* 267:381, 1962.
41. Schlesinger ER, Mazundar SM, Logrillo VM: The impact of placenta previa on survivorship of offspring to four years of age. *Am J Obstet Gynecol* 116:657, 1973.
42. Silver R, Depp R, Sabbagha RE, et al: Placenta previa: Aggressive expectant management. *Am J Obstet Gynecol* 150:15, 1984.
43. Laing FC: Placenta previa: Avoiding false-negative diagnoses. *J Clin Ultrasound* 9:109, 1981.
44. Aris F: Randomized trial on the use of cervical cerclage for the management of patients with placenta previa and significant bleeding before 30 weeks of gestation. Abstract No. 28, 7th Annual Meeting of the Society of Perinatal Obstetricians, Lake Buena Vista, Florida, February 5–7, 1987.
45. Read JA, Cotton DB, Miller FC: Placenta accreta: Changing clinical aspects and outcome. *Obstet Gynecol* 56:31, 1980.

Chapter 8

Additional Maternal and Fetal Indications

Gary D.V. Hankins, MD, and
Larry C. Gilstrap III, MD

In the preceding chapters, the common indications for abdominal delivery of the fetus have been discussed. This chapter will focus on additional indications for cesarean delivery, the majority of which are secondary to either maternal or fetal disease states. Prominent among the fetal indications for abdominal delivery are the possible acquisition of a herpes virus infection during passage through an infected birth canal, damage to an already existing congenital lesion such as hydrocephaly or a ventral wall defect, or birth trauma due to a maternal condition that can concomitantly compromise the fetus such as immune thrombocytopenic purpura. Maternal indications include the presence of a permanent cervical cerclage, mechanical obstructions of the birth canal, and malignancies involving the reproductive tract.

FETAL INDICATIONS

Herpes Simplex Virus

Because genital herpes is not a reportable disease, its exact incidence is unknown. In many areas of the United States, however, genital herpes is diagnosed more frequently than gonorrhea among women visiting private gynecologists and accounts for up to 5% of the diagnoses in women presenting to sexually transmitted disease clinics.[1] In 1979, the incidence of herpes simplex virus (HSV) infection in Rochester, Minnesota, was reported to be 128 cases per 100,000 population with an upward trend in the number of cases.[2] Infected females exceeded infected males by 50%. Moreover, these women were generally young (median age, 23 years) and in the reproductive age group. In general, these data are indicative of national trends.

During pregnancy, genital tract recovery of HSV has ranged from 0.65% to 5.7% prior to the onset of labor, with 1% as the generally accepted figure for virus recovery in asymptomatic pregnant women.[3–7] With a current birth rate of 3.6 million per year in the United States, this disease process will account for at least 36,000 abdominal deliveries per year if one uses a conservative estimate that only 1/100 women will require cesarean delivery for HSV. Depending upon the background cesarean section rate, HSV alone would account for 5%–10% of all cesarean deliveries.

Neonatal infections with HSV are relatively rare and are estimated to occur in 1/3,500 to 1/30,000 live births. The devastating nature of the neonatal infections, with up to 60% of those infected dying and 50% of the survivors having severe, permanent neurologic sequelae, has mandated an aggressive approach with regard to abdominal delivery. With intact membranes, it would appear that the fetus will rarely become infected.[7] Classically, the viral attack rate with continuous exposure of the fetus to the virus after rupture of the fetal membranes is quoted as 50%–55%. Abdominal delivery of the exposed fetus within 4 hours of membrane rupture has been shown, albeit with a limited number of patients, to reduce the frequency of neonatal infections from 55% to 7%.[6,8] Based upon these data, a recommendation was promulgated to deliver women with known or suspected active genital herpes abdominally if they presented within 4 hours of membrane rupture and to allow vaginal delivery if a longer period of time had elapsed.[6,8] The validity of this approach today must be questioned and informed consent is of paramount importance. Even with prolonged rupture of membranes, a woman with vulvar lesions has only a 1 in 3 chance of concurrent cervical virus shedding. Thus, in utero fetal exposure to HSV in many of these women would be very low and abdominal delivery might still be warranted. Balanced against such an aggressive approach towards cesarean delivery is the fact that Arvin and associates have shown that only 1.4% of women with a history of genital HSV will be shedding versus intrapartum and when shedding, 80% will have vulvar shedding only. Further, in addition to multiple reports documenting isolated deliveries of infants through the birth canal during episodes of viral shedding without subsequent neonatal infections, Prober and co-workers recently reported a series of 34 such exposed infants, none of whom became infected.[9] Based upon their data the maximal infection rate from exposure to HSV during recurrent maternal genital outbreaks or asymptomatic cervical shedding was 8%. Additionally, even with intact membranes, it would appear that the fetus can become infected during first episodes of genital herpes.[7] In the setting of ruptured membranes and suspected genital HSV infection, abdominal delivery is performed on an urgent basis, usually under general anesthesia to expedite the delivery. The type of uterine incision is determined at the time of surgery according to the usual obstetrical indications, ie, the degree of thinning of the lower uterine segment and the fetal presentation.

The fact that 50%–70% of neonatal HSV infections occur in asymptomatic women is not surprising because cervical infections are usually asymptomatic. Moreover, 1.4% to 14% of women with HSV will have asymptomatic shedding at some time during gestation. Formerly, weekly cervicovaginal cultures at 36 weeks gestation in all women with documented prior HSV infections combined with a thorough inspection of the external genital tract, as well as cultures of any other suspicious areas, was recommended. Women at risk for preterm delivery, ie, with preterm labor, a history of preterm rupture of fetal membranes, multiple gestations, or cervical cerclage placement, were recommended to have cultures instituted at each visit commencing at 32 weeks gestational age or earlier, depending on the clinical circumstances. The recent publication of several landmark papers on both primary and recurrent HSV infections during pregnancy has prompted a reevaluation of this management scheme.[7,9–11] First, the risk to the fetus/neonate is greatest when dealing with primary genital infections. In this setting negative genital tract HSV cultures should be a prerequisite for vaginal delivery. Second, reliance on weekly antenatal genital tract cultures has proved unreliable in predicting the status of viral shedding at delivery in women with recurrent episodes of HSV infections.[7] Accordingly, the Committee on Obstetrics: Maternal and Fetal Medicine of the American College of Obstetricians and Gynecologists has stated that current information does not clearly support the value of culturing asymptomatic women with histories of *recurrent* disease, however, such women with no active lesions during pregnancy should have at least one negative culture prior to vaginal delivery.[11] A subsequent ACOG Techinal Bulletin Update went on to further state that cesarean delivery cannot be justified even when no culture has been taken if no active lesions are present.[12] Accordingly, we have adopted a surveillance program in women with recurrent disease which consists of cervical and vulvar cultures at 36 weeks only followed thereafter by visual inspection for lesions and questioning for symptoms. Women at high risk for premature labor or premature rupture of membranes are followed similarly with the exception that the initial cultures are obtained at 32 weeks or timed to correspond with the onset of these complications during previous pregnancies.

IMMUNE THROMBOCYTOPENIC PURPURA

Immune thrombocytopenic purpura (ITP) is an immunologic disease state characterized by production of an IgG class of antibody directed against platelets.[13] Antibody-coated platelets are then rapidly cleared from the maternal circulation via the reticuloendothelial system, in particular by splenic macrophages. Clinically, the disease is characterized by exacerbations and remissions. During exacerbations, the patient may notice easy bruisability or bleeding from the gums. Platelet counts will be low ($<150,000/mm^3$), and on peripheral blood smears large platelets that are decreased in number are frequently seen. The increased size of the platelets will be reflected by an increase in the mean platelet volume as determined by the Coulter counter. The presence of normal to increased numbers of megakaryocytes on bone marrow biopsy confirms a consumption process as opposed to a production problem.

Pregnancy may be associated with exacerbations of ITP, and maternal platelet counts may plummet. Because the antibody involved is of the IgG class and can cross the placenta, the fetus is also at risk of developing a hemorrhagic diathesis.[14] Both fetal morbidity and fetal death during pregnancies complicated by ITP may actually occur before the onset of labor, and less than half of fetal deaths result from hemorrhage.[15]

Although standard therapeutic regimens such as steroids and splenectomy may produce a favorable response in terms of maternal platelet count and bleeding tendencies, the fetus receives little or no benefit from such treatment and fetal platelet counts often do not parallel those seen in the mother.[16–19] Moreover, the clinical utility of maternal antiplatelet antibody levels in predicting fetal involvement is controversial. Cines and colleagues found circulating antiplatelet antibody, but not platelet-associated antibody, useful in the identification of the fetus with severe thrombocytopenia.[20] However, Kelton et al found platelet-associated antibody to be the best predictor of neonatal thrombocytopenia and Scott et al found neither to be of value.[21,22] Thus, no maternal test seems to be of value in predicting the fetus at risk.

Direct assay of the fetus, in the form of fetal scalp sampling and platelet counts, has proved of value in determining the optimal route of fetal delivery. Scott and associates allow women with ITP to enter labor; once the cervix is dilated 2 to 3 cm and the fetal membranes have ruptured, fetal scalp blood sampling and a platelet count are performed.[22] To date, they have had excellent results and no untoward fetal outcomes by allowing vaginal delivery if the platelet count exceeds $50,000/mm^3$ and performing abdominal delivery for lower counts. They selected $50,000/mm^3$ as the safe level for vaginal delivery based on a literature review and their own data, which showed no serious neonatal hemorrhage at this level. With a platelet count of less than $50,000/mm^3$, however, 28% of the fetuses had serious hemorrhages. When performing the fetal scale platelet determination, we have found it useful to assay the platelet count by two independent methods. First, a visual estimate of platelets is performed from a Wright-stained scalp blood smear, followed by a platelet count utilizing a hemocytometer. The use of heparin-coated capillary tubes for scalp blood sampling can result in platelet clumping and falsely depressed values. More recently, fetal umbilical cord sampling has been used to determine the route of delivery.[23]

When undertaking an abdominal delivery in a fetus with a low platelet count, every effort must be made to prevent fetal injury.[24] This includes an adequate skin and uterine incision. If the lower uterine segment is poorly formed, with insufficient room to ensure an atraumatic delivery, a low vertical uterine incision, which can easily be extended, should be used. Cesarean delivery forceps may also be necessary in the atraumatic delivery of the fetal head. If the mother is to be exposed to the additional risk of a cesarean delivery, every effort must be made to ensure that the delivery is atraumatic for the fetus.

If the mother's platelet count is low, meticulous attention to surgical techniques and hemostasis will be required. With platelet counts below 20,000/mm^3 or with overt bleeding, platelet transfusions can be given. However, antibody will also attach to the donor platelets and hasten their clearance from the circulation. Steroids, if not previously used, will produce no measurable increase in platelets for at least a week or longer. Microfibrillar collagen may be of use in augmenting hemostasis in this setting, although data to either confirm or refute this conclusion are presently lacking. Topical thrombin can be used in areas of diffuse oozing, such as the bladder flap, and drains may also be placed in an attempt to prevent hematoma formation. Serial hematocrits should be obtained to detect hematoma formation and persistent bleeding. Broad-spectrum antibiotic coverage is instituted if an infected hematoma is suspected.

Congenital Anomalies

Operative delivery of the fetus with congenital anomalies may become necessary because of a labor dystocia and fear of maternal trauma. More frequently, operative delivery will be performed to minimize fetal trauma and deliver the newborn in the best possible condition. Antenatal sonographic evaluation[25] to define as completely as possible the magnitude of the defect(s) is of value for assembling the necessary support teams in the newborn period, as well as for parental counseling and decision making regarding the most appropriate route of delivery. The ultrasound examination can be supplemented by radiographic studies to include amniograms and computerized tomography (CT) scans if needed. Magnetic resonance imaging (MRI) may also be useful, especially in circumstances where sonography is limited by a paucity of amniotic fluid. MRI is also particularly good for visualizing fetal intracranial anatomy and fetal subcutaneous tissues.[26] Additionally, the fetus is not exposed to ionizing radiation. Amniocentesis also provides valuable information in the form of fetal karyotypes, virologic studies, fluid protein content, and a host of other data, depending upon the individual defect(s) suspected. The more data that are made available to both the physician and parents, the easier it will be to arrive at the best decision for all concerned. For example, the parents of a fetus with an isolated omphalocele might elect an aggressive

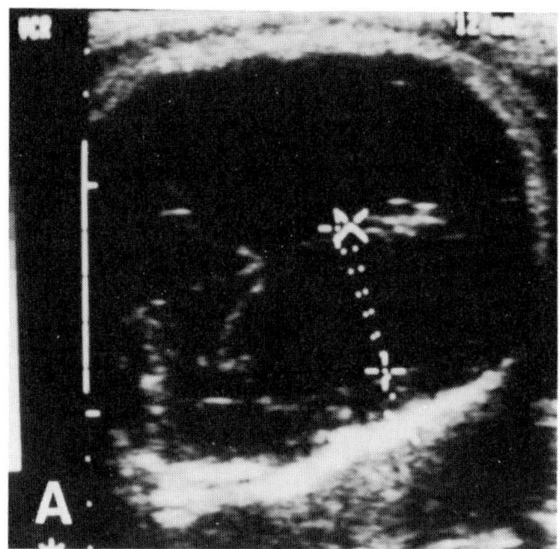

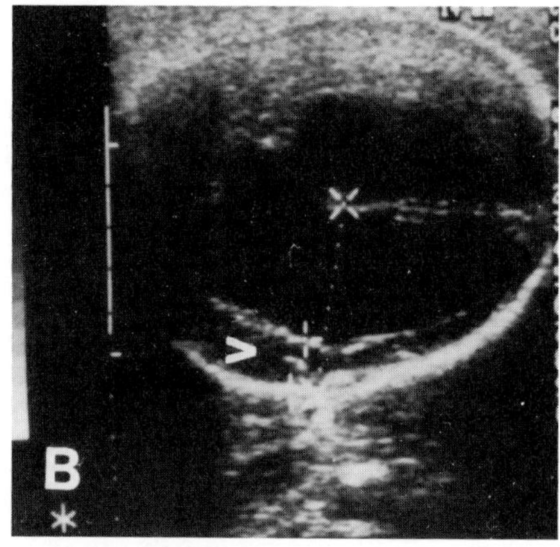

FIGURE 8.1 Sonographic diagnosis of fetal hydrocephaly. (A) Lateral ventricular wall to hemispheric width ratio (ratio = 0.73); (B) measurement of cortical thickness (13 mm).

management plan to include operative delivery and immediate surgical repair of the infant's defect. However, add to this same lesion a 47,XY + 13 karyotype, and the parents and physician may elect conservative management consisting of a vaginal delivery and a different postnatal management. The ethical and legal considerations regarding the peripartum management of such complex and emotionally charged issues do not permit ready solutions.

Hydrocephalus

Hydrocephalus occurs in approximately 1 in 2,000 pregnancies, ranging from 0.12 to 2.5 per 1,000 births.[27] Spinal bifida will complicate 25%–30% of the cases and is usually associated with a less favorable prognosis. Other factors associated with a poor outcome include (1) associated congenital anomalies, (2) absence of cerebral cortex—hydranencephaly, (3) shift of the midline—porencephaly, (4) head circumference greater than 50 cm, and (5) cortical thickness less than 10 mm.[25] The diagnosis of fetal hydrocephaly can be established with ultrasonography by determining the ratio of the lateral wall of the ventricle to the hemispheric width (Figure 8.1). Table 8.1 illustrates the normal ratios with advancing gestation. If ultrasound is unavailable, a fetogram may be helpful to confirm the presence of fetal hydrocephaly (Figure 8.2). In cases of isolated congenital hydrocephalus, the importance of the cortical thickness has recently been questioned by Lorber and others. In Lorber's series, infants with isolated hydrocephalus and a cortical thickness of less than 10 mm had an overall survival of 79%, and 82% of the survivors had intelligence quotients above 80.[28–30] The most important factor contributing to a poor prognosis was delay in treatment.[31] Survival rates and intellectual development

TABLE 8.1 Normal Values for the Lateral Ventricle to Hemispheric Width (LV/HW) Ratio at Selected Gestational Ages

Gestational Age (weeks)	LV/HW Ratio Percentile		
	10th	50th	90th
12	77	85	94
16	47	59	70
20	32	42	52
24	26	34	42
28	25	31	37
32	25	31	36
36	26	31	36
40	24	29	34

Source: Jeanty P, Romero R: Is this hydrocephaly?, in *Obstetrical Ultrasound.* New York, McGraw-Hill Book Co, 1984, p 101. Data reproduced with permission of the author.

were best in infants who received early shunting. Nonetheless, associated central nervous system anomalies, such as agenesis of the corpus callosum or cerebellum, porencephaly, and temporal lobe dysplasia, portended a dismal prognosis.[32]

Hydrocephaly with associated spina bifida is a more severe lesion and is almost always accompanied by significant physical impairment. High spinal canal lesions result in the severest loss of motor function and the lowest survival rates.[33] Severe hydrocephalus, defined as a cortical thickness of less than 15 mm in conjunction with spina bifida, is associated with only a 20%–46% survival rate and a 48%–60% rate of mental retardation. To assist the clinician with the management of these fetuses, Vintzileos and associates have proposed management and delivery plans for both isolated hydrocephaly and hydrocephaly with spina bifida. These recommendations are summarized in Figures 8.3 and 8.4.[33] To avoid the complications of prematurity, intervention should be delayed until at least 32 or preferably 34 weeks of completed gestation. This plan clearly is designed in favor of the fetus, as opposed to the mother, and entails the full support of the pediatricians and neurosurgeons for aggressive postnatal management. Moreover, the goal of surgical delivery is to avoid fetal trauma.

Ventral Wall Defects

Until recently, the majority of ventral wall defects remained undiagnosed prior to delivery. The increasingly frequent use of ultrasonography in obstetrics, and the routine maternal serum α-fetoprotein screening, will lead to the antenatal diagnosis of these lesions (Figure 8.5).[34] With increasing antenatal diagnosis, the question of the optimal route of delivery will become central to appropriate clinical management. Key considerations

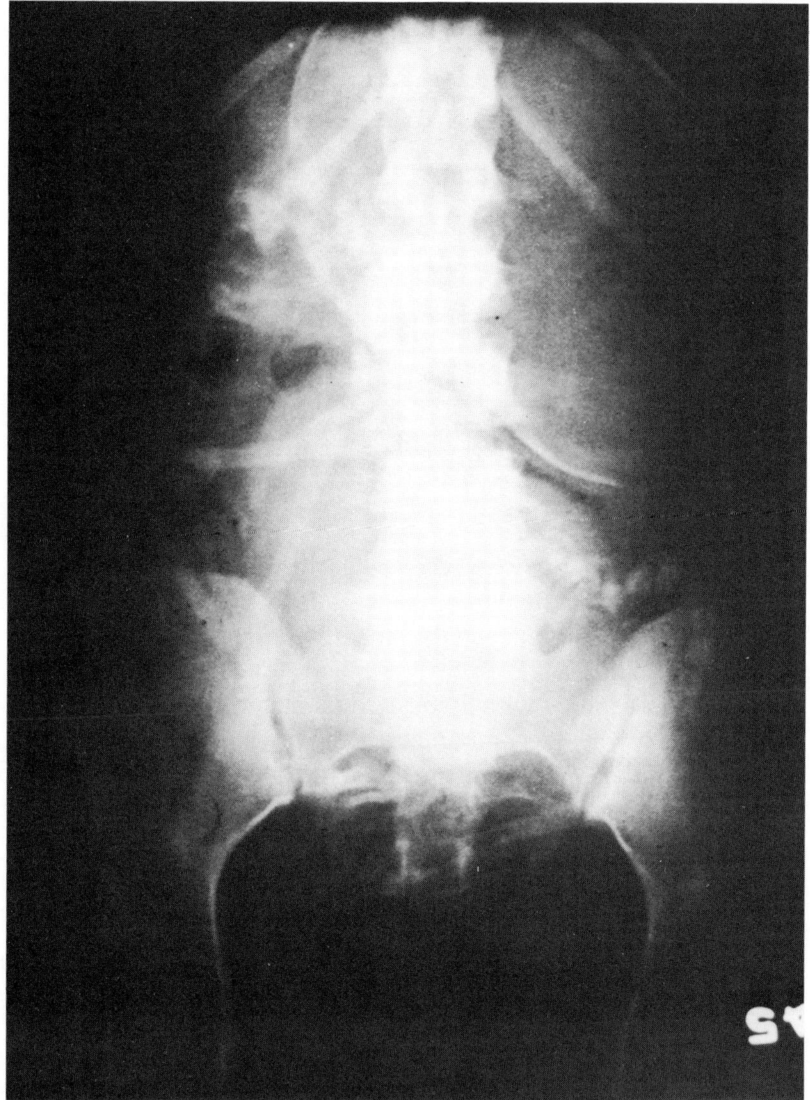

FIGURE 8.2 Fetogram illustrating a breech presentation with fetal hydrocephaly.

are the avoidance of trauma to the fetus, including contamination of the gut and abdominal contents with bacteria and subsequent infection.

Carpenter et al, in an 8-year review of ventral wall defects in the state of Maine, found that only 16% were diagnosed antenatally.[35] Gastroschisis accounted for 13 of the defects and one infant death. Only one infant with gastroschisis had additional congenital defects compared to 16 of the 25 infants who had an omphalocele. Associated defects in infants with omphaloceles included eight heart defects, four genitourinary defects, two neural tube defects, and three trisomies on karyotype. The severity of the defects is attested to by 10 neonatal deaths, 7 of which involved a

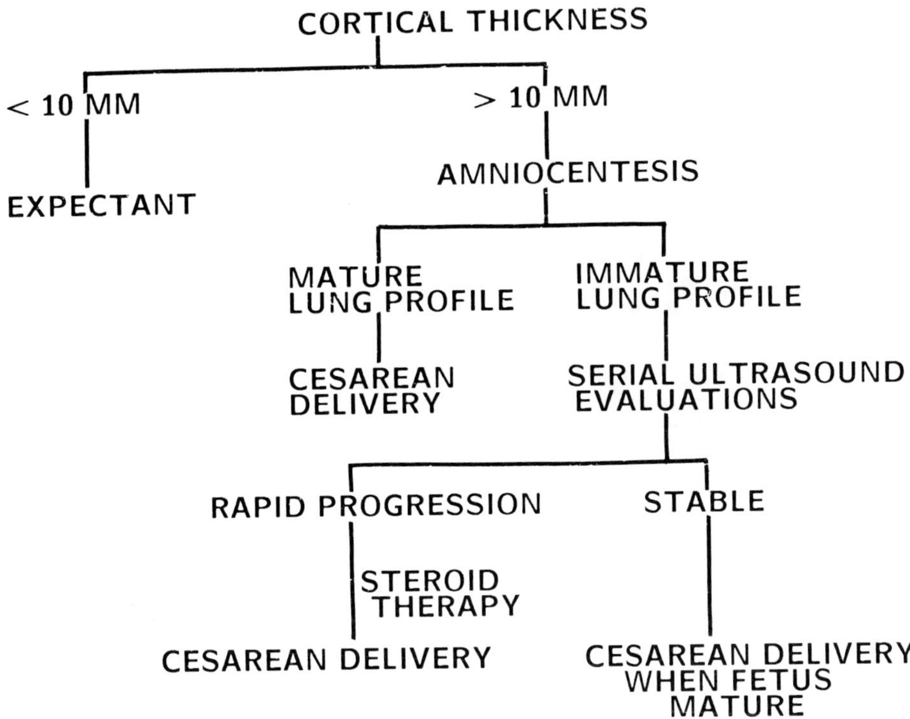

FIGURE 8.3 Management scheme for fetal hydrocephaly and associated spina bifida based on cortical thickness.

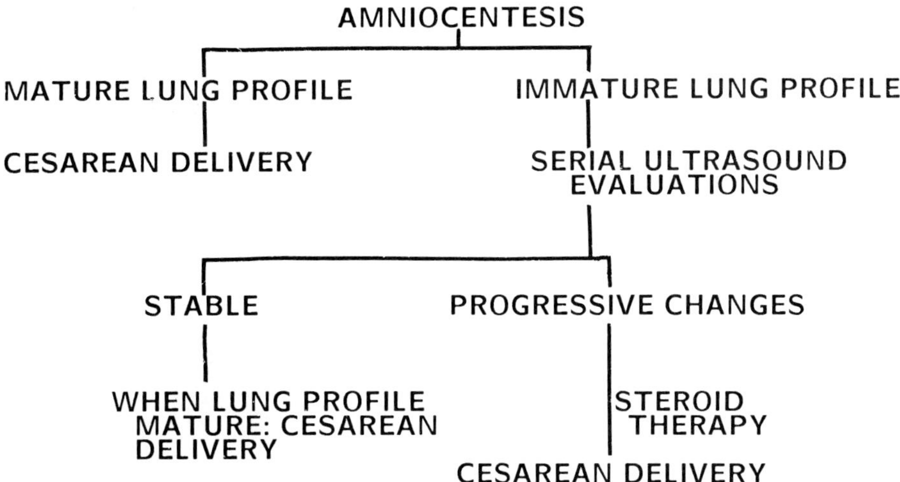

FIGURE 8.4 Management scheme of isolated idiopathic fetal hydrocephaly (L:S ratio, lecithin:sphingomyelin ratio).

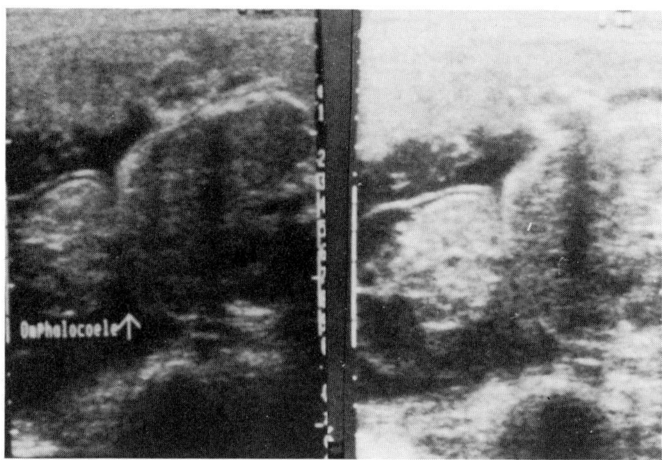

FIGURE 8.5 Ultrasound evaluation of a fetus with an omphalocele. (Note membrane around the extrophied viscera.)

cephalic fold omphalocele (which carried a 78% mortality). Of the 25 infants with an omphalocele, only 7 (28%) have had a repair and are considered to be without any significant impairment. By contrast, 92% of the infants with gastroschisis (Figure 8.6) had successful surgical repairs and 85% are without any impairment. In this series, the only instance of bowel injury occurred in the undiagnosed cases. One omphalocele sac was inadvertently ruptured during a cesarean section performed for fetal distress, and during a vaginal delivery one infant's umbilical cord was avulsed. A single infant delivered vaginally sustained intraperitoneal sepsis following surgical repair.

Despite the apparent lack of adverse effects from vaginal delivery in

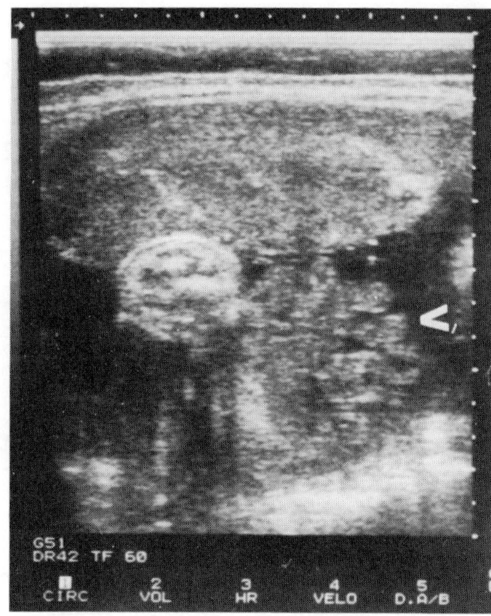

FIGURE 8.6 Ultrasound demonstrating a fetus with a gastroschisis at the arrow. (Note the absence of membrane around the extrophied viscera.)

the series reported by Carpenter and associates[35] and by Kirk and Wald,[34,36] there remain proponents of abdominal delivery.[37–39] Certainly an abdominal delivery could allow the fetus to be passed sterilely or at least less contaminated to a gowned and gloved pediatrician for immediate stabilization and preparation for initial surgical repair. If this approach is undertaken, infants with uncomplicated isolated defects would be the best candidates based on their excellent prognosis. Abnormal karyotypes or cephalic fold omphaloceles would indicate a less aggressive approach because both the short- and long-term prognoses for these fetuses are poor. Aggressive management requires more than an obstetrician and a sterile delivery atmosphere. To optimize fetal outcome, a pediatric surgeon should be available to repair the defect within a reasonable time.

MATERNAL INDICATIONS

In general, obstetrical indications, not maternal disease, will determine the route of delivery. Exceptions to this rule include, but are not limited to, permanent cervical cerclages, mechanical obstructions of the birth canal, and genital tract malignancy.

Cervical Cerclage

The presence of a permanent Schirodkar cerclage or a permanent cervicouterine cerclage that has been placed transabdominally will necessitate abdominal delivery.[40,41] A lower uterine segment transverse incision can usually be performed. Women who have had multiple attempts at cerclage placement may develop scarring in the area of the vesicouterocervical fascia, and development of the bladder flap may be difficult. When scarring is encountered, a low vertical uterine incision may be surgically necessary.

Mechanical Obstructions

Condylomata acuminata may attain such a size that the vaginal canal is physically obstructed. Alternatively, the vagina may be reduced to a rigid cylinder prone to extensive lacerations and profuse hemorrhage. Lesser degrees of condylomata acuminata are not an indication for an abdominal delivery, nor is the risk of the neonate subsequently developing laryngeal papillomatosis. Nonetheless, the patient should be advised of the potential risk of this complication.

Mechanical obstruction of the birth canal in the setting of lymphomas and Hodgkin's disease has also been an indication for abdominal delivery. Involved lymph nodes in the pelvis and vaginal side walls can attain a size of up to 7–8 cm within a brief period of time. Similarly, leiomyomata, either arising in the lower uterine segment and cervix or else pedunculated and prolapsed into the pelvis, can obstruct labor. Ovarian tumors may also mechanically obstruct vaginal delivery. Benign cystic teratomas and endometriomas are the most common.

Gynecologic Cancer

Gynecologic cancer is reported to occur once in 470 pregnancies.[42] Cervical cancer affects 1 in 664, vulvar 1 in 8,000, ovarian 1 in 9,000, and vaginal cancer 1 in 37,000 pregnancies.[43] Treatment of cervical carcinoma in situ can be deferred pending completion of the pregnancy. If microinvasive disease is suspected, however, a cone biopsy is required. Invasive cervical cancer diagnosed in the first or second trimester should be treated aggressively. Frequently, aggressive therapy results in loss of the pregnancy. If cancer is first diagnosed in the third trimester, the woman may elect to postpone treatment until there is evidence of fetal lung maturity (Chapter 9). Amniocentesis to evaluate the L:S ratio and the presence of phosphatidyl glycerol (PG) can be performed. In selected cases of documented fetal lung immaturity, steroids can be administered, with delivery in 48 hours. Because delivery is often performed before term and with an unfavorable cervix, abdominal delivery may be preferred and may be followed by surgical treatment or radiation therapy. Hacker and colleagues, in a large series of patients, found no difference in the 5-year survival rate of women treated immediately upon diagnosis in the third trimester compared to those who awaited fetal lung maturity and whose treatment was delayed for up to 8 weeks.[44] Theoretically, delivery of the fetus through an involved cervix could cause the spread of cancer during cervical dilatation.[45] Although classical cesarean delivery is advocated to avoid cutting into the tumor mass, data to support this approach are lacking.[44]

Experience with all other genital tract malignancies during pregnancy is limited and recommendations are similarly based. Ovarian cancer is generally treated, at least at the time of surgical diagnosis, no differently than if the patient were not pregnant but still desirous of fertility. Unilateral oophorectomy has often been performed if the tumor is unilateral, well encapsulated, associated with negative peritoneal cytology, and of low histologic grade.[43] Vaginal delivery is not contraindicated in these women. Similarly, women with vulvar cancer can undergo the usual surgical procedures even while pregnant and be allowed a vaginal delivery. Based upon limited experience in women with vaginal cancer, opinions favor an abdominal delivery. As in cervical cancer, treatment in the first and second trimesters should not be postponed, and in the third trimester the fetus should be delivered as soon as lung maturity is documented or induced so that maternal treatment can be instituted.

The opinions expressed in this chapter are those of the authors and not necessarily those of the United States Air Force or the Department of Defense.

REFERENCES

1. Corey L: The diagnosis and treatment of genital herpes. *JAMA* 248:1041, 1982.
2. Chuang T, Daniel WP, Perry HO, et al: Incidence and trend of herpes progenitalis: A 15-year population study. *Mayo Clin Proc* 58:436, 1983.

3. Bolognese RJ, Corson SL, Fuccilo DA, et al: Herpes virus hominis type II infection in asymptomatic pregnant women. *Obstet Gynecol* 48:507, 1976.
4. Scher J, Bottone E, Desmond E, et al: The incidence and outcome of asymptomatic herpes simplex genitalia in an obstetric population. *Am J Obstet Gynecol* 144:906, 1982.
5. Jacob AJ, Epstein J, Madden DL, et al: Genital herpes infection in pregnant women near term. *Obstet Gynecol* 63:480, 1984.
6. Nahmias A, Josey WE, Naib ZM, et al: Perinatal risk associated with maternal genital herpes simplex infection. *Am J Obstet Gynecol* 110:825, 1971.
7. Arvin AM, Hensleigh PA, Prober CG, et al: Failure of antepartum maternal cultures to predict the infant's risk of exposure to herpes simplex virus at delivery. *N Engl J Med* 315:796, 1986.
8. Amstey MS, Monif GRG: Genital herpes virus infection in pregnancy. *Obstet Gynecol* 44:394, 1974.
9. Prober CG, Sullender WM, Yasukawa LL, et al: Low risk of herpes simplex virus infections in neonates exposed to the virus at the time of vaginal delivery to mothers with recurrent genital herpes simplex virus infections. *N Engl J Med* 316:240, 1987.
10. Brown AZ, Vontver LA, Benedetti J, et al: Effects on infants of a first episode of genital herpes during pregnancy. *N Engl J Med* 317:1246, 1987.
11. ACOG Committee Statement: Perinatal herpes simplex virus infections. July, 1987.
12. ACOG Techinal Bulletin Update #102: Herpes simplex virus infections. July, 1987.
13. McMillan R: Chronic idiopathic thrombocytopenic purpura. *N Engl J Med* 304:1135, 1981.
14. Heys RF: Child bearing and idiopathic thrombocytopenic purpura. *J Obstet Gynaecol Br Commonwealth* 73:205, 1966.
15. O'Reilly RA, Taber BZ: Immunologic thrombocytopenic purpura and pregnancy. *Obstet Gynecol* 51:590, 1978.
16. Tancer ML: Idiopathic thrombocytopenic purpura and pregnancy. *Am J Obstet Gynecol* 79:148, 1960.
17. Heys RF: Steroid therapy for idiopathic thrombocytopenic purpura during pregnancy. *Obstet Gynecol* 28:532, 1966.
18. Jones RW, Asher MI, Rutherford CJ, et al: Autoimmune (idiopathic) thrombocytopenic purpura in pregnancy and the newborn. *Br J Obstet Gynaecol* 84:679, 1977.
19. Scott JR, Cruikshank DP, Kochenour NK, et al: Fetal platelet counts in the obstetric management of immunologic thrombocytopenic purpura. *Am J Obstet Gynecol* 136:495, 1980.
20. Cines DB, Dusak B, Tomaski A, et al: Immune thrombocytopenic purpura and pregnancy. *N Engl J Med* 306:826, 1982.
21. Kelton JG, Inwood MJ, Barr RM, et al: The perinatal prediction of thrombocytopenia in infants of mothers with clinically diagnosed immune thrombocytopenia. *Am J Obstet Gynecol* 144:449, 1982.
22. Scott JR, Rote NS, Cruikshank DP: Antiplatelet antibodies and platelet counts in pregnancies complicated by autoimmune thrombocytopenic purpura. *Am J Obstet Gynecol* 145:932, 1983.
23. Weiner C: Diagnostic umbilical blood sampling—initial two years experience. Abstract 37. Society of Perinatal Obstetricians, February 5–7, 1987.
24. Pritchard JA, MacDonald PC, Grant NF: Medical and surgical injuries during pregnancy and the puerperium, in *Williams Obstetrics*, ed 17. Norwalk, Conn, Appleton-Century-Crofts, Chapter 28.
25. Hobbins JC, Grannum PAT, Berkowitz RL: Ultrasound in the diagnosis of congenital anomalies. *Am J Obstet Gynecol* 134:331, 1979.
26. Lowe TW, Weinrib J, Santos-Ramos R, et al: Magnetic resonance imaging in human pregnancy. *Obstet Gynecol* 66:629, 1985.

27. Stein SC, Feldman JG, Apjel S, et al: The epidemiology of congenital hydrocephalus. A study in Brooklyn, NY, 1968–1976. *Child's Brain* 8:253, 1981.
28. Lorber J: Medical and surgical aspects in the treatment of congenital hydrocephalus. *Neuropaediatrie* 2:239, 1970.
29. Lorber J: Ethical problems in the management of myelomeningocele and hydrocephalus. The Milroy Lecture, 1975. *J Coll Physicians Lond* 10:47, 1975.
30. Lorber J: Ventriculo-cardiac shunts in the first week of life. *Dev Med Child Neurol* 20:13, 1969.
31. Lorber J: Results of treatment of myelomeningocele. *Dev Med Child Neurol* 13:279, 1971.
32. Raimond AJ, Soare P: Intellectual development in shunted hydrocephalic children. *Am J Dis Child* 127:664, 1974.
33. Vintzileos AM, Ingardia CJ, Nochimsom DJ: Congenital hydrocephalus: A review and protocol for perinatal management. *Obstet Gynecol* 62:539, 1983.
34. Wald NJ, Cuckle HS, Barlow RD, et al: Early antenatal diagnosis of exomphalos. *Lancet* 1:1368, 1980.
35. Carpenter MW, Curci MR, Dibbins AW, et al: Perinatal management of ventral wall defects. *Obstet Gynecol* 64:646, 1984.
36. Kirk EP, Wah RM: Obstetric management of the fetus with omphalocele or gastroschisis: A review and report of one hundred twelve cases. *Am J Obstet Gynecol* 146:512, 1983.
37. Leuke RR, Hatch EI: Fetal gastroschisis: A preliminary report advocating the use of cesarean section. *Obstet Gynecol* 67:395, 1986.
38. Jassani MN, Gauderer MWL, Fanaroff AA, et al: A perinatal approach to the diagnosis and management of gastrointestinal malformations. *Obstet Gynecol* 59:33, 1982.
39. Didolkar SM, Hall T, Phelan J, et al: The prenatal diagnosis and management of a hepatomphalocele. *Am J Obstet Gynecol* 141:221, 1981.
40. Benson RC, Durfee RB: Transabdominal cervicouterine cerclage during pregnancy for the treatment of cervical incompetency. *Obstet Gynecol* 25:145, 1965.
41. Olsen S, Tobiassen T: Transabdominal isthmic cerclage for the treatment of incompetent cervix. *Acta Obstet Gynecol Scand* 61:473, 1982.
42. Lutz MH, Underwood PB Jr, Rozier JC, et al: Genital malignancy in pregnancy. *Am J Obstet Gynecol* 129:536, 1977.
43. Donnegan WL: Cancer and pregnancy. *Ca* 33:194, 1983.
44. Hacker NF, Berick JS, Lagasse LD, et al: Carcinoma of the cervix associated with pregnancy. *Obstet Gynecol* 59:735, 1982.
45. Subrahmaniyam K, Pant GC, Sanyal B: Pregnancy complicated by cancer of the cervix—A study of 90 cases. *Indian J Cancer* 14:340, 1977.

Chapter 9

The Elective Cesarean
Timing of Delivery

Steven H. Golde, MD

When it becomes necessary to plan a cesarean electively, the major issue of concern to both the obstetrician and the patient is: "Is the fetus mature?" Though simple in concept, this question is complex and without a single answer. It presupposes that there is some standardized way to determine maturity and that there is general agreement on the definition of fetal maturity for all situations. Is gestational maturity required, or is fetal pulmonic maturity sufficient? How can each be measured, and with what degree of accuracy and safety? These are more than philosophic concerns because they are the source of much misunderstanding and confusion among the patient, obstetrician, and pediatrician and may form the basis of medicolegal action when outcomes are poor or costly. The preterm infant is particularly at risk for the development of hyaline membrane disease (HMD), which is responsible for 70% of early infant loss.[1] Affected infants are not only at risk for death but may also suffer permanent pulmonary damage and intellectual impairment. HMD is distinctly a process of fetal immaturity and thus is preventable if the accurate gestational date is known or accurate assessment of pulmonary status is provided. This chapter will examine these issues and provide guidelines for practical management.

The lung develops from anlage of the embryonic foregut during the fifth week of fetal life.[2] Growth of the bronchi and bronchioles proceed along with ingrowth of mesenchyme; the lung resembles a gland. No gas exchange surfaces are present during this phase.

By the 18th week, bronchiolar growth accelerates and invasion of blood vessels occurs in the surrounding mesenchyme. Terminal sacs form, lined predominantly with cuboidal epithelium. Limited gas exchange is possible but inefficient. This is the so-called cunicular phase of lung growth and lasts until about the 25th week. The terminal sacs formed by the terminal bronchioles expand, producing flattened epithelium resembling adult type I lung cells. Vascularity increases markedly during this period. By the 26th to 28th week, sufficient air sac formation has occurred to permit gas exchange in many cases. Actual alveolarization, the extreme flattening of pulmonary epithelium with bulging of lung capillaries into the air sac space, occurs near term, and remodeling continues until about the eighth year of life.

Maturation of lung support structures occurs in concert with alveolarization. This includes increasing rigidity of the chest wall, with growing muscularization and ossification of ribs. Fibrous support is also increased. Fetal chest wall compliance decreases as maturity approaches so that negative pressures can be maintained with exhalation.

Lung surfactant, detectable by the 18th week of gestation, undergoes accelerated formation by the 32nd week (80% gestation). This timing relationship holds true across most mammalian species studied. The enzymatic pathways may be stimulated by either fetal or maternal stress states. These include intrauterine growth retardation (IUGR), premature rupture of membranes (PROM), maternal hypertension, etc. A variety of endogenous hormones have been implicated; among these are glucocorticoid, prolactin, thyroid hormone, epithelial growth factor, and adrenal neuropeptides.

The role of surfactant is to lower surface tension at the air–liquid interface. This reduction allows the partially collapsed alveoli to retain a small residual volume of air, the functional residual capacity. This air volume prevents complete collapse with subsequent shunting and provides for lung inflation at lower pressures than would otherwise be possible. Surfactant is composed chiefly of phospholipid. The primary phospholipid produced is dipalmitoyl phosphatidylcholine (DPPC). Phosphotidylinositol (PI), another component of surfactant, increases in concentration and peaks at 35–36 weeks. After this PI peak, phosphatidylglycerol (PG) appears. PI apparently serves as a phosphate transfer point in the formation of PG. PG aids in the migration and dispersal of DPPC at the air–liquid interface. The appearance of surfactant components can be roughly related to the length of gestation. Approximately 50% of patients at 34 weeks gestation have lecithin:sphingomyelin (L:S) ratios of 2.0. L:S ratio maturation proceeds at an exponential rate steadily until term. PG usually does not appear until the 36th week and is always present at term in normal fetuses.

As the maturation of surfactant components, structural changes in alveolarization, and the stability of the external chest wall advance, the incidence of (RDS) steadily declines. Even at early gestation (28–30 weeks), the incidence of RDS is reportedly 50% or less. Immature levels of surfactant do not accurately predict the development of RDS because many other factors play important roles. The presence of mature surfactant levels, however, decreases this risk to almost zero. As gestation ad-

TABLE 9.1 Categories of Lung Maturation by the Lung Profile

Fully Mature		
	L/S ratio:	≥2.0
	PG present:	≥2%
Comment: These fetuses are mature and can be delivered with an extremely low risk of RDS. This includes fetuses of diabetic women.		
Transitionally Mature		
	L/S ratio:	≥2.0
	PG present:	<2%
Comment: These fetuses are generally mature and have a low risk of developing RDS unless they are a product of a diabetic pregnancy.		
Immature		
	L/S ratio:	<2.0
	PG present:	<2%
Comment: These fetuses should be considered at risk for the development of RDS.		

vances, the incidence of RDS declines precipitously. Less than a 5% risk has been observed at gestations above 34 weeks.

The rate of surfactant maturation accelerates after the 32nd week. Some pregnancies require more surfactant than others to sustain neonatal alveolar stability. This is especially true of the infant of the diabetic mother. Surfactant concentration and quality can be roughly categorized into three groups (Table 9.1).

The rate of anatomic maturation is the most important element in determining respiratory sufficiency at birth. Early lung development is thus not consistent with air breathing. Disease processes that restrict this maturation or impair sufficient formation of exchange surfaces are associated with neonatal respiratory embarrassment. Later in development, surfactants, which stabilize alveoli, become the limiting factor in maintaining pulmonary function. All of these processes, anatomic and physiologic, are linked to gestational age and the medical condition of the fetoplacental unit. Gestational age factors are usually more significant than stresses placed on the fetus, but these stresses may accelerate or retard either anatomic or biochemical maturation processes.

Is it possible to actually know gestational maturity with available obstetric techniques? Term pregnancy is defined as 37 or more weeks of completed gestation measured from the last menstrual period (LMP). In the aggregate, LMP is a reasonable estimate of the length of gestation. For the individual patient, however, inaccuracies often occur because of the fallibility of human recall, irregular cycle length, hormonal contraceptive use, and anovulatory cycles. Hertz et al[3] demonstrated that in women with early registration for obstetric care, pregnancy had to be continued to the 42nd week to fall within the 90th percentile confidence interval inclusive of a gestation at 38 weeks. Without early obstetric care, the reliability of LMP dating drastically declined. Late registrants had to be at least 46 weeks pregnant in this public service population before this degree of accuracy could be assured.

Two methods of recording ovulation events—basal body temperature recording and, more recently, luteinizing hormone peak determination kits—provide reliable clues that are potentially more precise determinants of in utero gestational age than other measures. It is rare, however, to find patients with accurate charting of these phenomena. When present, they constitute reliable evidence of gestational age and may be used to establish the actual maturity of a pregnancy.

Prenatal care should include efforts to achieve menstrual confirmation. Clinical markers include early pelvic examination, quickening, the auscultation of fetal heart tones by fetal stethoscope, and fundal growth measured by the MacDonald method. Recent policy statements by the American College of Obstetricians and Gynecologists[4] conclude that if all these factors are present and confirm the patient's dating by her regular last normal menstrual period, gestation can be reliably documented. Under such circumstances, elective cesarean in the documented nondiabetic patient may be safely performed after 38 weeks.

Surfactant may be measured by phospholipid analysis, usually performed by thin-layer chromatography, or by a variety of biophysical phenomena, depending on the natural properties of phospholipids.

Phospholipids in aqueous solutions behave much like detergents and foam when shaken. Ethanol is a competitive, nonfoaming surfactant and can be used to titrate the quantity and quality of phospholipid present in amniotic fluid. The shake test (foam stability test) is based on this principle. By titrating amniotic fluid with varying concentrations of ethanol, a semiquantification can be achieved. Commercial kits are available to perform this serial titration rapidly.[5]

Phospholipid complexes exist as membranous structures known as "lamellar bodies" in the amniotic fluid. Micron-sized small particles such as these scatter light much like a diffraction grating. This tendency to scatter light can be quantitatively assessed spectrophotometrically. The more surfactant present and the better its tendency to form lamellar bodies, the more light is scattered. Absorbance measured at 650 nm, termed the "OD650 test (or A650 test)," has proved to be a reliable index of fetal lung maturity based on these principles.[6] The test is simple to perform, and spectrophotometric equipment is available in all general clinical laboratories.

Other modalities that have been investigated rely on phase differences of fluorescent dyes dispersed throughout the lamellar body membranes.[7,8] Additional rapid methods have also been described.[9]

More recently, a sensitive immunologic test has been developed to determine the presence of PG. The slide test is highly specific for PG and will reliably detect it.[10] If it is positive (ie, if PG is detected), maturity of the surfactant system is highly likely. If the test is negative, it must be used in conjunction with another test of fetal lung maturity because other components of lung maturity may be present.

Tests of the type described above are rapid and require little investment in either time or money to be established in the standard clinical laboratory. They can be thought of as screening procedures, signifying fetal lung maturity if positive and the need for more extensive chemical investigation if negative. They have a high positive predictive value and a low false-positive rate, but all of them suffer from a moderate false-negative rate (ie, they underpredict the presence of fetal lung maturity). If these tests are negative, they should be followed with thin-layer chromatography to increase the negative predictive value.

Recent empiric observations of the association of various ultrasonic markers of advanced gestation have identified useful indices closely allied to the presence of lung maturation.[11,12] Though previous studies comparing sonographic markers of advanced gestation with L:S ratios have demonstrated discrepancies, prospective studies of neonatal outcome strongly support the use of ultrasound for this purpose.[13] An accurately measured biparietal diameter (BPD) of at least 9.2 cm carries less than a 0.5% chance of lung immaturity in nondiabetic patients undergoing cesarean section.[14] Similar relationships have been validated for femur lengths of at least 7.3 cm.[15] Curiously, the single ultrasonic variable, grade III placenta, for which published associations with mature L:S ratios exist, has demonstrated the poorest correlation with mature neonatal lung function.[16,17] The rationale behind the use of sonographic markers is based on the following arguments:

1. Amniocentesis is not without risk. Multiple studies have demonstrated the risks of this procedure, which vary from 3% to 15%. Often fetal or placental position prevents a safe tap.
2. The risk of RDS using ultrasonic markers is about the same as with the L:S ratio. This RDS risk is a function of gestational age. The more mature a fetus actually is, the less its inherent risk for HMD. This risk is about 5% at 34 weeks, dropping to 1% by 36 weeks. These figures are limited to nondiabetic patients. The risk in diabetic patients has been observed to be considerably higher.[18]
3. There is a 5% incidence of BPD of 9.2 cm at 34 weeks gestation. The actual risk of HMD with a BPD of 9.2 cm (in nondiabetic patients) is therefore the result of the risk of being 34 weeks pregnant, having a BPD of 9.2 cm (5%), and developing HMD at this gestation (also 5%). This equates with a risk of 0.25% and is close to the observed incidence found in studies addressing neonatal outcome.

Placental grading, on the other hand, is more subjective than caliper measurements. Some groups of patients exhibit accelerated placental maturation that lags behind fetal lung development. This seems particularly true in black women with hypertensive disease or in fetuses exhibiting

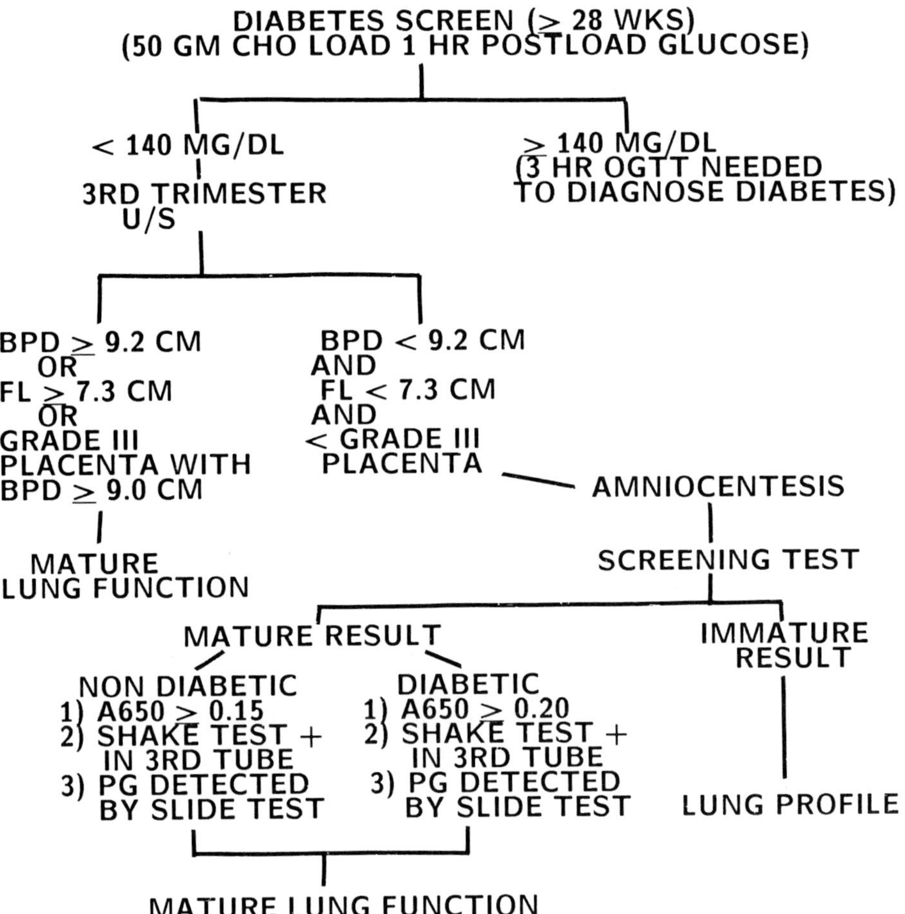

FIGURE 9.1 Flowchart of the fetal lung maturity testing sequence. OGTT, oral glucose tolerance test; U/S, ultrasound; BPD, biparietal diameter; FL, femur length; PG, phosphatidylglycerol.

growth retardation. The majority of predictive failures have occurred in this population.

A lung maturity determination protocol as outlined in this discussion has been found to be clinically useful. In brief, for nondiabetic patients, an ultrasound examination is performed initially and a search is made for any of the listed ultrasonic variables previously discussed. If any variable is mature, amniocentesis is not performed. Amniocentesis is reserved for those patients who do not meet ultrasound criteria. The amniotic fluid obtained is submitted for analysis by a battery of screening tests. For instance, the A650 test can be used and is easy to perform. If these tests indicate maturity, the testing sequence is complete. Lung profile testing should be reserved for those samples that are negative for all screening tests. Patients with diabetes are required to undergo amniocentesis. Cri-

TABLE 9.2 Criteria for Lung Maturation by Amniotic Fluid Analysis

Test	Criteria for Maturity
A650	0.150 (nondiabetics) 0.200 (diabetics)
Lumadex-FSI	Positive in 47% (nondiabetics) Positive in 50% (diabetics)
Shake test	Positive at 1:2 dilution (for all patients)
L:S ratio	2.0 (nondiabetics)
PG	(For all patients)
Amniostat	Positive (for all patients)

teria designated for diabetes are used in rapid screening tests. Table 9.2 presents the currently accepted criteria for lung maturity. If these markers fail to demonstrate lung maturity, a lung profile is performed. This sequence of testing, outlined in Figure 9.1, has eliminated the need for third trimester amniocentesis in more than 70% of patients. The need for lung profile analysis has been reduced by 85%. These savings have been achieved without sacrificing speed or accuracy of diagnosis.

In summary, elective intervention should be buttressed by the establishment of fetal pulmonary maturity. Conclusive evidence of fetal gestational maturity by multiple corroborative milestones is satisfactory but often not present. The use of other noninvasive tests such as ultrasound is satisfactory, provided carefully established guidelines are followed. Amniocentesis and analysis of amniotic fluid surfactant are necessary in a minority of cases. No fetus should be electively delivered, however, without some qualified test of maturity.

REFERENCES

1. Farrell PM, Wood RE: Epidemiology of hyaline membrane disease in the United States. *Pediatrics* 58:167, 1976.
2. Moore KL: *The Developing Human*, ed 3. Philadelphia, WB Saunders Co, 1982, pp 219–223.
3. Hertz RH, Sokol RJ, Knoke JD, et al: Clinical estimation of gestational age: Rules for avoiding preterm delivery. *Am J Obstet Gynecol* 131:395, 1978.
4. Report of a Consensus Development Conference Sponsored by the National Institute of Child Health and Human Development. Antenatal Diagnosis: II Predictors of Fetal Maturation. NIH Publication No. 79-1973. 1979.
5. Sher G, Statland BE, Freer DE, et al: Performance of the amniotic fluid foam stability-50 percent test. A bedside procedure for the prenatal detection of hyaline membrane disease. *Am J Obstet Gynecol* 134:705, 1979.
6. Sbarra AJ, Selvaraj RJ, Cetrulo CL, et al: Positive correlation of optical density at 650 nm with lecithin/sphingomyelin ratios in amniotic fluid. *Am J Obstet Gynecol* 130:788, 1978.
7. Golde SH, Vogt JF, Gabbe SG, et al: Evaluation of the FELMA microviscosimeter in predicting fetal lung maturity. *Obstet Gynecol* 54:639, 1979.

8. Golde SH, Mosley GS: A blind comparison study of the lung phospholipid profile, fluorescence microviscosimetry, and the lecithin/sphingomyelin ratio. *Am J Obstet Gynecol* 136:222, 1980.
9. Goldkrand JW, Varki AJIT, McClurg JE: Rapid prediction of pulmonary maturity by amniotic fluid lipid globule formation. *Obstet Gynecol* 50:191, 1977.
10. Garite TJ, Yabusaki KK, Moberg LJ, et al: A new rapid slide agglutination test for amniotic fluid phosphatidylglycerol: Laboratory and clinical correlation. *Am J Obstet Gynecol* 147:681, 1983.
11. Golde SH, Petrucha R, Meade KW, et al: Fetal lung maturity: The adjunctive use of ultrasound. *Am J Obstet Gynecol* 142:445, 1982.
12. Hayashi RH, Berry JL, Castillo MS: Use of ultrasound biparietal diameter in timing of repeat cesarean section. *Obstet Gynecol* 57:325, 1981.
13. Petrucha RA, Golde SH, Platt LD: The use of ultrasound in the prediction of fetal lung maturity. *Am J Obstet Gynecol* 144:931, 1983.
14. Golde SH, Platt LD: Use of ultrasound to predict fetal lung maturity in 247 consecutive elective cesarean deliveries. *J Reprod Med* 29:9, 1984.
15. Tahilrammaney MP, Golde SH, Platt LD: The use of femur length by ultrasound in the prediction of fetal lung maturity. *Am J Obstet Gynecol*, in press.
16. Quinlan R, Cruz A: Ultrasonic placental grading and fetal pulmonary maturity. *Am J Obstet Gynecol* 142:110, 1982.
17. Tabsh KMA: Correlation of real-time ultrasonic placental grading with amniotic fluid lecithin/sphingomyelin ratio. *Am J Obstet Gynecol* 145:504, 1983.
18. Mueller-Heubach E, Caritis SN, Edelstone DI, et al: Lecithin/sphingomyelin ratio in amniotic fluid and its value for the prediction of neonatal respiratory distress syndrome in pregnant diabetic women. *Am J Obstet Gynecol* 130:28, 1978.

Anesthesia for Cesarean Delivery

Chapter 10

The Uncomplicated Patient

Larry C. Gilstrap III, MD, and
Gary D.V. Hankins, MD

There has been a steady rise in the cesarean delivery rate in this country from 4%–5% two decades ago to the present rate of 20%–28%.[1] Although there is no unanimity of opinion regarding the exact cause of this increase in operative delivery in this country, there is general agreement that the four most common indications are dystocia, abnormal presentation, fetal distress, and repeat operations.[1–4] No doubt, the threat of litigation also plays some role, albeit difficult to measure, in this increasing rate of cesarean delivery.

Concomitantly with the increased rate of operative deliveries has been an increase in the number of anesthetic procedures performed in obstetric patients, creating a critical need for specially trained and qualified personnel in the field of obstetric anesthesia. Anesthesia, especially general anesthesia, for cesarean delivery still accounts for a significant proportion of the maternal mortality in this country.[5,6] Unfortunately, with the exception of large tertiary obstetric centers, there is a paucity of obstetric anesthesia services. Thus, it is of paramount importance that the practicing obstetrician have a basic understanding of the general principles and techniques of anesthesia for the pregnant woman.

GENERAL PRINCIPLES

Several principles must be kept in mind when choosing an anesthetic technique for cesarean delivery. Of central importance is that there are two "patients" involved, mother and fetus. An anesthetic technique considered ideal for one of them may be detrimental to the other. For example, although regional anesthesia generally causes less depressive effects on the neonate, it may be associated with significant complications in the mother with hematologic abnormalities induced by severe preeclampsia. On the

TABLE 10.1 Physiologic Changes in Pregnancy

Cardiovascular system	
Cardiac output	Increase
Blood volume	Increase
Heart rate	Increase
Blood pressure	Initial decrease[a]
Peripheral resistance	Decrease
Hematocrit	Decrease
Hematologic system	
Leukocytes	Increase
Fibrinogen (I)	Increase
Factors VII–X	Increase
Factor II	Slow increase
Factors XI, XIII	Decrease
Platelets	Unchanged
Prothrombin time, partial thromboplastin time	Slow decrease
Respiratory system	
Tidal volume	Increase
Vital capacity	Unchanged
Functional residual capacity	Decrease
Compliance	Unchanged
Minute ventilation	Increase
PCO_2	Decrease
HCO_3	Decrease
Renal system	
Serum creatinine	Decrease
Serum blood urea nitrogen	Decrease
Creatinine clearance	Increase
Gastrointestinal system	
Gastric emptying	Decrease
Cardiac valve competency	Decrease
Regurgitation	Increase

[a] Returns to prepregnancy levels by term.

other hand, in uncomplicated pregnancies, the mother may have less risk of an anesthetic-related death from a regional anesthetic, whereas the fetus with marginal uteroplacental reserve may be placed at increased risk by conduction anesthesia.

Another important principle to consider when choosing an appropriate anesthetic technique is the increased risk of aspiration in the obstetric patient.[5,6] The two major reasons for this are decreased gastric emptying in the pregnant woman and the fact that many women have recently eaten and are unprepared for surgery.

Many physiologic changes occurring in pregnancy are summarized in Table 10.1 and must also be taken into consideration. The most dramatic, and one of the most significant, is the increase in both plasma and red cell blood volumes, which begins early in pregnancy and continues until term.[7] The resultant increase in blood volume of approximately 1,500 mL will more than adequately compensate for the average blood loss at the time of cesarean delivery, estimated to be 1,000–1,100 mL.[8,9]

Blood pressure usually drops significantly from prepregnancy levels in the first half of pregnancy and returns to the prepregnancy level early in the third trimester. Although it is well documented that peripheral resistance decreases significantly during pregnancy, the exact mechanism of the blood pressure changes is unknown. Those providing both anesthesia and obstetrical care for the pregnant patient must be cognizant of the "supine hypotensive syndrome" associated with aorta and vena cava compression when the patient is supine. This, coupled with the hypotensive effects of various anesthetic techniques, can severely compromise uterine blood flow.

REGIONAL ANESTHESIA

Although there has been an increase in the use of regional anesthesia for cesarean delivery over the past two decades, general anesthesia is still used more frequently in most centers.[2,6,10] Regional anesthetic techniques suitable for cesarean birth in the uncomplicated patient are subarachnoid or spinal anesthesia and continuous lumbar epidural anesthesia.

Subarachnoid Block

A subarachnoid block is especially suited for cesarean delivery in the uncomplicated patient. The technique consists of injecting a local anesthetic into the subarachnoid space, utilizing a small needle (25- to 26-gauge). Tetracaine (Pontocaine), 1%, in a dose of approximately 8 mg usually provides satisfactory anesthesia for the cesarean. In very large women, up to 10 mg of tetracaine may be required to provide satisfactory anesthesia, with the goal of providing an anesthetic level of T-4 to T-8. In general, patients are more comfortable during the procedure when the anesthetic level is at T-4 (approximate nipple level). It should be noted that the 8- to 10-mg dose of tetracaine is twice the usual dose (usually 2 cc of 0.2% solution or 4 mg) utilized for subarachnoid block with vaginal delivery. With vaginal delivery, an anesthetic level of approximately T-10 is sought.

Tetracaine in the usual doses will provide anesthesia for 1.5 to 2 hours. Because of the longer duration of anesthetic effect with tetracaine, a popular alternative is 5% lidocaine (Xylocaine) in 7.5% glucose in a dose of 60–75 mg designed to achieve a T-4 block. The main advantage of 5% lidocaine is its rapid onset and relatively short duration of action. This latter characteristic may actually be a disadvantage in the technically difficult cesarean delivery. In the patient with several previous cesareans, especially with a transverse or pfannenstiel-type incision, the usual duration of lidocaine's effect, 45 minutes to 1 hour, may be insufficient.

More recently, bupivacaine (Marcaine) has gained popularity as the ideal agent for spinal anesthesia for cesarean delivery in the uncomplicated patient. The usual dose is 10–15 mg of a 0.75% solution in a hyperbaric dextrose solution. The duration of action is between 1.5 and 2 hours. With this relatively small dose of bupivacaine, very little drug enters the maternal circulation and, hence, very little reaches the fetus.

Less of the anesthetic agents used for spinal and epidural anesthesia are required to produce a given level of anesthesia in pregnant women than in the nonpregnant patient. The principal reason given for the smaller

TABLE 10.2 Complications of Subarachnoid Block

Hypotension
Spinal headaches
Total spinal block
Arachnoiditis
Meningitis
Bladder distension

dose requirement is that both the epidural and subarachnoid spaces are reduced in size because of engorgement of the peridural veins during pregnancy.

The major complications of subarachnoid block anesthesia are summarized in Table 10.2 The most common of these complications is maternal hypotension secondary to sympathetic blockade with resultant decreased intravascular volume. This hypotension may be further aggravated by aorta and vena cava compression from thc gravid uterus—the supine hypotensive syndrome. Unanimity of opinion regarding what level of blood pressure or blood pressure drop constitutes hypotension with spinal anesthesia is lacking.

It is not uncommon for the normal pregnant woman at term to have a systolic blood pressure between 90 and 100 mm Hg—a level that would be considered hypotension in many patients. Thus, it is difficult to use an absolute blood pressure level to define hypotension and, more importantly, to decide when to treat the patient. A drop in blood pressure of 15%–20% would be more clinically useful, as would signs of fetal distress appearing after injection of the anesthetic agent.

Several measures can be undertaken to reduce the incidence and severity of hypotension with spinal anesthesia. Prior to performance of the block, the patient should receive an intravenous infusion of 500–1,000 mL of balanced salt solution (dextrose free) over 20–30 minutes. Following subarachnoid block, the uterus should be displaced to the left to prevent aortic and vena cava compression. Blood pressure should be monitored every few minutes to detect hypotensive changes promptly. If significant hypotension does develop, it may be necessary to give the patient parenteral ephedrine, 10–15 mg, and to continue a balanced salt volume infusion. Some anesthesiologists may actually use ephedrine prophylactically prior to performing the block (Table 10.3).

Although vomiting with resultant aspiration is rare with a subarach-

TABLE 10.3 Prevention of Hypotension from Subarachnoid Block

Hydration	1,000 mL of balanced salt solution (sugar-free)
Left uterine	Displacement—continuous
Ephedrine	25–50 mg IM prophylactically or 10–15 mg IV if hypotension develops

TABLE 10.4 Complications of Epidural Anesthesia

Hypotension
Subarachnoid injection
Prolonged block
Intravascular injection
Epidural hematoma
Infection

noid block, it is still prudent to give the patient an antacid. It is also possible that a regional anesthetic will work only partially or not at all and that a general anesthetic may become necessary. Because small amounts of anesthetic agents are usually used with spinal anesthesia, central nervous system toxicity and resultant convulsions are rare.

Epidural Block

Peridural or epidural anesthesia is gaining popularity as the technique of choice for uncomplicated cesarean delivery. Utilizing a continuous technique via an indwelling catheter eliminates concern about the length of the operative procedure. Continuous lumbar epidural anesthesia is clearly the technique of choice in the technically difficult, but otherwise uncomplicated, cesarean.

The major disadvantage of epidural block is the large volumes of anesthetic agents required compared to spinal anesthesia. This larger amount of anesthetic agent, in turn, increases the chance of potential side effects for both mother and fetus. Complications of epidural anesthesia are summarized in Table 10.4 and mirror those of spinal anesthesia. The same precautions used to prevent and/or treat hypotension occurring with spinal anesthesia should be utilized with the peridural technique, including adequate preblock hydration, uterine displacement, and the use of ephedrine.

Inadvertent puncture of the dura usually occurs with the large-bore introducer and is usually immediately apparent prior to the injection of large amounts of anesthetic agents. However, the epidural catheter itself may puncture the dura[11] and, if unrecognized, large amounts of anesthetic agents may be injected into the subarachnoid space. This, in turn, will result in a total spinal block, which could rapidly prove fatal unless immediately and appropriately treated. Treatment consists of supporting respiration and correcting hypotension until the block wears off.

Another potentially serious complication of epidural anesthesia is the inadvertent injection of large volumes of anesthetic agents intravascularly. The epidural veins are large and engorged near term and are relatively easy to puncture with the epidural catheter.[12] The most serious effect of intravascular injection is central nervous system toxicity and resultant convulsions. The signs and symptoms of central nervous system toxicity are summarized in Table 10.5. This particular complication can usually

TABLE 10.5 Signs and Symptoms of Central Nervous System Toxicity Due to Local Anesthetic Agents

Slurred speech
Dizziness
Metallic taste in mouth
Ringing in ears
Paresthesia of mouth
Syncope
Seizures

be prevented by aspirating through the catheter prior to injection and by using a small test dose of anesthetic. The treatment of central nervous system toxicity is summarized in Table 10.6.

Hematoma formation in the epidural space resulting from epidural anesthesia is uncommon in the uncomplicated patient. However, both spinal and epidural anesthesia should be avoided in patients with defects in the coagulation system. These specific patients are discussed in more detail in Chapter 8. Fortunately, serious infection is a rare complication of epidural anesthesia.

There is no consensus of opinion as to the ideal anesthetic agent to use for epidural block. The three most commonly used agents are lidocaine, bupivacaine, and chloroprocaine (Nesacaine). Lidocaine is given in a 1%–2% concentration and has a 1- to 2-hour duration, depending upon the concentration. Bupivacaine is given in a concentration of 0.5%; the 0.75% concentration is not currently recommended for epidural anesthesia in the pregnant woman. Bupivacaine usually has a duration of 1.5–2.5 hours. Chloroprocaine is given in a 2%–3% concentration and has a 45- to 90- minute duration.

Regardless of the agent employed, patients are generally given a small test dose (1–2 mL), followed by a larger test dose several minutes later and then the full anesthetic dose. The use of epinephrine to delay systemic absorption is controversial.

Fetal Heart Rate Abnormalities

It is not uncommon to see fetal heart rate (FHR) abnormalities following the injection of a regional block. Characteristically, the FHR abnormality will be bradycardia of several minutes' duration. Although the bradycardia may be pronounced, the FHR rarely drops below 60 bpm. The etiology of this FHR abnormality is felt to be secondary to decreased uteroplacental

TABLE 10.6 Treatment of Central Nervous System Toxicity

Establish airway and support ventilation
Provide oxygen
Prevent/treat seizures—thiopental, diazepam
Correct hypotension—ephedrine, fluid, uterine displacement

blood flow, which, in turn, is probably secondary to maternal hypotension, albeit mild, due to the local anesthetic. Even more pronounced FHR bradycardia may occur with maternal seizures secondary to central nervous system toxicity. Key principles of treatment are to give the patient oxygen, turn her on her left side, correct hypotension with fluid and ephedrine, and prevent or treat seizures. Of importance is that the fetus is generally best served by conservative management, ie, no immediate delivery. If the infant is delivered immediately, it is at high risk for significant acidosis and central nervous system depression. On the other hand, if the maternal conditions leading to fetal distress (hypotension, seizures, or both) are corrected, the FHR will return to normal as the fetus is resuscitated in utero. Given time, the fetus will be born in good condition, barring any other catastrophic event.

Effects on Neonates

It is well established that the majority of drugs given to the pregnant woman cross the placenta and attain significant blood levels in the fetus and newborn. This is certainly true of the local anesthetics used for regional anesthetic techniques, especially epidural block,[13] and there has been obvious concern over the potential adverse effects on the neonate. Although some have reported neurobehavioral changes in newborns whose mothers received epidural anesthesia,[13–15] others have stated that the low doses of medication used for epidural anesthesia have minimal effects on the behavior of the newborn.[16] More importantly, the effects of these drugs on long-term outcome and neurobehavior in newborns have not been studied and are not clear. Thus, although these regional anesthetic techniques offer many advantages for use with cesarean delivery, the lowest possible effective dose should be utilized.

GENERAL ANESTHESIA

Although regional anesthesia, spinal and epidural, is the most commonly used technique for uncomplicated cesarean delivery, general anesthesia is still a frequent choice, especially for emergent cesarean delivery, in the United States. For example, Hicks et al, in a survey of 39 anesthesia training centers, reported that 43% of the patients received a general anesthetic.[17] Datta and Alper reported a similar general anesthetic rate (38%).[18] Reasons for the continued use of general anesthesia include reliability, expeditious induction, and avoidance of hypotension.[18] The major risk is pulmonary aspiration with attendant morbidity and mortality. Effects on the neonate, ie, neonatal depression, are usually minimal and uncommon, especially with the use of newer techniques and agents. It should be noted, however, that virtually all anesthetic agents cross the placenta readily and may achieve significant fetal levels.

TABLE 10.7 Balanced General Anesthesia[a]

Nitrous oxide
Oxygen
Thiopental
Succinylcholine

[a] Addition of a halogenated agent with less nitrous oxide and more oxygen is now standard procedure in many hospitals.

Nitrous Oxide

Of all the inhalational agents, nitrous oxide has been the mainstay of cesarean deliveries for many years and is the principle "anesthetic gas" in use in obstetrics today. Classically, nitrous oxide was given in combination with a fast-acting barbiturate (usually thiopental) and a muscle relaxant (usually succinylcholine) in what was frequently called "balanced general anesthesia" (Table 10.7). High concentrations of nitrous oxide (70%), along with 30% oxygen, were initially used. Recently there has been a trend toward the use of smaller nitrous oxide concentrations (50%) and higher oxygen concentrations (50%).[10] Several reasons have been given for this change in philosophy. Higher Apgar scores in newborns whose mothers received higher concentrations of oxygen (at least 50%) and lower concentrations of nitrous oxide have been reported.[19,20] Another concern has focused on the possible neurobehavioral changes associated with high (70%) nitrous oxide concentrations.[21,22]

A potential problem with the use of nitrous oxide as the sole inhalational agent for cesarean birth has been maternal awareness and recall of the operative procedure, especially with lower concentrations of nitrous oxide. For example, up to 25% of patients may experience some form of awareness when nitrous oxide is given in a concentration of 50% or less.[23–26] Even with higher concentrations (67%–70%), there may be a small percentage of patients with significant awareness of their cesarean birth.[20,24] Concern for the increased awareness associated with the use of nitrous oxide alone for cesarean delivery generated interest in finding a suitable anesthetic agent that could be given to supplement nitrous oxide. Moir reported excellent results with the addition of 0.5% halothane to 50% nitrous oxide and 50% oxygen.[20]

None of his patients who received halothane had recall or awareness as compared to 2 of 50 patients who received 70% nitrous oxide and 30% oxygen. Subsequently, others have reported ablation of recall and awareness following cesarean with the supplementation of nitrous oxide with a halogenated agent.[27–30] Thus, it is standard practice today to utilize one of the halogenated agents to supplement nitrous oxide (50%) and oxygen (50%). These potent agents have not been reported to depress the neonate and do allow for higher maternal oxygen concentrations with attendant benefit to the fetus. However, there is the potential side effect of increased bleeding in the mother, as discussed below.

TABLE 10.8 Halogenated Agents

Halothane (fluothane)
Methoxyflurane (penthrane)
Enflurane (ethrane)
Isoflurane (forane)

Halogenated Agents

These volatile anesthetics (Table 10.8) readily cross the placenta and may affect the fetus if given in sufficiently large doses. Although halothane concentrations range from 0.2% to 1.0%, low-dose regimens (0.2%–5.0%) are generally recommended. A common regimen utilizes nitrous oxide (50%), oxygen (50%), and halothane in a concentration of 0.5%.

Methoxyflurane, which was first introduced in the 1960s, has also been used to supplement nitrous oxide for cesarean delivery. However, large doses of this agent may be associated with nephrotoxicity secondary to metabolic products of this agent.[31] Thus, only small total doses and concentrations are recommended.

Enflurane has also been reported to be a satisfactory agent to supplement nitrous oxide for cesarean delivery.[32] It is very similar to halothane in its effects. Isoflurane, on the other hand, is relatively new, and there is little information in the literature regarding its efficacy and safety for cesarean delivery.

A major concern regarding the use of halogenated agents as supplements to nitrous oxide and oxygen for cesarean has been the potential for increased blood loss secondary to depressed uterine muscle contractility. There have been many reports on the in vitro depressant effect of halothane on uterine muscle contractility.[32–36] The other halogenated agents have also been reported to cause similar uterine muscle depressant effects.[35,37] With regard to the in vivo effects of halogenated agents in pregnant women undergoing cesarean, opinion is less than unanimous.

Although some studies have shown no increased risk of bleeding with halogenated agents,[20,32,38] others have reported an increased risk of hemorrhage.[10,39–42] In a recent report, Abboud and colleagues were unable to identify any increased risk of bleeding from halogenated agents in women undergoing "elective repeat cesarean delivery."[43] Gilstrap and colleagues, however, did report a significantly increased risk of bleeding in women undergoing cesarean for dystocia (failure to progress and/or cephalopelvic disproportion), breech presentation, and repeat operations.[10] The difference, when compared to the results with balanced general anesthesia without halogenated agents or to conduction anesthesia, was still significant when either repeat cesareans or breech categories were excluded. Of special note was the alarmingly high incidence of blood transfusions in women receiving a halogenated agent.[10]

One reason for disagreement in the studies concerning increased

TABLE 10.9 Prophylactic Steps for the Prevention of Aspiration

Fasting	10–12 hours prior to procedure
Antacids	20–40 minutes prior to procedure
Intubation	
Timely extubation	When protective reflexes have returned

blood loss is the various parameters used to gauge the amount of blood loss or hemorrhage. Many of the techniques used have been less than precise. In the study by Gilstrap et al, the endpoint of transfusion requirement, anemia, and predelivery to postdelivery hematocrit change were used. Another possible explanation for the difference in results is in the groups or categories of patients studied. For example, patients who are in labor and have a cesarean for dystocia may be more susceptible to the uterine relaxant effects of halogenated agents than patients who undergo an elective repeat cesarean.[10,43] The possible association of halogenated agents and postpartum hemorrhage or excessive blood loss is obviously not clear. However, the potential for such a maternal complication must be weighed against the theoretical benefit to the fetus, especially in view of the fact that fetal risks as assessed by all available and acceptable techniques are less than clear.

Aspiration Risk

Anesthesia-related deaths still account for a significant proportion of maternal mortality in both the United States and England, and aspiration plays a significant role in this mortality.[44]

There are several steps that should be followed or considered in all obstetric patients requiring anesthesia for cesarean delivery, especially general anesthesia. Aspiration prophylaxis is summarized in Table 10.9. Unfortunately, as previously mentioned, many obstetric patients do not fast prior to cesarean. Of all the prophylactic techniques listed, the one that has created the most contributions to the literature and discussion is the use of antacids. It is well established that the use of antacids will not prevent all cases of death from aspiration,[44,45] but it is the general consensus that antacids will reduce the risk of serious morbidity.[46–48] It is recommended that a clear antacid, such as sodium citrate, be utilized instead of colloidal antacids. Nevertheless, even under the best circuumstances, aspiration syndrome may occur. If it does happen, clinical management of the patient as outlined in Chapter 27 should be considered.

LOCAL ANESTHESIA

Of the various techniques available for cesarean delivery, the most infrequently used is the local block technique. Several reasons account for this situation. The first is the concern for the adequacy of anesthesia, ie, will the patient be comfortable? The availability of other techniques, general and regional, in the majority of hospitals also plays a significant role in the infrequent use of this technique. Perhaps the most important reason is that very few obstetricians are trained in this technique or have *any* experience with it, and are thus reluctant to use it. Even two decades ago, it was rare for the average resident to see local anesthesia, let alone use it.[49]

With the proven efficacy and relative safety of both inhalational and regional anesthesia, one could certainly question the need for knowledge of this technique. However, there is the rare patient in whom knowledge of this technique could be lifesaving, especially to the fetus. Such a patient would be one with obvious fetal distress and the unavailability of trained anesthesia personnel in a relatively short period of time. Local block technique would probably be less of a risk to both the mother and the fetus than a spinal block performed by the obstetrician who was also planning to do the cesarean. Local block anesthesia might also be useful in the setting of an inadequate or "patchy" regional block that was given in an emergency.

The largest recent series in which local block anesthesia was used for cesarean was that of Ranney and Stanage,[50] who reported the use of this technique in 218 patients. Their results led them to conclude that "local field block of the abdominal wall is the least complicated, most direct anesthetic technique which will provide the necessary relief from pain, yet least adversely modify the maternal–fetal physiology."[50]

Several techniques have been described for local block anesthesia for cesarean delivery.[49,50] The easiest technique for the inexperienced physician to remember is the one described by Busby.[49] The basis for this technique is a nerve block of the major branches supplying the abdominal wall, to include the 10th, 11th, and 12th intercostal nerves and the ilioinguinal and genitofemoral nerves. According to Busby, this former group of nerves can be located at a point midway between the costal margin and the iliac crest in the midaxillary line, and the latter group can be found at the level of the external inguinal ring (Figure 10.1). Amazingly, only one skin puncture is made at each of the four sites (right and left sides). At the intercostal block site, the needle is directed horizontally and injection is carried out down to the transversalis fascia, avoiding injection of the subcutaneous fat. According to the original technique, approximately 8 cc of an 0.5% lidocaine solution is injected. Probably 5–8 cc of a 1% solution would be just as efficacious. The procedure is then repeated at a 45° angle cephaloid and caudad at this one site. At the ilioinguinal and genitofemoral sites, the injection is started at a site 2–3 cm from the pubic tubercle at a 45° angle. And, finally, the skin overlying the planned incision is anesthetized by raising a "wheal."[49]

The technique described by Ranney and Stanage[50] differs from that

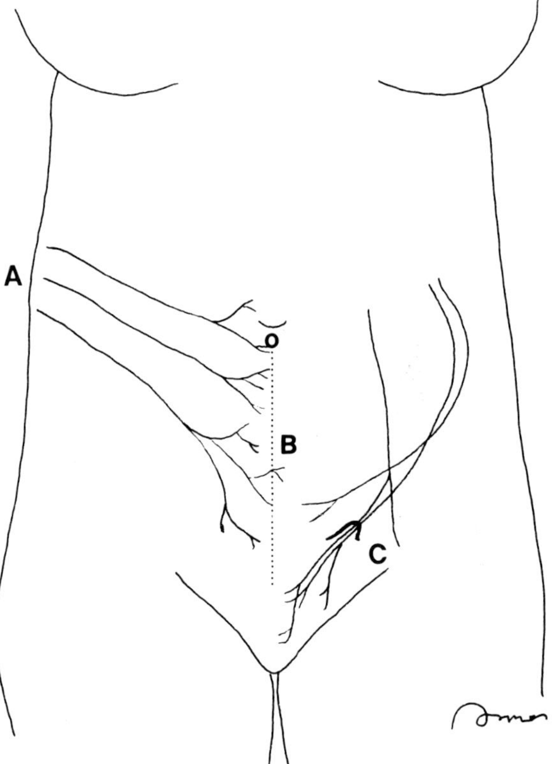

FIGURE 10.1 Local anesthetic block according to the method of Busby.[49] (A) Injection site halfway between costal margin and iliac crest in midaxillary line to block 10th, 11th, and 12th intercostal nerves. (B) Injection along line of proposed skin incision. O = injection site. (C) Injection at external inguinal ring to block genitofemoral and ilioinguinal nerves. (Drawn by M.O. Ahn, MD.)

of Busby[49] in that 12 separate puncture sites are utilized, four equally placed sites in the midline (longitudinally from just below the umbilicus to just above the symphysis) and four sites on either side of the midline (approximately 4 cm to the right and left of the umbilicus) (Figure 10.2). At each site, there are three separate injections of 1–2 cc of a 1% procaine solution—one at right angles to the skin and two at 45° angles to the right and left. The injection again is deep to the rectus fascia, and the subcutaneous fat is avoided. Attempts are also made to infiltrate the peritoneum. The bladder flap should also be infiltrated prior to incision. Great care must be taken to avoid undue tugging and pulling on the peritoneum and viscera, regardless of the technique used. The patient may require large doses of narcotic after the birth of the infant! For a more thorough description of these techniques, the reader is referred to the articles by Busby and Ranney and Stanage.[49,50]

In addition to these techniques, a different technique has been used by the authors and editors.[51] This technique is called the "diamond field block technique" (Figure 10.3) and is similar to that of Ranney and Stanage.[50] As demonstrated by Figure 10.3, five injections are required for adequate cesarean anesthesia. After abdominal field block, the procedures as outlined for anesthetizing the peritoneum and bladder flap by Ranney and Stanage should be followed.

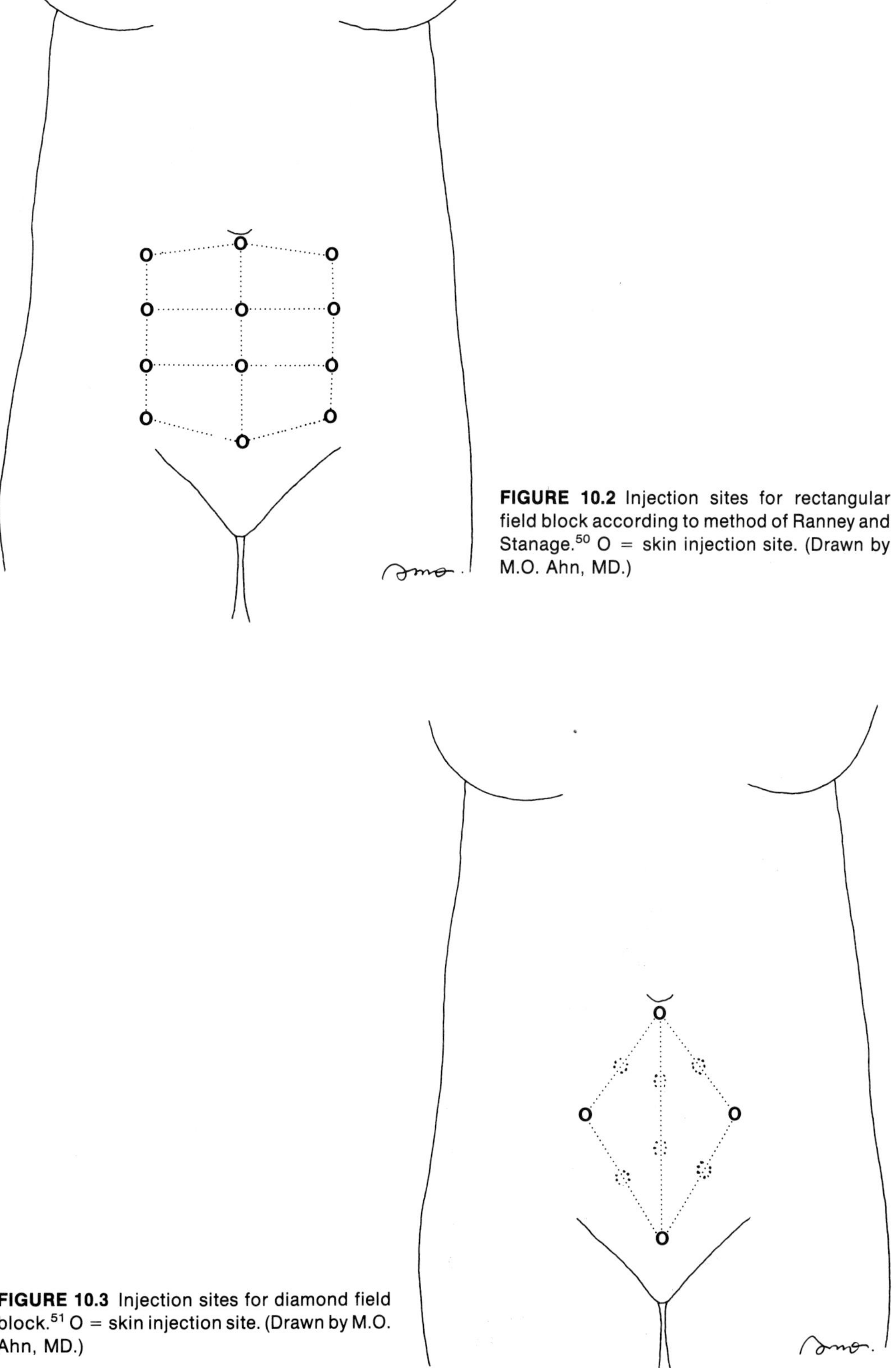

FIGURE 10.2 Injection sites for rectangular field block according to method of Ranney and Stanage.[50] O = skin injection site. (Drawn by M.O. Ahn, MD.)

FIGURE 10.3 Injection sites for diamond field block.[51] O = skin injection site. (Drawn by M.O. Ahn, MD.)

SUMMARY

The obstetrician must be familiar with the various anesthetic techniques available for cesarean delivery, especially with regard to potential complications and side effects. There is no ideal anesthetic technique for all sections, and each patient must be considered individually. General inhalation anesthesia is certainly efficacious (with minimal risk and complications) for the majority of patients undergoing cesarean delivery for the four most common indications—dystocia, repeat operation, abnormal presentation, and fetal distress. Regional block anesthesia, spinal and epidural, is efficacious for three of the four indications — dystocia, repeat surgery, and abnormal presentations. Regional techniques, however, are often not appropriate in the presence of overt signs of fetal distress because of the potential for hypotension and decreased uteroplacental blood flow. Moreover, unless a line is already in place (as in continuous epidural anesthesia), time may also play a significant limiting factor.

Local field block may have a role in the rare patient who needs an emergency cesarean at a time when there is little or no anesthesia support available.

Regardless of the technique used, all patients should be preoxygenated, have lateral displacement of the uterus, receive a preoperative dose of antacid, and be watched closely for signs of hypotension and aspiration. Anesthesia for complicated patients, as well as for uncommon indications, is covered in Chapter 11.

The opinions expressed in this chapter are those of the authors and not necessarily those of the United States Air Force or the Department of Defense.

REFERENCES

1. Gilstrap LC III, Hauth JC, Toussian S: Cesarean section: Changing incidence and indications. *Obstet Gynecol* 63:205, 1984.
2. Bottoms SF, Rosen MG, Sokol RJ: The increase in the cesarean birth rate. *N Engl J Med* 302:559, 1980.
3. Mann LI, Gallant J: Modern indications for cesarean section. *Obstet Gynecol* 135:437, 1979.
4. Hibbard CT: Changing trends in cesarean section. *Am J Obstet Gynecol* 125:798, 1976.
5. Shaw DB, Wheeler AS: Anesthesia for obstetric emergencies. *Clin Obstet Gynecol* 27:112, 1984.
6. Rubin G: Maternal death after cesarean section in Georgia. *Am J Obstet Gynecol* 139:681, 1981.
7. Chesley LC: Plasma and red cell volumes during pregnancy. *Am J Obstet Gynecol* 112:440, 1972.
8. Pritchard JA: Changes in the blood volume during pregnancy and delivery. *Anesthesiology* 26:393, 1965.
9. Ueland K: Maternal cardiovascular dynamics. VII. Intrapartum blood volume changes. *Am J Obstet Gynecol* 126:671, 1976.

10. Gilstrap LC III, Hauth JC, Hankins GDV, et al: Effect of type of anesthesia on blood loss at cesarean section. *Obstet Gynecol* 69:328, 1987.
11. Moir DD, Hesson WR: Dural puncture by an epidural catheter. *Anesthesia* 20:373, 1965.
12. Tahir AH, Adriani J, Naraghi M: Acute systemic toxicity from bupivacaine during epidural anesthesia in obstetric patients. *South Med J* 68:1377, 1975.
13. Scanlon JW, Brown WU, Weiss JB, et al: Neurobehavioral responses of newborn infants after maternal epidural anesthesia. *Anesthesiology* 40:121, 1974.
14. Standley K, Soule AB, Copans SA, et al: Local-regional anesthesia during childbirth: Effect on newborn behaviors. *Science* 186:634, 1974.
15. Rosenblatt DB, Belsey EM, Lieberman BA, et al: The influence of maternal analgesia on neonatal behavior. II. Epidural bupivacaine. *Br J Obstet Gynecol* 88:407, 1981.
16. Tronick E, Wise S, Als H, et al: Regional obstetric anesthesia and newborn behavior: Effect on the first ten days of life. *Pediatrics* 58:94, 1976.
17. Hicks JS, Levinson G, Shnider SM: Obstetric anesthesia training centers in the U.S.A.—1975. *Anesth Analg* 55:839, 1976.
18. Datta S, Alper MH: Anesthesia for cesarean section. *Anesthesiology* 55:152, 180.
19. Rorke MJ, Davey DA, Dutoit HJ: Fetal oxygenation during cesarean section. *Anesthesia* 23:585, 1968.
20. Moir DD: Anesthesia for cesarean section: An evaluation of a method using low concentrations of halothane and 50 percent of oxygen. *Br J Anaesth* 42:136, 1970.
21. Scanlon JW, Shea E, Alper MH: Neurobehavioral responses on newborn infants following general or spinal anesthesia for cesarean section. *Abstracts of Scientific Papers.* Annual Meeting, American Society of Anesthesiologists, Chicago, 1975, p 91.
22. Hodgkinson R, Bhatt M, Kim SS, et al: Neonatal neurobehavioral test following cesarean section under general and spinal anesthesia. *Am J Obstet Gynecol* 132:670, 1978.
23. Crawford JS: Anesthesia for cesarean section: A proposed method of evaluation with analysis of technique. *Br J Anaesth* 34:179, 1962.
24. Crawford JS: Awareness during operative obstetrics under general anesthesia. *Br J Anaesth* 43:179, 1971.
25. Wilson J, Turner DJ: Awareness during cesarean section under general anesthesia. *Br Med J* 1:280, 1969.
26. Abouleish E, Taylor FH: Effect of morphine-diazepam on signs of anesthesia, awareness, and dreams of patients under N_2O for cesarean section. *Anesth Analg* 55:702, 1976.
27. Crawford JS, Burton M, Davies P: Anaesthesia for section: Further refinements of a technique. *Br J Anaesth* 45:726, 1973.
28. Coleman AJ, Downing JW: Enflurane anesthesia for cesarean section. *Anesthesiology* 43:354, 1975.
29. Latto IP, Waldron BA: Anesthesia for cesarean section. *Br J Anaesth* 49:371, 1977.
30. Warren TM, Datta S, Ostheimer GW, et al: Comparison of the maternal and neonatal effects of halothane, enflurane, and isoflurane for cesarean delivery. *Anesth Analg* 62:516, 1983.
31. Mazze RI, Trudell RJ, Cousins MJ: Methoxyflurane metabolism and renal dysfunction: Clinical correlation in man. *Anesthesiology* 35:247, 1971.
32. Coleman AJ, Downing JW: Enflurane anesthesia for cesarean section. *Anesthesiology* 43:354, 1975.
33. Munson ES, Maier WR, Caton D: Effects of halothane cyclopropane and nitrous oxide on isolated human uterine muscle. *Obstet Gynaecol Br Commonwealth* 76:27, 1969.
34. Naftalin NJ, Phear WPC, Goldberg AH: Halothane and isometric contractions of isolated pregnant rat myometrium. *Anesthesiology* 42:458, 1975.

35. Munson ES, Embro WJ: Enflurane, isoflurane, and halothane and isolated human uterine muscle. *Anesthesiology* 46:11, 1977.
36. Naftalin NJ, McKay DM, Phear WPC, et al: The effects of halothane on pregnant and nonpregnant human myometrium. *Anesthesiology* 46:15, 1977.
37. Dolan WM, Eger EI, Margolis AJ: Forane increases bleeding in therapeutic suction abortion. *Anesthesiology* 36:96, 1972.
38. Galbert MW, Gardner AE: Use of halothane in a balanced technique for cesarean section. *Anesth Analg* 51:701, 1972.
39. Albert CA, Angerson G, Wallace W, et al: Flurothane for obstetric anesthesia. *Obstet Gynecol* 13:282, 1959.
40. Vasicka A, Kretchmer H: Effect of conduction and inhalational anesthesia on uterine contraction. *Am J Obstet Gynecol* 82:600, 1961.
41. Stallabrass P: Halothane and blood loss at delivery. *Acta Anaesthesiol Scand* 25:376, 1966.
42. Bosomworth P, Sikora F, Welch CM: Fetal ECG and obstetrical blood loss with halothane anesthesia. *Anesthesia* 23:140, 1962.
43. Abboud TK, Kim SH, Henriksen EH, et al: Comparative maternal neonatal effects of halothane and enflurane for cesarean section. *Acta Anaesthesiol Scand* 29:663, 1985.
44. Cohen SE: The aspiration syndrome. *Clin Obstet Gynecol* 9:235, 1982.
45. Peskett WGH: Antacids before obstetric anesthesia. *Anesthesia* 28:509, 1973.
46. Roberts RB, Shirley MA: Reducing the risk of acid aspiration during cesarean section. *Anesth Analg* 53:859, 1974.
47. Roberts RB, Shirley MA: The obstetrician's role in reducing the risk of aspiration pneumonitis. *Am J Obstet Gynecol* 124:611, 1976.
48. Gibbs CP, Schwartz DJ, Wynne JW, et al: Antacid pulmonary aspiration in the dog. *Anesthesiology* 51:380, 1979.
49. Busby T: Local anesthesia for cesarean section. *Am J Obstet Gynecol* 87:399, 1963.
50. Ranney B, Stanage WF: Advantages of local anesthesia for cesarean section. *Obstet Gynecol* 45:163, 1975.
51. Gilstrap LC, Phelan JP: Local anesthesia for cesarean delivery: The diamond field block technique (unpublished data).

Chapter 11

The High-Risk Patient

Larry C. Gilstrap III, MD, and
Gary D.V. Hankins, MD

Management of the pregnant patient with serious complications prior to delivery presents a significant challenge to both the obstetrician and the anesthesiologist. When operative delivery is required in patients with complications such as severe preeclampsia, heart disease, or diabetes, the anesthesiologist must have a thorough knowledge and understanding of how these various disease states affect the pregnant woman and her unborn child. Of paramount importance is communication and cooperation between the obstetrician and the anesthesiologist.

PREECLAMPSIA AND ECLAMPSIA

Preeclampsia is a disease state peculiar only to pregnancy. It is characterized by hypertension, proteinuria, and edema, and its primary pathophysiologic feature is widespread vasospasm. Preeclampsia can be classified as mild or severe. Pregnancy-induced hypertension (PIH) is a mild form of hypertension without the other features of preeclampsia, ie, proteinuria and edema. Eclampsia is simply the presence of seizures in a patient with preeclampsia. Chronic hypertension is hypertension in a patient that either existed prior to pregnancy or occurred prior to the 20th week of gestation. This classification of hypertension is summarized in Table 11.1.

Preeclampsia–eclampsia occurs predominantly in women pregnant for the first time (>20 weeks gestation). Others at high risk of developing preeclampsia include women with diabetes, chronic hypertension, multiple fetuses, and other chronic vascular diseases (such as systemic lupus erythematosus). Chronic hypertension is much more common in the multiparous patient, the elderly primigravida, and black women. Unlike preeclampsia, which is a pregnancy-specific event, chronic hypertension is a

TABLE 11.1 Classification of Hypertension during Pregnancy

Pregnancy-induced hypertension (PIH)
Preeclampsia
Mild
Severe
Eclampsia
Chronic hypertension

coexistent but otherwise unrelated occurrence, the primary determinants of which are age, race, and obesity.

When deciding on an anesthetic technique for cesarean delivery in patients with preeclampsia, one must consider the severity of the disease process. Mild preeclampsia is defined as a sustained systolic blood pressure of 140 mm Hg (but less than 160 mm Hg) or a diastolic blood pressure of 90 mm Hg (but less than 110 mm Hg), mild proteinuria (less than 5 g/24 hr or 1+ to 2+ on spot urine checks), and edema. PIH is defined in a similar way with regard to blood pressure changes but is not associated with proteinuria or significant edema.

Severe preeclampsia is defined as a systolic blood pressure of 160 mm Hg or greater or a diastolic blood pressure of 110 mm Hg or greater that is sustained. Other factors that would place the patient in the severe category include significant proteinuria (3+ or 4+ on a spot urine specimen or 5 g in a 24-hour urine collection), oliguria, cerebral or visual disturbances, hematologic or hepatic abnormalities, and heart failure with pulmonary edema (Table 11.2). Severe, unrelenting epigastric pain is also suggestive of worsening of the disease process.

There are significant changes in the cardiovascular system that must be considered in light of the effects of severe or long-standing preeclampsia. Of these, the most significant is the change in blood volume, which in the normal, nonpreeclamptic patient has been shown to increase to 50% above nonpregnant values.[1] In the patient with preeclampsia, especially severe preeclampsia, or eclampsia, however, the blood volume is decreased and approaches that of the nonpregnant state.[2]

Other changes in cardiovascular parameters, such as cardiac output, systemic vascular resistance, pulmonary capillary wedge pressure, and left ventricular stroke work index, depend on the point in the disease at which

TABLE 11.2 Clinical Features of Severe Preeclampsia

Hypertension—blood pressure ≥160/110 mm Hg
Proteinuria—3+ to 4+ on spot or ≥5 g per 24 hr
Cerebral/visual disturbance—headache, scotomata, blurred vision
Hematologic abnormalities—thrombocytopenia, anemia, hemoconcentration
Hepatic abnormalities—elevated serum glutamic oxaloacetic transaminase (SGOT), bilirubin
Renal abnormalities—oliguria (<500 cc per 24 hr), elevated blood urea nitrogen, creatinine, decreased creatinine clearance
Heart failure/pulmonary edema

these factors are monitored or the therapeutic manipulations that have been performed.[3] For example, Cotton et al,[4] as well as Groenendijk, et al,[5] reported that women with preeclampsia prior to the initiation of therapy had normal pulmonary capillary wedge pressures, high systemic vascular resistance, and essentially normal cardiac output. Both Benedetti and colleagues[6] and Hankins and associates[3] reported similar findings in women who had received magnesium sulfate and/or hydralazine therapy, with the exception of lower peripheral vascular resistance. The 13 patients managed by Phelan and Yurth[7] and Rafferty and Berkowitz[8] received vigorous fluid therapy and had the lowest vascular resistance and highest cardiac outputs reported. Other conditions, such as heart disease, chronic hypertension, and diabetes, as well as loss of vascular tone secondary to sympathetic blockade from conduction anesthesia, can also alter the cardiovascular changes associated with preeclampsia and eclampsia.[3]

Although hematologic abnormalities may certainly occur in patients with severe preeclampsia and eclampsia, notably thrombocytopenia and hemolytic anemia, overt disseminated intravascular coagulation (DIC) occurs only rarely.[9]

Anesthesia for Mild Preeclampsia/PIH

For the patients with mild forms of preeclampsia or PIH, either regional or general techniques are probably satisfactory, provided that there are no signs of significant hypovolemia and adequately trained anesthesiologists are available for such techniques. If there is any question about the severity of the disease, balanced general anesthesia is probably safer and preferable.

Anesthesia for Severe Preeclampsia and Eclampsia

As previously mentioned, patients with severe preeclampsia or eclampsia generally have a decreased blood volume similar to that of the nonpregnant woman.[2] The vascular tree is contracted but not underfilled. The contracted vascular tree, if dilated by conduction anesthesia and sympathetic blockade, must be filled with volume infusion of crystalloid solution to avoid hypotension and impairment of uteroplacental and maternal renal blood flow. Once delivered, the conduction anesthetic will be allowed to dissipate, and the preeclamptic woman may again develop severe vasospasm and hypertension. If the volume load required for the anesthetic has been excessive, the vascular tree may be relatively overfilled, with the subsequent development of pulmonary edema. In spite of these concerns, many investigators advocate the use of conduction techniques, primarily epidural block, for both analgesia and anesthesia in patients with severe preeclampsia and eclampsia in an attempt to control both pain and blood pressure.[10–16] Moveover, epidural block has been reported to actually increase uteroplacental blood flow.[15,17] Others (including the authors of this chapter) believe that the inherent risks of conduction anesthesia for either analgesia or anesthesia for cesarean delivery in the patient with severe preeclampsia or eclampsia outweigh the potential benefits. If conduction anesthesia is employed in these patients, extra caution is required to avoid or detect and promptly treat hypotension.

General anesthesia for cesarean delivery is also not without some risks to the woman with severe preeclampsia. The major risk is during intubation and extubation, when the blood pressure may show a transient but significant increase secondary to sympathetic stimulation.[18–20] Moreover, Hodgkinson et al[20] reported increases in pulmonary arterial pressure, pulmonary capillary wedge pressure, central venous pressure, and mean arterial pressure during both intubation and extubation in women with preeclampsia. Although theoretically this pressure response to endotracheal intubation may increase the risk of cerebral hemorrhage and/or edema, cardiac failure, and pulmonary edema, there is little documentation of this risk in the literature. Moreover, there is evidence that the hypertensive response to intubation can be dampened by appropriately administered antihypertensive agents such as nitroglycerin.[19,21] And finally, in a series of 245 cases of eclampsia, Pritchard and associates[22] confirmed the efficacy and safety of general anesthesia for women who required cesarean delivery. There were no cases of cerebral hemorrhage, pulmonary edema, or mortality in any of the patients from anesthetic complications. The technique utilized for patients requiring cesarean delivery in their series consisted of thiopental, succinylcholine, nitrous oxide, and oxygen.[22] Today most physicians would probably add a halogenated agent to the above regimen in an attempt to decrease the concentration of nitrous oxide and increase that of inspired oxygen.

Preoxygenation is especially important in these patients, as are left uterine displacement and preinduction antacids. Fluids should be kept at a minimum during surgery; however, close attention should be paid to blood loss. Many patients with severe preeclampsia cannot tolerate the normal 700- to 1,000-cc blood loss associated with cesarean section, and consideration should be given to earlier transfusion if blood loss is excessive. With regard to transfusion, immediate attention should be given to the patient with severe preeclampsia who becomes either normotensive or hypotensive during surgery, regardless of the estimated blood loss.

Chronic Hypertension

Patients with chronic hypertension and without evidence of superimposed preeclampsia can receive epidural or general anesthesia for cesarean delivery. With regard to epidural anesthesia, care must be taken to avoid significant hypotension, and, with general anesthesia, antihypertensive drugs such as nitroglycerin may be necessary to prevent significant blood pressure elevation from endotracheal intubation.

DIABETES

Diabetes mellitus is one of the most common medical complications of pregnancy. Fortunately, with recent advances in both perinatal and neonatal medicine, both maternal and neonatal mortality and morbidity have been significantly decreased. Cesarean is the most common method of delivery in pregnant women with insulin-dependent diabetes. The cesarean birth rate for diabetic women ranges from 55% to 81% in several series.[23–25] Thus, as with patients with preeclampsia, the obstetrician and anesthesiologist must communicate and cooperate in the management of the pregnant patient with insulin-dependent diabetes who requires a cesarean delivery.

Non-Insulin-Dependent Diabetes

Pregnant women who have gestational diabetes and who do not require insulin may receive either regional (spinal or epidural) or general anesthesia. However, when regional techniques are used, non-glucose-containing fluids should be utilized for preloading. The use of glucose-containing fluids can significantly raise the maternal glucose level and thus increase the risk of neonatal hypoglycemia.[26]

Insulin-Dependent Diabetes

In the ideal situation where the patient has had good prenatal care, the woman with insulin-dependent diabetes will have good control over blood sugar and will not have significant metabolic derangements prior to cesarean delivery. When a cesarean is planned, it should be scheduled as the first case in the morning and the usual morning dose of insulin should be withheld. Two intravenous lines are ideal—one for hydration with non-glucose-containing electrolyte solutions and one for glucose infusion. The glucose solution should not be given at a rate of more than 125–150 cc/hr. As previously mentioned, rapid infusion with glucose-containing fluid may raise the maternal blood sugar significantly.[26] Blood glucose should be monitored during prolonged surgery. If insulin is needed, small doses of regular insulin (rapid onset and short duration) can be given intravenously. If the patient is in poor metabolic control, appropriate therapy (ie, insulin, electrolyte solutions, potassium, or glucose) should be instituted and the patient brought under reasonable control prior to beginning anesthesia for the cesarean delivery.

Either regional or general anesthesia is acceptable for cesarean delivery in most diabetic women. An exception would occur in the diabetic

TABLE 11.3 Suggested Sliding Scale for Postcesarean Insulin Injection in the Diabetic Mother

Serum Glucose[a]	Regular Insulin (units)[b]
150	0
150–200	2
200–250	4
250–300	6
300–350	8
>350	Consider insulin infusion pump

[a] Checked every 4 hours.
[b] Given subcutaneously.

patient with fetal distress, in which case a general anesthetic would be preferable. It has been reported that diabetic mothers who received spinal anesthesia had infants with lower Apgar scores compared to those whose mothers received general anesthesia.[27] More recent evidence indicates that spinal anesthesia does not cause increased problems in the newborn if meticulous attention is paid to strict control of maternal sugar and the avoidance of hypotension.[28] If regional anesthetic techniques are chosen, prehydration with a nondextrose solution should be carried out and hypotension promptly treated if it occurs. Gibbs and associates have reported on the prevention of severe hypotension during regional anesthesia via hydration with 30 mL per kilogram of body weight of Ringer's lactate.[29]

For general anesthesia, a balanced technique utilizing nitrous oxide, oxygen, and halothane is usually satisfactory. As with all patients undergoing cesarean section, antacids should be given preoperatively to prevent aspiration.

Following delivery, close attention should be paid to insulin and glucose requirements. Since the half-life of human placental lactogen is only 20–30 minutes, many patients will not require large doses of insulin immediately after surgery or for the first few days postpartum. In fact, if long-acting insulin has been given on the morning of surgery, the patient must be watched closely for the development of hypoglycemia. A glucose infusion should continue during the immediate postpartum period, and regular insulin, in small doses, can be given according to a sliding scale if necessary (Table 11.3). It is probably safer to have the patient a little on the high side with regard to blood sugar than to have severe hypoglycemia. When the patient is able to tolerate oral feedings, she can resume long-acting insulin, beginning with one-third to one-half of the predelivery dose and adjusting as needed. Preparation for cesarean in the pregnant woman with diabetes is summarized in Table 11.4.

HEART DISEASE

The changes in the cardiovascular system during pregnancy have been described in Chapter 10. These changes, especially the increase in blood

TABLE 11.4 Protocol for Cesarean Delivery in the Diabetic Patient

First case in A.M.
Hold A.M. insulin
Two intravenous lines
Balanced electrolyte solution (for hydration)
Glucose-containing solution (125–150 cc/hr)
Preoperative antacids
Blood glucose and electrolytes prior to surgery
Regular insulin (5–10 units) IV as needed
Anesthesia
Regional[a]—spinal or epidural
General—nitrous oxide, oxygen, halogenated agent
Left lateral uterine displacement

[a] Unless significant maternal complications or fetal distress occur.

volume, can adversely affect pregnant women with significant heart disease. Thus, in general, women with heart disease are at increased risk of complications during pregnancy. Fortunately, the majority of such women tolerate pregnancy and delivery satisfactorily.

The incidence of heart disease in pregnancy has decreased from the early 1940s and 1950s and occurs in approximately 1% of pregnant women today.[30] Although there has been a decline in rheumatic fever in this country,[31] rheumatic heart disease is still the most common form of heart disease encountered in pregnancy. The incidence of congenital heart disease in pregnancy has increased over the past few decades,[32] however, secondary to improvement in medical and surgical therapy of these lesions.

There is no ideal anesthetic technique for pregnant women, and each must be individualized with special attention to both the patient's functional classification (New York Heart Association) and the actual anatomical defect present. Although the functional classification is helpful in predicting pregnancy tolerance, both functional capacity and the specific anatomical lesion are better predictors of anesthetic tolerance. For example, a pregnant woman with aortic stenosis may have only mild symptoms (class II) but may develop severe symptoms if significant hypotension occurs secondary to a regional anesthetic. The New York Heart Association's classification is based upon physical limitations and is summarized in Table 11.5. Class I patients have few, if any, symptoms, whereas patients with class IV disease experience symptoms at rest. General management should strive to decrease hemodynamic stress, and includes the prevention or treatment of hypotension and hypertension, supplemental oxygen, and meticulous fluid management in an attempt to prevent cardiac decompensation. Antibiotic prophylaxis for endocarditis (Table 11.6)

TABLE 11.5 Classification of Heart Disease According to Physical Restriction[a]

Class I	Asymptomatic
Class II	Symptomatic with exertion
Class III	Symptomatic with normal activities
Class IV	Symptomatic at rest

[a] New York Heart Association.

TABLE 11.6 Current Recommendations for the Prevention of Bacterial Endocarditis in Patients Undergoing Cesarean Delivery

Regimen 1[a]
Aqueous Penicillin G, 2 million units IV or IM, or ampicillin, 1–2 g IV or IM
plus
Gentamicin, 1.5 mg/kg IV or IM
This regimen is given 30–60 minutes before delivery and is repeated every 8 hours for 2 additional doses

Regimen 2[a]—penicillin-allergic patients
Vancomycin, 1 g IV over 60 minutes
plus
Gentamicin, 1.5 mg/kg IV or IM
This regimen is repeated in 12 hours

[a] These doses may need to be modified in patients with compromised renal function or in the event of obstetrical complications.

Source: Kaplan EL, Bisno A, Facklam R, et al: Prevention of bacterial endocarditis. *Circulation* 56:139A, 1977.

should be considered for patients with significant valvular lesions and ventricular septal defects. Specific cardiac conditions that place the patient at significant risk are listed in Table 11.7 and are individually discussed below.

Mitral Stenosis

With modern surgical techniques, pregnant women with severe mitral stenosis are uncommon. Pregnant women with moderate or severe stenosis are at increased risk from both hypotension and fluid overload. Thus preloading with balanced salt solutions prior to regional anesthesia may place these women at increased risk of pulmonary edema. Conversely, if hypotension does develop, it could cause significant deleterious effects. Although there is no unanimity of opinion, balanced general anesthesia may be safer in patients with class III or IV mitral disease when cesarean delivery is necessary unless invasive cardiac monitoring is readily available. Clark and associates recently reported detailed intrapartum data obtained via invasive monitoring in eight women with class III or IV mitral disease.[32] Spinal anesthesia should probably be avoided because of the increased risk of hypotension. Pregnant women who have atrial fibrillation of recent onset are at increased risk of mortality,[30,34] and cardioversion is recommended.[30]

TABLE 11.7 High-Risk Cardiac Conditions during Pregnancy

Mitral stenosis—New York Heart Association classes III and IV
Mitral stenosis and atrial fibrillation
Aortic stenosis
Artificial heart valves
Tetralogy of Fallot—uncorrected
Eisenmenger's syndrome
Pulmonary hypertension
Myocardial infarction

Aortic Stenosis

Fortunately, this is a rare lesion in pregnant women. Because of the risk of hypotension and hypovolemia secondary to sympathetic blockade from regional anesthesia, balanced general anesthesia is probably the safest anesthetic technique for cesarean delivery. One of the largest reviews of aortic stenosis in pregnancy was provided by Arias and Pineda.[35]

Septal Defects

The initial physiology with either ventricular or atrial septal defects is a left-to-right shunt. Most women with these entities have small lesions and tolerate pregnancy well. Either epidural or general anesthesia is appropriate for pregnant women with small lesions and left-to-right shunts who require a cesarean delivery. Women with long-standing lesions may develop life-threatening pulmonary hypertension and right ventricular failure. When pulmonary hypertension is severe enough to result in shunt reversal, the maternal mortality is tremendously increased.[36] The ideal anesthetic technique for these patients is unclear. Significant hypotension, however, should obviously be avoided, because in acute cases it can result in cardiovascular collapse.

Tetralogy of Fallot

Uncorrected tetralogy of Fallot is an uncommon condition in pregnancy. It is a congenital heart problem characterized by a ventricular septal defect with right-to-left shunting, pulmonary artery stenosis or outflow tract obstruction, right ventricular hypertrophy, and an overriding aorta. The risk of mortality is increased during pregnancy.[30] If cesarean delivery is required, balanced general anesthesia or epidural narcotic administration is preferred. Hypotension, which can be associated with standard conduction anesthesia, may be quite detrimental to these patients.

Eisenmenger's Syndrome and Primary Pulmonary Hypertension

Both of these conditions significantly increase the mortality risk for pregnant women.[36,37] Both are also characterized by markedly increased pulmonary vascular resistance. Because diminished venous return is especially dangerous in these patients, hypotension and hypovolemia should be avoided. Although conduction anesthesia has been used without adverse sequelae in patients with pulmonary hypertension,[38] general anesthesia may be safer for a cesarean delivery. Epidural narcotic administration has been reported in such patients and may represent the ideal anesthetic agent for the complicated cardiac patient.[39]

Prosthetic Valves

It has been amply documented that women with cardiac valve replacement can undergo successful pregnancies.[40] Because the majority of these women are on anticoagulant therapy, spinal and epidural anesthesia are contraindicated. Thus, general anesthesia is usually the method of choice for operative delivery in these patients.

Myocardial Infarction

There is little detailed information in the literature regarding the management of pregnant women with recent myocardial infarction, especially with regard to anesthesia for cesarean delivery. However, Hankins and colleagues recently reported on the use of epidural anesthesia in two women with myocardial infarction during pregnancy who delivered vaginally.[41] In both of these patients, extensive hemodynamic monitoring was carried out. Epidural anesthesia, as well as general anesthesia, would probably be satisfactory if cesarean delivery were necessary and time permitted their judicious institution.

Antibiotic Prophylaxis

Antibiotic prophylaxis should be utilized in pregnant women with valvular heart lesions, septal defects, or a history of endocarditis who undergo cesarean delivery. Ampicillin (or Penicillin G), in combination with an aminoglycoside (gentamicin or tobramycin), is sufficient to cover most patients. For women who are allergic to penicillin, vancomycin can be utilized.[42] The use of antibiotic prophylaxis in women with mitral valve prolapse is controversial and not yet settled. The risk of prophylaxis, however, would appear to be minimal.

OTHER CONDITIONS

Asthma

Pregnant women with well-controlled asthma who require a cesarean may receive either regional anesthesia (spinal or epidural) or balanced general anesthesia. If regional anesthesia is chosen, great care must be taken to avoid excessive traction on the peritoneum and abdominal and pelvic viscera in order to minimize the risk of nausea and vomiting. Patients with asthma may experience increasing symptoms during surgery under regional blockade.[43,44]

With general anesthesia, there is controversy regarding the best agent for induction of anesthesia and for muscle relaxation.[44] The usual doses of thiopental may contribute to bronchospasm during intubation;[45] for this reason, some have advocated the use of ketamine.[46,47] Succinylcholine may also cause bronchospasm, and pancuronium has been suggested as a suitable alternative.[44,48]

When general anesthesia is used, nitrous oxide and oxygen are usually supplemented with halothane. Halothane causes little or no bronchial irritation[49] and may actually cause bronchial relaxation. Although ether was formerly used because of its bronchodilatation effect, low concentrations are actually quite irritating to the bronchial tree and may actually contribute to bronchospasm.

Placental Abruption

The cesarean rate in patients with placental abruption is very high, especially if the fetus is still alive. Because the potential for fetal distress is markedly increased in these patients, regional anesthesia for patients with severe abruption is not recommended. The mother is also at significant risk of hypovolemia from hemorrhage, and sympathetic blockade from a regional block would exacerbate the hypovolemia and be deleterious. Moreover, there is the ever-present risk of coagulopathy in these patients, which adds to the increased risk of regional blockade.

Sickle Cell Disease

Patients with sickle cell disease who require cesarean delivery may receive either regional or general anesthesia. These patients should be well preoxygenated, and great care must be taken to prevent both hypotension and hypoxia.

SUMMARY

There is no ideal anesthetic technique suitable for all patients with various high-risk conditions. Each patient must be evaluated on an individual basis. Similarly, there is no anesthetic technique without risk. Therefore, it is of paramount importance for the anesthesiologist and obstetrician to communicate and work closely together when caring for the pregnant woman with a high-risk condition. If optimal care is to be provided to both mother and fetus, it is imperative that both the anesthesiologist and obstetrician have a sound basic understanding of both disciplines.

The opinions expressed in this chapter are those of the authors and not necessarily those of the United States Air Force or the Department of Defense.

REFERENCES

1. Pritchard JA: Changes in blood volume during pregnancy and delivery. *Anesthesiology* 26:393, 1965.

2. Pritchard JA, Stone SR: Clinical and laboratory observations on eclampsia. *Am J Obstet Gynecol* 99:754, 1967.
3. Hankins GDV, Wendel GD, Cunningham FG, et al: Longitudinal evaluation of hemodynamic changes in eclampsia. *Am J Obstet Gynecol* 150:506, 1984.
4. Cotton BD, Gonik B, Dorman KF: Cardiovascular alterations in severe pregnancy-induced hypertension: Acute effects of intravenous magnesium sulfate. *Am J Obstet Gynecol* 148:162, 1984.
5. Groenendijk R, Trimbos MJ, Wallenburg HCS: Hemodynamic measurements in preeclampsia: Preliminary observations. *Am J Obstet Gynecol* 150:232, 1984.
6. Benedetti TJ, Cotton BD, Read JC, et al: Hemodynamic observations in severe preeclampsia with a flow-directed pulmonary artery catheter. *Am J Obstet Gynecol* 136:465, 1980.
7. Phelan JP, Yurth DA: Severe preeclampsia. I. Peripartum hemodynamic observations. *Am J Obstet Gynecol* 144:17, 1982.
8. Rafferty TD, Berkowitz RL: Hemodynamics in patients with severe toxemia during labor and delivery. *Am J Obstet Gynecol* 138:263, 1980.
9. Pritchard JA, Cunningham FG, Mason RA: Coagulation changes in eclampsia: Their frequency and pathogenesis. *Am J Obstet Gynecol* 124:855, 1976.
10. Moir DD, Victor-Rodrigues L, Willocks J: Epidural analgesia during labor in patients with preeclampsia. *J Obstet Gynecol Br Commonwealth* 79:465, 1972.
11. Craig CJT: Eclampsia and the anaesthetist. *South Afr Med J* 46:248, 1972.
12. Speroff L: Toxemia of pregnancy: Mechanism and therapeutic management. *Am J Cardiol* 32:582, 1973.
13. Marx GF: Obstetric anesthesia in the presence of medical complications. *Clin Obstet Gynecol* 17:165, 1974.
14. Newsome L, Bramwell RS: Severe preeclampsia—hemodynamic effects of lumbar epidural anesthesia (abstract). *Anesth Analg* 63:175, 1984.
15. Jouppilla P, Jouppilla R, Hollmen A, et al: Lumbar epidural analgesia to improve intervillous blood flow during labor in severe preeclampsia. *Obstet Gynecol* 59:158, 1982.
16. Ramanathan J, Khalil M, Chauhan D, et al: Anesthetic management of "HELLP Syndrome" in severe preeclampsia—a retrospective study (abstract). *Anesth Analg* 65:5124, 1986.
17. Jouppilla R, Jouppilla P, Hollmen A, et al: Epidural and placental blood flow during labour in pregnancies complicated by hypertension. *Br J Obstet Gynaecol* 86:969, 1979.
18. Fox EJ, Sklar GS, Hill CH, et al: Complications related to the pressure response to endotracheal intubation. *Anesthesiology* 47:524, 1977.
19. Snyder SW, Wheeler AS, James FM: The use of nitroglycerin to control severe hypertension of pregnancy during cesarean section. *Anesthesiology* 51:563, 1979.
20. Hodgkinson R, Husain FJ, Hayashi RH: Systemic and pulmonary blood pressure during cesarean section in parturients with gestational hypertension. *Can Anaesth Soc J* 27:389, 1980.
21. Fahmy NR: Nitroglycerin as a hypotensive drug during general anesthesia. *Anesthesiology* 49:17, 1978.
22. Pritchard JA, Cunningham FG, Pritchard SA: The Parkland Memorial Hospital protocol for treatment of eclampsia: Evaluation of 245 cases. *Am J Obstet Gynecol* 148:951, 1984.
23. Gabbe SG, Mestman JH, Freeman RK, et al: Management and outcome of diabetes mellitus, Classes B-R. *Am J Obstet Gynecol* 129:723, 1977.
24. Leveno KJ, Hauth JC, Gilstrap LC, et al: Appraisal of "rigid" blood glucose control during pregnancy in overtly diabetic women. *Am J Obstet Gynecol* 135:793, 1979.

25. Schneider JM, Curet LB, Olson RW, et al: Ambulatory care of the pregnant diabetic. *Obstet Gynecol* 56:144, 1980.
26. Kenepp WB, Shelley CW, Juman S: Effects on newborn of hydration with glucose in patients undergoing cesarean section with regional anesthesia. *Lancet* 1:645, 1980.
27. Datta S, Brown WU: Acid-base status in diabetic mothers and their infants following general or spinal anesthesia for cesarean section. *Anesthesiology* 47:272, 1977.
28. Datta S, Naulty JS, Ostheimer GW, et al: Acid-base status in diabetic mothers and their infants following spinal anesthesia. *Anesthesiology* 55:A319, 1981.
29. Gibbs CP, Spohr L, Petrakis J, et al: Prevention of hypotension with hydration. *Anesthesiology* 55:A308, 1981.
30. Ueland K: Cardiovascular diseases complicating pregnancy. *Clin Obstet Gynecol* 21:429, 1978.
31. Land MA, Bisno AL: Acute rheumatic fever: A vanishing disease in suburbia. *JAMA* 249:895, 1983.
32. Clark SL, Phelan JP, Greenspoon J, et al: Labor and delivery in the presence of mitral stenosis: Central hemodynamic observations. *Am J Obstet Gynecol* 152:984, 1985.
33. Kaplan EL, Bisno A, Facklam R, et al: Prevention of bacterial endocarditis. *Circulation* 56:139A, 1977.
34. Szekely P, Snaith L: Atrial fibrillation and pregnancy. *Br Med J* 1:1407, 1961.
35. Arias F, Pineda J: Aortic stenosis and pregnancy. *J Reprod Med* 20:229, 1978.
36. Jones AM, Howitt G: Eisenmenger's syndrome in pregnancy. *Br Med J* 1:1627, 1965.
37. McAnulty JH, Metcalfe J, Ueland K: General guidelines in the management of cardiac disease. *Clin Obstet Gynecol* 24:773, 1981.
38. Spinnato JA, Krayhack BJ, Cooper MW: Eisenmenger's syndrome in pregnancy: Epidural anesthesia for elective cesarean section. *N Engl J Med* 304:1215, 1981.
39. Abboud TK, Raya J, Noueihed R, et al: Intrathecal morphine for relief of labor pain in a parturient with severe pulmonary hypertension. *Anesthesiology* 59:477, 1983.
40. O'Neill H, Blake S, Surgrue D, et al: Problems in the management of patients with artificial valves during pregnancy. *Br J Obstet Gynecol* 89:940, 1982.
41. Hankins GDV, Wendel GD, Leveno KJ, et al: Myocardial infarction during pregnancy: Pathophysiologic considerations. *Obstet Gynecol* 65:139, 1985.
42. Kaplan EL, Anthony BF, Bisno A, et al: Prevention of bacterial endocarditis. *Circulation* 56:139A, 1977.
43. Gold MI, Helrich M: A study of the complications related to anesthesia in asthmatic patients. *Anesth Analg* 42:283, 1963.
44. Brown WN: Respiratory problems, in James FM, Wheeler AS (eds): *Obstetric Anesthesia: The Complicated Patient.* Philadelphia, FA Davis Co, 1982, pp 103–121.
45. Aviado DM: Regulation of bronchometer tone during anesthesia. *Anesthesiology* 42:68, 1975.
46. Corssen G, Gutierrez J, Reves JG, et al: Ketamine in the management of asthmatic patients. *Anesth Analg* 51:588, 1972.
47. Hirshman CA, Downes H, Farboud A, et al: Ketamine block of bronchospasm in experimental canine asthma. *Br J Anaesth* 51:713, 1979.
48. Duvaldestin P, Demetriou M, Henzel D, et al: The placental transfer of pancuronium and its pharmacokinetics during cesarean section. *Acta Anaesth Scand* 22:327, 1978.
49. Gold ML: Anesthesia for the asthmatic patient. *Anesth Analg* 49:881, 1970.

Operative Techniques

Chapter 12

Opening and Closing the Abdomen

Donald G. Gallup, MD

Abdominal incisions and their closure for the obstetric patient vary tremendously with the urgency for operative intervention and the prior experience of the surgeon. Unfortunately, incisions are only infrequently individualized. Some techniques, in certain instances, may be superior to others. Incisions should meet certain basic criteria, including reasonably quick entry, adequate exposure, and a closure that will leave minimal chance of infection or dehiscence. This chapter is designed to allow the surgeon to compare classic techniques with some recently reported modifications.

In the young obstetric patient, incisions resulting in an excellent cosmetic scar are desirable, although not always feasible. In addition, abdominal wound infections, and occasionally the resulting dehiscence occurring after obstetrically related operative procedures, are a psychological and economic problem for the patient and prolong hospitalization and convalescence. Factors negatively affecting proper wound healing include diabetes, malnutrition, prior irradiation, older age, alcoholism, preoperative shaving, duration of the preoperative stay, duration of the operation, the use of Penrose-type drains, ascites, immunosuppression (including long-term corticosteroid therapy), and obesity.[1–4] Other factors noted to increase wound complication rates in obstetric patients include associated anemia, premature rupture of the membranes, prolapsed cord, and meconium staining. Wound infection rates associated with cesarean delivery range from 2.5% to 16.1%.[2] Other factors in wound disruption include the choice of suture material, closure techniques, and occurrence of excessive coughing due to pulmonary disease or vomiting.[5] These issues are discussed in more detail in Chapter 25.

In general, abdominal incisions for obstetric patients can be divided into vertical and transverse incisions. Regardless of the incision chosen,

TABLE 12.1 Commonly Used Sutures

Suture Type	Tissue Reaction (1–4)	Relative Strength (1–4)
Absorbable		
Plain gut	4	2
Chromic gut	3	2
Polyglycolic acid (Dexon)	2	3
Polygalactia 910 (Vicryl)	2	3
Nonabsorbable		
Natural (silk, cotton)	4	2
Polypropylene monofilament		
Surgilene	1	4
Prolene	1	4
Braided synthetics (Dacron, Mersilene, Ti-Cron, Ethibond)	2	4
Metal	4	4

wound complications can be avoided by adhering to certain basic principles:

1. Preoperative showering, with careful cleansing of the umbilicus, should be done in all elective cases.
2. Clip preparation of pubic and abdominal hair is preferable to shave preparation when elective surgery is planned.
3. An iodophor skin preparation is preferable. There is no evidence that plastic adhesive drapes are more effective in preventing wound infection.[6] In fact, they may prove harmful if they lift from the skin.
4. Drains should be liberally used, particularly when there is preoperative infection or when a large wet potential space is left. Patients with defects in blood coagulation should have incisions drained. Closed drainage systems such as the Jackson-Pratt or Hemovac system through a separate stab wound are preferred. A Penrose-type drain should never be brought out through the principal surgical incision.
5. Prophylactic antibiotics should be considered in selected patients and are discussed in Chapter 20.
6. Fascia should not be closed with chromic catgut. The choice of suture should be based, at least partially, on the type of incision and the condition of the patient (ie, the presence of infection). Although handling of the suture may be based on the individual surgeon's preference, the strength and reaction of sutures should be considered (Table 12.1).
7. Subcutaneous Penrose drains should be avoided. Subcutaneous spaces should be drained with a closed system if the patient is obese or if the area lacks hemostasis.
8. The skin can be closed with suture or by the use of a skin stapler. A delayed closure (ie, pack open for 5–7 days) is recommended for pa-

tients with gross contamination (eg, the presence of gross pus or enterotomy in a patient with an unprepared bowel).[7]

9. Cautery should not be used to incise the skin or the fascia.

TRANSVERSE INCISIONS

The best cosmetic incision is the transverse incision. Depending on the circumstances, some patients may not be candidates (eg, emergency cesarean delivery) for this incision. Proponents of transverse incisions have suggested that these incisions are as much as 30 times stronger than midline incisions. For instance, Mowat and Bonnar[8] noted that abdominal wound dehiscence after cesarean delivery was eight times more common with a vertical incision compared to a transverse incision. However, other studies either show an advantage of midline incisions over transverse incisions in avoiding dehiscence or else show no evidence to support either method.[7,9] Transverse incisions result in less pain and less chance of respiratory infection due to splinting. On the other hand, transverse incisions do have certain disadvantages: the division of multiple layers of fascia and muscle, with formation of potential spaces; the division of nerves and muscles; and longer operating time.

The Pfannenstiel Incision

This is an excellent cosmetic incision and is indicated in nonobese women when the extra speed of delivery afforded by a vertical incision is not essential. It should not be used when exposure is critical, eg, in reoperating on a patient for hemorrhage.

Exposure of the pregnant uterus is often marginal, particularly in the obese patient. Rapid extension of the incision is difficult and the incision is usually wet, necessitating a subfascial closed drainage system in some patients. Regarding fascial closure, a running suture can be utilized in patients with clean wounds. In assessing the use of running versus interrupted polyglycolic acid sutures in *midline* incisions, Fagniez et al[10] noted no difference in dehiscence rate in a randomized prospective trial of 3,135 patients. Drains should be used in the subfascial space if complete hemostasis is unattainable. Subcutaneous sutures are unnecessary, and the skin may be closed with staples or a subcuticular suture.

A modified Pfannenstiel incision has been advocated. Once the transverse subcutaneous incision is carried to the aponeurosis of the external oblique muscle and anterior sheath of the recti, the fascia is cleansed cephalad and caudad from the umbilicus to the symphysis in the midline. A vertical incision is then made in the linea alba. This modified incision is not expedient, and subcutaneous closed drainage may be indicated.

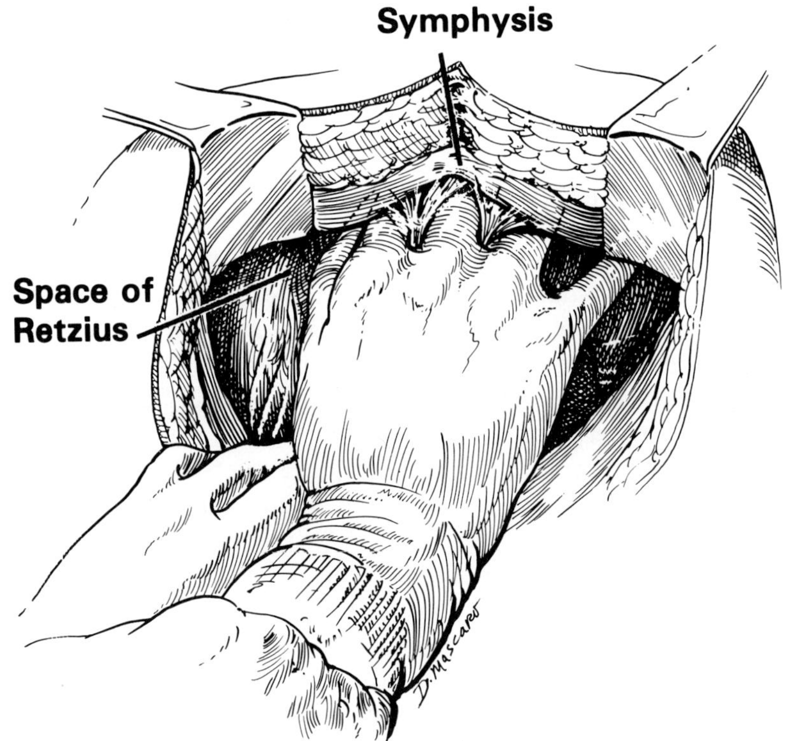

FIGURE 12.1 Developing the space of Retzius for mobilization of the bladder. Cephalad traction with the opposite hand of the surgeon on the peritoneum will aid in exposure of the space.

The Cherney Incision

Occasionally, the surgeon who makes a low transverse abdominal incision will be surprised to find the incision inadequate to deliver the infant safely and expediently, or not large enough to obtain adequate exposure for hemostasis or to deal with associated abnormal conditions. Under these circumstances, the safe approach is not to "half-transect" the recti, but rather to perform a modified Cherney incision. This incision also affords excellent exposure of the pelvic sidewall when needed, ie, in patients who require hypogastric artery ligation. The incision is about 25% longer than a midline incision from the umbilicus to the symphysis.[11]

In patients who have the peritoneum already opened, it is useful to develop the space of Retzius by blunt dissection prior to incising the recti. This can be easily accomplished by the use of traction and in the relatively bloodless midline (Figure 12.1). Thus, the inferior epigastric vessels can be easily located, and injury is avoided. The pyramidalis muscles are sharply dissected. The fibrous, tendinous recti are then sharply dissected from their insertion into the pubis. The peritoneal incision can be extended laterally, about 1 finger breadth cephalad to the bladder.

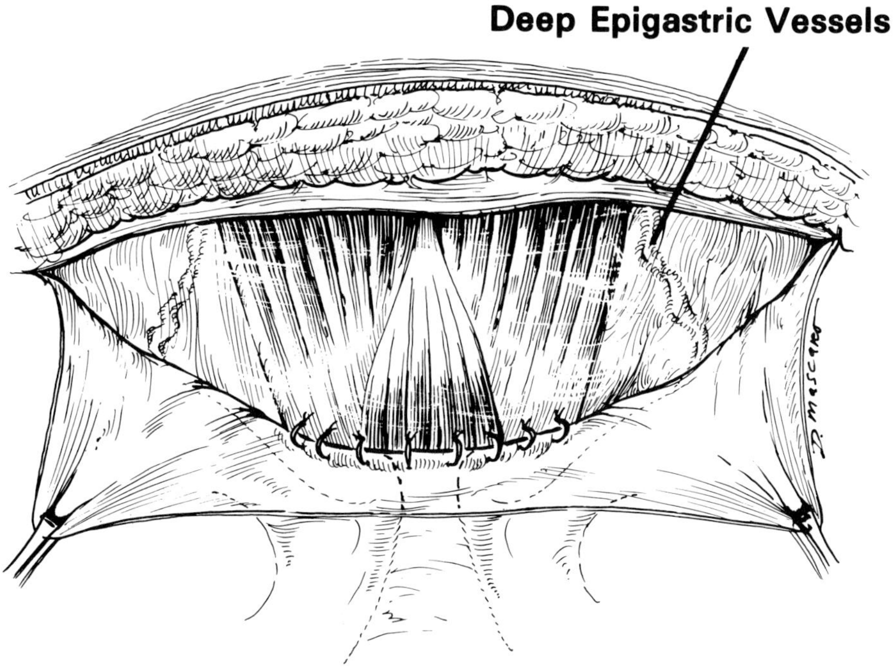

FIGURE 12.2 The Cherney incision involves incising the tendinous recti sharply at their insertion into the pubis. The recti are united by the use of interrupted sutures.

After closure of the peritoneum, the rectus tendons are united to the lower flap of the rectus sheath (Figure 12.2). The remaining portion of the incision can be closed as noted above. Drainage of the subfascial space may be necessary.

The Maylard Incision

The true transverse muscle-cutting incision, the Maylard or Maylard-Bardenheuer incision, is a poor incision for cesarean deliveries because of the time it requires.[12] It does afford excellent exposure of the pelvis and is used by many physicians for radical pelvic surgery, including exenterations and removal of large adnexal masses. For the obstetric patient, this incision can be used for exploration for postpartum bleeding and possible hypogastric artery ligation or hysterectomy. It is an excellent incision for the patient who is treated by radical hysterectomy for cervical cancer in the first trimester of pregnancy. It may be used for pregnant patients with adnexal masses; however, exposure of the upper abdomen is limited.

Some feel that a Pfannenstiel incision can be converted into a Maylard incision simply by incising the recti and avoiding the inferior (deep) epigastric vessels. These vessels, which are located lateral and posterior to the muscles, must be identified and ligated prior to incising the recti in

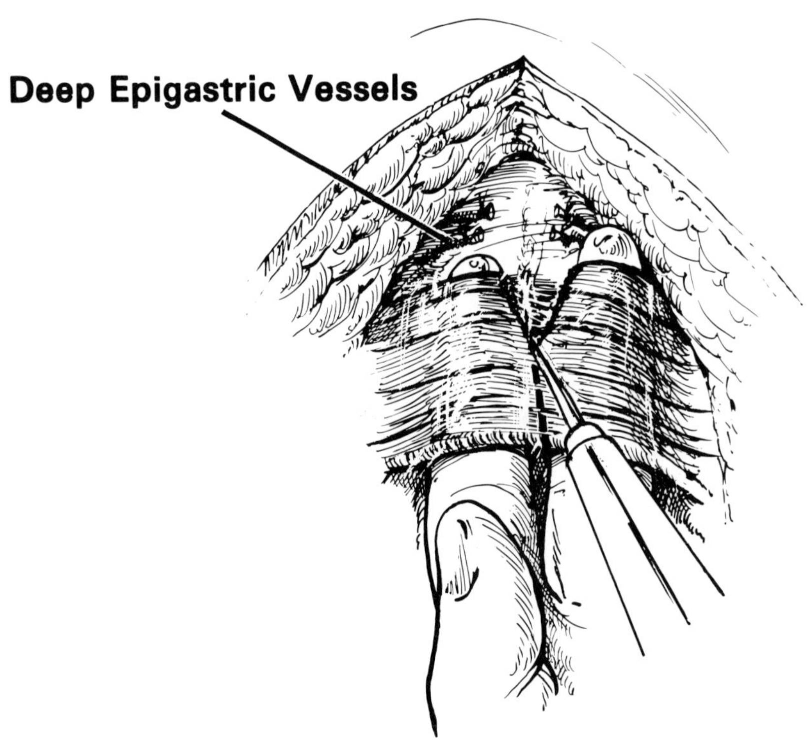

FIGURE 12.3 The Maylard incision incising the recti with cautery. The hand of the surgeon is withdrawn as the muscle is cut. The inferior epigastric vessels have been previously isolated, ligated, and sectioned.

order to avoid vessel retraction and hematoma formation (Figure 12.3). This approach has the disadvantage of transecting the fascia that has been denuded of its muscular blood supply. If a Pfannenstiel incision must be widened, conversion to a Cherney incision is preferable.

The recti are not easily approximated when closing. However, if they are first sutured to the overlying fascia, fascial closure will result in reapproximation of the muscles. A running technique, as with the Pfannenstiel incision, is preferred. Subfascial drains are often necessary.

VERTICAL INCISIONS

When exploratory laparotomy is needed and the diagnosis is uncertain, a vertical incision is indicated. For instance, trauma in the pregnant patient demands a vertical incision. Vertical incisions can be divided into two types—midline and paramedian.

The Paramedian Incision

Paramedian incisions have been advocated because of their allegedly greater strength. However, Guillou et al,[13] in a prospective study, found

TABLE 12.2 Possible Indications for Midline Incisions in Obstetric Patients

Acute fetal distress
Prolapsed cord without a monitor
Shock, hypovolemia
Prior midline incision
Ovarian tumor highly suspicious for malignancy
Trauma
Obesity

little difference in respiratory complications, wound infections, and dehiscence when comparing midline, medial paramedian, and lateral paramedian incisions. None of the patients with lateral paramedian incisions developed incisional hernias. Hernia occurrence in midline and medial paramedian incisions was essentially the same. Increases in bleeding, infection rates, and operating time, as well as the possibility of atrophy of the rectus muscle, are arguments against the use of paramedian incisions. The abdominal area caudad to the arcuate line, or the lower half of the lower abdominal wall, is relatively weak. Most hernias associated with vertical incisions occur in this area. However, in a large series of high-risk patients who had midline incisions closed with modified suture techniques, no incisional hernias were noted.[7] One possible remaining indication for a right paramedian incision in the pregnant patient is suspected appendicitis.

The Midline Incision

A midline incision is rapid, easy to perform, relatively bloodless, and may be useful in the obstetric situations described in Table 12.2. In general, the lower midline incision is made from the umbilicus to the symphysis and can be extended around the umbilicus and more cephalad as needed. Because of the naturally occurring diastasis of the recti in pregnancy, there is little need to separate the muscles, thus affording rapid access to the peritoneal cavity.

The obese patient presents a special problem. Pitkin noted a 4% wound complication rate in nonobese women undergoing hysterectomy as compared to a 29% wound complication rate in obese patients.[14] In 1977, Morrow et al[15] suggested modifications of preoperative care, intraoperative techniques, and postoperative care in obese patients and noted a 13% wound infection rate. By modifying their technique, the wound infection rate in a group of 97 obese patients managed by us was 3%, compared to 42% in an obese group not operated on by our protocol.[7] Krebs and Helmkamp[16] suggested a periumbilical transverse incision in massively obese patients and noted a 24% wound infection rate. Because muscle cutting may be needed with this approach, the incision time is too lengthy for most cesarean deliveries. If any transverse incision

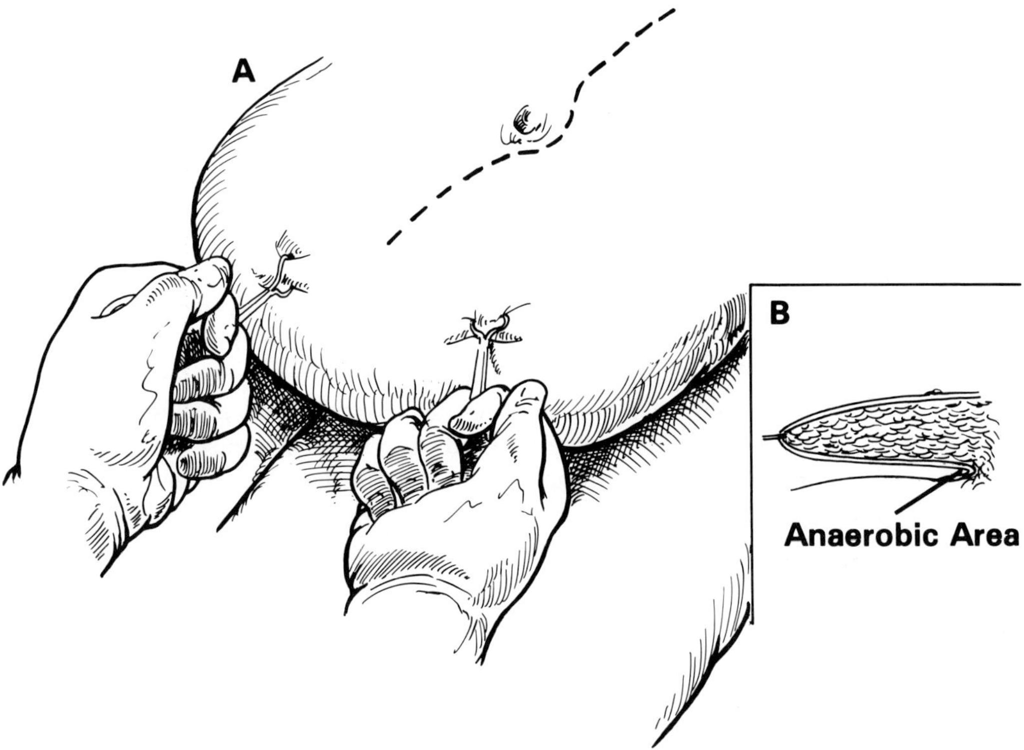

FIGURE 12.4 Midline incision in an obese patient. The panniculus is retracted inferiorly (A), and the incision avoids the moist anaerobic environment (B) beneath the subpanniculus fold.

is chosen for obese patients, it should be away from the subpanniculus fold.

The Technique for Midline Incisions in the Obese Patient

When time permits, preoperative care should include pHisohex showers and thorough cleansing of the umbilicus. Clip removal of abdominal hair is preferred. The midline incision is made by first retracting the panniculus caudad, below the superior margins of the symphysis, in order to avoid the "land of the anaerobes" (Figure 12.4). When a hysterectomy is necessary, a wound protector is used to improve exposure in the pelvis.

Midline incisions may be closed with interrupted or figure-eight sutures using polyglycolic acid or one of the more delayed absorbable sutures such as monofilament polyglyconate or polydioxanone. The bites in the fascia should be at least 1.5 cm from the edge. Because obese patients are at high risk for dehiscence and later incisional hernias, a Smead Jones internal retention suture using monofilament polypropylene has been suggested.[5,7,15] Layered catgut closure should not be used, as dehiscence rates are too high.[17] Investigators publishing in the general surgical literature

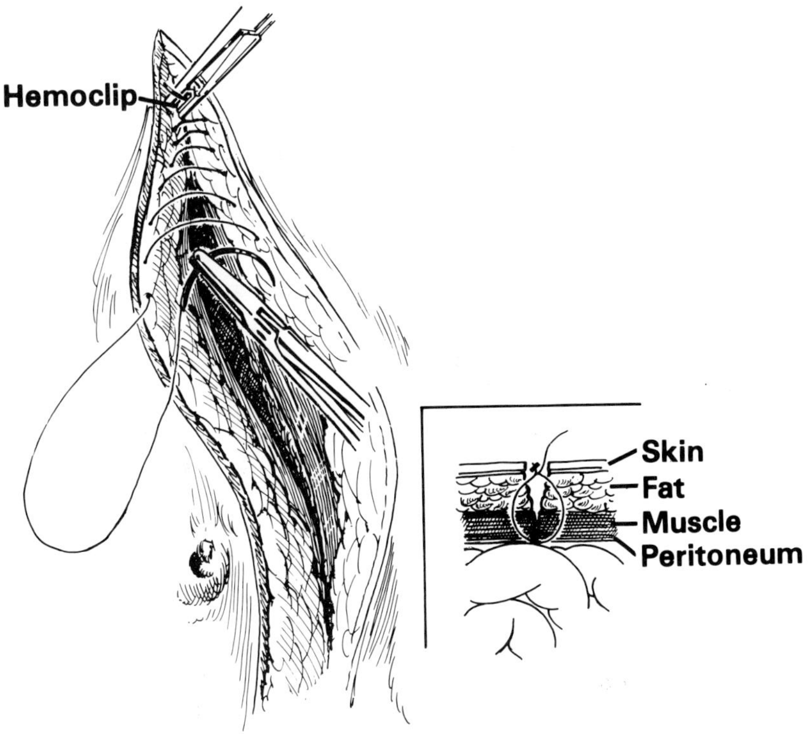

FIGURE 12.5 Running the fascia and peritoneum using No. 2 Surgilene (Davis and Geck, Danbury, CT) on a large CT needle.

strongly support the use of a running continuous suture of large-bore monofilament polypropylene in midline incision.[18–22] Shepherd et al[23] have reported over 200 cases of high-risk gynecology patients in whom a mass closure technique with running monofilament polypropylene was used, and no wound dehiscences were noted. Large, closely spaced (about 1.5 cm apart) bites that are at least 2 cm lateral to the cut edge of the fascia are recommended. This running technique distributes tension equally over a continuous line. The closure is expedient and cost effective, and has the additional advantage of relative minimization of foreign material in the wound. Interlocking continuous suture may slow the healing process by decreasing vascularization. To prevent untying, a clip on the short end of the suture is used. A large needle also aids in closure (Figure 12.5). In relatively thin patients, the knot may be buried beneath the fascia.

Subcutaneous sutures may be used, but a closed drainage system is placed anterior to the fascia. Drains should be left in place for at least 72 hours or until the output is less than 20 cc in 24 hours. The skin is closed with a suture stapler. Staples are left in place for 2 weeks. A nasogastric tube should be inserted during the operative procedure and left in place for 24 hours to avoid distention.

SECONDARY CLOSURE

A few patients should not have primary incision closure at the time of cesarean delivery. Such patients have contaminated wounds, including those with a ruptured appendix or intraabdominal abscess or an injury to an unprepared bowel. In these cases, following closure of the fascia, a bridge consisting of rolls of gauze can be used to support loosely tied, interrupted 3-0 monofilament polypropylene sutures of the skin.[24] These sutures can be placed using a mattress technique, about 2 cm apart. Dressing sponges (4 × 8 in) are laid in the wound, posterior to the sutures, and are changed periodically following wound cleansing. In 5–7 days the dressing gauze is removed, and the previously placed sutures are simply tied to approximate the skin edges. In obese patients, a closed drainage system is placed in the subcutaneous space. Steristrips may be used for further support.

COLOSTOMY INCISIONS

Rarely, the distal colon is injured during cesarean delivery. This is discussed in greater detail in Chapter 19. In the presence of gross fecal contamination due to colon injury, surgical consultation is frequently required. A diversion of the fecal stream is often indicated. When large rents occur, a temporary loop colostomy is usually needed. Loop colostomy is applicable only to those parts of the colon with mesentery long enough to permit the colon to be mobilized outside the abdominal cavity, while preserving the blood supply. The sigmoid and transverse colons are usually used for loop colostomies.[25]

The colostomy loop may be placed at the upper end of a midline incision; however, a separate oblique or vertical incision, about 5 cm long, over the rectus muscle may be preferable. Using a separate incision prevents fecal drainage from contaminating the suture line of the original laparotomy incision. After teasing the colon through the incision by placing an umbilical tape or vessel loop through an avascular portion of the mesentery and exerting gentle traction, a glass rod with connecting rubber tubing is placed through the mesentery. Retraction of the loop is thus prevented. The loop and surrounding skin are covered with petroleum gauze. In 24–72 hours the colostomy can be opened with a longitudinal 3-cm incision along the tinea.

REFERENCES

1. Cruse PJE: Infection surveillance: Identifying the problem and the high-risk patient. *South Med J* 70(suppl 1):40, 1977.
2. Mead PB: Managing infected abdominal wounds. *Contemp Obstet/Gynecol* 14:69, 1979.

3. Cruse PJE, Foord R: A five year prospective study of 23,649 surgical wounds. *Arch Surg* 107:206, 1973.
4. Dineen P: A critical study of 100 conservative wound infections. *Surg Gynecol Obstet* 113:91, 1961.
5. Wallace D, Hernandez W, Schlaerth JB, et al: Prevention of abdominal wound disruption utilizing the Smead-Jones closure technique. *Obstet Gynecol* 56:26, 1980.
6. Alexander JW, Aerni S, Plettner JP: Development of a safe and effective one-minute preoperative skin preparation. *Arch Surg* 120:1367, 1985.
7. Gallup DG: Modification of celiotomy techniques to decrease morbidity in the obese gynecologic patient. *Am J Obstet Gynecol* 150:171, 1984.
8. Mowat J, Bonnar J: Abdominal wound dehiscence after cesarean section. *Br Med J* 2:256, 1971.
9. Greenburg G, Salk RP, Peskin GW: Wound dehiscence. Pathophysiology and prevention. *Arch Surg* 114:143, 1979.
10. Fagniez PL, Hay JM, Lacaine F, et al: Abdominal midline incision closure. *Arch Surg* 120:1351, 1985.
11. Cherney LS: A modified transverse incision for low abdominal operations. *Surg Gynecol Obstet* 72:92, 1941.
12. Maylard AE: Direction of abdominal incision. *Br Med J* 2:895, 1907.
13. Guillou PJ, Hall TJ, Donaldson DR, et al: Vertical abdominal incisions—a choice? *Br J Surg* 67:359, 1980.
14. Pitkin RM: Abdominal hysterectomy in obese women. *Surg Gynecol Obstet* 142:532, 1976.
15. Morrow CP, Hernandez WL, Townsend DE, et al: Pelvic celiotomy in the obese patient. *Am J Obstet Gynecol* 127:335, 1977.
16. Krebs HB, Helmkamp F: Transverse periumbilical incision in the massively obese patient. *Obstet Gynecol* 63:241, 1984.
17. Goligher JC, Irvin TT, Johnston D, et al: A controlled clinical trial of three methods of closure of laparotomy wounds. *Br J Surg* 62:823, 1975.
18. Knight CD, Griffen FD: Abdominal wound closure with a continuous monofilament polypropylene suture. Experience with 1,000 consecutive cases. *Arch Surg* 118:1305, 1983.
19. Archie JP, Feldtman RW: Primary abdominal wound closure with permanent continuous running monofilament sutures. *Surg Gynecol Obstet* 153:721, 1981.
20. Kratzer GL: Intestinal anastomosis and abdominal wound closure using monofilament Prolene polypropylene suture. *Dis Colon Rectum* 21:342, 1978.
21. Dale WA: Closure of abdominal wounds, in O'Leary JP, Woltering EA (eds): *Techniques for Surgeons.* New York, John Wiley & Sons, Inc, 1985, pp 31–33.
22. Richards PC, Balch CM, Aldrete JS: Abdominal wound closure: Randomized prospective study of 571 patients comparing continuous vs interrupted suture techniques. *Ann Surg* 197:238, 1983.
23. Shepherd JH, Cavanagh D, Riggs D, et al: Abdominal wound closures using a nonabsorbable single layer technique. *Obstet Gynecol* 61:248, 1983.
24. Menendez MA: The contaminated closure, in O'Leary JP, Woltering EA (eds): *Techniques for Surgeons.* New York, John Wiley & Sons, Inc, 1985, pp 36–37.
25. Carey LC, Fabri PJ: The intestinal tract in relation to gynecology, in Mattingly RF, Thompson JD (eds): *Operative Gynecology*, ed 6. Philadelphia, JB Lippincott Co, 1985, pp 449–479.

Chapter 13

Cesarean Delivery
The Extraperitoneal Approach

Richard P. Perkins, MD

In an era when cesarean section is increasingly employed to improve the welfare of the newborn, a greater number of women inevitably develop serious puerperal infection. Because of antimicrobials, the modern parturient is not frequently faced with death from infection, but rather with the discomfort and financial liabilities associated with prolonged hospitalization.

DePalma et al, *Obstetrics and Gynecology*

Until the middle of the 20th century, primary cesarean delivery after prolonged labor was performed relatively infrequently and with considerable trepidation. Under these conditions, the morbidity and mortality from infectious complications of cesarean birth were formidable; to avoid this necessity, earlier generations of obstetricians were carefully schooled in the intricacies of midpelvic forceps applications. A much greater tolerance for prolonged labor and suboptimal progress also existed in order to skirt the hazards of invading the uterus following protracted labor, because, under these circumstances, surgery often resulted in major morbidity, occasional loss of future fertility, and even death.

Since those early days, many changes and advances in obstetric management and the control of infectious disease have occurred. The gradual restriction of the classic cesarean delivery to selected, appropriate cases reduced some elements of morbidity. An opportunity also occurred to exclude the hysterotomy incision from the peritoneal cavity (at least postoperatively) when the low segment transverse incision became the standard of practice. The use of and necessity for cesarean hysterectomy progressively declined, and is now largely reserved for cases of intractable hemorrhage.

The most significant advance contributing to a liberalization of attitudes regarding cesarean delivery was the advent of effective antibiotic therapy. With the initial availability of penicillin, the later discovery of the aminoglycosides, and the more recent introduction of other broad-spectrum agents, concerns originally prompted by the morbidity of prior generations gradually waned. As stated by DePalma et al at the beginning of this chapter, concern no longer centers primarily on the risk of death from overwhelming sepsis, but rather on issues of expense, inconvenience, and prolonged hospitalization. With the advent of every new, more expensive, and more highly touted broad-spectrum antibiotic, we are constantly reminded that obstetric infection is still unconquered. Current practices appear to be moving toward the routine use of prophylactic antibiotics with any increased risk of infection. Although the observed results appear to justify this trend, the inevitable emergence of resistant strains of microorganisms will undoubtedly perpetuate the quest for new therapeutic alternatives.

THE ORIGINS OF EXTRAPERITONEAL CESAREAN DELIVERY

Soon after advances in anesthesia rendered major surgery feasible, the problem of serious postoperative obstetric morbidity came sharply into focus. This was a time when the classic cesarean delivery incision was utilized regularly. It was speculated, with considerable justification, that many of the serious complications resulted from peritoneal contamination, both at the time of surgery and continuing into the postoperative period. As the low segment approach gained acceptance, it was noted that the ability to extraperitonealize this incision by covering it with the bladder appeared to be associated with a decrease in generalized abdominal morbidity. Without antibiotics, however, considerable serious disease remained, especially that of abscess formation requiring one or more subsequent operative procedures. It was speculated that if soiling the abdominal cavity at the time of surgery could be avoided, perhaps these serious sequelae could be reduced.

Various operative approaches were designed. Ultimately, two general alternatives remained following the use and study of available options. One approach, popularized by Waters,[1] involved the extraperitoneal approach to the lower uterine segment by the supravesical route. Considerable technical difficulty was encountered with this method, centering primarily on the successful separations of the peritoneal reflection and urachus from the dome of the bladder. Because of the tenacious adherence of the peritoneal reflection at this point, attempts to gain the retrovesical space frequently resulted in multiple inadvertent peritoneal entries. The frustrated surgeon attempting to learn this technique frequently abandoned it, feeling that such inadvertent entry would undoubtedly nullify the desired advantage. Although subsequent experience has not proven this pessimism to be entirely justified, the Waters operation, highly de-

TABLE 13.1 Historical Results of Extraperitoneal Procedures

Author	Type of Procedure	Number of Cases	Average Labor (hr)	Average Hours Ruptured Membranes	Peritoneal Entry(%)	Bladder Injury (%)	Wound Infection
Waters[1]	Supravesical	32	53	38½	26	—	19
Norton[3]	Paravesical	160	42.6	29.8 (w/labor)	27.5	5	—
Levine[4]	Paravesical	35	59	30	8.5	5.7	—
Keettel[5]	Supravesical	56	40	30	39	2	30 with transverse abdominal incision, 0 with vertical
Stansfield[6]	Combined	52	85% (>36 hr) 63% (>48 hr)	—	4	2	4
Atherton[7]	Supravesical Paravesical	37 31	32	24	21	7.4	28
Paternite[8]	Paravesical	93	86% (>24 hr)	88% (>12)	33	2	3.2
Durfee[9]	Paravesical	125 48 pri 77 sec	(Elective cases only)	—	4	0	—

sirable in its anatomic result, failed to gain popularity because of its technical difficulty.

Latzko,[2] and later Norton,[3] popularized an approach to the lower uterine segment by skirting the bladder laterally. In exchange for the increased facility in dissection, however, the paravesical approach yielded a smaller operative site through which to perform hysterotomy and deliver the fetus. Experience with the technique and proper case selection tended to minimize this disadvantage, but it nonetheless persists as a potential drawback.

In the United States, the use of this approach reached its peak from the 1930s to the early 1950s. By 1960, however, in spite of evidence that the peritoneal exclusion concept had considerable merit, the meteoric rise in antibiotic use began to take its toll. As a generation of physicians trained to perform this procedure reached the autumn of their academic careers, enthusiasm for the procedure was dampened by the lack of trained and objective instructors. Despite the persistence of postoperative infectious complications (which persist to the present day), extraperitoneal cesarean surgery was relegated to the status of a surgical novelty. The voices of

Table 13.1 (*continued*)

Febrile Morbidity Overall (%)	Drained?	Febrile before Surgery (%)	Average Hospital Stay (days)	Perinatal Mortality (%)	Maternal Mortality (%)	Comments
81	Yes	44	18	3	0	20/26 morbid postoperative were afebrile by fourth day; average operating times—54 min; good display of operative technique.
61	Yes	6.7	—	5.6	1.87	24.4% of babies over 3,800 g; good display of operative technique.
17	Yes?	17	—	8.6	0	
60 after labor, 50 with no labor	No	30	12	5.4	0	Average operating time, 97 min; ileus in 36%, 11% requiring nasogastric suction; excellent review of older series; antibiotics to many
17	Yes	20	—	7.6	0	Fetal distress in 65%
—	—	78	14	19	0	Almost all treated with antibiotics; 20% pure endometritis; 7.4% ileus postoperatively.
—	Most	52	—	—	0	Average time to baby: 30–35 min; endometritis = 8.6%, UTI = 2.2%
2	No	0	—	—	0	Four failures; good display of operative technique

those few remaining experienced obstetric surgeons who continued to support the procedure as a viable alternative were diminished to a whisper, and the merits of the extraperitoneal surgical approach were shouted down by a coalition of detractors, most of whom had never seen, much less performed, it. Finally, the operation fell into disuse, and references to it, even as a facet of obstetric surgical history, began to disappear from newer editions of standard textbooks within the specialty.

Most published series extolling the virtues of extraperitoneal cesarean delivery suffered from a serious lack of appropriate control subjects.[1–9] Because the operation was chosen only in circumstances of extreme risk, those reporting their results could not, in good conscience, have subjected their patients to the manifestly more morbid alternative of the transperitoneal operation. As the decline in the popularity of the operation was precipitous, no carefully controlled series to prove its validity appeared before the end, despite at least two attempts.[7,10] Only recently have any new efforts been made to provide comparative data upon which the scientific merits of the operation might be judged.[11,12]

Prior larger series on extraperitoneal surgery are summarized in Table

13.1. As can be seen, the morbidity sometimes associated with the procedure, even in the hands of experienced surgeons, was considerable. It must be recognized that the circumstances under which such surgery was contemplated were extreme. Perinatal complications of this order of magnitude in a modern context would be unacceptable. In order to see these data in their true light, one must have a sense of how disastrous would have been the results in a control group, had one been utilized. Waters' experience with more than 2,000 cases yielded only seven maternal deaths. This maternal mortality rate of 350 per 100,000 cesarean deliveries, although extravagant by modern standards, was highly admirable for the times.

Results with the paravesical extraperitoneal cesarean delivery were reported by Norton.[3] The maternal death rate of 1.87%, although intimidating, must be compared to the rates of 5% or more under the circumstances that characterized the times. The advantage of experience was evident in this report, for out of 9 bladder injuries (5.6%), 8 occurred in the first 53 cases performed and only 1 in the last 107. Postoperative morbidity associated with peritoneal entry approached that of the series as a whole, suggesting that although this event was comparatively frequent (27.5% of all procedures), it did not influence the results substantially.

Keettel and Randall[5] reported on their experience at the University of Iowa with the Waters procedure. Their report noted the prolonged operating time intrinsic to this procedure prior to the delivery of the baby and the adverse effects that can be observed under these circumstances with general anesthesia. (This has also been a factor in choosing the paravesical approach, which is usually faster.) A single bladder injury was reported, but a 39% incidence of peritoneal entry occurred. Postoperative morbidity was similar to that reported by Norton, despite the fact that some procedures were performed electively.

One study that attempted to provide control data was reported by Gilbert and colleagues in 1953.[10] This review was intended to present the operation in the context of "modern antibiotic therapy." Although not successful in providing legitimate statistical analysis, these authors did note a shorter total operating time with elective extraperitoneal operations compared to the traditional low cervical cesarean delivery. These authors did not drain the extraperitoneal space, however, which most current proponents of the operation suggest as a requirement. They concluded that the operation has merit in patients who have been in prolonged labor.

Stansfield and Drabble[6] reported a modification of the Waters operation as promoted by Bourgeois and Phaneuf.[13] This technique involved *bilateral* paravesical dissection prior to attempting to free the bladder from the peritoneal reflection. The result was a markedly enhanced exposure of the lower uterine segment. They also utilized drainage of the retrovesical space and antibacterial instillations at the time of surgery, a concept currently enjoying renewed popularity in transperitoneal procedures.

A negative report on the effectiveness of the peritoneal exclusion procedure came from Atherton and Williamson,[7] who attempted to compare the extraperitoneal to the standard operation in the presumably infected patient. A comparison of supravesical and paravesical techniques was attempted, with a moderate number of technical errors and an associated increase in overall morbidity. They concluded, as did Douglas and Landesman,[14] that the operation had little merit.

Paternite and Bachand[8] published an analysis of 93 consecutive operations without comparable controls. Their results were similar to those of other series regarding minor complications, but the overall results in terms of morbidity were highly satisfactory. They also suggested that the merits of the procedure lay primarily in its use in the high-risk patient.

Prior to more modern times, the last two reports on the use of this operation came from Durfee[9] and from Ellis and DeVita.[15] The former presented results of a modified Norton procedure and the latter those of a Phaneuf-style operation. In 1961, Ellis and DeVita observed that "every obstetrician should be able to perform an extraperitoneal cesarean delivery to be considered a well-rounded practitioner of the specialty."

Illustrative of the clinical circumstances of the time and the sorts of problems faced in earlier days were the criteria proposed by Dieckmann[16] for choosing the extraperitoneal operation. Among these were:

1. Labor for more than 24 hours
2. Membranes ruptured for more than 24 hours
3. Attempts at delivery by forceps or by version
4. Induction of labor by bag, bougie, or pack
5. Evidence of uterine infection
6. More than six vaginal examinations
7. More than 12 rectal examinations
8. Dead or damaged fetus

Similar high-risk circumstances are not unknown in modern practice. Although current antibiotic therapy has created a climate of relative complacency, in contrast to the high anxieties of the past, the desire to retain all options for avoidance of maternal compromise when cesarean delivery is required should remain paramount in importance to all obstetric surgeons.

THE POTENTIAL ROLE OF EXTRAPERITONEAL CESAREAN DELIVERY

To place the peritoneal exclusion operation in perspective, one must consider the potential advantages of this operation over the transperitoneal procedure and emphasize any unique features of this technique. For many, no argument favoring this approach will succeed, and the issue may appear drawn to an extreme to support a concept with few merits. To those willing to consider the matter objectively, however, some of the potential benefits may appear worthy of further consideration.

Although it is true that the operation was originally designed at a time when the problem of the seriously infected patient could best be characterized as desperate, those who performed the operation skillfully noted that definite benefits were derived. A large number of patients not only survived serious infection that otherwise might have cost them their lives, but also maintained their fertility and ovarian function. Because these considerations rarely apply in the modern era, one must look to more subtle benefits in order to justify recommending the operation.

Comparatively few modern studies report the frequency of pelvic abscess formation. It is likely that this complication has been substantially reduced and, in many cases, eliminated by antibiotic therapy. A small number of such complications continue to appear; however, these series frequently involve the care of indigent patients.[17,18] In many of these instances, reoperation one or more times is required for appropriate resolution of these serious sequelae, sometimes involving distant abdominal sites and sometimes resulting in sterility, castration, or other consequences. Ledger, however, showed that the incidence of such serious sequelae was not reduced by the administration of prophylactic antibiotics.[19]

No modern proponent of the extraperitoneal procedure has accumulated enough cases on which to base a positive statement regarding the effectiveness of this approach in preventing abscess formation. However, no such complication occurred in our high-risk population at the University of Colorado. One should also recognize, however, that the majority of these patients were given antibiotic therapy prior to surgery. Nonetheless, in the series by DePalma et al,[17] 6% of patients treated prophylactically prior to the onset of surgery by traditional transperitoneal methods suffered the occurrence of either a pelvic abscess or "phlegmon."

Data regarding our experience[12] with extraperitoneal cesarean deliveries, in comparison to deliveries in normal patients and patients with risk factors similar to those in the extraperitoneal group, are reproduced in Table 13.2. It should be noted that out of the 93 extraperitoneal operations reported, fewer than 10 were performed by the faculty members involved in the study; the vast majority were done by supervised senior house officers who had performed no more than 2–3 such procedures in the past. By comparison, although a faculty member was not always part of the surgical team in the two control groups, one was regularly present to influence directly the surgical technique. In general, however, the level of experience of the operating surgeon in the other two groups was somewhat lower than that of the operating surgeon in the extraperitoneal population.

It can be seen from Table 13.2 that the preoperative status of the extraperitoneal patients was similar to or placed them at higher risk than

TABLE 13.2 Preoperative Data on Patients Undergoing Extraperitoneal Cesarean Section and Control Patients

Group	No.	Membranes Ruptured >24 hr (%)	Labor (mean hr)	Febrile before Surgery (%)	Preoperative Antibiotics (%)
I. Extraperitoneal cesarean section[a]	93	50.5	17.2	67.7	83.9
II. Normal controls[b]	50	6[c]	7[c]	12[c]	24[c]
III. Abnormal controls[b]	50	52	11.3	24[d]	44[c]

[a] Data on the additional 43 patients courtesy of W. A. Bowes, Jr, MD.
[b] Data from Perkins.[12]
[c] Incidence significantly different from I ($P > 0.005$).
[d] Incidence significantly different from I ($P > 0.05$).
Source: Perkins RP: Role of extraperitoneal cesarean section. *Clin Obstet Gynecol* 23:583, 1980. Reproduced with permission of Harper and Row, Publishers.

that of the normal and abnormal controls. There were no differences among the three groups in mean values for maternal age, parity, or fetal weight, except that mean parity in group II was higher because of the predominance of elective repeat cesarean deliveries. The incidence of ruptured membranes for more than 24 hours, duration of labor, fever prior to surgery, and the use of preoperative antibiotics differed significantly between groups I and II, and significant differences were noted between groups I and the other groups in the incidence of fever before surgery.

In Table 13.3, the mean time of anesthesia from induction to delivery, duration of surgery, and mean decrease in postoperative hematocrit were all similar among the three groups. Mean 1-minute Apgar scores in groups II and III, and 5-minute Apgar scores in group III, differed significantly from those of group I. This was thought to be explained in part by the somewhat higher frequency of low-birth-weight babies in the extraperi-

TABLE 13.3 Operative Data on Patients Undergoing Extraperitoneal Cesarean Section and Control

Group	No.	Mean Time (min)		Mean Decrease in Hematocrit (%)	Mean Apgar Scores	
		Anesthesia, Induction to Delivery	Operation		1 min	5 min
I. Extraperitoneal cesarean section[a]	93	11.6	67.4	5.6	4.7	7.7
II. Normal controls[b]	50	11.2	61.3	5.2	6[c]	7.8
III. Abnormal controls[b]	50	11.6	70.8	6.5	5.8[c]	8.3[c]

[a] Data on the additional 43 patients courtesy of W. A. Bowes, Jr, MD.
[b] Data from Perkins.[12]
[c] Differs from I ($P < 0.05$).
Source: Perkins RP: Role of extraperitoneal cesarean section. *Clin Obstet Gynecol* 23:583, 1980. Reproduced with permission from Harper and Row.

TABLE 13.4 Postoperative Data on Patients Undergoing Extraperitoneal Cesarean Section and Control Patients

Group	No.	Positive Cultures (%)		Febrile (>37.5°C) >3 days (%)	Hospitalized >8 days (%)
		Pathogens	Anaerobes		
I. Extraperitoneal cesarean section[a]	93	52.9	32.9	38	16.3
II. Normal controls[b]	50	24[c]	14[c]	42	16
III. Abnormal controls[b]	50	40[c]	26	48	28

[a] Data on the additional 43 patients courtesy of W. A. Bowes, Jr., MD.

[b] Data on groups II and III are from Perkins.[12]

[c] Differs from I ($P < 0.05$).

Source: Perkins RP: Role of extraperitoneal cesarean section. *Clin Obstet Gynecol* 23:583, 1980. Reproduced with permission from Harper and Row.

toneal group, as well as by the impression of a more prolonged interval from hysterotomy to delivery of the baby in this group. This factor, related to anatomic restrictions at the operative site, has been shown to have an adverse effect on 1-minute Apgar scores[20] and remains a minor disadvantage of the extraperitoneal procedure.

Table 13.4 provides postoperative data and bacteriologic information on the three groups. Significant differences are seen in the frequencies of positive cultures for potential pathogens and anaerobes among the populations. This should be noted in spite of the high incidence of preoperative antibiotic administration. Despite these differences, the incidence of prolonged hospitalization and febrile morbidity did not differ among the three groups.

One factor not reported statistically in this population was the rate of return of normal bowel function and the ability of the patient to tolerate a regular diet. Because of exclusion of operative manipulation within the peritoneal cavity, extraperitoneal patients regularly return to satisfactory bowel function at a more rapid rate than do others. However, because the point at which a patient receives a regular diet is largely determined by the person prescribing management, this factor may be as much a reflection of the prescribing physician as the status of the patient.

What one may conclude from the data in Table 13.4 is that, despite the manifestly higher risks observed in the patients subjected to extraperitoneal cesarean in contrast to the other two comparison groups, the postoperative courses were similar. The significantly more frequent utilization of preoperative antibiotics may, however, be a factor confounding satisfactory interpretation of the benefits of the operation. The additional fact of diminished Apgar scores in the extraperitoneal group, even with the consideration of the higher frequency of low-birth-weight babies, is another detracting factor despite its generally benign implications.

Other considerations must be offered in order to evaluate objectively the potential merits of extraperitoneal cesarean delivery. All such procedures reported here involved drainage of the retrovesical and subfascial spaces for at least 2–3 days postoperatively. Naturally, this is not a routine feature of transperitoneal section. In order to provide adequate control groups for the assessment of the influence of this factor, a series of comparable patients operated on transperitoneally and provided with the potential benefits of drainage of these spaces should be studied.

Additional advantages of the extraperitoneal operation are the theoretical lack of contamination of the peritoneal cavity by the types of organisms shown experimentally and clinically to result in abscess formation.[21] There were no such complications observed in this series. Prior to the establishment of extraperitoneal cesarean as an alternative to transperitoneal surgery at the University of Colorado in 1973, there were one or more such serious complications per year requiring reoperative procedures.

Prior series on the use of this procedure have commented extensively upon the frequency of peritoneal entries, bladder injuries, and trauma to neighboring normal vital structures.[1–10] In our series, there were only two inadvertent bladder injuries (2.2%), only one of which occurred during a procedure begun under faculty supervision. Ways of avoiding this complication will be discussed in the following section on operative technique. Our frequency (of approximately 25%) of one or more inadvertent peritoneal entries compares favorably to that of other series. In almost every case, the fenestration was recognized prior to hysterotomy and quickly closed. In those cases in which fenestration was not noted before delivery of the baby, a search for such entries resulted in identification and closure afterward. It is felt that small, unrecognized peritoneal defects are occluded during the process of delivery and that major (and, more importantly, continuing) soiling of the peritoneal cavity through these entries is thus prevented. In comparing postoperative morbidity between those with and without peritoneal entry, no differences could be demonstrated. None of these entries was sufficient to constitute an anatomical circumstance tantamount to a standard transperitoneal operation.

It is not known what role contamination by particulate or foreign matter may play in the development of pelvic abscess formation. As has been shown, extensive meconium contamination of the abdominal cavity, if not properly removed, can result in a granulomatous response, with resultant fibrous adhesions and abdominal pain.[22] Of course, the extraperitoneal operation would preclude this rare development. Whether or not vernix, decidual, or trophoblastic material could result in additional morbidity is unknown.

In two cases in our series, the extraperitoneal approach had to be abandoned because of technical difficulties. In one instance, the patient had had a previous attempt at extraperitoneal operation at another institution. Substantial anatomic alteration and fibrous tissue formation prevented appropriate identification and handling of the local anatomy on the repeat attempt. In the other case, inadequate filling of the bladder prior to the attempted dissection rendered the procedure technically unsatisfactory, resulting in extensive inadvertent entry into the peritoneal reflection. In contrast, several patients initially operated on by these means have undergone a subsequent elective transperitoneal operation. Surgical dissection of the anatomy by the customary approach was in no way compromised by the prior extraperitoneal operation, and from the surgeon's point of view, it was frequently difficult to discern that any prior surgical procedure had occurred in this area. This author has had no experience in attempting a repeat *extraperitoneal* operation, but philosophically, there would seem to be no pressing reason to perform elective repeat operations by this approach in the absence of clinical indications similar to those prompting the extraperitoneal approach.

INDICATIONS FOR EXTRAPERITONEAL CESAREAN DELIVERY

If one is favorably inclined toward the choice of the extraperitoneal cesarean delivery, the following considerations constitute legitimate indications. Others more liberally inclined toward the procedure may consider lesser indications as appropriate[23,24]:

1. Patients who have been in labor for more than 12 hours prior to delivery
2. Patients with ruptured membranes for more than 6–12 hours, especially if labor has begun
3. Patients with suspected or clinically established intrauterine infection
4. Patients who have undergone multiple examinations
5. The absence of any pressing contraindications, as listed in the next section
6. The presence of a surgeon competent to perform or adequately supervise the procedure

CONTRAINDICATIONS TO EXTRAPERITONEAL CESAREAN DELIVERY

Although some advocates insist that all operations may be attempted extraperitoneally because the conversion to a transperitoneal procedure is technically simple, certain clinical circumstances may present difficulties that render the operation impractical. Some of these include:

1. A low-lying, predominantly anterior placenta previa or another unusual anatomic variation
2. A prior cesarean, particularly one utilizing the classic incision
3. A vertex-presenting baby estimated to weigh more than 4,000 g with-

out preceding labor or a baby weighing more than 3,500 g in an abnormal lie or presentation without preceding labor

4. A baby of any size in a back-down, transverse lie
5. A need for coincident adnexal surgery or evaluation, abdominal exploration, or sterilization
6. The presence of established, acute fetal distress demanding expedient delivery (such as umbilical cord prolapse)
7. The absence of a qualified supervising or operating surgeon

THE TECHNIQUE OF EXTRAPERITONEAL CESAREAN DELIVERY (MODIFIED NORTON METHOD)

The patient should be properly selected and prepared. As part of the preparation and obtaining of consent for the operation, the patient should be informed that the customary approach to this operation involves a left paramedian incision. This approach facilitates dissection at the left side of the bladder and provides more nearly optimal exposure than the midline vertical incision. Some surgeons choose to utilize a transverse lower abdominal incision. If this is chosen, it is highly likely that a muscle-dividing (Cherney) incision will be required for adequate operative exposure (Chapter 12). The traditional Pfannenstiel incision, although successful in some cases, will frequently cause considerable mechanical difficulty for the operating team. In addition, the necessity to utilize two drains for adequate evacuation of the operative site should be explained to the patient and to the nursing staff, so that undue concern regarding the appearance of the drains will not trouble the patient, and the abundant efflux of serosanguineous drainage will not be alarming to the nursing staff and be interpreted as evidence of incipient evisceration. Also, the necessity to utilize drains ideally through sites other than the surgical wound further limits the feasibility of choosing a transverse incision.

With the presence of an experienced surgeon, the type of anesthesia utilized for this procedure is optional. If it is felt that an excessive amount of time may be required prior to delivery of the baby, such as with an inexperienced surgeon under direct instruction, the use of epidural anesthesia may be preferred.

With the patient positioned on the operating table in the left lateral tilt position, a standard Foley catheter or, alternatively, a triple-lumen catheter is placed in the bladder. Then 300–500 mL of solution is infused through the catheter into the bladder in order to distend it for better definition of the operative planes. The tubing leading to the collection bag should then be firmly occluded by a clamp. It is helpful to inject one 10-mL ampule of methylene blue into the infusion solution so that, if the bladder is approached too closely, the mucosa can be identified prior to complete fenestration of the bladder during the operation. This also provides the additional benefit of assisting in the diagnosis of unrecognized bladder entry prior to the conclusion of the operation, as well as utilizing the antibacterial effect of the dye. The infusion is begun rapidly at the beginning of the operation, is monitored, and ultimately is turned off by the circulating nurse once the desired anatomic effect has been achieved.

The surgeon operates from the patient's right side. Either a left paramedian or transverse abdominal incision is made. The peritoneum, peritoneal reflection, distended bladder with overlying transversalis fascia, and their respective anatomic relationships can be defined.

The transversalis fascia overlying the bladder is opened at approximately the midpoint between the symphysis and the dome of the bladder. Our preference is to bluntly extend this incision vertically up to (but not through) the peritoneal reflection at the dome. Other authors prefer a transverse incision. Once this has been done, the bladder will bulge forth, covered only by serosa. At this point, we prefer to begin the paravesical dissection prior to deflation of the bladder, as persisting inflation tends to maintain elevation of the peritoneal reflection, which drops below and behind the dome of the bladder for a variable distance. This facilitates dissection down to the uterine surface.

Dissection is carried out largely in a blunt manner, laterally and inferiorly displacing the fatty tissue gently while attempting to retract the bladder to the patient's right side (Figure 13.1). The left paravesical approach is chosen in preference to the right because of the higher incidence of uterine dextrorotation, which facilitates the definition and utilization of this space as opposed to that on the right.

In order to prevent inadvertent excursion into the vessels lying lateral to the uterus at this point, the surgeon is advised to palpate the uterine surface continually. If one attempts gently to dissect the fatty tissue laterally and the bladder medially from this surface, the likelihood of success is maximized.

Once the uterine surface has been identified and reached, with the peritoneal reflection above and the bladder retracted gently to the right, the bladder may be deflated.

It is *critical* to recognize that there is a thin layer of fascia overlying the uterus, separating the anterior lower uterine segment from the bladder. This must be entered sharply, extended carefully in a cephalocaudal direction, and retained on the uterine surface of the bladder. Failure to recognize the existence of this layer and preserve its integrity predisposes to inadvertent bladder entry. The achievement of the appropriate plane may be confirmed by minor bleeding occurring from the uterine surface.

Once this vesicouterine space is entered, it is developed bluntly with the finger to achieve the greatest amount of operating space. It will be noted that the bladder retracts more readily in its midportion than at the level of the left superior portion, where it remains firmly adherent to the peritoneal reflection. It is in this area that the obliterated umbilical arterial

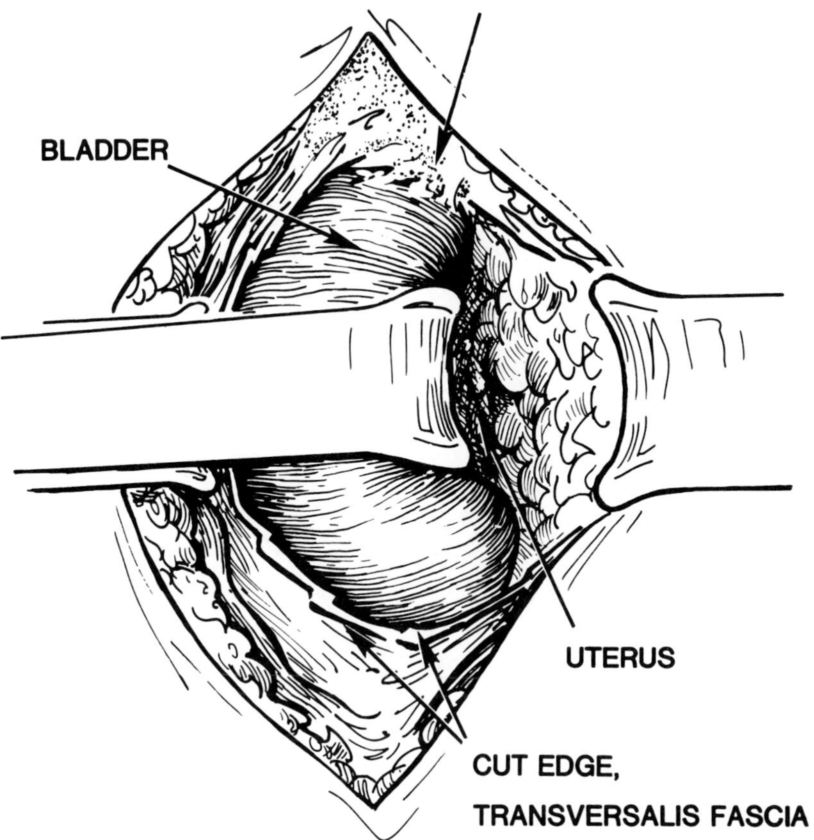

FIGURE 13.1 Bladder exposed and partly retracted to the patient's right after division of the transversalis fascia; paravesical "chicken fat" can be seen laterally. (Drawing by Michael Norviel.)

ligament can sometimes be identified. It will be noted that a greater space behind the bladder and on the anterior surface of the uterus can be developed bluntly than can be exposed and utilized readily for performing the hysterotomy. It is these anatomic restrictions that frequently make extraction of the baby somewhat more difficult than with the standard transperitoneal approach (Figure 13.2).

With the bladder elevated and retracted firmly to the right, a standard transverse lower uterine segment incision is made approximately 2–3 cm below the peritoneal reflection. The operator is warned that making the incision too low in the space, especially when the cervix has previously achieved an advanced state of effacement and dilatation, may result in entry into the cervix or the anterior fornix. It should be noted that this entire operative approach results in a somewhat more caudal anatomic

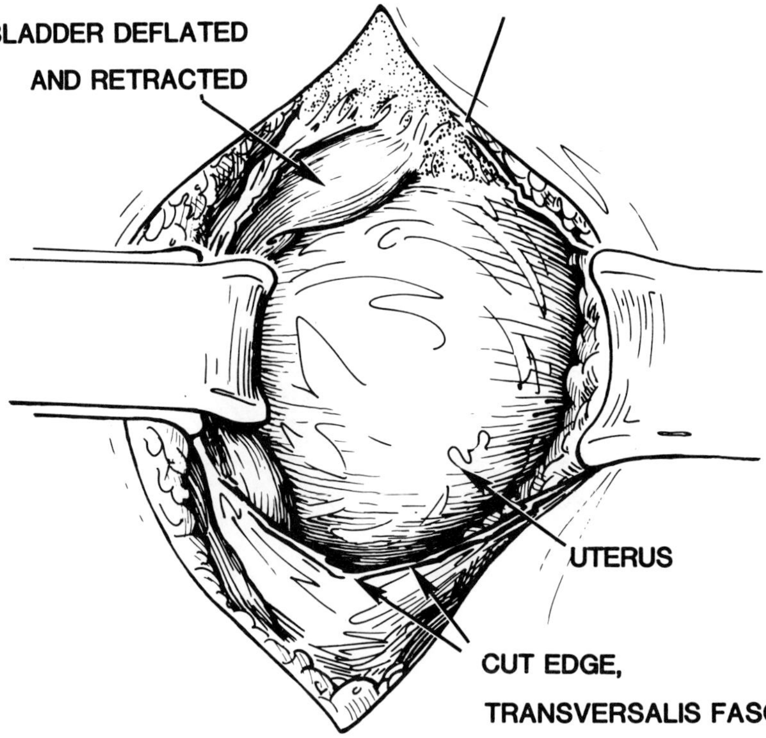

PERITONEAL REFLECTION

BLADDER DEFLATED AND RETRACTED

UTERUS

CUT EDGE, TRANSVERSALIS FASCIA

FIGURE 13.2 Bladder fully deflated and retracted following identification and dissection of the vesicouterine fascia (still adherent to the bladder); uterine surface exposed, ready for hysterotomy. (Drawing by Michael Norviel.)

location than one customarily visualizes with transperitoneal surgery. The right-hand portion of the hysterotomy incision must be extended underneath the displaced bladder. The baby may then be delivered through this space. It is suggested that standard cesarean forceps be present on the operating table in case undue difficulties in extracting the baby are encountered. Alternatives include Kielland forceps or a nonmetallic vacuum extractor apparatus.

Following delivery of the baby, the placenta is manually removed or expressed by fundal massage. Obviously, the uterus cannot be exteriorized during extraperitoneal surgery. It is often noted, however, that bleeding from the uterus following removal of the placenta is less than that commonly observed at transperitoneal surgery. The reasons for this are obscure, but may relate to the lack of broad ligament venous compression from exteriorization of the uterus. At this time, the peritoneal reflection should be reidentified and carefully examined for inadvertent entries. Any entries found should be closed with continuous suture of rapidly absorbable material. The hysterotomy incision can then be repaired in a standard manner.

Once the hysterotomy incision is closed, the surgeon may elect to infuse more of the methylene blue solution into the bladder to check for inadvertent entries. If any entries are identified, they should be repaired in the customary fashion. If none is found, preparations should be made for placement of the retrovesical drain.

A stab wound is made in the patient's left lower quadrant, ideally near the lateral margin of the rectus muscle at the bottom of the incision. Care should be taken to avoid perforation of the vessels lateral to the rectus. Through this is drawn a ¾-in Penrose drain (or, alternatively, a catheter from a vacuum evacuation drainage system), which is placed along the hysterotomy incision underneath the bladder to its most lateral extreme on the right side. Thereafter, the bladder is repositioned to close off the left paravesical defect, using rapidly absorbable suture materials. This is done in an attempt to exclude this space from the subfascial space, although, of course, this is not entirely possible.

A stab wound is made on the patient's right side corresponding anatomically to that on the left. A similar drain is drawn through this incision, extreme care being taken not to injure or puncture the bladder or vulnerable vessels. This drain is laid under the fascial incision. No specific attempts are made to close the transversalis fascia over the bladder. The rectus fascia ventral to the muscle is closed with interrupted sutures of absorbable material, the subcutaneous tissues are closed as per the operator's preference, and the skin is closed.

The drains should remain undisturbed for at least 48 hours, with the expectation that there will be substantial efflux of fluid for at least the first 24 hours.

The bladder catheter may be removed the following morning. If inadvertent bladder entry has occurred, the catheter may remain for 7–10 days. Under these circumstances, it can also serve as a convenient route for irrigation or removal of clot and prevention of infection.

Should circumstances dictate the necessity for conversion of this operation to the standard transperitoneal variety, this can be readily accomplished by incising the peritoneal reflection superior to the bladder.

One modification of the extraperitoneal cesarean procedure promoted by Bourgeois and Phaneuf[13] involves *bilateral* paravesical dissection and separation of the bladder from the lower uterine segment from both sides. Subsequently, having defined the lateral extents of the bladder and having carefully separated them from the uterine surface, one may approach the peritoneal reflection differently. This may facilitate the safe removal of the reflection from the dome of the bladder. One must also remember that the urachus is also in this location and may make the dissection more difficult. On occasion, the urachus may be patent.

Another modification of this concept was presented by Ricci.[25] This involves the standard midline abdominal approach to the peritoneum, which is then incised above the dome of the bladder, entering the peritoneal cavity in a transverse fashion. The bladder is then dissected off the uterine surface in the customary fashion, and the superior portion of parietal peritoneum is resutured to the visceral peritoneum on the uterine surface, thereby excluding the peritoneal cavity again prior to hysterotomy. The rationale behind this approach remains the same as for the others, and space may be enhanced for delivery. The placement of drains with this approach is more difficult.

POSTOPERATIVE ADVANTAGES

As stated earlier, extraperitoneal surgical patients frequently experience a return of normal bowel function and appetite more rapidly than those who have experienced transperitoneal surgery. Although the point at which alimentation is permitted in the postsurgical patient is largely a matter of individual physician judgment, using the customary criteria for arriving at such decisions frequently reveals the extraperitoneal patient to be advantaged. This frequently results in the potential for earlier discharge from the hospital than with the transperitoneal cesarean.

The drains may be advanced or removed whenever drainage is minimal. It is strongly advised that they not be removed before the fourth postoperative day. Although some have voiced concerns regarding the introduction of infection by the presence of these foreign bodies, we have seen no clear evidence of this in any patient offered the advantage of drainage in any surgical procedure. We also do not advocate any attempt to utilize the lumen of a Penrose drain by perforation of the material or packing of the lumen by other substances. It is our opinion that the Penrose drain functions most usefully by the egress of materials along its outer surface. Naturally, these drains must be secured either to the skin edge or by the utilization of a safety pin in order to prevent the drain from disappearing into the wound. Once the drains are removed, the skin incision, if small enough, can be allowed to close spontaneously or can be sutured or taped secondarily.

We believe that the properly chosen extraperitoneal candidate will have had a sufficiently high risk of infection that the prophylactic use of antibiotic treatment is logical. Given this view, we believe that beginning antibiotic treatment after cord clamping (at the latest) is most rational. Judging from the data on transperitoneal operations, it is likely that three doses of the appropriately selected antibiotic regimen from the time before surgery to a point 8–12 hours postoperatively should suffice in the patient without established clinical infection. If the patient is clinically infected, the duration of therapy is determined by criteria customarily applied by the responsible surgeon.

The material in this chapter was taken in large part from Perkins RP: Extraperitoneal cesarean section: Part I. Background and bacteriologic considerations; Part II. Indications and description. *Mediguide to OB/GYN* 1985; 4(2), 4(3), New York, Lawrence DellaCorte Publications for Miles Laboratories, with the kind permission of the editor.

REFERENCES

1. Waters EG: Supravesical extraperitoneal cesarean section. *Am J Obstet Gynecol* 39:423, 1940.
2. Latzko W: Uber den extraperitonealen Kaiserschmtl. *Zentralbl Gynaekol* 33:275, 1909.
3. Norton JF: A paravesical extraperitoneal cesarean section technique. *Am J Obstet Gynecol* 5:519, 1946.
4. Levine W, Weiner S: Late dystocia treated by the Norton extraperitoneal cesarean section. *Am J Obstet Gynecol* 54:1013, 1947.
5. Kettel WC, Randall JH: Experience with extraperitoneal cesarean section at the University of Iowa Hospitals. *Am J Obstet Gynecol* 58:510, 1949.
6. Stansfield FR, Drabble LWD: As assessment of extraperitoneal cesarean section. *Lancet* 1:74, 1951.
7. Atherton HE, Williamson PJ: A clinical comparison of extraperitoneal cesarean section and low cervical cesarean section for the potentially or frankly infected parturient. *Am J Obstet Gynecol* 68:1091, 1954.
8. Paternite CJ, Bachand MS: Extraperitoneal cesarean sections: Analysis of 93 consecutive operations. *Obstet Gynecol* 3:282, 1954.
9. Durfee RB: Elective extraperitoneal cesarean section. *Surg Gynecol Obstet* 110:173, 1960.
10. Gilbert CRA, Valdares J, Kaltreider DF, et al: Extraperitoneal cesarean section vs. the laparotrachelotomy in the era of modern antibiotic therapy. *Am J Obstet Gynecol* 66:79, 1953.
11. Imig JR, Perkins RP: Extraperitoneal cesarean section: A new need for old skills. *Am J Obstet Gynecol* 125:51, 1976.
12. Perkins RP: The merits of extraperitoneal cesarean section: A continuing experience. *J Reprod Med* 19:154, 1977.
13. Bourgeois GA, Phaneuf LE: The surgical anatomy of extraperitoneal cesarean section. *Am J Obstet Gynecol* 57:237, 1949.
14. Douglas RG, Landesman R: Recent trends in cesarean section. *Am J Obstet Gynecol* 59:96, 1950.
15. Ellis GJ, DeVita MR: Extraperitoneal cesarean section: A simplified technique. *Am J Obstet Gynecol* 82:695, 1961.
16. Dieckmann WJ: Discussion of the Cosgrove paper. *Am J Obstet Gynecol* 52:237, 1946.
17. DePalma RT, Leveno KJ, Cunningham FG, et al: Identification and management of women at high risk for pelvic infection following cesarean section. *Obstet Gynecol* 55(suppl):185S, 1980.
18. Gibbs RS, Hunt JE, Schwarz RH: A follow-up study on prophylactic antibiotics in cesarean section. *Am J Obstet Gynecol* 117:419, 1973.
19. Ledger WJ: The problem patient: Failure of surgical prophylaxis. *Hosp Pract* 14:165, 1979.
20. Batta S, Ostheimer GW, Weiss JB, et al: Neonatal effect of prolonged anesthetic induction for cesarean section. *Obstet Gynecol* 58:331, 1981.

21. Onderdonk AB, Bartlett JG, Louie T, et al: Microbial synergy in experimental intra-abdominal abscess. *Infect Immun* 13:22, 1976.
22. Freedman SI, Ang EP, Herz MG, et al: Meconium granulomas in post-cesarean section patients. *Obstet Gynecol* 59:383, 1982.
23. Perkins RP: The role of extraperitoneal cesarean section. *Clin Obstet Gynecol* 23:583, 1980.
24. Haesslein HC, Goodlin RC: Extraperitoneal cesarean section revisited. *Obstet Gynecol* 55:181, 1980.
25. Ricci JV, Marr JP: *Principles of Extraperitoneal Cesarean Section*. Philadelphia, Blakiston Co, 1942.

Chapter 14

Cesarean Delivery
The Transperitoneal Approach

Jeffrey P. Phelan, MD, and
Steven L. Clark, MD

During the past decade the cesarean delivery rate has risen dramatically. By 1984, cesarean delivery had become the number one in-hospital operative procedure in the United States[1] and accounted for more than 20% of all live births. This higher rate has been attributed to the performance of elective repeat cesareans and primary cesareans for fetal distress and breeches.[2] Although not as dramatic, the cesarean birth rate has also increased at the Los Angeles County–University of Southern California Medical Center (Table 14.1) since 1970, rising 55%. This rate would be 30% higher if vaginal birth after cesarean was not an available option for the obstetrical patients at the Medical Center.[3]

A primary reason for the rise in cesarean births is that there is no single indication for a cesarean. Chapters 2–8 discussed the multiple indications for cesarean delivery. At the same time, investigators have focused on various methods of reducing the cesarean delivery rate (Chapter 30). These include vaginal birth after cesarean (Chapters 31–35), external cephalic version of the breech or transverse lie (Chapter 36), vaginal delivery of the breech presentation (Chapter 3), and new techniques to assess fetal acid-base status (Chapter 5). But, as a rule, cesarean delivery is necessary whenever vaginal delivery cannot be safely accomplished without compromising the mother or the fetus.

The focus of this chapter is on the performance of cesarean and the reasons or underlying rationale for the various uterine incisions available. Thus, the decision has already been made to perform a cesarean, anesthesia has been administered (Chapters 10 and 11), and the abdomen has been opened (Chapter 12).

TABLE 14.1 Frequency of Cesarean Delivery at Los Angeles County–University of Southern California Medical Center, 1970–1986

Year	Total Deliveries	Cesareans
1970	9,775	910 (9.3%)
1971	9,425	822 (8.7%)
1972	9,421	910 (9.7%)
1973	10,434	1,068 (10.2%)
1974	11,584	1,078 (9.3%)
1975	11,629	1,166 (10.0%)
1976	13,780	1,468 (10.6%)
1977	13,303	1,653 (12.4%)
1978	12,538	1,549 (12.4%)
1979	13,213	1,624 (12.3%)
1980	13,297	1,687 (12.7%)
1981	14,712	1,632 (11.1%)
1982	14,871	1,751 (11.8%)
1983	16,660	1,828 (11.0%)
1984	16,557	2,006 (12.1%)
1985	18,143	2,319 (12.9%)
1986	17,147	2,465 (14.4%)

Source: RH Paul, unpublished data.

TYPES OF UTERINE INCISIONS

The choice of which uterine incisions to make is largely dictated by the clinical conditions at the time of the cesarean. Table 14.2 illustrates the usual reasons for the various types of uterine incisions. It must be emphasized that these are not absolutes but merely serve as a guide to the clinician. At times, a different type of uterine incision may be necessary.

The low transverse or Kerr uterine incision[4] is the most common uterine incision and is used in over 90% of all cesareans.[5] This incision (Figure 14.1) offers many advantages to the patient. It is easier to repair,

TABLE 14.2 Usual Indications for the Three Types of Uterine Incisions

Uterine Incision	Indication
Low transverse (Kerr)	Vertex presentation
Low vertical (Kronig)	Breech presentation (premature)
	Undeveloped lower uterine segment
Classical	Back-down transverse lie
	Anterior placenta previa
	Rapid delivery required
	Lower segment exposure technically not feasible
	Elective cesarean hysterectomy

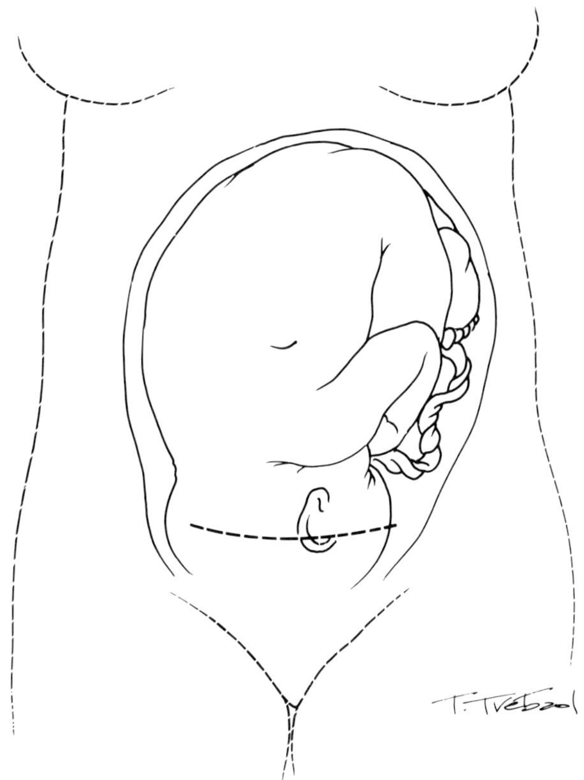

FIGURE 14.1 A low transverse uterine incision in a patient with a vertex presentation.

and adhesion formation and blood loss are reduced. Its greatest advantage is that it is associated with a low probability of dehiscence and/or rupture in a subsequent pregnancy.[5] Thus, patients with a low transverse uterine incision can be considered candidates for a subsequent trial of labor.

The disadvantages of the low transverse incision are few. If this incision is used in patients with an undeveloped lower uterine segment (eg, a premature breech), there is a greater chance of a lateral extension into the major vessels. This complication not only results in increased blood loss but may also necessitate hysterectomy. When an undeveloped lower uterine segment is encountered, a low vertical uterine incision may be prudent. Another disadvantage of a low transverse incision is that if more room is needed, the incision must be extended to either a J or T incision in order to deliver the baby.

The low vertical or Kronig incision[6] (Figure 14.2) is also a lower segment incision. The advantages of this incision are similar to those of the low transverse incision; it is preferred in patients with an undeveloped lower uterine segment. When it is used in these circumstances, there is a lower risk of lateral extension into the vessels. In addition, the Kronig

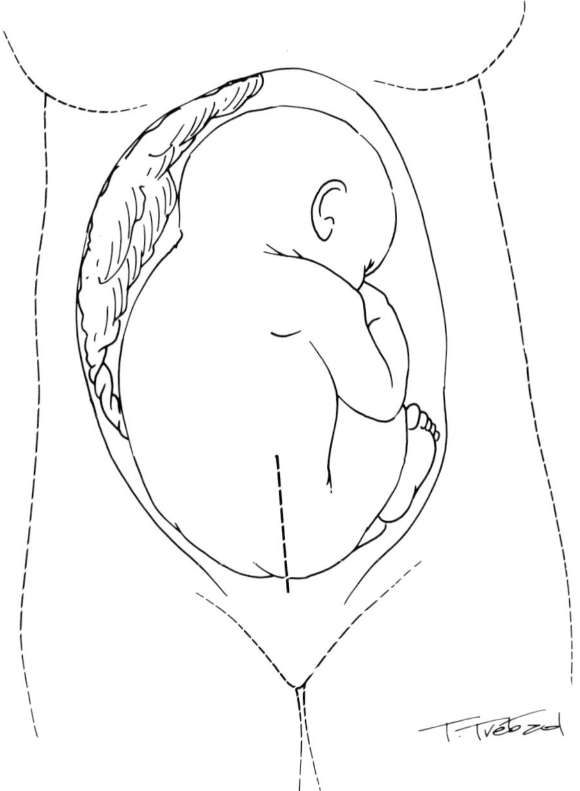

FIGURE 14.2 A low vertical uterine incision in a patient with a breech presentation.

incision is indicated if a contraction ring needs to be cut in order to deliver the infant. If more room is needed for delivery, adequate space can be easily obtained by extending the incision superiorly into the upper uterine segment. As in the patient with a low transverse uterine incision, patients whose low vertical incision is confined to the lower uterine segment have a low probability of dehiscence and/or rupture in a subsequent pregnancy[5] and can be considered candidates for a subsequent trial of labor.

The major advantages of the Kronig incision are similar to those of the low transverse uterine incision. A primary disadvantage of the low vertical uterine incision is the possibility of downward extension of the incision, which might tear the cervix, vagina, or bladder. This may occur despite a degree of bladder mobilization that would have been more than adequate for a low transverse incision. Finally, an extension of the incision into the upper uterine segment will preclude a subsequent trial of labor.

The classic uterine incision or vertical upper segment uterine incision is rarely required in contemporary obstetrics (Figure 14.3). As illustrated in Table 14.2, its use is limited to situations where the lower uterine segment cannot be adequately exposed, where elective cesarean hyster-

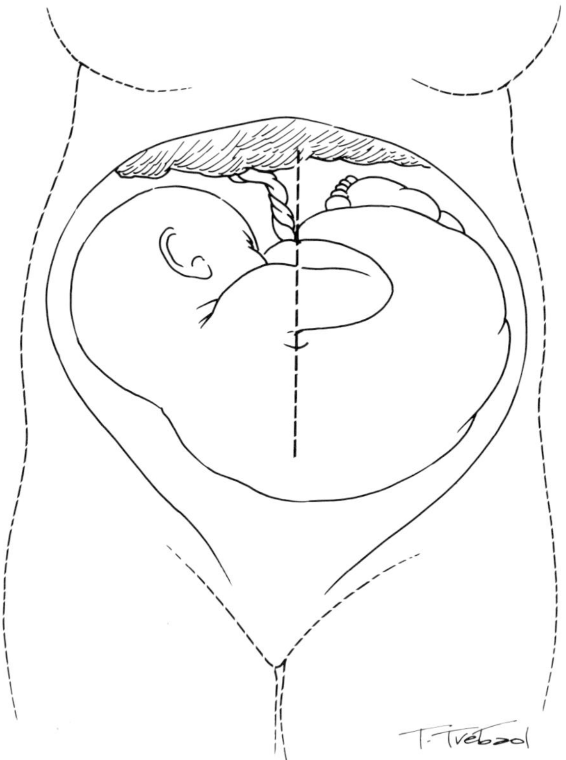

FIGURE 14.3 A classic cesarean incision in a patient with a back-down transverse lie.

ectomy is planned, or in the presence of a back-down transverse lie that cannot be converted to a cephalic or breech presentation.

There are a few advantages to this incision, including a decreased risk of bladder injury because the bladder is not taken down. Its primary advantage is that it allows rapid delivery when circumstances dictate such a need. Additionally, such an incision may allow the surgeon to avoid entering the uterus through an anterior placenta previa, thus decreasing the potential for significant fetal and maternal bleeding.[7] However, if the surgeon utilizes a low transverse or vertical incision, he can often dissect around the placenta rather than going through it, thus obviating the need for a classic uterine incision.

The disadvantages of the classic uterine incision are many, resulting in limited use of this incision in modern obstetrics. In addition to the difficulties associated with repair, adhesion formation is more common and infection rates are higher. This incision is also associated with a greater risk of rupture in a subsequent pregnancy.[5,8] As a result, patients with a classic uterine incision are cautioned against a subsequent trial of labor and are advised to undergo elective repeat cesarean delivery when fetal lung maturity has been documented (Chapter 10).

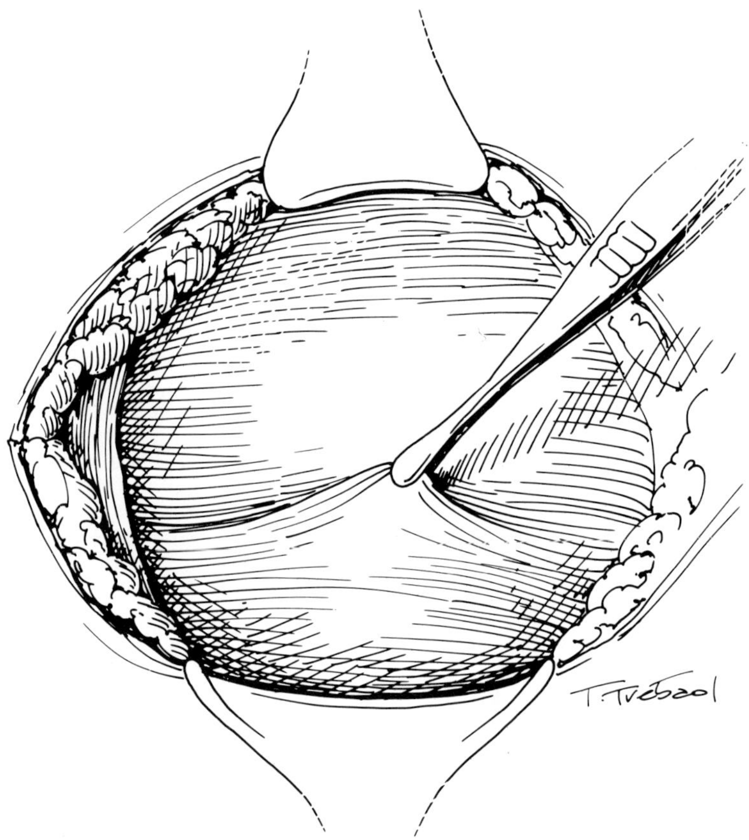

FIGURE 14.4 The vesicouterine serosa is grasped with forceps in the midline. The bladder has been retracted caudad.

LOW TRANSVERSE CESAREAN DELIVERY

Because the low transverse uterine incision is the most common type of cesarean delivery, it will serve as the basis for illustrating the technique of cesarean delivery. After the abdomen has been opened (Chapter 12), the surgeon will frequently find that despite the left lateral tilt of the mother, the uterus is frequently dextrorotated. This places the left round ligament closer to the midline. For diagrammatic purposes this is not demonstrated, but the surgeon must remember that dextrorotation will shift the uterine midline. Thus, proper identification of the uterine position prior to making an incision is the first important step.

Once the position of the uterus has been determined, a loose reflection of vesicouterine serosa that overlies the uterus is grasped with forceps in the midline, as illustrated (Figure 14.4). The vesicouterine serosa is then incised with either a scalpel or scissors and opened transversely at the upper margin of the bladder (Figure 14.5).

When opening transversely, the scissors are directed laterally and

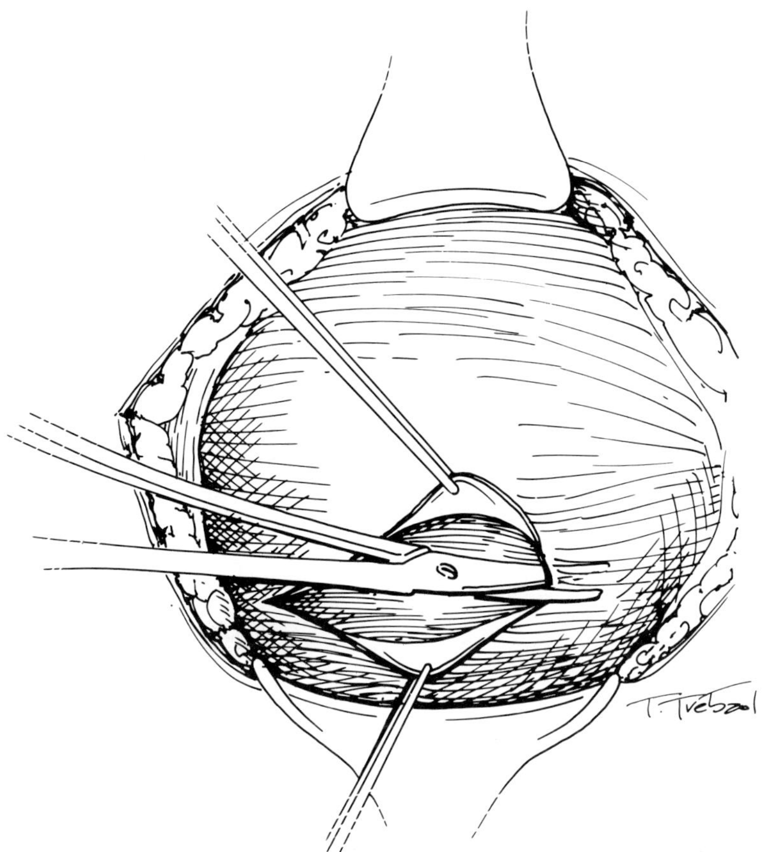

FIGURE 14.5 The vesicouterine serosa is incised and opened transversely with scissors.

slightly upward toward the margins of the uterus. After the vesicouterine serosa has been opened, the lower portion of the visceral peritoneum is grasped with forceps and the bladder is reflected free of the underlying lower uterine segment (Figure 14.6). Either sharp or blunt dissection may be used, depending upon the clinical circumstances. When using blunt dissection, pressure is applied to the lower uterine segment (as opposed to the bladder) in the midline. Once free in the midline, a sweeping motion can be used cautiously to free up the bladder laterally. With a low transverse uterine incision, the bladder flap does not need to be taken down as far as is necessary with a low vertical uterine incision.

With the bladder reflected free of the underlying myometrium, a bladder retractor is placed in the incision to keep the bladder out of the operative field. A small uterine incision (Figure 14.7) is made above the detached bladder. During this time, suction is used to keep the field clear and to minimize the risk of fetal laceration.[9] The incision is carried through the myometrium to the fetal membranes or, on occasion, into the uterine cavity. This is the point of greatest risk for fetal laceration (an uncommon

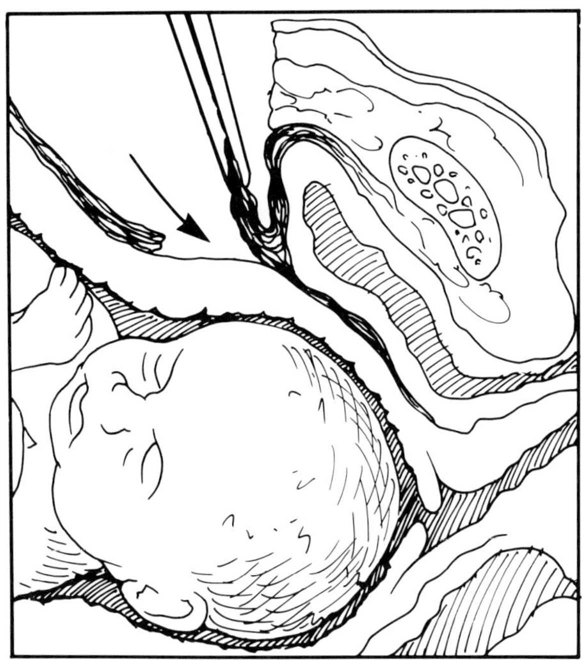

FIGURE 14.6 On cross section, the bladder is reflected free of the lower uterine segment with either sharp or blunt dissection. The arrow illustrates the direction of the dissection. The forceps are on the vesicouterine serosa that contains the bladder.

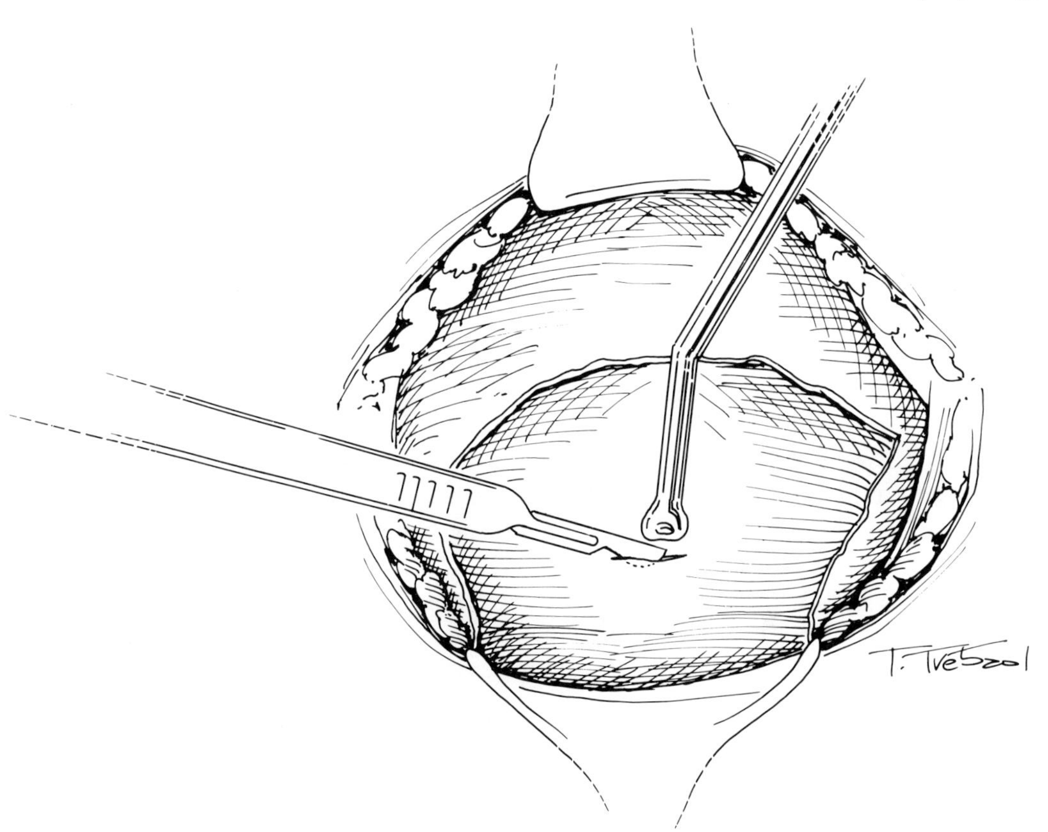

FIGURE 14.7 With a bladder retractor in place to keep the bladder out of the field, a small incision is made in the lower uterine segment. Suction is used to keep the field clear.

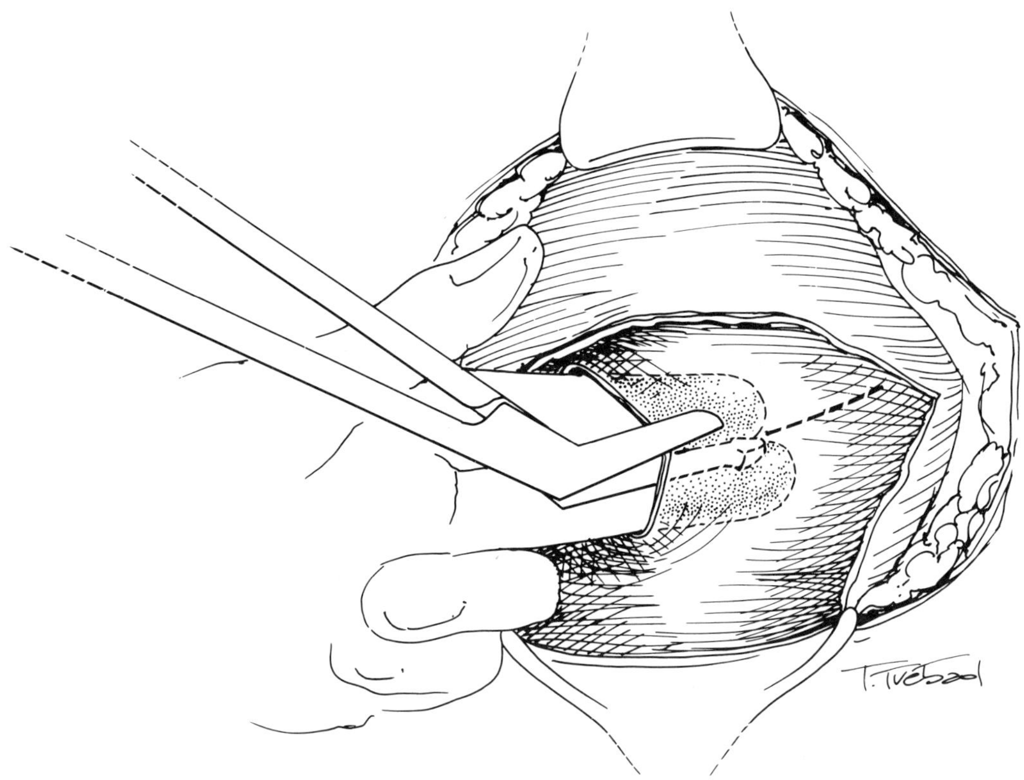

FIGURE 14.8 Once the uterus is entered, the uterine incision is extended laterally and upward with bandage scissors. Fingers are inserted to protect against fetal injury.

complication), which may occur even in expert hands, especially when the lower uterine segment is extremely thin or when rapid delivery is mandatory.

Once the uterus has been entered, the incision can be extended transversely, using bandage scissors (Figure 14.8) or the surgeon's index fingers. Either approach protects the fetus from injury. If bandage scissors are used, a Richardson retractor is often necessary for lateral retraction and adequate visualization of the incision. This approach permits better control of the incision and enables the surgeon to curve the incision upward and avoid the uterine vessels. In contrast, the use of the surgeon's index fingers is a quicker technique. This approach involves hooking the index fingers in the uterine incision. While applying pressure laterally and *upward*, the fingers are pulled apart and the myometrium is split.

DELIVERY OF THE INFANT AND PLACENTA

Prior to the delivery of the fetal head, it is important to assess the adequacy of the uterine and abdominal incisions. This will help avoid a trapped fetal head with a breech delivery or shoulder dystocia with a macrosomic fetus. In addition, an adequate uterine incision reduces the risk of an extension into the broad ligament and the uterine vessels. If there is inadequate space to deliver the infant through the transverse uterine incision, the incision can be converted either to a J incision by extending the transverse uterine incision along the lateral edge of the uterus or to a T or Anchor incision by an upward midline extension into the upper uterine segment. Under both of these circumstances, a subsequent trial of labor would not be indicated because of a greater risk of uterine rupture[5,8]; however, such an incision is preferable to a traumatic delivery through an inadequate uterine incision. If the abdominal incision seems inadequate, a Cherney incision (Chapter 12) will permit adequate exposure. After adequate exposure has been obtained, the retractors are removed and a hand is inserted into the uterine cavity. The fetal head is gently elevated with the hand and through the uterine incision. If the head is deep in the maternal pelvis, short-handled Simpson forceps can be used to elevate it. When the head is wedged in the maternal pelvis, upward pressure by an assistant using a sterile glove should help dislodge it. When elevating the fetal head wedged in the maternal pelvis, the surgeon's wrist should be kept straight to avoid using the lower uterine segment as a fulcrum; such technique minimizes the risk of a uterine laceration. Under certain circumstances, such as an unengaged vertex during an elective cesarean, a vacuum extractor, as illustrated in Figure 14.9, may be helpful in delivering the fetal head.[10] But the vacuum extractor may not be helpful in all circumstances. For instance, its use is associated with a longer interval between the uterine incision and the delivery.[11] In situations such as fetal distress, the use of the vacuum extractor could delay delivery and potentially aggravate any underlying fetal compromise. In the case of a breech or transverse lie, the vacuum is not indicated and the infant must be manually extracted.

Once the infant's head is delivered, the nasal and oral pharynxes are suctioned with a bulb syringe or, if meconium is present, with a Delee trap. With the help of an assistant, fundal pressure is applied transabdominally and the remainder of the body is delivered. At this time, a dilute intravenous infusion of oxytocin (20 units/L) is administered through the intravenous line to stimulate uterine contractions, reduce blood loss, and enhance placental separation. The umbilical cord is doubly clamped while the infant is kept at the level of the maternal abdominal wall. Once the cord is clamped and cut, the infant is handed to the resuscitation team. Then a blood sample is obtained from the placental end of the cord for further analysis.

If the need for umbilical cord gases is indicated from the patient's clinical circumstances, they should also be obtained at this time. The use of cord gases would appear to be beneficial in confirming not only the presence of fetal distress but also the degree and basis of any fetal acidosis.[12] Cord gases are obtained by doubly clamping a 10-cm length of

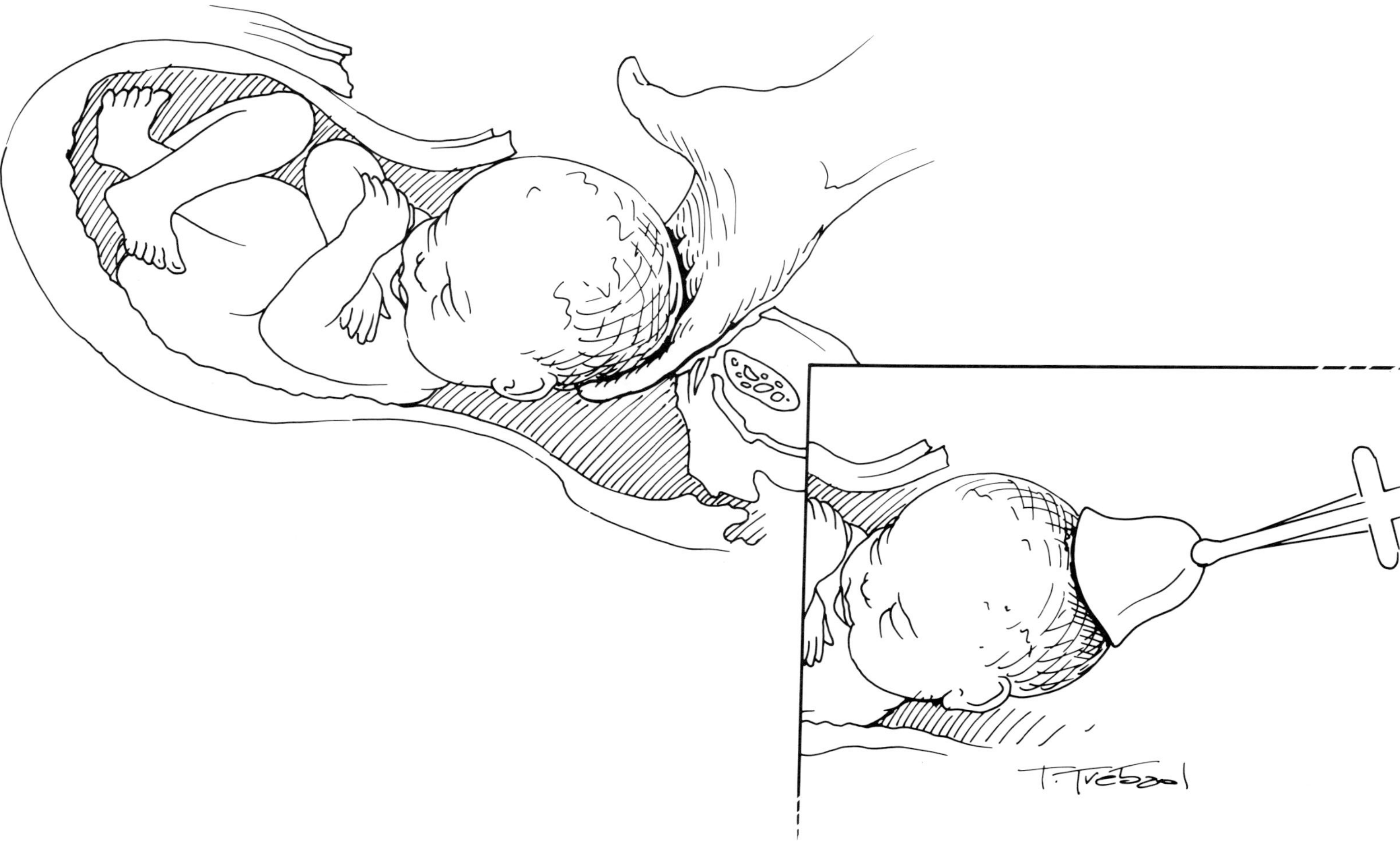

FIGURE 14.9 On cross section, the infant's head is delivered through the transverse lower uterine incision with the hand. *In the lower panel* a vacuum extractor is used to deliver the head.

cord. Using two separate syringes, blood is aspirated from an umbilical artery with one syringe and from the umbilical vein with the other syringe. The blood is placed on ice and sent to the laboratory for analysis.

The uterine incision is immediately inspected for any bleeding sites. Significant bleeding vessels are clamped with ring forceps or a similar instrument. If bleeding is minimal, the placenta can be delivered with gentle traction of the umbilical cord or manually. Once removed, the placenta is inspected to determine whether any fragments are missing. The uterine cavity is then inspected and wiped clean with a moist laparotomy sponge to remove any remaining fetal membrane, placental fragments, or vernix. If the patient has not been in labor, a ring forcep or pean clamp can be used to determine cervical patency. If the cervix is closed, it can be *cautiously* dilated with either instrument to ensure lochia drainage. The contaminated instrument should then be removed from the operating field.

REPAIR OF THE UTERINE INCISION

After the delivery of the infant and the placenta, the uterus may be delivered onto the maternal abdominal wall. Exteriorization of the uterus does not expose the mother to greater morbidity, and it seems to facilitate uterine repair and to reduce blood loss.[13] A moist laparotomy sponge can be used to drape the uterus in order to keep it moist and to afford better traction for repair of the incision. Uterine massage is also carried out simultaneously. Under most circumstances, uterine bleeding is encountered at the angles of the incision and may be dealt with by the placement of ring forceps or similar instruments. A third ring forcep can also be used to grasp the lower portion of the lower uterine segment in the midline. This will permit better visualization and allow easier repair of the uterine incision.

The uterine incision can be closed with one or two layers of continuous chromic suture. Figure 14.10 illustrates the first layer of a two-layer closure of a low transverse uterine incision. It is important to begin the closure with the initial stitch just beyond the angle of the incision. In Figure 14.10, the first layer is closed with a continuous locking stitch of absorbable suture through the myometrium. Interrupted stitches are also acceptable (Figures 14.13). If possible, avoid bringing the needle back out once it has been inserted to reduce the possibility of bleeding.

Previous reports[14,15] have expressed concern that a suture that incorporated the decidua would increase the probability of endometriosis in the scar. These investigators suggested that to avoid this complication, the suture should be placed only through the myometrium, not through the endometrial lining. However, this complication is relatively rare,[16] and

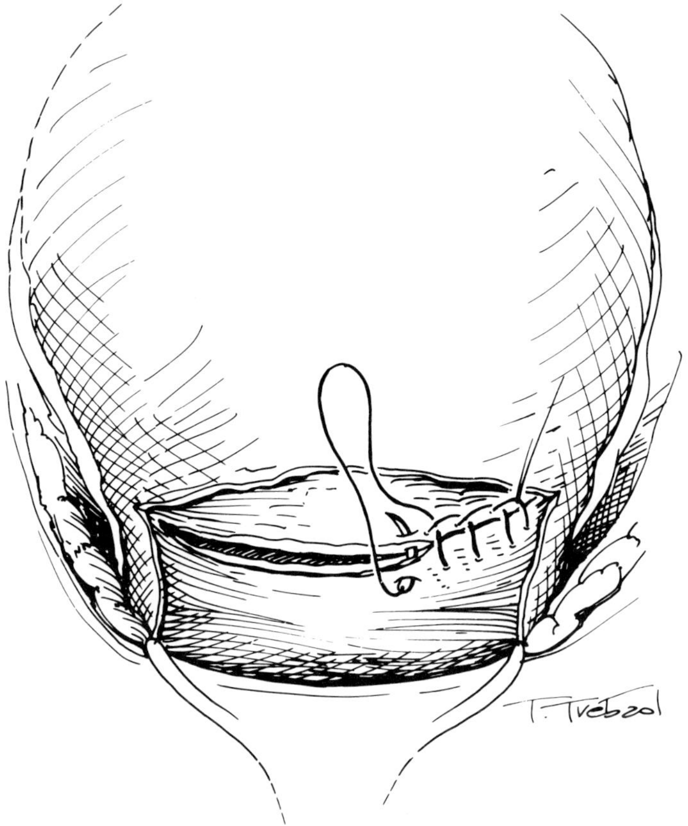

FIGURE 14.10 A continuous running lock stitch of absorbable suture is used to close the first layer of the uterine incision.

the additional time spent attempting to avoid endometrial incorporation probably exposes the patient to unnecessary operating and anesthesia time.

On occasion, a two-layer closure may be unnecessary.[17] This is especially true in patients with thin lower uterine segments in whom reapproximation with one layer has been achieved and hemostasis is adequate. However, many physicians routinely elect to close the uterus with two layers. A second inverted layer can be closed using a continuous Lembert's or Cushing's stitch of chromic suture (Figure 14.11). This may be achieved with either a vertical or horizontal stitch. The latter approach is frequently reserved for situations in which there is insufficient room to place a stitch without injuring the bladder. Once repaired, the incision site is inspected for any bleeding points. If any are present, a figure-eight stitch is usually sufficient to stop the bleeding.

With adequate hemostasis of the repaired lower uterine segment and any lacerations or extensions, the vesicouterine serosa is reapproximated

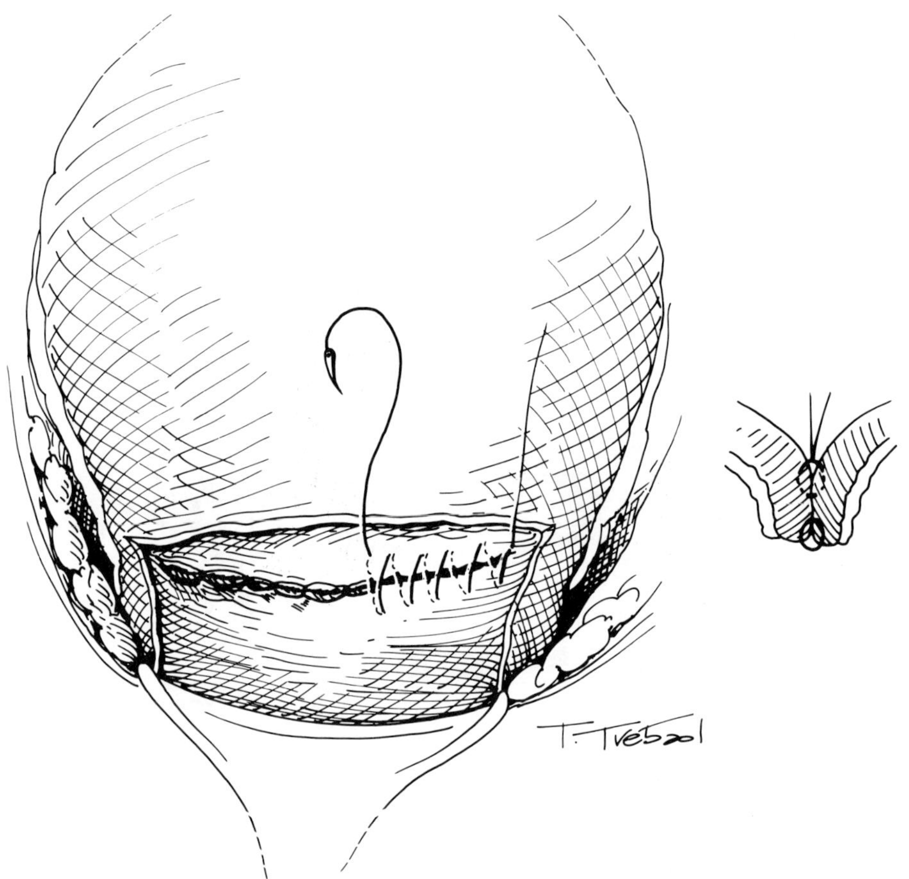

FIGURE 14.11 A second layer closure. In this case, a vertical imbricating stitch is used to invert the raw edge of the uterus.

with a running suture of 00 chromic (Figure 14.12). The uterus, fallopian tubes, and ovaries are inspected for evidence of any pathology. Prior to uterine replacement, surgical sterilization and/or incidental procedures such as cystectomy or oophorectomy (Chapter 17) can be performed. Once they are completed, the uterus is returned to the peritoneal cavity.

Before abdominal closure is started, the incision site should be reinspected for evidence of bleeding. If no further bleeding is evident, blood and amniotic fluid are suctioned from the paracolic gutters and cul-de-sac. After a correct needle and sponge count, the abdominal wall is closed as outlined in Chapter 12.

LOW VERTICAL INCISION

An alternative to the low transverse uterine incision, the low vertical incision (Figure 14.2), requires the bladder to be taken down further than

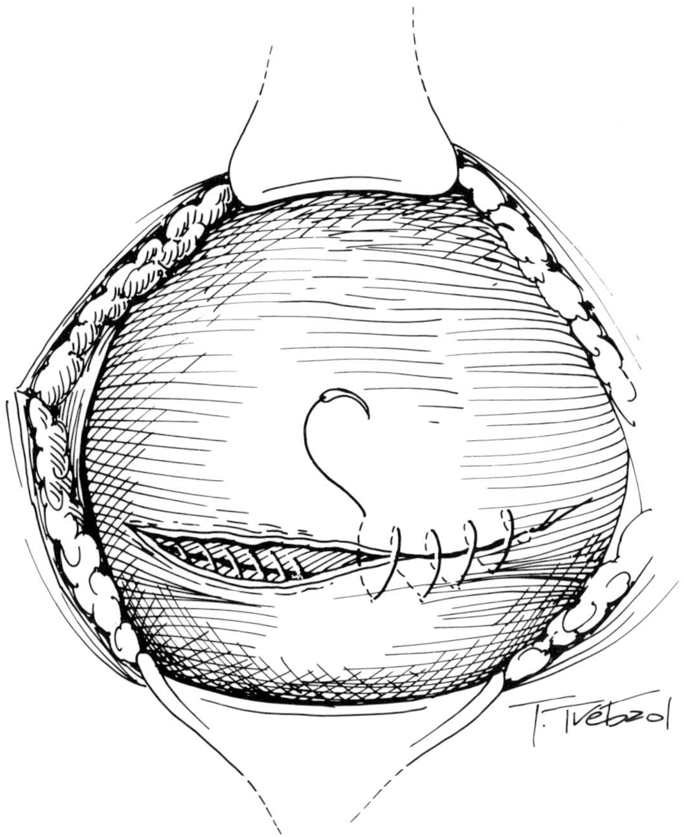

FIGURE 14.12 The vesicouterine serosa and bladder flap are reapproximated using a continuous stitch of absorbable suture.

with the low transverse incision. This incision is initiated in the lowest point of the exposed myometrium and is extended cephalad. Whether the incision needs to be extended into the upper uterine segment will depend upon the circumstances of the individual case. Any apparent or suspected extension into the upper segment needs to be carefully documented in the chart and the operative report. As an additional safeguard, it is helpful to inform the patient and review with her the potential risk and complications of such an incision on any subsequent pregnancy. Patients whose low vertical incision is confined to the lower uterine segment may be candidates for a subsequent trial of labor. In contrast, incisions that involve the upper uterine segment are more likely to rupture, and patients with such an incision are not considered candidates for a subsequent trial of labor.

The two-layer repair of a low vertical uterine incision (Figure 14.13) is similar to that of a low transverse incision. For ease of repair, the initial stitch should be placed beyond the inferior edge of the incision. From there a running stitch of absorbable suture (Figure 14.13), a running lock

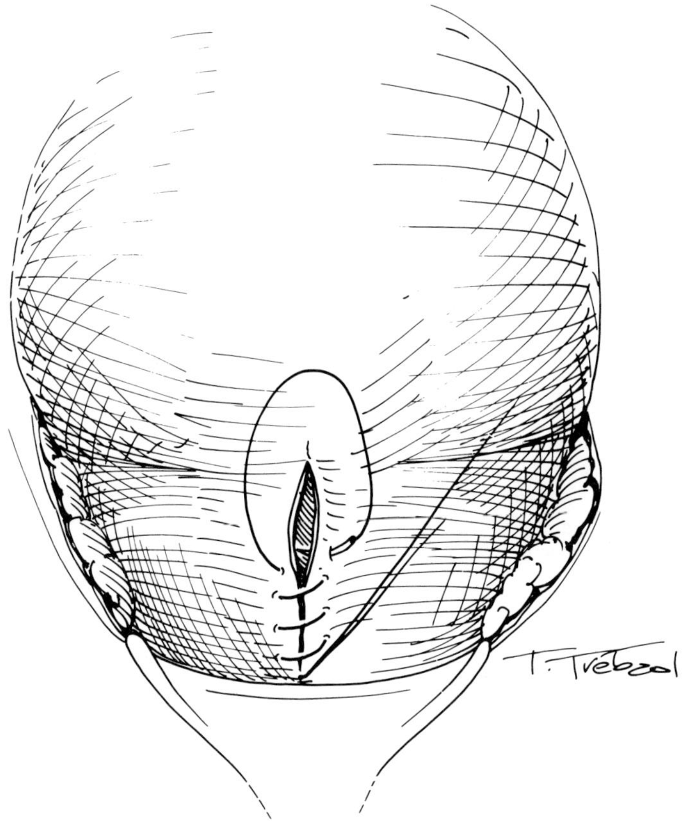

FIGURE 14.13 A first layer closure of a low vertical incision using a continuous stitch of absorbable suture. Note that the first stitch is placed beyond the inferior edge of the incision.

stitch (Figure 14.10), or others, as previously discussed, can be used to close the incision.[17] Once the low vertical incision is repaired, the cesarean is completed as outlined in the preceding section on the closure of the low transverse incision.

CLASSIC CESAREAN INCISION

Though rarely necessary, the classic cesarean incision is made through the anterior wall of the uterus and extended from near the top of the uterine fundus to above the level of the bladder (Figure 14.3). The uterus is initially incised with a scalpel and the incision is extended with bandage scissors. Following the delivery of the infant and the placenta, the uterine incision is closed with absorbable suture similar to that used with the low transverse incision. But due to the thickness of the uterine wall, a three-layer closure is frequently necessary. As an additional precaution, it is suggested that the final layer be inverted to eliminate any raw surface areas and thus

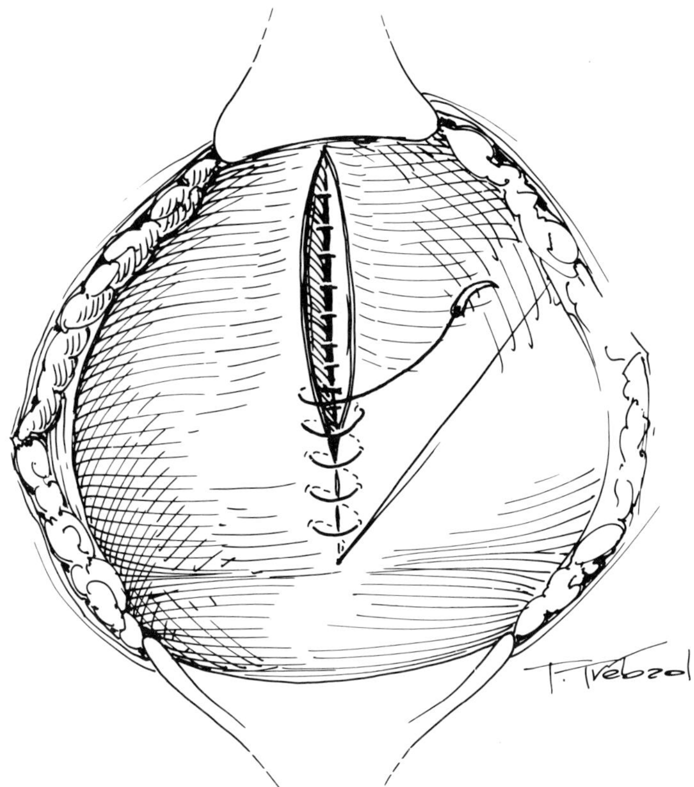

FIGURE 14.14 The final layer of a classic cesarean incision is closed.

reduce the potential for adhesion formation (Figure 14.14). A three-layer closure may not always be necessary. For instance, Potter and Elton[18] have suggested that interrupted sutures placed in the outer third of the uterus are sufficient for adequate uterine closure. As with the low vertical incision that extends in the upper segment, a classical incision needs to be documented in the medical records and the patient fully informed, because patients with upper segment uterine incisions are not considered candidates for a subsequent trial of labor.[5,8]

REFERENCES

1. Rutkow I: Obstetric and gynecologic operations in the United States, 1979 to 1984. *Obstet Gynecol* 67:755, 1986.
2. Shiono PA, McNellis D, Rhoads GS: Reasons for the rising cesarean delivery rates. *Obstet Gynecol* 69:696, 1987.
3. Phelan JP, Clark SL, Diaz F, et al. Vaginal birth after cesarean. *Am J Obstet Gynecol* 157:1510, 1987.
4. Kerr JMM: The technic of cesarean section with special reference to the lower uterine segment incision. *Am J Obstet Gynecol* 12:729, 1926.

5. Tahilramaney MP, Boucher M, Eglinton GS, et al: Previous cesarean section and trial of labor. Factors related to uterine dehiscence. *J Reprod Med* 29:17, 1984.
6. Kronig B: Transperitonealer Cervikaler Kaiser-Schnitt, in Doderlein A, Kronig B (eds): *Operative Gynakologie.* 1912, p 879.
7. Pritchard JA, McDonald PC, Gant NF (eds): *Williams Obstetrics,* ed 17. Norwalk, Conn, Appleton-Century-Crofts, 1985, p 411.
8. Pedowitz P, Schwartz RM: The true incidence of silent rupture of cesarean section scars: A prospective analysis of 403 cases. *Am J Obstet Gynecol* 74:1071, 1957.
9. Gerber AH: Accidental incision of the fetus during cesarean delivery. *Int J Gynaecol Obstet* 12:46, 1974.
10. Boehm FH: Vacuum extraction during cesarean section. *South Med J* 78:1502, 1985.
11. Arad I, Linder N, Bercovici B: Vacuum extraction at cesarean section neonatal outcome. *J Perinatol Med* 14:137, 1986.
12. Wible JL, Petrie RH, Koons A, et al: The clinical use of umbilical cord acid-base determinations in perinatal surveillance and management. *Clin Perinatol* 9:387, 1982.
13. Hershey DW, Quilligan EJ: Extraabdominal uterine exteriorization at cesarean section. *Obstet Gynecol* 52:189, 1978.
14. Sortor RF, Brines OA: Endometriosis involving cesarean section abdominal scar. Report of a case. *Obstet Gynecol* 10:425, 1957.
15. Kale S, Shuster M, Shangold J: Endometrioma in a cesarean section scar: Case report and review of the literature. *Am J Obstet Gynecol* 111:596, 1971.
16. Chatterjee SK: Scar endometriosis: A clinicopathologic study of 17 cases. *Obstet Gynecol* 56:81, 1980.
17. Hibbard LT: Cesarean section and other surgical procedures, in Gabbe SG, Niebyl JR, Simpson JL (eds): *Obstetrics—Normal and Problem Pregnancies.* New York, Churchill Livingstone, 1986, pp 517–546.
18. Potter MG, Elton NW: An improved method of closure in high classical cesarean section. *Am J Obstet Gynecol* 43:303, 1942.

Chapter 15

Cesarean Hysterectomy

David L. Barclay, MD

EVOLUTION OF THE OPERATION

Until the latter half of the 19th century, maternal mortality associated with cesarean birth approached 100% in some large maternity hospitals. Cesarean delivery was an operation of last resort performed under unsterile conditions; the uterus was often infected after protracted labor and prolonged rupture of the fetal membranes. Prior to 1882, when Max Sanger introduced closure of the uterine incision with multiple sutures, the uterus, with a gaping wound, was returned to the peritoneal cavity. Maternal death was the result of intraperitoneal hemorrhage and spillage of infected uterine contents. Cesarean hysterectomy was developed as a heroic operation of necessity in an attempt to reduce the exceptional maternal mortality rate of cesarean delivery.[1]

The period 1768–1869 should be considered the era of speculation. In 1768, Joseph Cavallini successfully excised the uteri of pregnant dogs and sheep, proving that the organ was not essential to life. Although several authors suggested that removal of the uterus at the time of cesarean delivery might reduce the mortality rate, Horatio Robinson Storer of Boston, in 1868, was the first to perform the operation.[2] In his patient, a tumor blocked the pelvis to such a degree that vaginal delivery was impossible, even with craniotomy. Tumors in the uterine wall prevented uterine contraction, and there was severe hemorrhage. A constrictor was placed around the lower uterine segment, the corpus amputated, and the cervical stump seared by hot iron and exteriorized through the lower pole of the abdominal closure. The patient survived the 3-hour operation under chloroform anesthesia but died on the third postoperative day, probably from sepsis and hemorrhage.

Eduardo Porro of Pavia, Italy, planned for and performed the first successful cesarean hysterectomy in 1876.[2] Prior to that time no woman in that city had ever survived a cesarean birth. The patient was a dwarf who had obvious pelvic deformity, resulting in absolute cephalopelvic disproportion. She underwent an early operation after only 6 hours of labor and rupture of the membranes. Operating time was 30 minutes, and a wire Cintrat's constrictor was used around the cervical stump to secure hemostasis. After incision of the uterus and removal of the infant, the uterus was delivered from the abdominal cavity. A snare was placed over the uterine fundus and both ovaries and snugged securely; the uterus and adnexa were excised. Peritoneal toilet was accomplished and a drain was placed through the cul-de-sac. The cervical stump was exteriorized through the lower pole of the abdominal incision to prevent intraperitoneal spillage, and the incision was closed with silver wire. The snare was removed on the fourth postoperative day and a gangrenous portion of the cervical stump sloughed off. The original Porro operation, therefore, consisted of a subtotal hysterectomy and bilateral salpingo-oophorectomy.

In 1878, Muller suggested the first major modification in the operation.[3] He delivered the uterus through the abdominal incision and constricted the lower uterine segment with an elastic tube, after which the uterus was incised, delivery effected, and the corpus amputated. The operation required a long incision, but the peritoneal cavity was protected from contamination. However, placement of the constrictor caused asphyxia of the child. The Porro-Muller operation had many advocates. In 1880, Isaac Taylor of New York performed the first Porro-type cesarean hysterectomy in the United States. He returned the cervical stump to the abdominal cavity after securing hemostasis, and no drains were employed. Unfortunately, his patient died on the 26th postoperative day from a pulmonary embolus. This unfortunate outcome, probably unrelated to the operative procedure, retarded acceptance of the technique of returning the cervical stump to the peritoneal cavity.

In 1880, Harris of Philadelphia reported the results of the first 50 cases of "cesarean ovaro-hysterectomy" in the world literature.[4] There were 29 maternal and 7 fetal deaths. Twenty-three of the operations had been performed in Italy and 11 in Australia. In 1881, E. Richardson performed the first successful cesarean hysterectomy in the United States; he used the Porro-Muller technique. Spencer Wells, in 1881, performed the first total cesarean hysterectomy, for cancer of the cervix. Goodson, in the United Kingdom in 1884, not only performed the first such operation in that country but used a transverse incision that was extended laterally by traction; this was the first reference to the low segment operation. In addition, he summarized 134 Porro operations. Intraperitoneal placement of the cervical stump was associated with a 77% mortality compared to a 53% mortality for extraperitoneal placement.[3]

Other contributors to evolution of the operations were Tait (1890), Moller (1892), and Von Waerz (1892). The last author introduced specific vessel ligation and returned the cervix to the peritoneal cavity in uninfected patients; otherwise, it was exteriorized. Otto Weiss, in 1900, reinforced interest in "dropping the stump" back into the peritoneal cavity in uninfected patients and described the operative technique in detail. In 1901, it was reported that of the 1,097 operations that had been performed to that date, the overall maternal mortality was 24.8%.[3]

In the United States during the first three decades of the twentieth century, the major indication for cesarean hysterectomy was intrauterine infection. Low cervical or extraperitoneal cesarean delivery subsequently became the procedure of choice in the presence of intrauterine infection.[1] J.W. Harris, in 1922, reported the John Hopkins Hospital experience: 64 subtotal hysterectomies in 223 cesareans, with a maternal mortality of 4.68%.[5] Eighteen operations were performed for sterilization. Lash and Cummings, in 1935, listed their indications for cesarean hysterectomy and included sterilization.[6]

Until the early 1940s, the major indications for surgery were hemorrhage, infection, and uterine pathology such as ruptured uterus or uterine fibroids. Little emphasis was placed on elective sterilization. In 1945, Wilson reported that 8.7% of all cesarean sections performed at the University of Rochester included a hysterectomy.[7] Indications were hemorrhage, uterine pathology, intrapartum infection, and sterilization. Reis and DeCosta, in 1947, summarized the literature from that era and concluded that in the United States, about 2.54% of cesareans were terminated by hysterectomy, with a maternal mortality of 5.2% in contrast to 3.42% for cesarean birth; no attempt was made to separate the results of elective operations from those of lifesaving procedures performed to prevent death from hemorrhage.[8] In 1948, Dieckman et al reported 153 cases of cesarean hysterectomy performed since 1931.[9] Again, the primary indications were uterine pathology and infection; some operations were performed for sterilization.

Increased availability of antimicrobial drugs and the introduction of blood banking procedures in the early 1940s expanded indications for all elective operations, including elective cesarean hysterectomy. In 1951, Davis advocated total cesarean hysterectomy for elective sterilization at the time of cesarean, removal of a diseased uterus, or removal of the uterus no longer functionally useful for a woman near the climacteric.[9] From July 1, 1947, to April 1, 1951, 140 of 700 cesareans performed at the Chicago Lying-In Hospital were terminated by hysterectomy. In 1953, Dyer et al reported 84 cases of total hysterectomy following cesarean or in the immediate puerperal period, performed in New Orleans.[10] He emphasized the fact that cesarean hysterectomy was the method of choice for surgical removal of a diseased uterus. The concept of total cesarean hysterectomy was strongly supported by that report. Because the dilated cervix is difficult to identify, he proposed passing a finger into the vagina, through the cervical canal, to identify the lower limits of the cervix. The last subtotal operation on the Tulane Service, Charity Hospital, in New Orleans, was performed in 1951.[11] This policy decision was predicated on reoperation and postoperative death among three patients who had undergone the subtotal operation for a ruptured uterus that extended into the cervix and vaginal fornix, resulting in postoperative hemorrhage. In 1955, Bradbury described refinements of the operative technique of total hysterectomy.[12] During the remainder of the 1950s, cesarean hysterectomy was openly advocated as a sterilization procedure, and indications for most operations were considered to be elective.[13–24] Complications of the operation were deemphasized. Brunschwig and Barber, in 1958, reported a radical cesarean hysterectomy and pelvic lymphadenectomy for treatment of cancer of the cervix.[25]

During the 1960s, there were a number of publications concerning cesarean hysterectomy primarily for elective reasons.[26–41] In 1963, Pletsch and Sandberg reviewed 1,819 cesarean hysterectomies reported in the American literature between 1950 and June 1962.[34] The question was raised of whether or not cesarean hysterectomy should replace cesarean delivery and tubal ligation for sterilization. Weed questioned the fate of the postcesarean uterus, and others were concerned about the "post-tubal ligation syndrome."[42] One-half of the September 1969 issue of *Clinical Obstetrics and Gynecology* was devoted to articles on the subject.[41] The first 1,000 consecutive operations performed between January 1, 1938, and September 1, 1959, at the Charity Hospital in New Orleans were reviewed.[11] Operations were included for review only if performed after 28 weeks gestation and following abdominal delivery; hysterectomies performed after vaginal delivery were excluded from the series. The operations were classified as either elective or emergency; the latter designation included only those operations performed as a lifesaving procedure to prevent exsanguination from profuse hemorrhage. Indications for hysterectomy were considered separate and distinct from those for cesarean section. In the case of uterine rupture with expulsion of the fetus into the abdominal cavity, the case was included as abdominal delivery and emergency hysterectomy. All cesareans were obstetrically indicated; none were performed merely to allow hysterectomy for sterilization. There were 800 elective and 200 emergency hysterectomies. During the last 8 months of the study, 25.9% of cesareans performed at the Charity Hospital were terminated by hysterectomy compared to 15.3% for the entire series.

During the 1970s, in addition to other publications,[43–48] three review articles were published.[49–51] The hysterectomies performed at the Tulane Service Charity Hospital in New Orleans were abstracted from the previous series published from that institution and updated to December 31, 1967.[51] A total of 866 cesarean hysterectomies were included in that series, using the same definitions used in the previous study. Starting in 1938, the operations were further analyzed by 7-year intervals, except for the last interval, which consisted of 9 years. The analysis provided an interesting insight into the changing indications and modifications of the operative procedure, particularly the discontinuance of the subtotal operation in 1951. Two additional papers described the use of primary cesarean hysterectomy to accomplish delivery and removal of the uterus for carcinoma in situ of the cervix.[52,53] The first paper comparing the characteristics of elective cesarean hysterectomy with cesarean birth, with or without tubal ligation, was presented.[54] Although the operation remained quite popular during the 1970s, notes of caution were mentioned in the discussions, particularly of the paper of Haynes and Martin.[49] It was noted that the incidence of cesarean hysterectomy was decreasing throughout the country. Although enthusiasm remained in private institutions, teaching services were losing interest.

Papers published between 1980 and 1985 reflect the changing attitude toward the operation.[55–69] One short paper discussed elective cesarean hysterectomy and another sterilization by cesarean hysterectomy, but the remainder discussed primarily operations performed for uncontrollable hemorrhage and uterine pathology.[55,65] The latter was only a relative indication, depending upon the experience of the surgeon. Concern was voiced about the loss of surgical skills and the adequacy of residency training. The obstetrician could, at any time, be confronted with a need for an emergency postpartum hysterectomy, perhaps without requisite previous training.[66] If the surgeon has had sufficient surgical training, is it not cost effective to remove a diseased uterus at the time of an obstetrically indicated cesarean? In a recent update tape,[69] Clark, from the University of Southern California, indicated that, in his institution, a cesarean hysterectomy is performed in roughly 1 out of 200 cesareans, primarily for control of hemorrhage. Dr. Plauché, from Louisiana State University in New Orleans, stated that hysterectomy is performed there in conjunction with every 100 cesareans, which is approximately 1 per 1,000 deliveries. These comments fairly summarize the current consensus concerning this operation.

INDICATIONS FOR CESAREAN HYSTERECTOMY

Emergency Hysterectomy

By definition, an emergency cesarean hysterectomy is a lifesaving procedure performed to control hemorrhage. Causes of hemorrhage fall into roughly four categories: uterine atony, placental disorders, ruptured uterus, and extension of the cesarean incision into the uterine vessels. In the Tulane series extending from 1938 through 1967, 31.6% of emergency operations were performed for uterine atony, which was considerably lower than the 67% incidence reported by O'Leary.[50,64] In current obstetrics the Couvelaire uterus is seldom encountered, and hysterectomy would be an option of last resort considering the associated hematologic problems. Significant uterine fibroids in a patient who has undergone an obstetrically indicated cesarean may be removed by hysterectomy, but the indication would be defined as elective. However, uterine fibroids may interfere with uterine contractility, causing hemorrhage. A submucous fibroid may be enucleated if the tumor mass interferes with adequate closure of the uterine incision.

Bleeding from the placental site is usually associated with a low-lying placenta involving the noncontractile lower uterine segment. The lower uterine segment is also less resistant to penetration by the placenta. As a result, hemorrhage from placenta previa is usually associated with placenta accreta, increta, or precreta; the last may result in laceration of the uterine vessels when the placenta is removed. Clark and colleagues identified the emergence of placenta accreta as a major indication for hysterectomy, much in excess of that noted in the older literature.[64] Placenta accreta is often associated with a uterine scar, suggesting that the sharp rise in the cesarean section rate in this country during the past decade may account for the increase.[70]

Uterine rupture is currently the third most common indication for emergency hysterectomy. Spontaneous rupture of the unscarred uterus frequently results from extension of an old cervical laceration; therefore, total hysterectomy is mandatory, and one must not overlook an associated vaginal laceration that could result in postoperative hemorrhage. Frank rupture of a prior classical uterine incision is a catastrophic event, often resulting in expulsion of the fetus into the abdominal cavity and near inversion of the uterus. Separation of a low segment scar is less traumatic and seldom results in either fetal loss or bleeding. It is not surprising that a wound in an involuting organ does not heal well, even in the less muscular, fibrous lower uterine segment. These scars can usually be repaired, although in the older literature this was a prime indication for elective removal of the uterus.[51] An exception is a low segment scar that has been penetrated by a low-lying placenta. Spontaneous rupture of an intact uterus is infrequent and can be associated with blunt trauma to the abdomen that compresses the uterus against the sacral promontory, lacerating the posterior wall.[71]

Extension of a low transverse incision into the uterine vessels is an uncommon occurrence. Although hemorrhage may be profuse, the necessity for hysterectomy must be tempered by the parity and desires of the patient. Ligation of the anterior division of one or both hypogastric arteries may decrease pulse pressure in the uterine artery, but bleeding may not be completely controlled.[72] It is usually necessary to develop the pararectal and paravesical spaces for identification and ligation of the uterine artery at its origin. However, the pelvis is very vascular in pregnancy, and venous bleeding remains a problem. Clark et al and Pelosi et al have both found hypogastric artery ligation to be frequently unsuccessful in controlling bleeding.[64,73] The ureters are in close proximity to the uterine vessel laceration and must be identified by palpation or visualized prior to placing ligatures.[74]

Elective Cesarean Hysterectomy

Indications for elective cesarean hysterectomy can be categorized into three groups: elective sterilization, medically indicated sterilization, and uterine pathology such as uterine fibroids, carcinoma in situ, or occasionally intrauterine infection. Primary cesarean birth performed to facilitate a hysterectomy has not been recommended, with the exception of the occasional patient who has elected to undergo hysterectomy at the time of delivery for uterine pathology, particularly carcinoma in situ of the cervix. Early cancer of the cervix may be treated with a primary cesarean delivery and radical hysterectomy with pelvic lymphadenectomy.[75,76]

A series of 242 elective cesarean hysterectomies were reported in 1976.[54] Of these operations, 68% were performed strictly for sterilization, usually after a repeat cesarean birth. In 1980, Britton reported 112 elective cesarean hysterectomies, of which 74 were planned and performed for sterilization; the remaining patients underwent hysterectomy for uterine or other gynecologic pathology or for medically indicated sterilization.[55] Plauché, in 1981, reported 108 cesarean hysterectomies performed in a private practice setting; 46.3% were for the purpose of sterilization.[61] Despite the enthusiasm for elective sterilization by cesarean hysterectomy evidenced by the literature of the preceding two decades, there is little current support for this method of sterilization in the absence of associated uterine or pelvic pathology.

In most series, uterine pathology has been described as carcinoma in situ of the cervix, uterine fibroids, or severe intrauterine infection. Since the advent of improved antibiotics, infection has seldom been reported as an indication, although, in advanced pelvic sepsis, it is an important adjunctive form of therapy. Carcinoma in situ of the cervix can usually be accurately diagnosed during pregnancy by colposcopy. If invasive disease has been excluded, vaginal delivery is allowed. However, some patients cannot be relied upon to return for completion of treatment, and others wish to complete treatment at the time of delivery. In 1977, 32 patients treated by cesarean hysterectomy were reported, with a satisfactory fetal and maternal outcome.[53] Adequate removal of the cervix was accomplished without difficulty because the operations were planned and performed prior to the onset of labor.

Uterine leiomyomata do not necessitate cesarean delivery unless there is interference with the labor and delivery process. If a cesarean birth is obstetrically indicated and the surgeon is experienced with the operation, cesarean hysterectomy may be considered.

In the older literature, a "thin uterine scar" was often listed as an indication for hysterectomy.[51] Most low segment scars can be repaired, but a defective vertical scar extending into the corpus or a T incision may not heal well. Most of these operations were performed in hospitals where tubal ligation was prohibited.

Uterine prolapse and vaginal relaxation in a patient undergoing an obstetrically indicated cesarean delivery may be an indication for definitive surgery at that time. However, a suprapubic urethrovesical suspension and plication of the uterosacral ligaments should be included to treat associated stress urinary incontinence and as prophylaxis for a postoperative enterocele.[54]

THE SURGICAL PROCEDURE

No special preparation is required for the patient who is to undergo an elective cesarean hysterectomy. Consent to sterilization forms are completed. Two units of packed red cells are prepared. Vaginal preparation is not routinely carried out. Antibiotic prophylaxis is the same as that ordinarily used by the surgeon for a cesarean delivery.

A cesarean hysterectomy is different from hysterectomy in the nonpregnant patient. The tissues are soft and pliable, and the uterine and paravesical veins are markedly distended. The basic surgical principles to be discussed are as follows:

1. The skin incision may be vertical or transverse.
2. The bladder is dissected from the lower uterine segment before delivery.
3. The uterine incision may be vertical or transverse in the lower segment.
4. Tissue tension is constant.
5. Sharp dissection is used throughout.
6. Ligation of vascular pedicles is delayed until the uterine vessels have been secured.
7. The ureters are identified.
8. The lower limits of the cervix are identified by palpation.

The operation may be performed under either general or conduction anesthesia, whichever is ordinarily used for cesarean delivery.[44,67] The abdomen can be entered through either a vertical or a low transverse incision. A low cervical cesarean is performed in the usual manner, except that the bladder flap is completely developed prior to incising the uterus; the presence of prior adhesions often requires sharp dissection. If a vertical incision is used, it can be extended into the uterine fundus to facilitate delivery of the infant, and the finger of an assistant can be placed in the upper pole of the incision to maintain constant traction on the uterus throughout the procedure. Constant traction on the uterus throughout is a key to maintaining anatomical relationships and decreasing blood loss. The uterus is delivered from the abdominal cavity. The placenta is removed

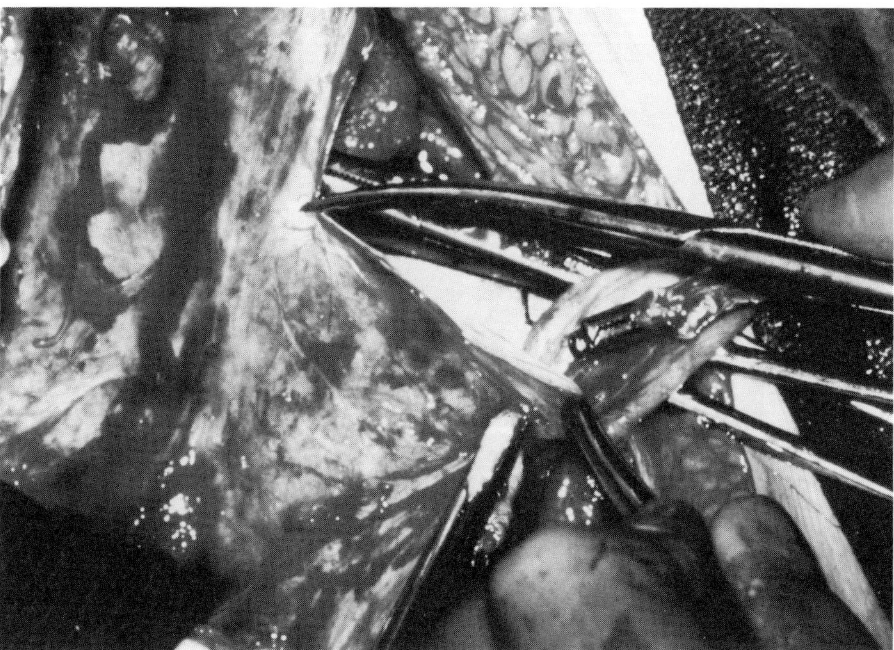

FIGURE 15.1 The uterine vessels are skeletonized by sharp dissection. Upward traction on the uterus markedly attenuates the uterine vessels. Clamps in the foreground are on the round ligament and utero-ovarian pedicles.

if it separates easily; otherwise, one proceeds immediately to secure the major vascular pedicles. If the edges of the uterine incision bleed, they can be secured with large sutures or simply clamped with small ring forceps. A self-retaining retractor is placed, and gauze sponges are packed into the cul-de-sac.

The ovaries are inspected and, if oophorectomy is not indicated, the operation is begun on one side by placing a clamp on the round ligament, which is cut; the anterior leaf of the broad ligament is incised to join the bladder flap incision. The avascular space in the broad ligament is penetrated, and the utero-ovarian ligament and fallopian tube are doubly clamped. One clamp is placed across the proximal pedicle of the utero-ovarian and round ligaments to prevent back bleeding. The broad ligament is incised sharply with a scissors and the uterine vessels are skeletonized (Figure 15.1). It is important that the assistant provide constant upward traction on the uterus to maintain anatomical relationships and place tension on the uterine vessels, particularly the uterine veins.

Dissection progresses so easily that the vessels can be skeletonized to the cardinal tunnel, jeopardizing the ureter. Before placement of a clamp on the uterine vessels, the angle of the bladder must be clearly identified and the location of the ureters established by palpation. The tissues are soft and pliable, and the ureter can be readily rolled between the thumb

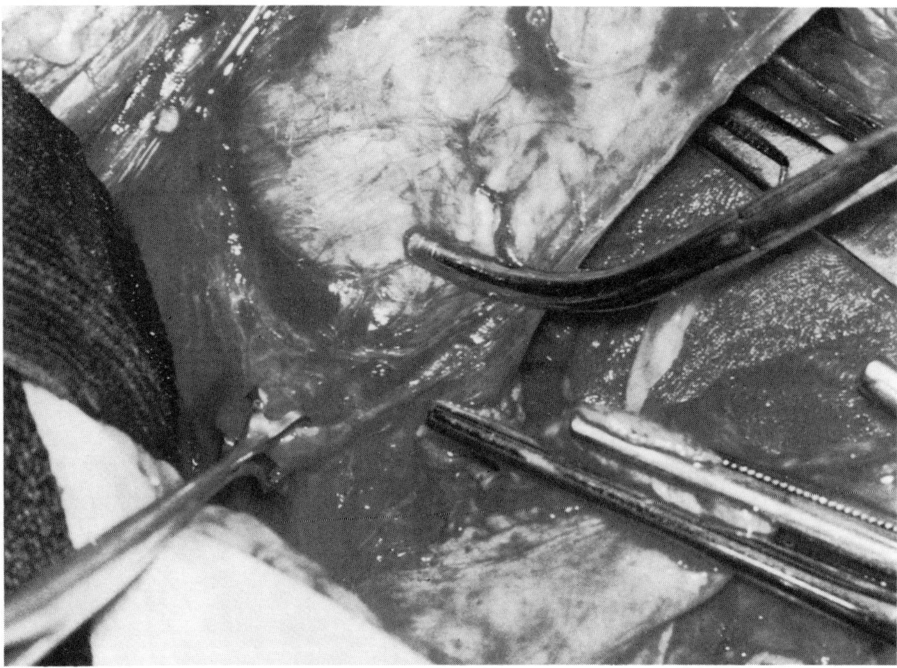

FIGURE 15.2 A Babcock clamp has been placed on the distal ureter for demonstration purposes. The angle of the bladder has been retracted and the uterine vessels have been clamped.

and forefinger for precise identification prior to placing the clamp on the uterine vessels (Figure 15.2).

A similar dissection is performed on the opposite side of the uterus. At this point, the major vascular pedicles have been secured with clamps, including a clamp on the uterine side of the uterine vascular pedicle to minimize back bleeding. The uterine vascular pedicles and the round ligaments are secured with stick ties. The utero-ovarian-fallopian tube pedicle is quite large and requires a free tie followed by a distal stick tie to be secured. However, if the pedicle is taken too close to the ovary, the ties tend to cut through the ovary, resulting in intraoperative or postoperative bleeding. For that reason, about 6%–10% of patients receive a unilateral salpingo-oophorectomy. On occasion, the utero-ovarian pedicle may be secured separately.

At this point, a hand is placed around the cervix, and the cervix and upper vagina are compressed between the thumb and forefinger, which tends to "milk" the uterine cervix upward for identification (Figure 15.3). If necessary, the bladder is advanced further on the upper vagina. An additional pedicle is usually required at the base of the cardinal ligament. A straight Kocher or Haney clamp is allowed to slide off the lateral portion of the cervix and grasp the base of the cardinal ligament. The bladder reflection from the anterior surface of the vagina is retracted away from

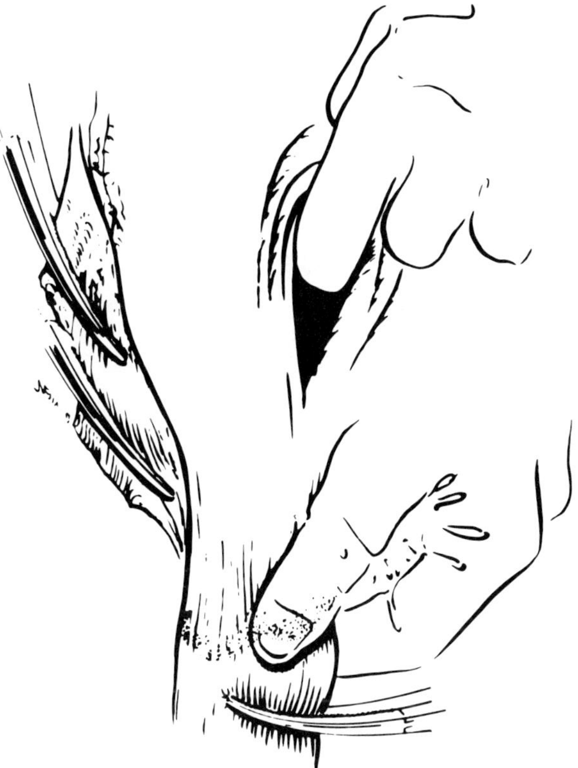

FIGURE 15.3 A vertical incision is used for traction. Compression of the upper vagina assists in identification of the cervix.

the tip of the clamp. A wedge-shaped pedicle is cut with a knife and is tied with a suture ligature, which may include and retie the adjacent uterine vascular pedicle. The bladder reflection from the upper vagina is again assured and the cervix identified by palpation (Figure 15.4). A curved Haney clamp can then be placed on each angle of the vagina, the vagina incised, and the specimen removed (Figure 15.5).

The anterior and posterior edges of the vaginal cuff are grasped with Kocher clamps. A suture ligature is placed on each angle and the remainder of the vaginal cuff is closed with figure eight sutures, taking care that the mucosal edge has not retracted. An alternative is simply to run the edge of the vaginal cuff with a locking suture. The pelvis is thoroughly inspected and irrigated, and hemostasis is secured. The vaginal cuff that is left open is probably functionally closed within 24–48 hours but is easy to open if there is a pelvic hematoma. The ovarian pedicle is secured to the adjacent round ligament and not attached to the vaginal cuff. If prophylactic antibiotics are used, drainage may not be necessary, although the use of a transvaginal T-tube or extraperitoneal drain is acceptable. The pelvis is usually reperitonealized with a continuous suture; however, the need for reperitonealization of the pelvis after hysterectomy is a debatable issue.

The surgical technique described is that preferred by the author.[77]

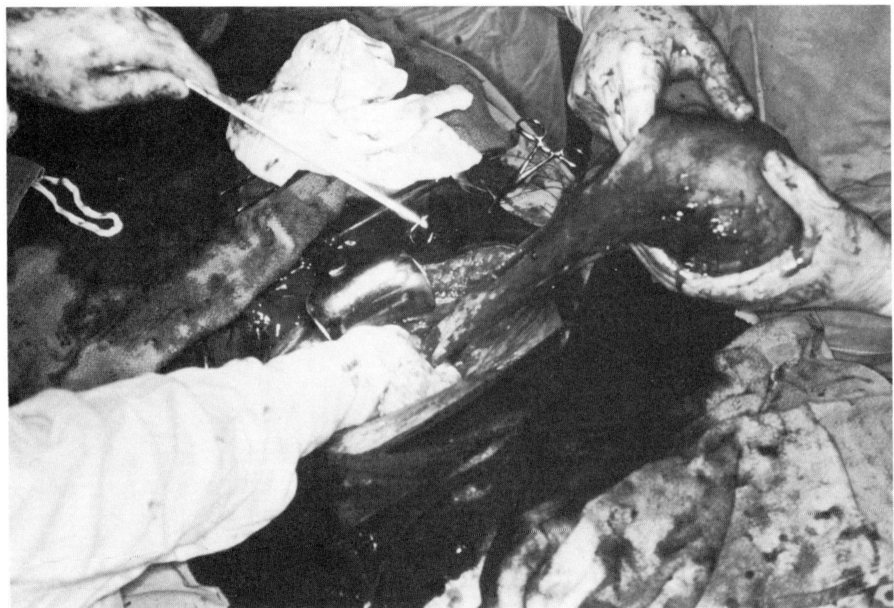

FIGURE 15.4 The upper vagina has been compressed to identify the cervix.

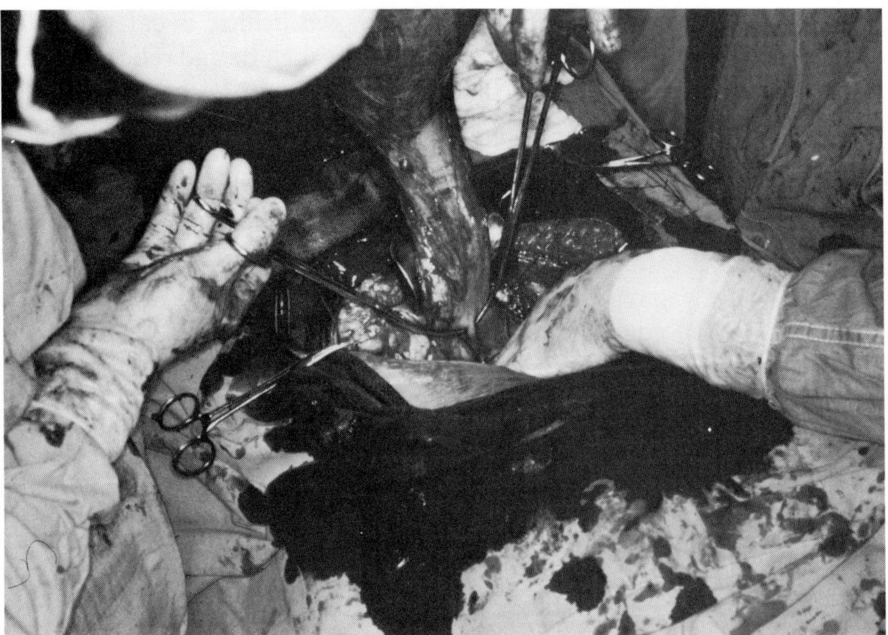

FIGURE 15.5 The vaginal angles have been secured.

There are, however, variations that should be mentioned.[61,68] Some surgeons prefer the low transverse uterine incision to decrease blood loss. Others delay dissection of the vesicouterine space until absolutely necessary because of the distended venous system. If there is some question about definite identification of the ureters by palpation, the uterine vessels may be taken at a higher level, which requires several pedicles along each side of the uterus close to the cervix. An alternative method of identifying the lower limits of the cervix is to incise the cervix anteriorly or enter the vagina posteriorly. Both methods lead to additional contamination of the operative field, and with a well-effaced cervix, delineation of cervix from vagina may still be difficult. Plauché has suggested that extrusion of mucus from cervical glands may assist in identifying the lower edge of the cervix.[69] In most reported series of emergency cesarean hysterectomies, a variable number of patients have retained a remnant of cervix. Absorbable polyglycolic acid or chromic catgut suture is used throughout the operation.

The technique of subtotal hysterectomy has not been discussed; the author has never done one. There is a role for supracervical hysterectomy, particularly in an emergency situation, in the hands of a surgeon who has had little experience with the operation. The principles of the operation are the same, and the cervical stump is simply closed after ligation of the uterine vessels and amputation of the corpus. One must be certain, however, that a uterine tear has not extended into the cervix or fornix of the vagina.

Operative Complications

In 1976, the author reported a 5-year review of abdominal deliveries in one institution and compared the operative characteristics of cesarean delivery, cesarean delivery and tubal ligation, and cesarean hysterectomy.[54] The mean operating time for cesarean hysterectomy was approximately 90 minutes, which was 38 minutes longer than for cesarean delivery and 33 minutes longer than for cesarean delivery with tubal ligation. During the last 2 years of the study, the operating time for cesarean hysterectomy was reduced to 75 $\pm$ 20.7 minutes. The operations were performed by residents under the supervision of staff physicians. Plauché reports an average operating time of about 2 hours.[63] Clark et al, reporting on emergency operations, has about a 3-hour operating time; much of this time was spent attempting to stop bleeding before a decision was made to remove the uterus.[64]

The incidence and quantity of blood transfusions depend upon the indications for the operation—whether emergency or elective and whether or not the elective operations were performed for uterine pathology such as large uterine fibroids. In addition, an indigent patient population has a lower average blood count prior to operation. A cesarean hysterectomy performed after a cesarean for a bleeding complication, such as placenta previa, obviously increases the need for blood replacement. In most reports from charity institutions, elective cesarean hysterectomy is associated with an approximately 20% incidence of blood transfusion.[51] In the author's series, approximately 20% of the patients undergoing elective cesarean hysterectomy received a transfusion but 4% of those undergoing cesarean delivery with or without tubal ligation were transfused.[54] The mean preoperative hematocrit in patients undergoing cesarean hysterectomy was 35.6% ± 3.5%. Of the 47 transfused patients, 13 were admitted to the hospital with a hematocrit of 30% or less and 1 had undergone a cesarean delivery for bleeding. Plauché reported 108 cesarean hysterectomies from a private practice, of which 86 were performed for elective reasons.[61] Among the elective operations, 11.8% of the patients received a transfusion. Approximately 25% of the patients receiving a transfusion were given only 1 unit of blood, which was the amount necessary to stabilize the vital signs. Fluid administration during the operation can often maintain vital sign stability until equilibration in the recovery room necessitates transfusion. For a planned, elective cesarean hysterectomy, it may be reasonable for the patient to store 1 unit of her own blood several weeks preoperatively.[78] Pritchard et al have demonstrated that a gravida at term can lose 1 L of blood with little or no hemodilution in the postpartum period.[79] In a series of 71 elective cesarean hysterectomies performed during 1 year, the incidence of transfusion was 7%.[51]

Elective ligation of the anterior division of the hypogastric artery prior to hysterectomy has proved to have little influence on the amount of blood loss or the incidence of transfusion.[73,80] Clark and associates have also found this to be true during emergency hysterectomy for hemorrhage.[64] However, if a uterine vessel retracts into the cardinal ligament adjacent to the ureter, or if excessive bleeding occurs for other reasons, one should open the pararectal and paravesical spaces, and place a clip on the anterior division of the hypogastric artery and on the uterine artery at its origin. Burchell demonstrated that although ligation of the anterior division of the hypogastric artery does not completely control bleeding from the uterine artery, it does decrease the pulse pressure and assist in defining the site of bleeding.[72] Compression of the aorta may provide temporary assistance.

Bladder entry, postoperative vesicovaginal fistula, and ureteral injury are recognized complications of cesarean hysterectomy. In the author's series, 4 of 390 patients undergoing repeat cesarean section without hysterectomy sustained bladder entry and repair with satisfactory healing.[51] Four of 242 patients undergoing elective cesarean hysterectomy sustained bladder entry; all occurred among the 114 patients undergoing a repeat cesarean birth. There was one unrecognized bladder injury among these patients; a vesicovaginal fistula was recognized on the fifth postoperative day and a successful early repair accomplished according to the method of Collins.[81] Bladder entry is ordinarily recognized, repaired, and heals uneventfully. Some authors have recommended that the bladder be partially distended with methylene blue or sterile milk prior to or after the hysterectomy to detect an unrecognized entry.[69] Most fistulas, however, probably result from inadvertent inclusion of bladder wall in closure of the vaginal cuff or separation of bladder muscle so that the adjacent mucosa undergoes subsequent necrosis. Leakage of urine usually occurs within the first 10 postoperative days.

Ureteral injury is a greater risk during cesarean hysterectomy than during abdominal or vaginal hysterectomy in the nonpregnant patient. The author's technique of cesarean hysterectomy can be used only if the surgeon is confident that the course of the ureter can be identified by palpation. If there is a question of ureteral injury, one can open the bladder extraperitoneally, identify the ureteral orifice, and place a retrograde ureteral catheter. Another alternative is to perform a linear ureterostomy at the pelvic brim and thread a ureteral catheter into the bladder. Partial severance of a ureter may be detected by injection of methylene blue into the ureteral lumen at the pelvic brim. In the author's series of 242 elective cesarean hysterectomies, there was injury to one ureter that was recognized, repaired, healed satisfactorily, and did not prolong the hospital stay.[54] In the Tulane series of 866 cesarean hysterectomies performed over a 30-year period, there were four ureteral injuries. Three of these were recognized, repaired, and healed satisfactorily, and one was repaired during the postoperative period. One ureteral injury occurred in 1959 and three during 1 year under the supervision of the same group of senior residents.[51] Plauché reported no ureteral injuries in a series of 108 elective and emergency operations performed in a private hospital.[61] Mickal and Plauché reported 808 consecutive operations from the Louisiana State University service at the Charity Hospital in New Orleans; there were 30 bladder entries, 7 vesicovaginal fistulas, and 2 ureteral fistulas.[68] Birch, on the other hand, reported in a verbal communication that cesarean hysterectomy is the gynecologic operation most commonly associated with ureteral injury in the state of Georgia.

Postoperative Complications

The primary postoperative complications are febrile morbidity secondary to infection of the operative site and bleeding. In the author's series, febrile morbidity after cesarean hysterectomy was 31%, compared to 55% after cesarean and 34% after cesarean delivery and tubal ligation.[54] By and large, cesarean tubal ligation and cesarean hysterectomy patients underwent a planned operation prior to the onset of labor. In addition, this study was performed in an era when prophylactic antibiotics were not used. In most studies, the incidence of febrile morbidity is less following cesarean hysterectomy than following cesarean delivery. This is particularly true if there has been prolonged labor or evidence of intrauterine infection. Although vaginal cuff infection is the most common source of febrile morbidity, urinary tract infection, pulmonary atelectasis, wound infection, thrombophlebitis, and breast inflammation must all be considered. Prophylactic antibiotics will undoubtedly reduce the incidence of infection.[69]

A special cause of postoperative febrile morbidity in the cesarean hysterectomy patient is ovarian abscess. The author reviewed 12 cases of postoperative ovarian abscess and found that 6 had occurred after cesarean hysterectomy. The latent period between the operation and the appearance of acute symptoms was as long as 300 days. The ovary in pregnancy is particularly susceptible to infection. The sutures on the utero-ovarian ligament may cut through the ovarian cortex sufficiently to allow entry of organisms.

After elective cesarean hysterectomy, one can expect a 4% incidence of postoperative bleeding, and half of these patients will undergo abdominal reentry. Vaginal cuff and incisional hematomas are managed in the usual manner. The ovarian pedicle and uterine vessels are the most common sites of intraabdominal bleeding and are treated like operative hemorrhage. The incidence of postoperative bleeding after cesarean hysterectomy should be compared with an incidence of approximately 0.7% after abdominal and 2% after vaginal hysterectomy in the nonpregnant patient.[82–85]

Addition of hysterectomy to cesarean delivery should increase the average hospital stay by 1 day or less.[54,69]

REFERENCES

1. Young JH: *Cesarean Section. The History and Development of the Operation from Earliest Times*. London, Lewis and Company, Ltd, 1944, pp 93–107.
2. Speert H: Eduardo Porro and cesarean hysterectomy. *Surg Gynecol Obstet* 106:245, 1958.
3. Durfee RB: Evolution of cesarean hysterectomy. *Clin Obstet Gynecol* 12:575, 1969.
4. Harris RP: Results of the first fifty cases of "cesarean ovaro-hysterectomy", 1869–1880. *Am J Med Sci* 80:129, 1880.
5. Harris JW: A study of the results obtained in sixty-four cesarean sections terminated by supravaginal hysterectomy. *Bull Johns Hopkins Hosp* 33:318, 1922.
6. Lash AF, Cummings WG: Porro cesarean section. *Am J Obstet Gynecol* 30:199, 1935.
7. Wilson KM: The role of Porro cesarean section in modern obstetrics. *Am J Obstet Gynecol* 50:761, 1945.
8. Reis RA, DeCosta EJ: Cesarean hysterectomy. *JAMA* 134:775, 1947.
9. Davis ME: Complete cesarean hysterectomy; logical advance in modern obstetric surgery. *Am J Obstet Gynecol* 63:838, 1951.
10. Dyer I, Nix FG, Weed JC: Total cesarean hysterectomy at cesarean section and in the immediate puerperal period. *Obstet Gynecol* 65:517, 1953.
11. Barclay DL: Cesarean hysterectomy at the Charity Hospital in New Orleans—1000 consecutive operations. *Clin Obstet Gynecol* 12:635, 1969.
12. Bradbury WC: Cesarean hysterectomy. *West J Surg* 63:232, 1955.

13. MacKenzie RA: Use of cesarean hysterectomy. *Am J Obstet Gynecol* 61:1309, 1951.
14. Dodek SM, Friedman JM, Treichler HP, et al: Cesarean hysterectomy (a review of 46 cases). *Med Ann Distr Columbia* 22:235, 1953.
15. Siegel IA: Total hysterectomy at time of cesarean section and in the puerperium. *Bull School Med Univ Md* 40:40, 1955.
16. Weigle EH: Cesarean section—total hysterectomy. *West J Surg* 63:123, 1955.
17. Davis JT, Ward SV: Cesarean hysterectomy. *J Louisiana Med Soc* 108:286, 1956.
18. Dyer I: Total cesarean and puerperal hysterectomy; a report of 205 cases. *Obstet Gynecol* 9:696, 1957.
19. Siegel IA: Total hysterectomy at time of cesarean section and in the puerperium. *South Med J* 50:195, 1957.
20. Hallat J, Hirsh H: Total hysterectomy for sterilization following cesarean section. *Am J Obstet Gynecol* 75:396, 1958.
21. Sandberg EC: Sterilization by cesarean hysterectomy. *Obstet Gynecol* 11:59, 1958.
22. Meyer H, Countiss EH: Cesarean hysterectomy. *Am J Obstet Gynecol* 77:1240, 1959.
23. Montague CF: Cesarean hysterectomy; its value as a sterilization procedure. *Obstet Gynecol* 14:28, 1959.
24. Reis RA: Cesarean hysterectomy. *Clin Obstet Gynecol* 2:977, 1959.
25. Brunschwig A, Barber HR: Cesarean section immediately followed by radical hysterectomy and pelvic node excision. *Am J Obstet Gynecol* 76:199, 1958.
26. Alford CD, Miller AC, Simpson JW: Cesarean section hysterectomy: A 10 year review. *Am J Obstet Gynecol* 82:664, 1961.
27. Dees DB Jr: Should hysterectomy replace routine tubal sterilization? *Am J Obstet Gynecol* 82:572, 1961.
28. Buell JI: Cesarean sections and cesarean section sterilizations at a private teaching hospital. *West J Surg* 70:79, 1962.
29. Larsson E: Evaluation of cesarean section hysterectomy. *J Am Med Wom Assoc* 17:720, 1962.
30. Morton JH: Cesarean hysterectomy. *Am J Obstet Gynecol* 83:1422, 1962.
31. Powell LC Jr: Cesarean section sterilization—hysterectomy or tubal ligation? *Obstet Gynecol* 19:387, 1962.
32. Riley FJ: Cesarean hysterectomy. *Trans N Engl Obstet Gynecol Soc* 16:13, 1962.
33. Soderstrom RM, Stipp CG: Cesarean hysterectomy—a safe procedure. *West J Surg* 70:150, 1962.
34. Pletsch TD, Sandberg EC: Cesarean hysterectomy for sterilization. *Am J Obstet Gynecol* 85:254, 1963.
35. Zeigler RF, Owen JC: Cesarean hysterectomy: Analysis of 61 cases. *Am Surg* 29:385, 1963.
36. Boyd A, Hofmeister FJ: Cesarean section and associated surgery. *Obstet Gynecol* 24:533, 1964.
37. O'Leary JA, Steer CE: A 10 year review of cesarean hysterectomy. *Am J Obstet Gynecol* 90:227, 1964.
38. Ward SV, Smith AH: Cesarean hysterectomy: Combined section and sterilization. *Obstet Gynecol* 26:858, 1965.
39. Fons JW, Brennan JJ: Multiple cesarean section. *Obstet Gynecol* 29:287, 1967.
40. Webb CF, Gibbs JV: Preplanned total cesarean hysterectomies. *Am J Obstet Gynecol* 101:23, 1968.
41. Symposium: Cesarean hysterectomy. *Clin Obstet Gynecol* 12:652, 1969.
42. Weed JC: The fate of the post cesarean uterus. *Obstet Gynecol* 14:780, 1960.
43. Tweedale PG, Sherline DM: Tubal ligation vs cesarean hysterectomy (letter). *Obstet Gynecol* 42:628, 1973.
44. LaPlatney DR, O'Leary JA: Anesthetic considerations in cesarean hysterectomy. *Anesth Analg* 49:328, 1970.

45. Patterson SP: Cesarean hysterectomy. *Am J Obstet Gynecol* 107:729, 1970.
46. Schneider GT, Tyrone CH: Cesarean hysterectomy. *Surg Gynecol Obstet* 130:502, 1970.
47. Howard P, Grubbs T: Cesarean section and cesarean hysterectomy—a five year evaluation at a nonuniversity teaching hospital. *J Tenn Med Assoc* 65:323, 1972.
48. Schneider GT, Mickal A: Cesarean hysterectomy for sterilization. *J Reprod Med* 15:117, 1975.
49. Haynes DM, Martin BJ Jr: Cesarean hysterectomy: A twenty-five-year review. *Am J Obstet Gynecol* 134:393, 1979.
50. O'Leary JA: Cesarean hysterectomy: A 15 year review. *J Reprod Med* 4:231, 1970.
51. Barclay DL: Cesarean hysterectomy—thirty years' experience. *Obstet Gynecol* 35:120, 1970.
52. Abitbol MM, Benjamin F, Gastillo N: Cesarean hysterectomy in the treatment of carcinoma in situ of the cervix diagnosed during pregnancy. *Am J Obstet Gynecol* 117:909, 1973.
53. Barclay DL, Frueh DM, Hawks BL: Carcinoma in situ of the cervix in pregnancy: Treatment with primary cesarean hysterectomy. *Gynecol Oncol* 5:357, 1977.
54. Barclay DL, Hawks BL, Frueh DM, et al: Elective cesarean hysterectomy: A 5 year comparison with cesarean section. *Am J Obstet Gynecol* 124:900, 1976.
55. Britton JJ: Sterilization by cesarean hysterectomy. *Am J Obstet Gynecol* 173:887, 1980.
56. Cesarean hysterectomy, in Ingram JM (ed): *Collected letters of the International Correspondence Society of Obstetricians/Gynecologists.* Dean M. Laux, No. 20, 1980.
57. Hill DJ, Beischer NA: Hysterectomy in obstetric practice. *Aust NZ J Obstet Gynecol* 20:151, 1980.
58. Park RC, Duff WP: Role of cesarean hysterectomy in modern obstetric practice (review). *Clin Obstet Gynecol* 23:601, 1980.
59. Perkins RP: Role of extraperitoneal cesarean section. *Clin Obstet Gynecol* 23:583, 1980.
60. Diebel ND: Cesarean hysterectomy for sterilization (letter). *Am J Obstet Gynecol* 140:351, 1981.
61. Plauché WC, Gruich FG, Bourgeois MO: Hysterectomy at the time of cesarean section: Analysis of 108 cases. *Obstet Gynecol* 58:459, 1981.
62. Bukovsky I, Schneider D, Weinraub Z, et al: Sterilization at the time of cesarean section: Tubal ligation or hysterectomy? *Contraception* 28:349, 1983.
63. Plauché WC, Wycheck JG, Iannessa MJ, et al: Cesarean hysterectomy at Louisiana State University, 1975 through 1981. *South Med J* 76:1261, 1983.
64. Clark SL, Yeh S-Y, Phelan JP, et al: Emergency hysterectomy for obstetric hemorrhage. *Obstet Gynecol* 64:376, 1984.
65. McNulty JV: Elective cesarean hysterectomy—Revisited. *Am J Obstet Gynecol* 149:29, 1984.
66. Chestnut DH, Eden RD, Gall SA, et al: Peripartum hysterectomy: A review of cesarean and postpartum hysterectomy. *Obstet Gynecol* 65:365, 1985.
67. Chestnut DH, Redick LF: Continuous epidural anesthesia for elective cesarean hysterectomy. *South Med J* 78:1168, 1173, 1985.
68. Mickal A, Plauché WC: *Cesarean Hysterectomy. Mediguide to Ob/Gyn.* Miles Pharmaceuticals, Vol. 4, No. 1. Lawrence DellaCorte Publications, Inc, 1985.
69. Barclay DL, Clark SL, Plauché WC: Cesarean hysterectomy. Update tape. *Am College Obstet Gynecol* 11: 1986.
70. Read JA, Cotton DB, Miller FC: Placenta accreta: Changing clinical aspects and outcome. *Obstet Gynecol* 56:31, 1980.
71. Dyer I, Barclay DL: Accidental trauma complicating pregnancy and delivery. *Am J Obstet Gynecol* 83:907, 1962.

72. Burchell CR: Physiology of internal iliac artery ligation. *J Obstet Gynecol Br Commonwealth* 75:642, 1968.
73. Pelosi M, Langer A, Hung C: Prophylactic internal iliac artery ligation at cesarean hysterectomy. *Am J Obstet Gynecol* 121:394, 1975.
74. Eisenhop SM, Richman R, Platt LD, et al: Urinary tract injury during cesarean section. *Obstet Gynecol* 60:591, 1982.
75. Sall S, Rini S, Pineda A: Surgical management of invasive carcinoma of the cervix in pregnancy. *Obstet Gynecol* 118:1, 1974.
76. Thompson JD, Caputo TA, Franklin EW III, et al: The surgical management of invasive cancer of the cervix in pregnancy. *Am J Obstet Gynecol* 121:853, 1975.
77. Barclay DL: *Current OB/Gyn Techniques,* Vol 1, No. 3. Surgical Communications, Inc. Ortho Pharmaceutical Corp, 1976.
78. Chestnut DH: Autologous blood for elective cesarean hysterectomy (letter). *Am J Obstet Gynecol* 150:796, 1984.
79. Pritchard JA, Baldwin RM, Dickey JC, et al: Blood volume changes in pregnancy and the puerperium. II. Red blood cell loss and changes in apparent blood volume during and following vaginal delivery, cesarean section and cesarean section plus total hysterectomy. *Am J Obstet Gynecol* 84:1271, 1962.
80. Evans S, McShane P: The efficacy of internal iliac artery ligation in obstetric hemorrhage. *Surg Gynecol Obstet* 160:250, 1985.
81. Collins CG, Barclay DL, Holmes JS: Urinary incontinence. *Clin Obstet Gynecol* 6:236, 1963.
82. Amirikio H, Evans TN: Ten year review of hysterectomies: Trends, indications and risks. *Am J Obstet Gynecol* 134:431, 1979.
83. Pratt JH: Common complications of vaginal hysterectomy. *Clin Obstet Gynecol* 19:645, 1976.
84. Dicker RC, Greenspan JR, Strauss LT, et al: Complications of abdominal and vaginal hysterectomy among women of reproductive age in the United States. *Am J Obstet Gynecol* 144:841, 1982.
85. Easterday CL, Grimes DA, Riggs JA: Hysterectomy in the United States. *Obstet Gynecol* 62:203, 1983.

Chapter 16

Uterine and Hypogastric Artery Ligation

Steven L. Clark, MD

Ligation of the uterine and hypogastric (internal iliac) arteries is an important part of the obstetrician's surgical armamentarium. At times, these techniques may be lifesaving. At other times, the ability to perform these procedures quickly and skillfully may allow control of otherwise intractable obstetric hemorrhage and permit uterine conservation. Unfortunately, both the uterine and hypogastric arteries lie in close proximity to other vital pelvic structures. Ligation of these vessels is therefore not without risk and requires meticulous surgical technique, especially in the case of hypogastric artery ligation. The indications for these procedures, listed in Table 16.1, are discussed in detail in Chapter 18. This chapter will focus upon the technical aspects of uterine and hypogastric artery ligation.

UTERINE ARTERY LIGATION

Ligation of the uterine arteries is not technically difficult. If properly performed, this technique is not associated with a significant incidence of major complications. In a review of over 200 women undergoing bilateral uterine artery ligation for postcesarean hemorrhage, O'Leary found this procedure effective in 95% of cases.[1] Uterine atony was the major indication for this procedure. The incidence of significant complications was low (1%) and appeared to be associated with operator inexperience. Urologic injury was not seen. Given the high success rate and the low rate of complications, uterine artery ligation is a logical first step in the control of hemorrhage of any etiology following failure of more conservative medical therapy.[2] (See Chapter 18.)

Technique

Uterine artery ligation is performed using a large Mayo needle and No. 1 chromic suture (Figure 16.1). The uterus and tube are elevated, exposing

TABLE 16.1 Common Indications for Uterine and Hypogastric Artery Ligation

Uterine atony
Placenta accreta
Lacerations of
Uterus
Broad ligament
Vagina

and flattening the broad ligament. The suture is placed so as to ligate the ascending uterine artery and accompanying veins at a level just below the site of the standard transverse lower uterine segment incision. The suture is placed into the myometrium from anterior to posterior approximately 2 cm medial to the lateral margin of the uterus. The needle is extracted from the posterior myometrium and redirected from posterior to anterior through an avascular space in the broad ligament. The suture is then securely tied and the procedure repeated on the opposite side. Depending on the surgeon and his/her position at the operating table, uterine artery ligation may be easier to do by first going anterior through an avascular space in the broad ligament and then through the posterior myometrium.

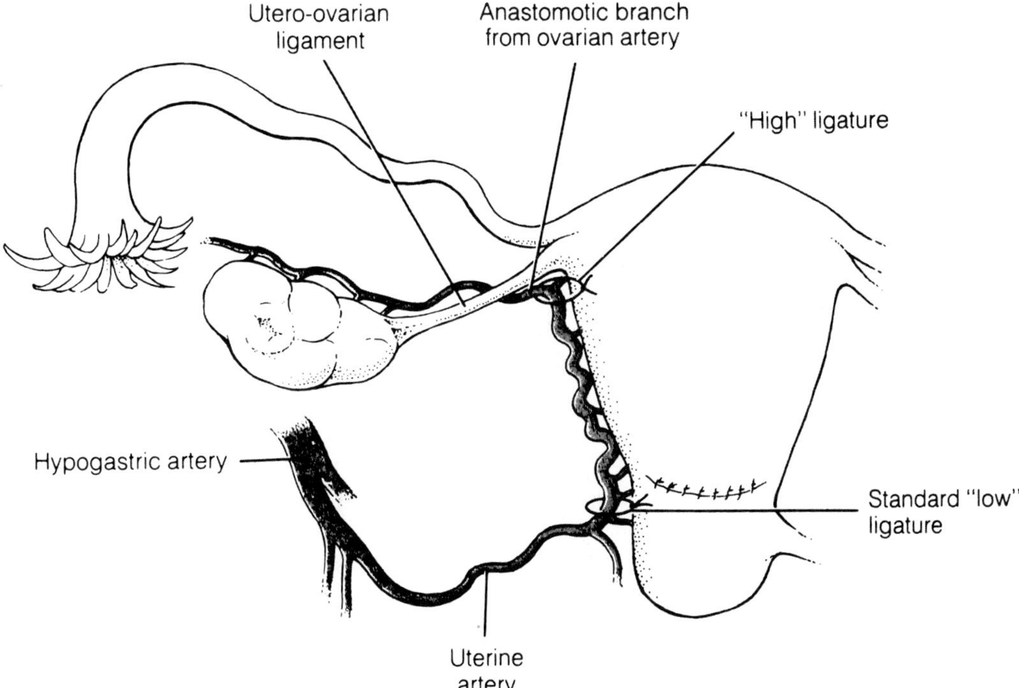

FIGURE 16.1 Technique of uterine artery ligation. Sutures are placed to encompass the ascending uterine arteries, as well as anastomotic branches from the ovarian arteries. (From Clark SL, Phelan JP: *Contemp OB-GYN* 24:70, 1984, with permission from Medical Economics Books, Oradell, NJ.)

TABLE 16.2 Efficacy of Hypogastric Artery Ligation in Avoiding Hysterectomy for Obstetric Hemorrhage

Indication	No. of Patients	Success	Percentage
Atony	21	9	43
Placenta accreta	7	4	57
Lacerations	8	1	13
Other	4	4	100
Total	41	18	44

Source: Data from Clark SL, Phelan JP, Yeh SY, et al: Hypogastric artery ligation for obstetric hemorrhage. *Obstet Gynecol* 66:353, 1985; Bruce SL, Paul RJH, Van Dorsten JP: Control of postpartum uterine atony by intramyometrial prostaglandin. *Obstet Gynecol* 59:47, 1982; Evans S, McShane P: The efficacy of internal iliac artery ligation in obstetric hemorrhage. *Surg Gynecol Obstet* 160:250, 1985.

Occasionally, anastomoses may exist between branches of the ovarian and uterine arteries in the area of the utero-ovarian ligament. In order to prevent collateral backflow to the uterine artery from such ovarian artery anastomoses, a second "high" ligature is often useful.[2] This ligature is placed at the utero-ovarian ligament–uterine junction. In placing this high ligature, care must be taken to avoid compromise to either extrauterine or interstitial portions of the fallopian tube.

HYPOGASTRIC ARTERY LIGATION

In the United States, hypogastric artery ligation was first performed in the late nineteenth century by Howard Kelly to control bleeding associated with carcinoma of the cervix. He described this technique as "the boldest procedure possible for checking the bleeding."

Branches of the anterior division of the internal iliac (hypogastric) artery provide the major blood supply to organs of the female pelvis. In an effort to avoid hysterectomy, ligation of these vessels has been recommended for control of otherwise intractable obstetric hemorrhage.[3,4] Reports of term pregnancy after bilateral ligation of both hypogastric and ovarian arteries attest to the abundant collateral blood supply of the female pelvis.[5] Unilateral hypogastric artery ligation reduces distal ipsilateral blood flow by only 48%. A more important clinical effect is an 85% diminution of pulse pressure distal to the site of ligation.[6] Thus, the hemodynamics of the distal arterial system are changed to resemble more closely those of a venous system amenable to hemostasis via simple clot formation. Several recent reports have examined the efficacy of bilateral hypogastric artery ligation in controlling obstetric hemorrhage and avoiding hysterectomy.[3,4,7] Reported success rates have ranged from 25% to 57%. A compilation of data from three recent series is presented in Table 16.2. These combined data indicate that hypogastric artery ligation is successful in avoiding hysterectomy in approximately half of the cases associated with uterine atony and placenta accreta and is far less successful when a uterine/broad ligament laceration is encountered. However, the number of subjects in each of these subgroups is small, and occasional success may be seen when ligation is performed for a broad ligament laceration; in some cases, identification and ligation of the lacerated vessels are facilitated by first performing hypogastric artery ligation.

Clark et al examined 19 patients undergoing bilateral hypogastric artery ligation for the control of otherwise intractable obstetric hemorrhage. These investigators found an increased incidence of ureteral injury and cardiac arrest due to blood loss in patients undergoing unsuccessful hypogastric artery ligation followed by hysterectomy compared to patients undergoing hysterectomy without prior hypogastric artery ligation.[3] In both cases, the ureteral injuries appeared to have been surgically related to the hysterectomy rather than to the hypogastric artery ligation itself. These authors concluded that the prolonged operative time and extensive blood loss after unsuccessful hypogastric artery ligation may have led to less meticulous surgical technique during the subsequent hysterectomy, resulting in ureteral injury. Thus, complications associated with unsuccessful hypogastric artery ligation appear to be associated with delay in instituting definitive therapy (hysterectomy) rather than with the surgical procedure itself. In a similar manner, Evans and McShane reported a low incidence of serious complications associated with hypogastric artery ligation.[4] Although extensive collateral circulation generally prevents ischemic complications, these investigators reported one patient with central pelvic ischemia, breakdown of the perineal skin and episiotomy site, and postischemic lower motor neuron damage with weakness in the lower extremities. Although this patient presumably had atypical collateral circulation resulting in this extremely rare complication, the possibility of ischemic sequelae must be kept in mind when evaluating the appropriateness of hypogastric artery ligation.

Technique

The first step in hypogastric artery ligation is to enter the retroperitoneal space (Figures 16.2, 16.3). This may be done either anteriorly, between the round and infundibulopelvic ligaments, or posteriorly in the posterior leaf of the broad ligament medial to the infundibulopelvic ligament and lateral to the external iliac artery. Next, the ureter is identified and retracted medially. The external iliac artery is then located and its course traced proximally to the bifurcation of the common iliac artery. At the bifurcation, the internal iliac (hypogastric) artery is found and its course traced distally; a tonsil tip sucker is helpful in this blunt dissection. Next, the areolar tissue surrounding the hypogastric artery is carefully dissected to free it from the adventitia for a distance of 2–3 cm. A right angle clamp is passed beneath the artery. The artery is doubly ligated with No. 0 silk

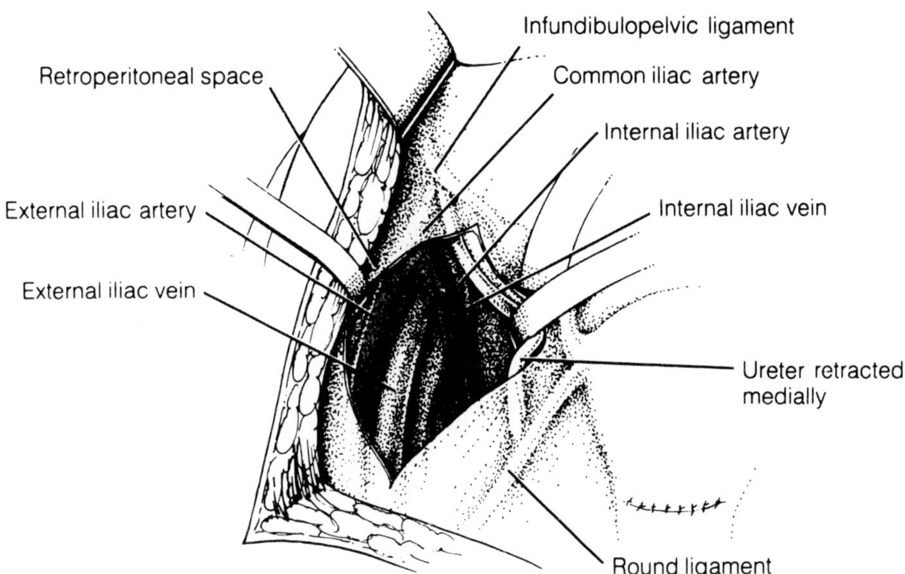

FIGURE 16.2 The retroperitoneal space has been opened, the ureter retracted medially, and the hypogastric artery exposed. (From Clark SL, Phelan JP: *Contemp OB-GYN* 24:70, 1984, with permission from Medical Economics Books, Oradell, NJ.)

suture, and the retroperitoneal space is closed with No. 3-0 polyglycolic acid suture. The ligation should be performed at a point distal to the origin of the posterior division of the internal iliac artery to avoid distal reversal of blood flow through vessels, comprising iliolumbar–lumbar and lateral sacral–middle sacral anastomoses.

Four potential pitfalls may be encountered when performing hypogastric artery ligation.

1. Misidentification and accidental ligation of the external iliac artery. This is an extremely serious complication and, if unrecognized, can lead to ischemia and loss of the ipsilateral leg. To avoid this complication, careful dissection and identification of anatomic landmarks, and palpation of femoral pulses before and after internal iliac artery ligation are essential.
2. Laceration of the internal or external iliac veins. These thin-walled structures lie immediately adjacent to the external iliac artery and may be easily lacerated if retroperitoneal dissection has been too vigorous or if the right angle clamp is improperly passed beneath the internal iliac artery. Such lacerations are often difficult to repair and may result in life-threatening hemorrhage. To avoid this complication, the tip of the clamp should be kept against the artery and passed from lateral to medial to avoid injuring the underlying and somewhat laterally placed external iliac vein. Elevation of the artery with a large Babcock clamp is also helpful (Figure 16.3).

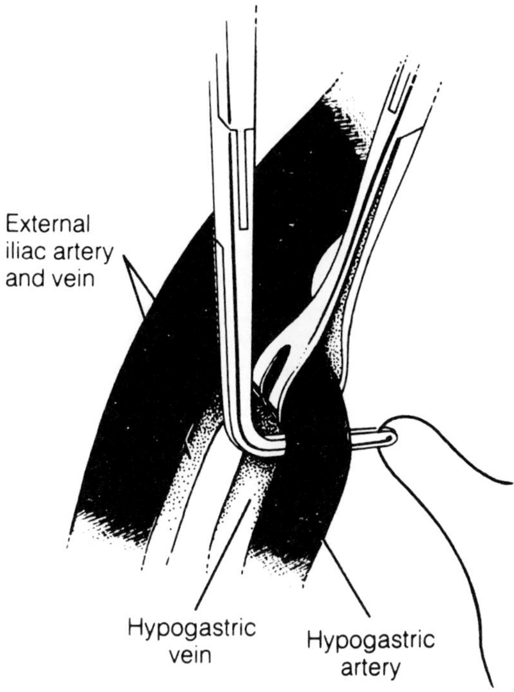

FIGURE 16.3 The hypogastric artery is elevated with a large Babcock clamp and the suture passed from lateral to medial. (From Clark SL, Phelan JP: *Contemp OB-GYN* 24:70, 1984, with permission from Medical Economics Books, Oradell, NJ.)

3. Ureteral injury. This may be avoided by promptly identifying the ureter and retracting it immediately after entering the retroperitoneal space.
4. Retroperitoneal hematoma. This complication may be encountered if hemostasis in the retroperitoneal space has been inadequate. Meticulous surgical technique is essential to avoid this complication. Small hemostatic clips are extremely helpful in controlling small bleeding vessels within the retroperitoneal space.

In conclusion, bilateral hypogastric artery ligation following the failure of other methods of achieving hemostasis is sometimes effective in controlling hemorrhage and avoiding hysterectomy. The overall success rate, however, is probably not greater than 50%, and the risk of serious complications associated with the failure of hypogastric artery ligation and subsequent hysterectomy is relatively high. Such a risk/benefit ratio is probably acceptable only in the hemodynamically stable patient of very low parity in whom future childbearing is of overwhelming concern. Patients meeting these criteria should first undergo bilateral uterine artery ligation following the failure of more conventional attempts to control hemorrhage (Chapter 18). If this procedure is ineffective, hypogastric artery ligation may be performed. However, in patients who do not meet these criteria, the relatively low success rate combined with the relatively high morbidity associated with failed hypogastric artery ligation and subsequent hysterectomy suggests that hypogastric artery ligation is best eliminated and hysterectomy promptly performed.[8]

REFERENCES

1. O'Leary JA: Stop obstetric hemorrhage with uterine artery ligation. *Contemp OB/GYN* 28:13, 1986.
2. Clark SL, Phelan JP: Surgical control of obstetric hemorrhage. *Contemp OB/GYN* 24:70, 1984.
3. Clark SL, Phelan JP, Yeh SY, et al: Hypogastric artery ligation for obstetric hemorrhage. *Obstet Gynecol* 66:353, 1985.
4. Evans S, McShane P: The efficacy of internal iliac artery ligation in obstetric hemorrhage. *Surg Gynecol Obstet* 160:250, 1985.
5. Mengert WF, Burchell RC, Blumstein RW, et al: Pregnancy after bilateral ligation of the internal iliac and ovarian arteries. *Obstet Gynecol* 34:669, 1969.
6. Burchell RC: Physiology of internal iliac artery ligation. *J Obstet Gynaecol Br Commonweath* 75:642, 1968.
7. Bruce SL, Paul RJH, Van Dorsten JP: Control of postpartum uterine atony by intramyometrial prostaglandin. *Obstet Gynecol* 59:47, 1982.
8. Clark SL, Yeh SY, Phelan JP, et al: Emergency hysterectomy for obstetric hemorrhage. *Obstet Gynecol* 64:376, 1984.

Chapter 17

Surgical Sterilization and Incidental Procedures—Appendectomy, Cystectomy

William L. Koontz, MD

The performance of a laparotomy gives the operator an opportunity to do procedures other than that for which the peritoneum was primarily opened. This is certainly the case with cesarean delivery. However, much controversy surrounds the performance of additional procedures at the time of abdominal delivery. Although tubal sterilization as a part of the operation is widely accepted and performed, there is much debate about the technique used, and little data exist regarding efficacy and complication rates. Other surgical procedures at the time of cesarean birth arouse even more controversy, with little agreement and even less data. This chapter will discuss these problems and make recommendations for dealing with them.

TUBAL STERILIZATION

Tubal sterilization is the most commonly performed additional procedure at the time of cesarean delivery. Approximately 14% of tubal sterilizations performed in the United States in 1980 were done at this time.[1]

Although the short-term risks have not been well documented, the consensus seems to be that they are determined primarily by factors involving the cesarean procedure itself, with little risk added by performance of the sterilization. Because of the probably very low morbidity involved in tubal sterilization and the great variety of factors influencing cesarean delivery–related morbidity, definitive data comparing the morbidity of the various techniques will probably never become available.

There are four major considerations involved in examining the long-term sequelae of tubal sterilization at the time of cesarean delivery: (1) increased risk of subsequent menstrual disturbances, (2) increased risk of

TABLE 17.1 Failure Rates of Tubal Sterilization Procedures Performed at the Time of Cesarean Delivery

Method	Percent of Failure
Pomeroy	0.25[11]–1.75[10]
Uchida	0.00[15]
Parkland[a]	0.25[9]
Irving[a]	0.00[10,14]
Madlener	7.32[10]

[a] Includes cases of puerperal sterilization not done at the time of cesarean delivery.

subsequent hysterectomy, (3) risk of regret, and (4) risk of sterilization failure.

The existence of a "posttubal ligation syndrome" involving pelvic discomfort, ovarian cyst formation, and increased menstrual flow remains controversial. Large studies of women who underwent sterilization by laparoscopic techniques have demonstrated no increase in menstrual disturbances after 2 years of follow-up.[2] There are no conclusive data showing an increased risk of menstrual disturbances following pregnancy-associated sterilization,[3] but the question remains unresolved.

Any sterilization procedure carries with it the risk of subsequent regret. For this reason, thorough counseling prior to the procedure is recommended. One study found that women undergoing sterilization at the time of cesarean delivery have a much higher incidence of regret at 2 years of follow-up than women undergoing interval procedures.[4] Others have described similar findings. Murray[5] found a preponderance of pregnancy-associated procedures among a group of women requesting reversal of sterilization. Emens and Olive[6] demonstrated that women undergoing sterilization at the time of cesarean delivery and in the immediate postpartum period had a much higher incidence of dissatisfaction than women undergoing interval procedures. They felt that a major factor in the increased incidence of regret was that many more of the pregnancy-related procedures had been initially recommended by the physician rather than requested by the patient. This underlines the importance of thorough discussion prior to the operation, with the physician providing nondirective information and the patient being completely comfortable with the final decision.

The failure rate of tubal sterilization done at the time of cesarean delivery (Table 17.1) has long been a source of controversy. In particular, the failure rate relative to that of interval procedures has been debated. The standard obstetrical textbooks of the 1960s[7–9] stated that tubal sterilization at the time of cesarean was associated with a much higher failure rate than procedures performed at other times. This conclusion was based primarily on the study of Prystowsky and Eastman.[10] In reviewing a series

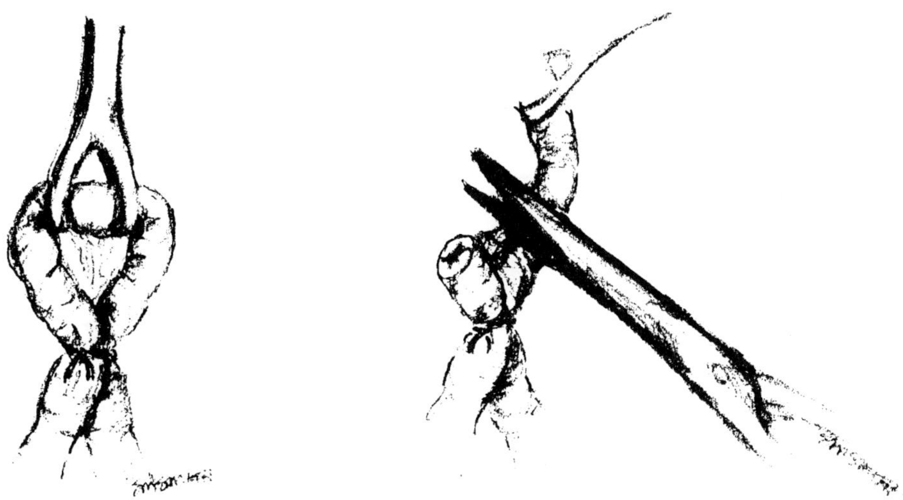

FIGURE 17.1 Pomeroy partial salpingectomy.

of 400 patients sterilized by the Pomeroy technique at the time of cesarean delivery, these authors found that at least 7 of these patients later became pregnant, a failure rate of at least 1 in 57. Pathologic findings in the failures were not described. Husbands et al,[11] on the other hand, found only one failure in a series of exactly the same size, and felt that this failure rate was comparable to that obtained with similar procedures performed following vaginal delivery.

The low failure rates of all of the commonly performed sterilization procedures and the difficulties inherent in long-term studies make comparison of the efficacy of the various techniques very difficult. Definitive data concerning this question are unavailable and are likely to remain so.

The most commonly performed sterilization procedure done at the time of cesarean delivery is the Pomeroy partial salpingectomy (Figure 17.1). This involves simple ligation of a knuckle of fallopian tube, including its mesosalpinx, and tight ligation of the loop with plain catgut. The loop of tube above the ligature is then excised, and the cut ends are observed for hemostasis. It is generally considered critical to use rapidly absorbable suture for this procedure, as this promotes scarring and closure of the tube. It also allows separation of the cut ends, theoretically reducing the incidence of recanalization. Advantages of this technique include (1) ease of learning; (2) very short operating time; (3) no dissection, thereby minimizing the risk of hemorrhagic complications; (4) a generally positive record of efficacy; and (5) relative ease of reversibility, should the need arise.

The Parkland procedure (Figure 17.2), as described by Pritchard and co-authors,[12] involves identification of an avascular area in the mesosalpinx, which is perforated and bluntly separated from the tube for a dis-

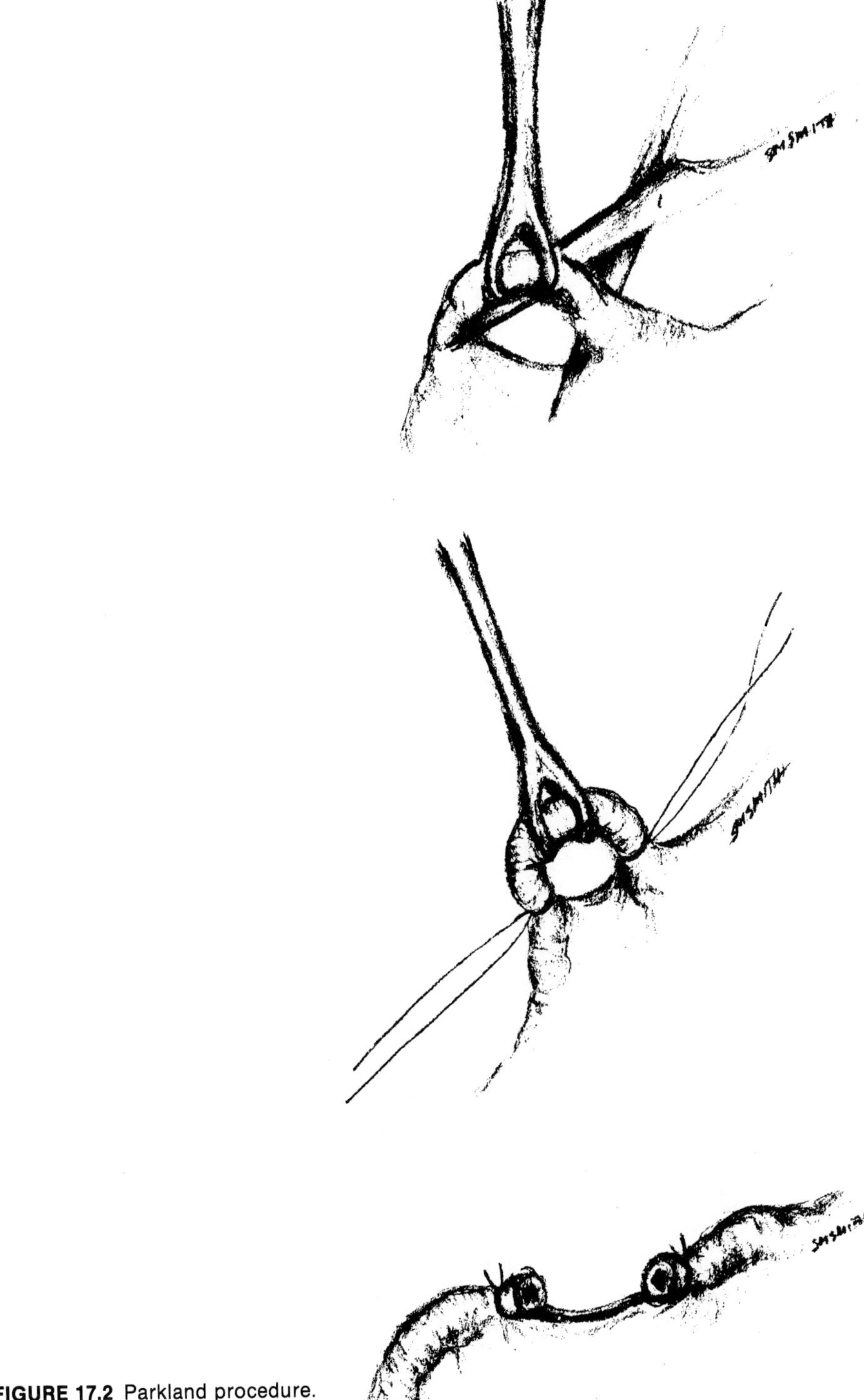

FIGURE 17.2 Parkland procedure.

tance of 2.5 cm. The tube is then ligated at each end of the freed area and the intervening portion is excised. The failure rate has been found to be approximately 1 in 400 procedures when the tube has actually been resected. This is also a relatively simple procedure that can be accomplished quickly and with minimal morbidity.

The Irving procedure[13] involves resection of a 2-cm portion of tube, followed by burial of the proximal stump in a subserosal pocket created on the anterior surface of the uterus (Figure 17.3). The distal cut end is then buried between the leaves of the broad ligament. Although this procedure requires more dissection and operating time than the two previously discussed, it is favored by some because of its extremely low failure rate. Irving[14] found no failures in 814 procedures performed at the Boston Lying-In Hospital between 1916 and 1949. In the previously mentioned study of Prystowsky and Eastman,[10] which described a relatively high failure rate for Pomeroy procedures, no failures were found after 206 Irving procedures.

The Uchida tubal sterilization procedure[15] requires subserosal injection of a dilute solution of epinephrine, incision of the serosa (Figure 17.4), and ligation and resection of a 5-cm length of the muscular portion of the tube. The proximal end is allowed to retract beneath the serosa, and the distal portion of the tube, including the fimbria, is completely resected (Figure 17.5). The Uchida fimbriectomy procedure appears to be extremely effective. Its developer has reported over 20,000 cases without a known failure. Of these cases, 1,195 were done at the time of cesarean delivery. While this series was being collected, the author saw 61 pregnancies following sterilization by other techniques. In spite of these excellent results, however, this procedure has not achieved great popularity in this country, and its ease and efficacy remain to be evaluated by numerous operators on a large scale.

Whatever the technique chosen for tubal sterilization at the time of cesarean delivery, there are several principles that must be rigidly observed. Detailed counseling that ensures thorough understanding of the procedure by the patient is essential. It may be appropriate to include the patient's spouse or significant other in these discussions. Because of the possible higher rate of regret following pregnancy-related procedures, it is critical that the patient not be talked into the procedure, and that it not be done if doubts are expressed. The permanence of the procedure should be stressed, thereby eliminating the widely held misconception that the tubes "come untied" after a certain number of years.

Although it seems too obvious to mention, one of the most common causes of sterilization failure remains error in identification of the fallopian tube. Although this is more likely to be a problem at the time of postpartum sterilization, it must not be overlooked at the time of cesarean delivery. The fimbriae should always be identified, and excised tissue should always be submitted for pathologic confirmation. When bilateral

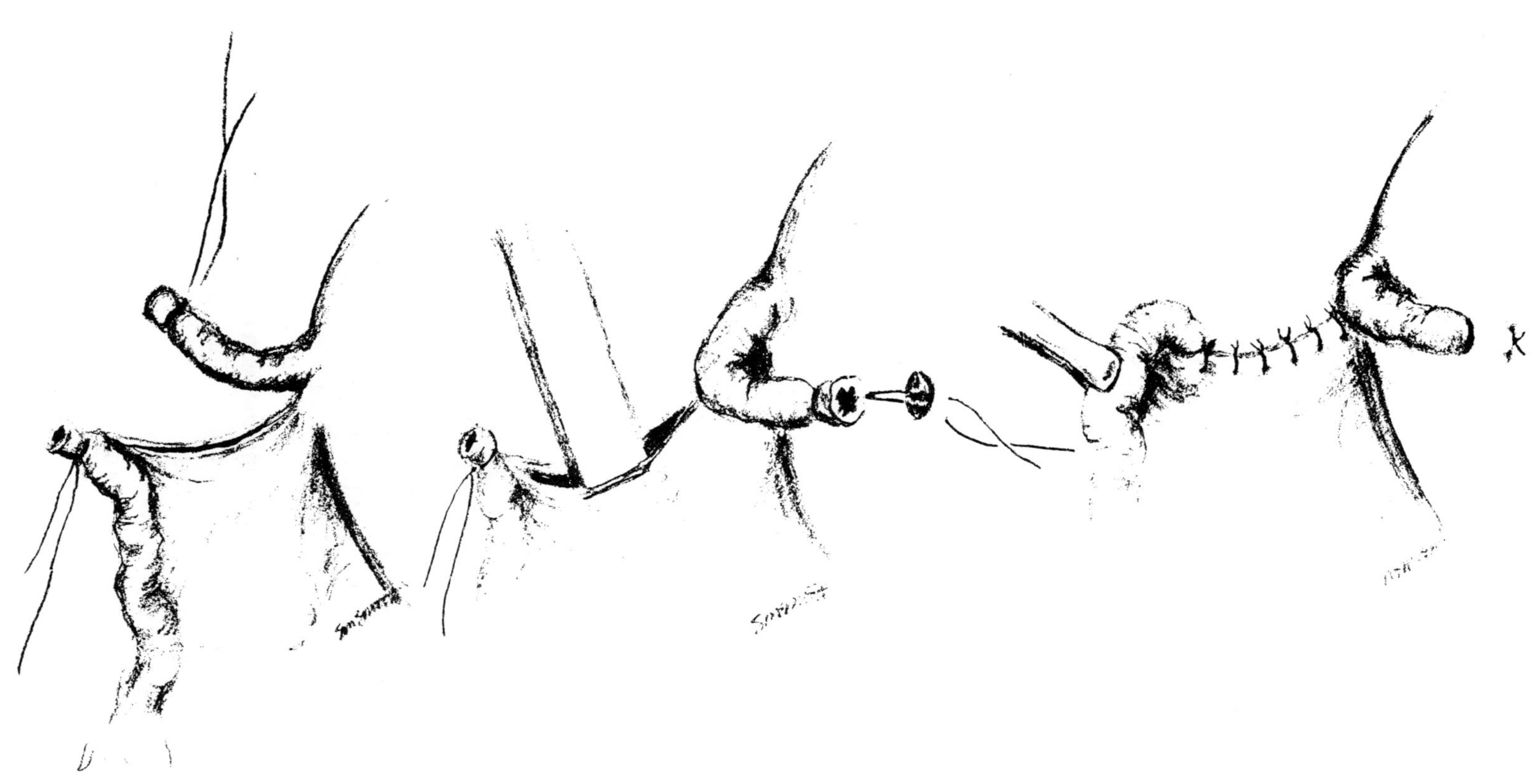

FIGURE 17.3 Irving procedure. (Adapted from Mattingly RF, Thompson JD [eds]: *TeLinde's Operative Gynecology*, ed 6. Philadelphia, JB Lippincott Co, 1985, with permission.)

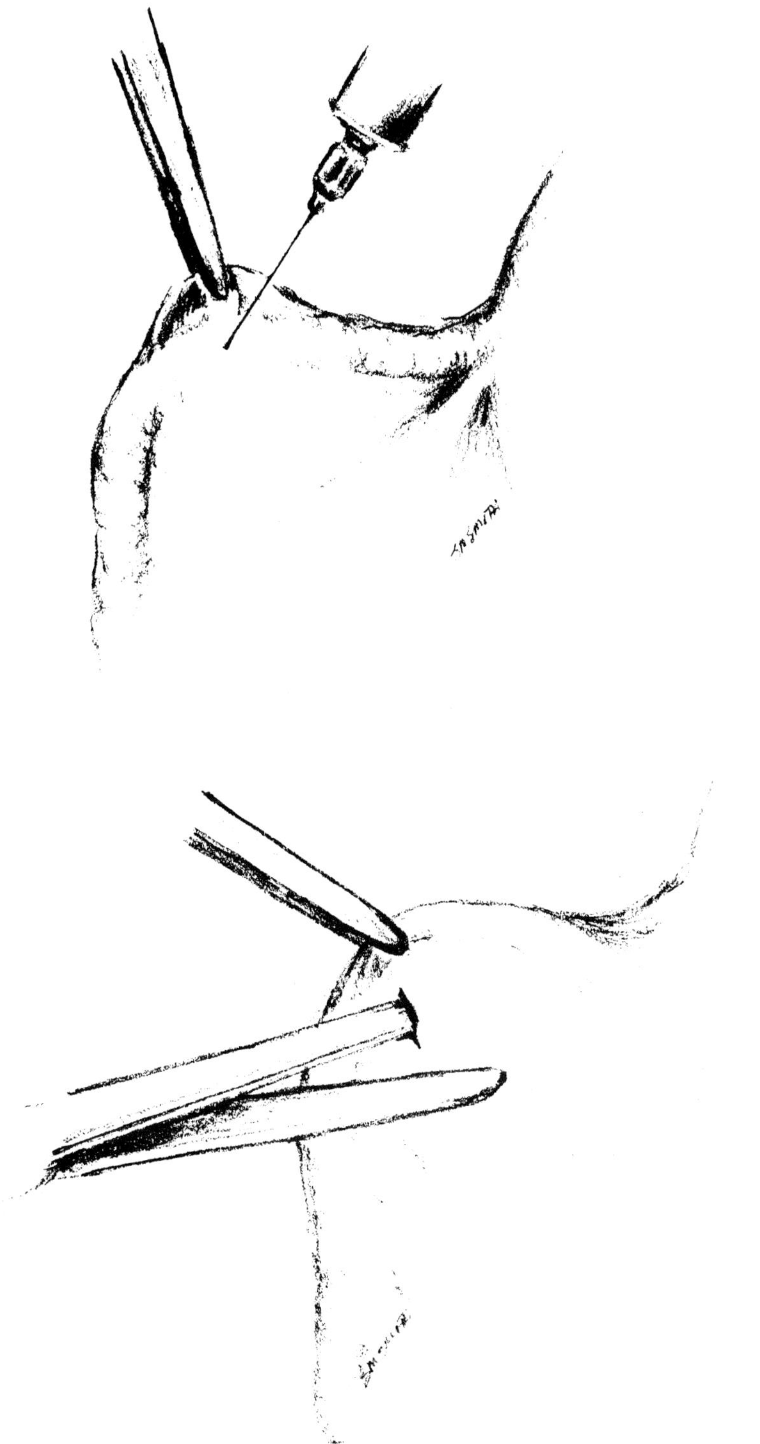

FIGURE 17.4 Uchida procedure—step 1. (Adapted from Mattingly RF, Thompson JD [eds]: *TeLinde's Operative Gynecology,* ed 6. Philadelphia, JB Lippincott Co, 1985, with permission.)

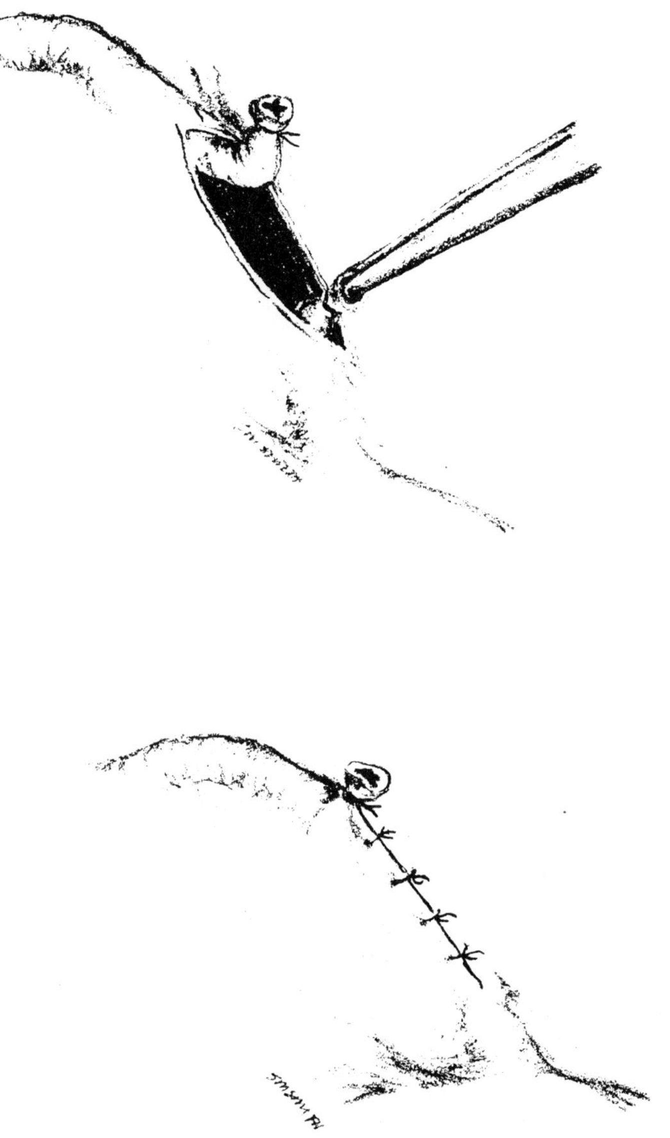

FIGURE 17.5 Uchida procedure—step 1. (Adapted from Mattingly RF, Thompson JD [eds]: *TeLinde's Operative Gynecology*, ed 6. Philadelphia, JB Lippincott Co, 1985, with permission.)

tubal segments are not identified, follow-up studies to evaluate the patient's fertility potential are indicated.

Because of the greatly increased vascularity of the pelvic organs during pregnancy, great care must be exercised in handling the tissues. Specifically, the veins in the mesosalpinges may easily be lacerated, and excessive traction and manipulation of this area must be avoided.

Presently, inadequate data exist to allow exclusive recommendation of one tubal sterilization technique over the others. Although the Uchida and Irving procedures appear to be very effective, the Pomeroy and Parkland procedures are also effective and are simpler to perform. Because the definitive data required to answer this question are unlikely to become available, the choice of procedure will probably depend on the preference and experience of the individual operator.

EXPLORATION OF THE ABDOMEN

In the discussion of cesarean delivery technique, the current edition of *Williams' Obstetrics*[12] recommends that the abdominal cavity be "systematically palpated" prior to closure of the peritoneum. Specifics of the technique are not described, and it is recommended only with the use of general anesthesia. Unacceptable levels of patient discomfort may occur when abdominal exploration is carried out under conduction anesthesia.

Although no data exist on the subject, many obstetricians feel that extensive abdominal exploration, especially careful examination of the bowel, will result in an unacceptable degree of patient discomfort and a high incidence of postoperative ileus. Personal experience indicates that exploration at the time of cesarean delivery is generally limited to the uterus and adnexae. It seems reasonable to extend this exploration when the patient has had symptoms referable to other intra-abdominal organs that could be evaluated by inspection and palpation.

INCIDENTAL APPENDECTOMY

Controversy regarding the advisability of incidental appendectomy at the time of cesarean has existed for many years. It was long taught that incidental appendectomy was absolutely contraindicated in the bloody, potentially infected environment of cesarean operations. The first series on the combined procedure was published by Larson in 1954.[16] She began performing appendectomy at the time of cesarean after one of her patients developed acute appendicitis within a few months of cesarean delivery. In addition to her own totally uncomplicated series of 20 patients, she reported personal communications from surgeons who had performed 764 combined procedures without mishap.

Despite the favorable initial report and several others that followed it,[17–19] philosophy and practice have not enthusiastically adopted the combined procedures as routine. In a 1957 editorial, Israel and Roitman[20] stated that sufficient evidence had accumulated to document the safety and advisability of the combined procedure. Waters[21] still found it necessary to make the same points 20 years later. The prevalence of incidental appendectomy at the time of cesarean delivery is not known, but it is probably quite low. Many years of experience seem to indicate that the procedure is not contraindicated at the time of uncomplicated cesarean delivery.

PROCEDURES ON THE ABDOMINAL WALL

Boyd and Hofmeister[19] reported 45 procedures performed on the abdominal wall at the time of cesarean delivery. These consisted of umbilical, ventral, and inguinal herniorrhaphies. No complications were noted. The authors concluded that because of the lack of problems and the avoidance of a separate surgical procedure, these procedures are indicated.

A recent study has described increased morbidity when extensive abdominal plastic procedures have been done at the time of total abdominal hysterectomy.[22] It seems obvious that these procedures should not be contemplated at the time of cesarean delivery.

SURGICAL PROCEDURES OF THE UTERUS

Most uterine abnormalities are better left alone when recognized at the time of cesarean delivery. Boyd and Hofmeister[19] listed 23 myomectomies performed during cesarean operations in their series and described no complications. Details of size, location, and criteria for removal were not given. Logic dictates that pedunculated myomas should be removed, given both the potential for torsion and the ease of the procedure. Subserosal myomas are unlikely to cause pregnancy problems and may regress significantly in the postpartum period. In addition, their removal may be associated with excessive blood loss. For these reasons, they should generally not be removed. Myomas in close proximity to the major vessels and other organ systems should definitely be left alone at the time of cesarean delivery.

In general, corrective procedures for uterine anomalies should not be undertaken at the time of cesarean delivery. An exception may be made when a small rudimentary uterine horn can be removed easily and without excessive blood loss. If some degree of failure of Mullerian duct fusion is noted, the anatomical details should be carefully noted and recorded in the patient's record. Because of the frequent association of uterine and renal anomalies, careful evaluation of the kidneys should be performed. Uterine anomalies may not always cause serious reproductive problems, and their attempted correction in a recently pregnant uterus may invoke massive blood loss. For these reasons, uterine unification procedures and excision of uterine septa should not be done at the time of cesarean delivery.

SURGICAL PROCEDURES OF THE ADNEXA

Careful inspection and palpation of the adnexae should be an integral part of all cesarean procedures. Abnormalities and the results of any previous pelvic surgical procedures, such as adhesions or missing organs, should be carefully noted. Often the history given by the patient concerning a

TABLE 17.2 Pathology of Procedures Done on the Ovaries at the Time of Cesarean Delivery in the Series of Boyd and Hofmeister[19]

Endometriosis	5
Serous cystadenoma	5
Cystic teratoma	4
Pseudomucinous cystadenoma	3
Decidual change	2
Follicular cyst	1
Granulosa cell cyst	1

prior surgical procedure is contradicted by the objective findings at surgery.

It seems clear that any ovarian lesion that may be neoplastic should be biopsied or removed for pathologic examination. Immediate frozen section examination should be requested when appropriate. Pathologic findings in 20 ovarian lesions removed at the time of cesarean delivery in the series of Boyd and Hofmeister[19] are listed in Table 17.2. When ovarian malignancy is documented, complete evaluation and surgical therapy should be carried out just as if the patient were not pregnant. If these skills are beyond the training and experience of the surgeon, consultation should be obtained. Paraovarian (hydatid) cysts have no malignant potential, but they may be a potential cause of adnexal torsion and may be easily removed.

OTHER PROCEDURES

Although theoretically any possible abdominal surgical procedure may be performed at the time of cesarean delivery, very few are performed in actual practice. If severe problems with a specific organ (e.g., gallbladder) predate the cesarean procedure, combined procedures may be considered. However, subjecting the patient to two simultaneous major surgical procedures, especially when she will soon be responsible for the care of a newborn infant, should be rare.

Although some authorities[23] have recommended a routine search for and removal of Meckel's diverticula during gynecologic procedures, no such recommendation exists for cesarean delivery. Indeed, unless the bowel is carefully examined, diagnosis of Meckel's diverticulum will be unusual. If a Meckel's diverticulum is seen that is unusually large, narrow-necked, inflamed, or suspected of containing heterotopic gastric or pancreatic elements, appropriate consultation should be obtained.

CONCLUSIONS

Tubal sterilization is the most commonly performed additional procedure done at the time of cesarean delivery. Although doubts exist concerning the best procedure, all of the widely used techniques are reasonably effective and are associated with very low morbidity. The suggestion that these procedures may be associated with a high incidence of later regret obligates the surgeon to provide detailed counseling prior to the procedure.

Although no consensus exists as to the proper extent of abdominal exploration at the time of cesarean, it is imperative that the adnexae be carefully examined. Possible ovarian neoplasia must be thoroughly evaluated and treated whenever it is encountered.

Most studies of incidental appendectomy at the time of cesarean delivery have indicated that it is a safe combined procedure. Performance depends on the operator's training and personal preference. In most cases, major procedures on the uterus and other organs should be avoided.

REFERENCES

1. Centers for Disease Control: Surgical sterilization surveillance; tubal sterilization and hysterectomy in women aged 15–44, 1979–1980. September 1983.
2. De Stefano F, Greenspan JR, Dicker RC, et al: Complications of interval laparoscopic tubal sterilization. *Obstet Gynecol* 61:153, 1983.
3. De Stefano F, Perlman JA, Peterson HB, et al: Long-term risk of menstrual disturbances after tubal sterilization. *Am J Obstet Gynecol* 152:835–841, 1985.
4. Grubb GS, Peterson HB, Layde PM, et al: Regret after decision to have a tubal sterilization. *Fert Steril* 44:248, 1985.
5. Murray J: A review of women requesting reversal of tubal sterilization. *Aust NZ J Obstet Gynaecol* 20:211, 1980.
6. Emens JM, Olive JE: Timing of female sterilization. *Br Med J* 2:1126, 1978.
7. Greenhill JP: *Obstetrics,* ed 13. Philadelphia, WB Saunders Co, 1965.
8. Taylor ES: *Beck's Obstetrical Practice,* ed 8. Baltimore, Williams & Wilkins Co, 1966.
9. Eastman NJ, Hellman LM (eds): *Williams' Obstetrics,* ed 13. New York, Appleton-Century-Crofts, 1966.
10. Prystowsky H, Eastman NJ. Puerperal tubal sterilization: Report of 1830 cases. *JAMA* 158463, 1955.
11. Husbands ME, Pritchard JA, Pritchard SA: Failure of tubal sterilization accompanying cesarean section. *Am J Obstet Gynecol* 107:966, 1970.
12. Pritchard JA, MacDonald PC, Gant NF: *Williams' Obstetrics,* ed 17. Norwalk, Conn, Appleton-Century-Crofts, 1985.
13. Irving FC: A new method of insuring sterility following cesarean section. *Am J Obstet Gynecol* 8:335, 1924.
14. Irving FC: Tubal sterilization. *Am J Obstet Gynecol* 60:1101, 1950.
15. Uchida H: Uchida tubal sterilization. *Am J Obstet Gynecol* 121:153, 1975.
16. Larsson E: Elective appendectomy at the time of cesarean section. *JAMA* 154:549, 1954.
17. Sweeney WJ: Incidental appendectomy at cesarean section. *Obstet Gynecol* 14:589, 1959.
18. Powell DV, Holmes DE, Beath DH, et al: Incidental appendectomy in obstetrics and gynecology. *Obstet Gynecol* 12:727, 1958.
19. Boyd A, Hofmeister FJ: Cesarean section and associated surgery. *Obstet Gynecol* 24:533, 1964.

20. Israel SL, Roitman HB: Cesarean section and prophylactic appendectomy: The passing of a prejudice. *Obstet Gynecol* 10:102, 1957.
21. Waters EG: Elective appendectomy with abdominal and pelvic surgery. *Obstet Gynecol* 50:511, 1977.
22. Voss SC, Sharp HC, Scott JR: Abdominoplasty combined with gynecologic surgical procedures. *Obstet Gynecol* 67:181, 1986.
23. Buchsbaum HJ: Meckel's diverticulum. *Obstet Gynecol* 45:311, 1975.

Intraoperative Complications

Chapter 18

Uterine Hemorrhage

Steven L. Clark, MD

Postpartum hemorrhage is classically attributable to one of three conditions: lacerations, atony, or retained placenta. This triad is as applicable to uterine hemorrhage following cesarean delivery as it is following vaginal delivery. Fortunately, in most instances, the source of the bleeding is readily apparent following a cesarean. Persistent bleeding will almost invariably be due to uterine atony; uterine, upper vaginal, or broad ligament laceration; or placenta accreta. The management of each of these conditions will now be considered in detail.

ATONY

Atony remains a major indication for emergency cesarean hysterectomy.[1,2] There is no one treatment that is uniformly effective in all cases of severe uterine atony. For this reason, any physician who performs a cesarean must have clearly defined a preestablished sequence of maneuvers designed to reverse uterine atony.[3,4] Such a sequence should be reviewed often, as hemorrhage from atony can be massive and leave little time for decision making (Table 18.1).

Step 1 involves rapid repair of the uterine incision accompanied by manual pressure on the exteriorized uterus. Prior to uterine closure, a rapid inspection of the uterine cavity is essential to rule out retained products of conception, which may contribute to the underlying atony. As manual pressure is being applied, a dilute solution of oxytocin, 40 units/L, is rapidly infused intravenously. An intravenous bolus of oxytocin may lead to profound hypotension, even in the absence of hypovolemia, and is unacceptable. Next, methergotamine maleate 0.2 mg, may be administered intramuscularly. In the absence of hypertension, it is at times appropriate to cautiously administer this drug intravenously. If the patient

TABLE 18.1 A Stepwise Approach to the Control of Uterine Atony

1. Apply bimanual pressure
2. Infuse oxytocin, 40 units/L
3. Administer methergine 0.2 mg IM or IV
4. Administer 15 mg PGF_2, 1.0–1.5 mg IM
5. Perform uterine artery ligation
6. Consider hypogastric artery ligation
7. Perform hysterectomy

fails to respond to these initial maneuvers, the next step involves the administration of 15 methyl prostaglandin F_2 alpha (PGF_2) (Prostin). This agent has been demonstrated to be effective both when administered intramuscularly and when injected directly into the myometrium.[5–7] Currently, there is no good evidence to support one route of injection over the other. Doses are administered in increments of 250 μg up to a total dose of 1–1.5 mg.

Should the uterus continue to be atonic and bleed following administration of oxytocin, methergine, and PGF_2 alpha, bilateral uterine artery ligation is indicated. This procedure is described in detail in Chapter 16. It is important to note here, however, that for maximal effect, the standard "low" ligation of the ascending uterine artery should be accompanied by the placement of an additional suture at the point of potential anastomoses between tubal branches of the ovarian artery and the uterine artery (Figure 18.1) in the vicinity of the utero-ovarian ligament.

When these measures have failed to reverse uterine atony, a rapid clinical decision is necessary. Hypogastric artery ligation is successful in stopping hemorrhage and avoiding hysterectomy in less than half of these cases.[8] Further, it is evident that the risk of serious maternal complications (including cardiac arrest) is high among patients who undergo unsuccessful hypogastric artery ligation for the control of obstetric hemorrhage and then proceed to emergency hysterectomy.[8] If the patient is clinically stable, of low parity, and highly desirous of future childbearing, hypogastric artery ligation may be attempted. However, if these conditions are not met, hypogastric artery ligation is best omitted and hysterectomy promptly initiated.[8] The details of hypogastric artery ligation are presented in Chapter 16.

When faced with severe atony, it is important to avoid undue delay in initiating definitive surgical therapy. It is notable that emergency hysterectomies performed for atony have a higher rate of complication, infectious morbidity, and operating time than those performed for any other indication.[1] This may, in part, be attributed to surgical indecision and delay in initiating hysterectomy in an effort to preserve fertility. In a large series of patients undergoing hysterectomy for atony, the mean blood loss *following* the decision for hysterectomy was 2,000 cc.[1] Thus, it is vital to accomplish the above maneuvers and make the decision for uterine con-

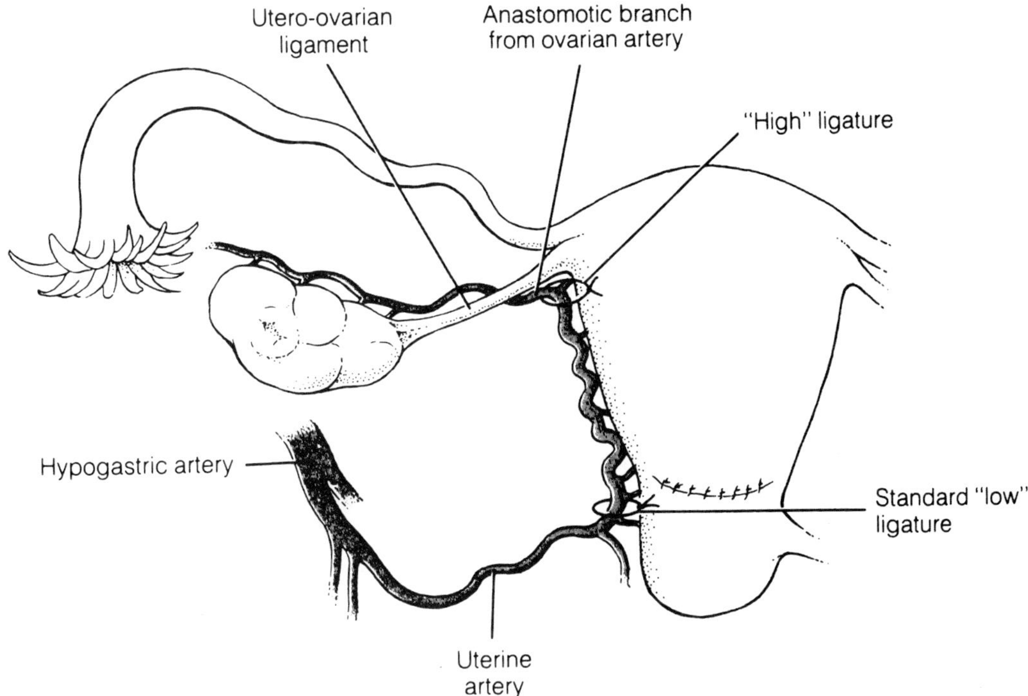

FIGURE 18.1 Technique of uterine artery ligation. Sutures are placed to encompass the ascending uterine arteries and the anastomotic branches from the ovarian arteries. (From Clark SL, Phelan JP: *Contemp OB-GYN* 24:70, 1984, with permission from Medical Economics Books, Oradell, NJ.)

servation or removal as expeditiously as possible. The decision to perform hysterectomy should be based upon the failure of available conservative methods rather than on an arbitrarily defined blood loss.

Total hysterectomy remains the procedure of choice after failure of conservative measures. However, removal of the cervix itself is often as time-consuming as an entire supracervical hysterectomy. In many cases of atony, the bulk of bleeding myometrium is in the fundus, and supracervical hysterectomy may be efficacious and appropriate, especially if the patient is hemodynamically unstable.

Risk factors for the development of severe postcesarean atony include the use of magnesium sulfate, oxytocin augmentation of labor, preoperative amnionitis, fetal macrosomia, and cesarean delivery for labor arrest.[1] When performing cesarean delivery in conjunction with any of these clinical conditions, the clinician would be wise to anticipate possible hemorrhage from atony.

PLACENTA ACCRETA

Placenta accreta is the second most common indication for emergency hysterectomy for obstetric hemorrhage.[1] Its incidence appears to be increasing.[9] This is due, in large part, to the well-documented association of placenta accreta with placenta previa and previous cesarean delivery, both of which have been increased by the recent trend toward more liberal indications for cesarean delivery. In a recent review of the subject, it was found that 25% of patients undergoing cesarean for placenta previa in the presence of one or more uterine scars subsequently underwent cesarean hysterectomy for placenta accreta.[9] This risk appears to increase directly with the number of previous uterine incisions.

Some authors have reported an unacceptably high mortality rate for patients with placenta accreta treated by procedures other than hysterectomy.[10] This conclusion, however, has not been borne out by recent studies.[9,11] In one recent review, 45% of patients with clinical placenta accreta were treated with measures other than hysterectomy, with no maternal mortality.[9] When the accreta is focal, simple excision of the site of trophoblast invasion, oversewing the area with several figure eight sutures, or sharp curettage may occasionally be effective. Nevertheless, except in cases of focal accreta in the young patient for whom future childbearing is of major concern, hysterectomy appears to remain the procedure of choice and should be initiated as soon as the diagnosis of placenta accreta is made.

Unlike uterine atony, in which most of the bleeding myometrium is in the fundus, many cases of placenta accreta (especially when associated with placenta previa) involve the lower uterine segment/cervical region. For this reason, in contrast to uterine atony, a supercervical hysterectomy may prove ineffective in controlling the bleeding, and total abdominal hysterectomy is almost always necessary.[1,9] Fortunately, the need for hysterectomy is usually evident before blood loss is massive, thus allowing a total hysterectomy to be performed with safety.

LACERATIONS

Lacerations following cesarean delivery may involve the uterus, vagina, or broad ligament. A low transverse uterine incision is more likely to be accompanied by lacerations following either the delivery of a macrosomic infant or the use of improper delivery technique. Whether the infant's head is delivered manually or with the aid of an instrument, it is of the utmost importance to try to avoid using the lower uterine segment as a fulcrum against which to gain a mechanical advantage.

Lacerations involving uterine tissue are usually sutured easily. When the laceration extends vertically into the vagina or laterally into the broad ligament, the situation becomes more complex. Lacerations extending inferiorly into the area of the lateral vagina generally are not associated with as significant a blood loss as those extending directly laterally into the broad ligament. Because of the potential proximity of such lacerations to the ureters, however, extreme care is mandatory in their repair. First, the distal apex of the incision must be carefully and conclusively identified, and the suture begun at or just beyond that point. In many cases, this point will only be millimeters away from the ureters. In such cases, it is essential that the broad ligaments be opened and the position of the ureters identified prior to placing the sutures. The placement of a No. 8 French ureteral catheter may aid the clinician in identifying the course of the ureter, especially in the area just proximal to the ureterovesical junction. Such placement may be easily accomplished in a retrograde manner by opening the bladder in a vertical fashion extraperitoneally, visualizing the ureteral orifices, and advancing a ureteral catheter up the appropriate ureter with the aid of a right-angle clamp. Following removal of the catheter, the bladder is repaired with an initial running and a second imbricating layer of 2-0 chromic. Failure to identify with certainty the course of the ureter or the position of the bladder during repair of vaginal or broad ligament lacerations may result in ureteral or bladder damage and/or fistula formation.

Most troublesome are lateral extensions of a low transverse incision into the broad ligament. Because of laceration of the uterine vessels, such extensions are often extremely bloody. In addition, to avoid ureteral injury when suturing within the broad ligament, a time-consuming and meticulous dissection may be necessary to isolate and ligate the bleeding vessel safely. For this reason, hysterectomies performed after lateral extensions result in more blood loss than those performed for any other indication.[1] As with vaginal lacerations, the first step in dealing with bleeding lacerations into the broad ligament involves meticulous dissection of the broad ligament, with identification of the iliac vessels and ureter. There is no place for blind suturing in this area. At times, it may be necessary to decrease uterine artery pulse pressure by ipsilateral hypogastric artery ligation prior to identification and repair of the bleeding uterine vessel, especially if it is torn near its origin from the hypogastric artery.[8,12] Occasionally the laceration may be so extensive that hysterectomy greatly facilitates exposure and hemostasis. When dealing with lacerations of the ascending uterine artery, it is well to keep in mind the course of the uterine artery after it exits from the internal iliac artery. It is often much more effective to identify the course of the bleeding vessel inferior to the laceration and ligate it than to make repeated attempts to apply figure eight sutures directly at the point of laceration.

In the presence of intractable hemorrhage following cesarean in the young patient, the decision of whether to perform uterine conservation or hysterectomy is one of the more difficult decisions encountered in obstetrics. For this reason, it is essential that the possibility of hysterectomy be discussed with any patient undergoing cesarean delivery, and in particular detail with patients who have any of the risk factors mentioned above. Only if the surgeon has complete understanding of the patient's desire for future childbearing can the proper decisions be promptly made.

Further, it is clear that the control of uterine hemorrhage following cesarean often mandates additional emergency procedures including ligation of the uterine arteries and hypogastric arteries, and cesarean hysterectomy. In the presence of such a condition, there is often insufficient time to call in a consultant. For this reason, physicians who undertake cesarean deliveries should be familiar with and have privileges for the performance of such additional procedures.

REFERENCES

1. Clark SL, Yeh S-Y, Phelan JP, et al: Emergency hysterectomy for the control of obstetric hemorrhage. *Obstet Gynecol* 64:376, 1984.
2. Chestnut DH, Eden RD, Gall SA, et al: Peripartum hysterectomy: A review of cesarean and postpartum hysterectomy. *Obstet Gynecol* 65:365, 1985.
3. Clark SL, Phelan JP: Surgical control of obstetric hemorrhage. *Contemp OB-GYN* 24:70, 1984.
4. Hayashi RH: Heading off disaster in postpartum hemorrhage. *Contemp OB-GYN* 22:91, 1982.
5. Hayashi RH, Castillo MS, Noah ML: Management of severe postpartum hemorrhage due to uterine atony using an analogue of prostaglandin F_2. *Obstet Gynecol* 58:426, 1981.
6. Bruce SL, Paul RH, Van Dorsten JP: Control of postpartum uterine atony by intramyometrial prostaglandin. *Obstet Gynecol* 59:475, 1982.
7. Tagaki S, Yoshida T, Togo Y, et al: The effects of intramyometrial injection of prostaglandin F_2 on severe postpartum hemorrhage. *Prostaglandins* 12:565, 1976.
8. Clark SL, Phelan JP, Yeh SY, et al: Hypogastric artery ligation for the control of obstetric hemorrhage. *Obstet Gynecol* 66:353, 1985.
9. Clark SL, Koonings PP, Phelan JP: Placenta previa—accreta and previous cesarean section. *Obstet Gynecol* 66:89, 1985.
10. McHattie TJ: Placenta previa accreta. *Obstet Gynecol* 40:795, 1972.
11. Read JA, Cotton DB, Miller FC: Placenta accreta: Changing clinical aspects and outcome. *Obstet Gynecol* 56:31, 1980.
12. Burchell RC: Physiology of internal iliac artery ligation. *Obstet Gynecol Br Commonwealth* 75:642, 1968.

Chapter 19

Management of Urinary and Gastrointestinal Tract Injuries

Carl V. Smith, MD, and
Donald G. Gallup, MD

The importance of a fundamental knowledge of surgical anatomy and precise surgical technique cannot be overemphasized for the obstetrician who performs a cesarean delivery. The intimate relationships between the urinary, gastrointestinal, and genital tracts require a pelvic surgeon to have more than a passing knowledge of their anatomy. However, even the most experienced surgeon may encounter distortions of anatomy, difficult dissections, and adhesions that predispose to injury. Prompt recognition and repair of the majority of these conditions result in no long-term functional sequelae. A discussion of the anatomic interrelationships, principles of recognition, and surgical repair is vital to a discussion of cesarean delivery.

URINARY TRACT INJURIES

The Urinary Bladder

The incidence of injury to the urinary bladder at the time of cesarean delivery is quite variable.[1–5] Older reports, in which midline abdominal and uterine incisions predominated, contain a lower incidence than those in recent years, in which a Pfannenstiel skin incision preceded a low transverse uterine incision.[6] In the course of normal pregnancy, the urinary bladder becomes an abdominal rather than a pelvic organ, which consequently places the bladder at higher theoretic risk at the time the parietal peritoneum is incised. Pfannenstiel incisions and entry into the peritoneal cavity at a more caudal level further increase the risk. Prior cesarean delivery, with resultant scarring and obliteration of the vesicouterine space, are additional risk factors.

As with many surgical complications, the best outcomes are associated with prevention of the injury. Injuries to the dome of bladder can be minimized by (1) preoperative catheterization of the bladder and (2) careful entry into the peritoneal cavity as far cephalad as possible. Careful palpation and assurance of transparency are critical factors prior to incision of what is thought to be the parietal peritoneum. Injuries to the base of the bladder are most frequent during a repeat procedure. As discussed above, clear tissue planes do not always exist in this circumstance. The pelvic surgeon should avoid blunt dissection of the bladder with a sponge stick or gauze-covered finger. Instead, meticulous sharp dissection reduces blood loss, as well as the possibility of inadvertent blunt entry into the bladder. Occasionally, sharp entry into the bladder will occur, but this is usually recognized promptly. When a blunt cystotomy occurs, it is frequently accompanied by bleeding that may obscure the cystotomy site or delay the diagnosis beyond the time when immediate repairs can be safely accomplished.

Another group of patients who appear to be at increased risk of bladder injury are those undergoing cesarean hysterectomy. Mickal and colleagues reported an inadvertent cystotomy rate of 5.2% in patients undergoing this procedure.[7] A similar rate was noted by Barclay—4.1% in 1,000 consecutive cesarean hysterectomies.[8] The majority of these injuries occur at the bladder base. Care must be exercised when mobilizing the bladder from the underlying lower uterine segment. Except in the case of elective cesarean hysterectomy, most patients have undergone labor, with resultant ballooning of the lower uterine segment and dilatation and effacement of the cervix. Consequently, distortion of the vesicouterine anatomy may be present. Careful sharp dissection of the bladder as caudal as possible is recommended. When the dissection has been carried below the level of the cervix, sharp entry into the vagina and identification of the cervix may be preferable to the more standard cross-clamping technique. Lastly, supracervical hysterectomy may prevent inadvertent bladder injury and is the procedure of choice when dealing with emergency hysterectomy in a hemodynamically unstable patient. Similarly, it should be considered when the surgeon is faced with a difficult dissection that may result in protracted operating time and increased blood loss.

With the increasing use of cesarean delivery and avoidance of difficult operative vaginal procedures, bladder injuries from the latter are rarely seen today. However, the potential for bladder injury exists in midpelvic vaginal delivery (vacuum extraction or midforceps rotation), with version and extraction of the second twin, and in difficult vaginal breech deliveries. McCausland et al in 1960 reported that 65% (15 of 23) pregnancy-related vesicovaginal fistulas resulted from forceps delivery.[9] In contrast, Dunlop, in 1969, reported on 292 midforceps deliveries without a single urinary tract injury.[10] For reasons previously stated, the experience of the latter author more closely approximates the realities of modern obstetrics. Fortunately, those injuries are rare today, in contrast to previous times, when recognition was not infrequently delayed and the subsequent fistulization rate appeared higher.

A final and even rarer time at which the bladder may be injured is at the time of uterine rupture, particularly of the scarred uterus. In older investigations, the rates of bladder injury associated with uterine rupture are between 10% and 14%.[11,12] Recent experience with uterine rupture or dehiscence in prior cesarean patients allowed a trial of labor suggests a much lower incidence.[13,14] Because the risk is present, the integrity of the bladder should be ascertained in patients suffering a lower uterine segment rupture or scar separation.

Recognition of Bladder Injury

Entry into the urinary bladder is usually recognized immediately. When entry into the peritoneum or mobilization of the bladder flap has been difficult or the operative field is bloody, the abdomen should not be closed until the integrity of the bladder is verified.

Transurethral instillation of methylene blue–colored saline aids in the diagnosis. Sterile milk may also be used and has the advantage of being nonstaining. However, methylene blue has wider availability in the operating suite and is probably the most common solution used. Leakage of fluid identifies the cystotomy site; repair may take place immediately or may be delayed until after delivery of the neonate. This technique may also be of value when extensive anterior vaginal lacerations complicate vaginal delivery. With the patient in the reverse Trendelenberg position, spillage of milk or colored saline should be evident.

Repair of Bladder Injuries

Full-thickness bladder lacerations should be repaired with a two-layer closure with 2-0 or 3-0 chromic. Continuous or interrupted sutures appear to function equally well in achieving a watertight closure. Whether or not to incorporate the mucosa in the suture line is controversial.[6,15,16] After repair, reinflation of the bladder to ensure a watertight closure seems reasonable.

Of major importance is the site of the cystotomy. A laceration of the bladder dome and its subsequent repair are rarely management problems. The blood supply to this area is excellent, and the tissue planes are more clearly defined. Alternatively, the bladder base appears to heal more slowly, is thinner, and receives less blood flow. More important is the possibility of a laceration in the trigone. Consequently the trigone should be visualized before a laceration to the bladder base is repaired. If the laceration is within 1 cm of the ureteral orifice, ureteral catheters should be inserted. If difficulty is encountered, an intentional cystotomy in the bladder dome is helpful and allows repair of the laceration under direct visualization.

Postoperative Bladder Drainage

It is evident that after a bladder laceration, catheter drainage of the bladder is required. Less clear, however, are the optimal duration and route of this drainage. If a literature consensus exists, it is that 7–10 days of bladder drainage is recommended. Eisenkop and colleagues found a mean length of 8.8 days of drainage (range, 4–15 days) in 52 patients sustaining either intentional or inadvertent cystotomy at the time of cesarean delivery.[14] At least 1 month's follow-up was obtained in 44 of these patients, and no evidence of fistula formation or bladder dysfunction was manifest. Clearly, some patients had shorter periods of decompression without adverse sequelae, but it is difficult to recommend lesser periods based on these data. Everett and Mattingly recommend the more traditional 7 days and note no fistulas in 77 patients so managed.[2]

Although no well-designed study has demonstrated a clear advantage of suprapubic catheterization, it does possess theoretic advantages over the transurethral route. The former technique allows the patient to void if she feels the urge. Similarly, by clamping the catheter in the final days, tone may be restored to an otherwise atonic bladder. In this fashion, repeat catheterization and its attendant risk of infection may be largely eliminated. However, the most important principle is to avoid overdistention of the bladder and potential disruption of the suture line. This may be readily accomplished by either method.

Incidence of Fistula Formation

The key to avoiding this rare complication of obstetrics is early recognition and repair of the cystotomy. The two studies cited above report a fistula rate of 0% after recognition, repair, and adequate drainage.[2,14] With meticulous surgical technique, the majority of patients with this complication today should have a similar outcome. Although the diagnosis and management of fistulas are discussed in Chapter 29, the appearance of clear liquid in the vagina should raise the suspicion of fistula. Prompt and complete bladder drainage in these cases has been reported to result in closure of the fistula in a percentage of the patients.[6,17] Although the majority of fistulas are vesicovaginal, injuries of the bladder base may lead to vesicouterine fistulas. Finally, a recent case of vesical endometriosis after bladder injury has been described.[18]

Ureteral Injury

Injury to the ureter is one of the most feared complications of a pelvic operation. Fortunately, its occurrence at the time of cesarean delivery is indeed rare. In most larger series of ureteral injury, the majority occur during abdominal hysterectomy. However, Eisenkop et al reported 7 ureteral injuries in 7,527 patients undergoing cesarean delivery.[14] Reviewing this extensive experience allows some insight into the mechanism of and means to avoid ureteral injury. Five of these patients experienced injury as the surgeon was attempting to control bleeding from extension of the uterine incision. In two of these patients, the injury was unrecognized intraoperatively. However, the diagnosis was made by pyelography within 48 hours of the operation. Both patients subsequently underwent reexploration with ureteroneocystostomy without complication. In another report, Nielsen and Hokegard found no ureteral injuries in 1,319 patients undergoing cesarean delivery.[4] These reports underscore the importance of establishing the integrity of the urinary tract before closing the abdomen if the clinical suspicion of injury exists.

To reduce the likelihood of ureteral injury, it is axiomatic that the pelvic surgeon should always be aware of the location of the ureter in relation to the operative field. This is particularly true when repairing extensions of the uterine incision into the vagina or broad ligament. Controlling hemorrhage with direct pressure while identifying the course of the ureter allows accurate suture placement and reduces the potential for ureteral injury.[4]

As with inadvertent cystotomy, the risk of ureteral injury increases when cesarean delivery is combined with hysterectomy. Barclay reported 4 such injuries in 1,000 consecutive cesarean hysterectomies.[8] A similar rate of 0.2% was noted by Mickal and colleagues.[7] At the time of cesarean hysterectomy, the procedures causing ureteral injury are similar to the nongravid procedures. Ligation of the infundibulopelvic ligament, clamping of the uterine vessels, and cross-clamping of the vaginal cuff are the most frequent procedures. In difficult cases, opening the retroperitoneal space and identifying the ureter prior to ligation of the infundibulopelvic ligament may be helpful. This can be accomplished by elevating the parietal peritoneum over the bifurcation of the common iliac arteries and incising longitudinally. Gentle blunt dissection of the loose areolar tissue should allow prompt identification of the ureter on the medial leaf. Similar attention to the course of the pelvic ureter and careful clamp placement at the cervical isthmus should reduce the potential for incorporation of the ureter into the vascular pedicles. Finally, wide mobilization of the bladder, taking small bites with clamps, should allow the ureter to be displaced laterally away from the vaginal angle. A final occasion of potential ureteral compromise is during reperitonealization of the pelvic floor, when it may undergo kinking. The surgeon should attempt to restore the anatomy to a near-normal condition with sutures placed superficially in the visceral peritoneum. A final intraoperative technique to prevent injury is the passage of ureteral stent, either cystoscopically or through a ureterotomy incision.[15] This procedure may assist the surgeon in locating the ureter, but it does not absolutely protect against injury and may, in fact, result in intimal damage or perforation. Similarly, if it is performed through a ureterotomy incision, the potential for a ureteral fistula exists; if this procedure is felt to be clinically warranted, it may be wise to do it in a retrograde fashion through a cystotomy.

Recognition of Ureteral Injury

Once a ureteral injury is suspected, the abdomen should not be closed until the injury is ruled out or recognized and repaired. The various methods by which to assess ureteral integrity will now be discussed. Intravenous injection of 10 cc indigocarmine may result in the extravasation of dye at the site of ureteral transection. This technique has the advantage of being rapid and noninvasive. Failure of dye to appear in the Foley bag or within the peritoneal cavity may suggest bilateral ureteral ligation. In the absence of these findings, one cannot definitely state that the ureter has not been injured. Ligation, kinking, or crush injuries may be overlooked.

An alternative technique is injection of the ureter directly with indigocarmine or methylene blue. As described by O'Leary and O'Leary, the retroperitoneal space is entered, and the ureter is elevated and injected with 0.5 cc methylene with a small-gauge needle.[19] Prompt appearance of dye in the catheter drainage system confirms ureteral patency. This technique, however, is useful only to detect complete unilateral obstruction. Ureteral kinking or bilateral injury should be evaluated by a different method.

More invasive techniques should be considered when evaluating the potential for the latter injury. Ureterotomy and antegrade passage of a ureteral stent may be of diagnostic value. The retroperitoneal space is entered and a small (0.5-cm) longitudinal incision is made in the ureter, through which a No. 5–8 French ureteral catheter or pediatric feeding tube is placed. It is then threaded down the length of the ureter into the bladder. If the catheter passes freely, potency is confirmed and it may be removed. The ureterotomy incision is closed with interrupted simple seromuscular sutures of 4–5 0 chromic. It is probably unnecessary to drain the site, but if this is desired, a soft Jackson Pratt-type closed suction system is appropriate.

If the passage of retrograde ureteral catheters is desired, the bladder is distended with saline or with clamping of the Foley catheter in order to elevate the bladder dome away from the trigone. A vertical incision is made in the dome, and the ureteral orifices are identified. Methylene blue or indigocarmine is then injected intravenously, and prompt spillage of dye should be evident. In the absence of these findings, retrograde catheterization of the ureter should be performed. If resistance is felt, the pelvic ureter should be inspected for obstruction. If the catheter passes freely, it

TABLE 19.1 Indications for Postoperative Pyleography

Flank pain or costovertebral angle tenderness
Unexplained fever or ileus
Evidence of copious amounts of clear fluid in the vagina
Oliguria unrelated to hypovolemia
Abdominal or flank mass

is removed, and a double-layered closure of the bladder is performed, as described earlier.

A final method of assessment of ureteral integrity is intravenous pyelography (IVP). Table 19.1 lists commonly accepted indications for an IVP. If the IVP is not diagnostic, consideration should be given to cystoscopy and retrograde pyelography or ureteral catheterization.

Repair of Ureteral Injuries

Without exception, injuries recognized at the time of operation should be immediately repaired. Much controversy, however, exists as to the management of injuries whose recognition is delayed. When the ureter is clamped or ligated, immediate delegation and close inspection are warranted.[20–23] A ureteral stent is positioned and is left in place for 7–10 days. The use of a retroperitoneal soft drain brought out through a separate stab wound and located away from any repair site is recommended. Active, closed system devices such as the Jackson-Pratt may be preferred.

The treatment of a complete or partial ureteral transection depends on the level of the injury. In general, injuries to the distal 5 cm of the ureter are best repaired by ureteroneocystostomy.[1,15,24] The precise technique with which to accomplish this repair is controversial. Specifically, is the use of an antireflux technique, such as the creation of a submucosal tunnel, necessary? When one examines the normal anatomy of the ureterovesical junction, it is apparent that there is a 3-mm intramural ureteral segment and a 7-mm submucosal segment.[5,15] Some appear to favor the antireflux technique.[5,15,16,25] Tunneling is time-consuming in an emergency and may be unnecessary in adults. Figure 19.1 demonstrates the principal components of the procedure. The distal ureter is ligated with permanent suture. The free proximal end is tagged with a suture to facilitate its placement within the bladder. A vertical incision in the dome is made, as described earlier. A small incision is made in the bladder mucosa, through which a clamp is inserted. A submucosal tunnel is created, the length of which should be two to three times the width of the ureter. The tagged end of the ureter is placed in the clamp and drawn inside the bladder. The free ureteral end should be spatulated and sewn to the edges of bladder mucosa with 0000 chromic suture. Performance of this anastomosis may be facilitated by the placement of a No. 5–8 French stent. The serosal side of the anastomosis should be supported by additional

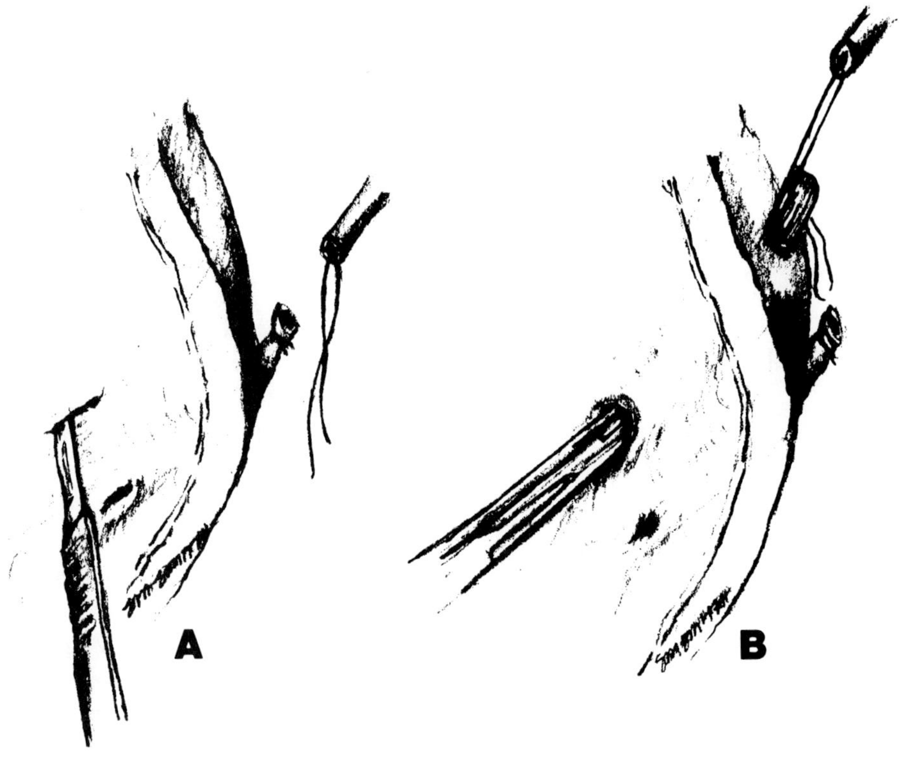

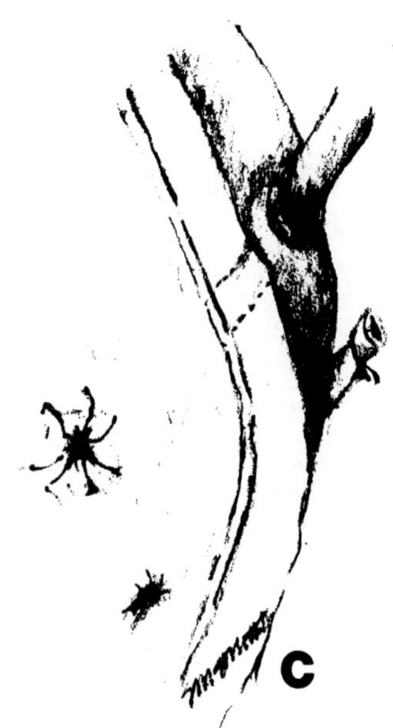

FIGURE 19.1 Technique of ureteroneocystostomy. (A) The distal end of the ureter is ligated with permanent suture, and the free distal end is tagged with a suture. A new incision in the bladder mucosa is made in the trigone after vertically incising the bladder dome. (B) A submucosal tunnel is created through which the distal end is drawn. (C) The distal end is spatulated and a mucosal–mucosal anastomosis is performed with 0000 chromic suture. (Adapted from Mattingly RF [ed]: *TeLinde's Operative Gynecology.* Philadelphia, JB Lippincott Co, 1977, with permission.)

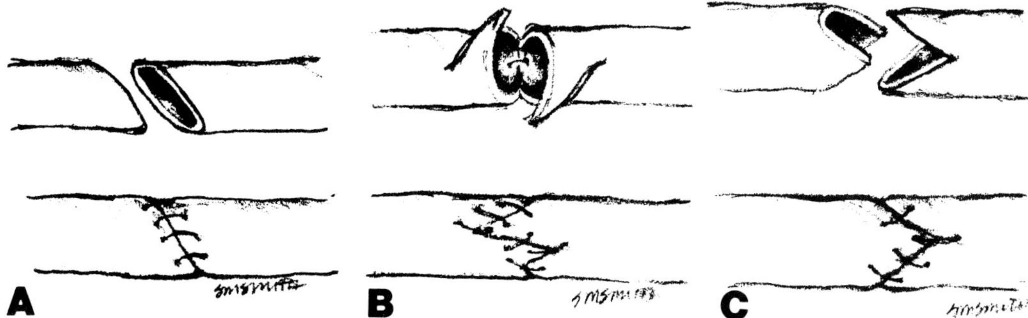

FIGURE 19.2 Techniques of ureteroureteral anastomosis. (A) Spatulation, (B) Z-plasty, (C) oblique. (Adapted from Mattingly RF [ed]: *TeLinde's Operative Gynecology.* Philadelphia, JB Lippincott Co, 1977, with permission.)

sutures of 0000 chromic. The bladder is then closed with standard double-layer closure, as described earlier. The ureteral stent should be left in place for 10–14 days and the bladder continuously drained for 7–14 days. A critical factor that should improve the outcome of this procedure is to avoid tension on the anastomotic site. This may be accomplished by suturing the bladder wall to the musculature of the pelvic wall, as described by Prout and Koontz.[26]

More difficult technical problems arise when the ureter is damaged between 5 and 10 cm from the ureterovesical junction. Two procedures exist with which to reimplant the ureter into the bladder. The first, described by Harrow, is also referred to as the "psoas muscle hitch."[27] In brief, it consists of placing a series of seromuscular sutures in the bladder and attaching them to the belly of the psoas muscle. The bladder, being a mobile, distensible organ, lends itself well to this procedure and, consequently, reduces tension on the anastomotic site. The construction of a Boari flap in an attempt to re-create the distal ureter is done as a last resort to restore continuity of the urinary tract.[28,29] It is technically more difficult, and few individuals have had vast experience with it.

Injury to the ureter at or above the pelvic brim is most likely to occur at hysterectomy. This is indeed a rare site of injury at cesarean delivery. When it occurs, ureteroureterostomy is the procedure of choice. It is performed over a ureteral stent. A technique to minimize compromise of the ureteral lumen should be selected. The repair should be accomplished with 0000 chromic interrupted sutures, avoiding the mucosa. Oblique repairs, Z-plasty, or spatulation will provide a watertight anastomosis without compromise of the lumen (Figure 19.2). Reperitonealization should be performed and the retroperitoneal space drained. Finally, with extensive distal ureteral damage, transureteral reanastomosis may be the procedure of choice. Cutaneous ureterostomy is rarely indicated.

Delayed Recognition of Ureteral Damage

The management of ureteral injury recognized in the immediate postoperative period is controversial. The appearance of clear fluid from the vagina is the usual presentation. Regardless of whether or not immediate repair is effected, immediate decompression is warranted in order to preserve renal function. Percutaneous nephrostomy, or, more rarely, open nephrostomy is the procedure of choice. Beland reported on five patients with seven ureteral injuries who underwent a variety of repairs, with a postoperative discovery range of 1–30 days.[20] All had excellent results. A similar experience was reported by Kamholz et al.[23] The traditional approach, however, is to perform urinary diversion and subsequent repair usually after 4–6 weeks[3,6,16] if the injury is recognized more than 72 hours after the initial operation. Within the first 72 hours, immediate reoperation is appropriate. The reasons for this approach are primarily related to extensive tissue edema and reaction.

Postoperative Considerations and Outcome

Bladder drainage and the maintenance of ureteral stent drainage should be considered for 7–14 days following the repair of ureteral injuries. During the postoperative period, evidence of pyelonephritis, flank pain, or fever should raise the clinical suspicion of infection or reobstruction. Appropriate cultures and pyelography should be performed. As with bladder injuries, the recognition of ureteral injury and early definitive repair are associated with an exceedingly low rate of fistula formation (approaching zero). Unfortunately, when ureteral injury is diagnosed postoperatively, the prognosis is not as favorable. Consequently, careful surgical technique with aggressive investigation to establish the integrity of the ureter are the obstetrician's chief methods of preventing the occurrence of long-term sequelae. The definitive repair of most bladder injuries should be within the province of the obstetrician, but urologic consultation is also suggested. In the case of ureteral injury, liberal consultation with a urologist or a gynecologic oncologist should be considered.

GASTROINTESTINAL TRACT INJURIES

Damage to the gastrointestinal tract during cesarean delivery is rare. Nielsen and Hokegard reported 1 such injury in 1,319 cesarean deliveries.[4] Risk factors include prior abdominal operations and a history of pelvic infection, which may lead to adhesion formation. Such adhesions predispose the patient to bowel injuries, particularly at the time the peritoneum is incised. Sharp incision through only the transparent layer of the peritoneum should reduce the incidence of this injury. No particular diagnostic strategies are required, as the injury is usually evident. During cesarean delivery, the small bowel is more commonly injured than the colon. At cesarean hysterectomy, the sigmoid may also be injured. As management techniques differ, injuries to the small and large bowel will be discussed separately.

SMALL BOWEL INJURY

In patients requiring lysis of adhesions during cesarean delivery, the small bowel may inadvertently be entered. Sharp dissection of those adhesions with the scissor tips pointed away from the bowel will help avoid this complication. Small, isolated defects in the serosa may be closed with interrupted silk sutures on an atraumatic needle. Alternatively, multiple small defects that do not involve the mucosa may safely be left without repair.

Full-thickness lacerations should be repaired. A double-layered closure should be utilized. The mucosa is incorporated in the first layer and repaired with running or interrupted sutures of 000 or 0000 chromic. A seromuscular layer of similar-sized silk suture is then utilized. In order not to narrow the lumen, a transverse closure of the longitudinal defect is advised.[30]

When multiple enterotomy sites or a long single site are encountered, consideration should be given to a small bowel resection and reanastomosis.[31,32] Figure 19.3 demonstrates the surgical technique for a resection and two-layered reanastomosis. First, the enterotomy site is clamped with Kocher clamps to isolate the site and reduce peritoneal soiling with intestinal contents. A V-shaped wedge of mesentery is removed after the vessels have been carefully clamped and ligated. Traction sutures of 000 to 0000 silk are utilized at the margin of the resection. The tissue between the jaws of the clamps is then sharply removed. Placement of an atraumatic intestinal clamp such as a Glassman clamp on either side of the anastomosis will reduce the loss of gastrointestinal contents until the anastomosis is completed. First, the mucosal layer is closed with a running or interrupted layer of 000 or 0000 chromic. Next, a seromuscular layer of interrupted silk sutures is used, placed 0.5 cm apart.

An alternative to this technique is the single-layered Gambee anastomosis. Experience with this technique in gynecologic surgery was reported by Wheeless.[33] In brief, a single-layered closure is used, beginning in the mucosa of one side and ending in the mucosa of the other. This technique is faster than the double-layered technique.

With either technique, the mesenteric defect is closed with interrupted or running sutures to prevent the possibility of herniation. After the completion of the anastomosis, the lumen should be palpated to ensure adequacy. Pitfalls with any type of reanastomosis include incorrect suture placement, interference with mesenteric blood supply, and compromise of the lumen.

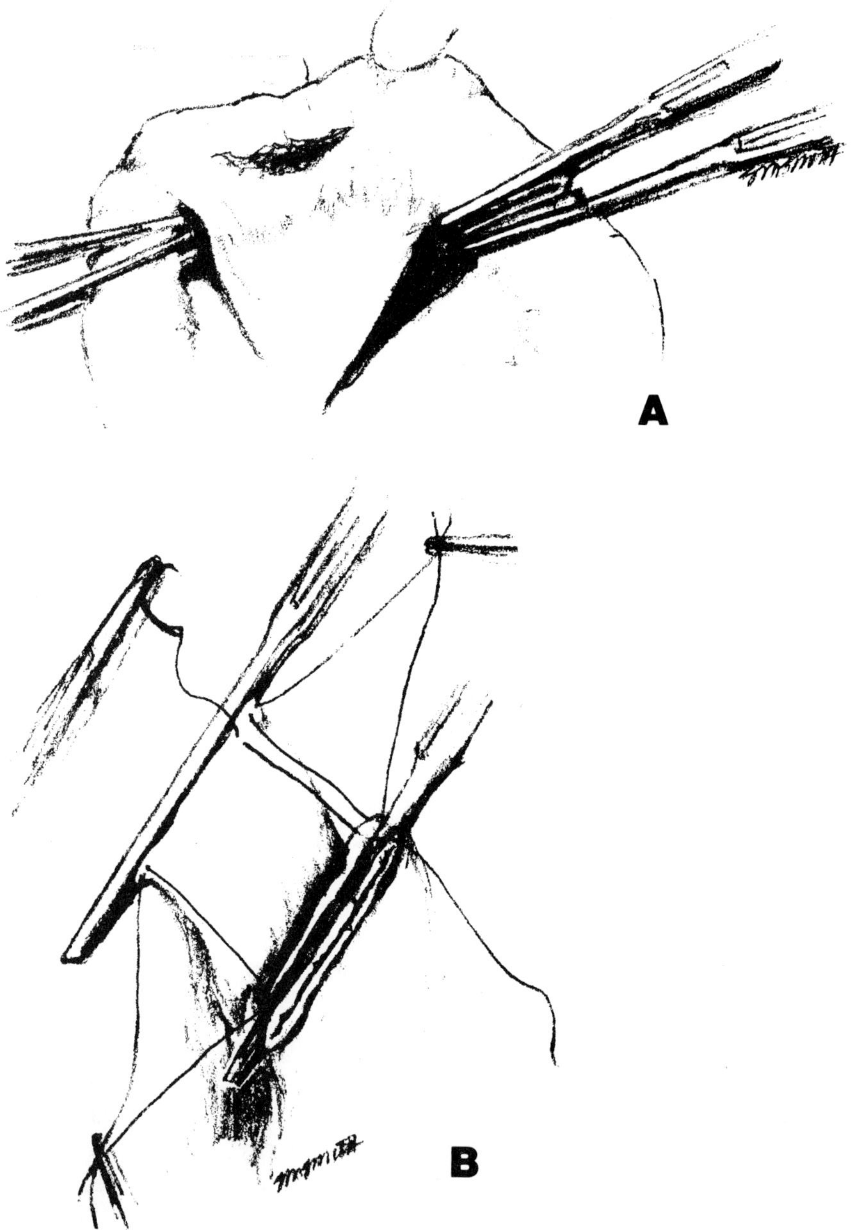

FIGURE 19.3 Small bowel resection and reanastomosis. (A) The enterotomy site is doubly clamped with Kocher clamps to reduce peritoneal soilage. A V-shaped wedge of mesentery is removed, with ligation of individual vessels. (B) Seromuscular traction sutures are placed at the margin of the resection. (C,D) The posterior row of seromuscular sutures with 00 silk has been placed, and the tissue crushed by the clamps is sharply excised. (E) The mucosal anastomosis is completed with interrupted chromic sutures. (F) The final seromuscular layer of sutures is placed. (Adapted from Mattingly RF, Thompson JD [eds]: *TeLinde's Operative Gynecology.* Philadelphia, JB Lippincott Co, 1985, with permission.)

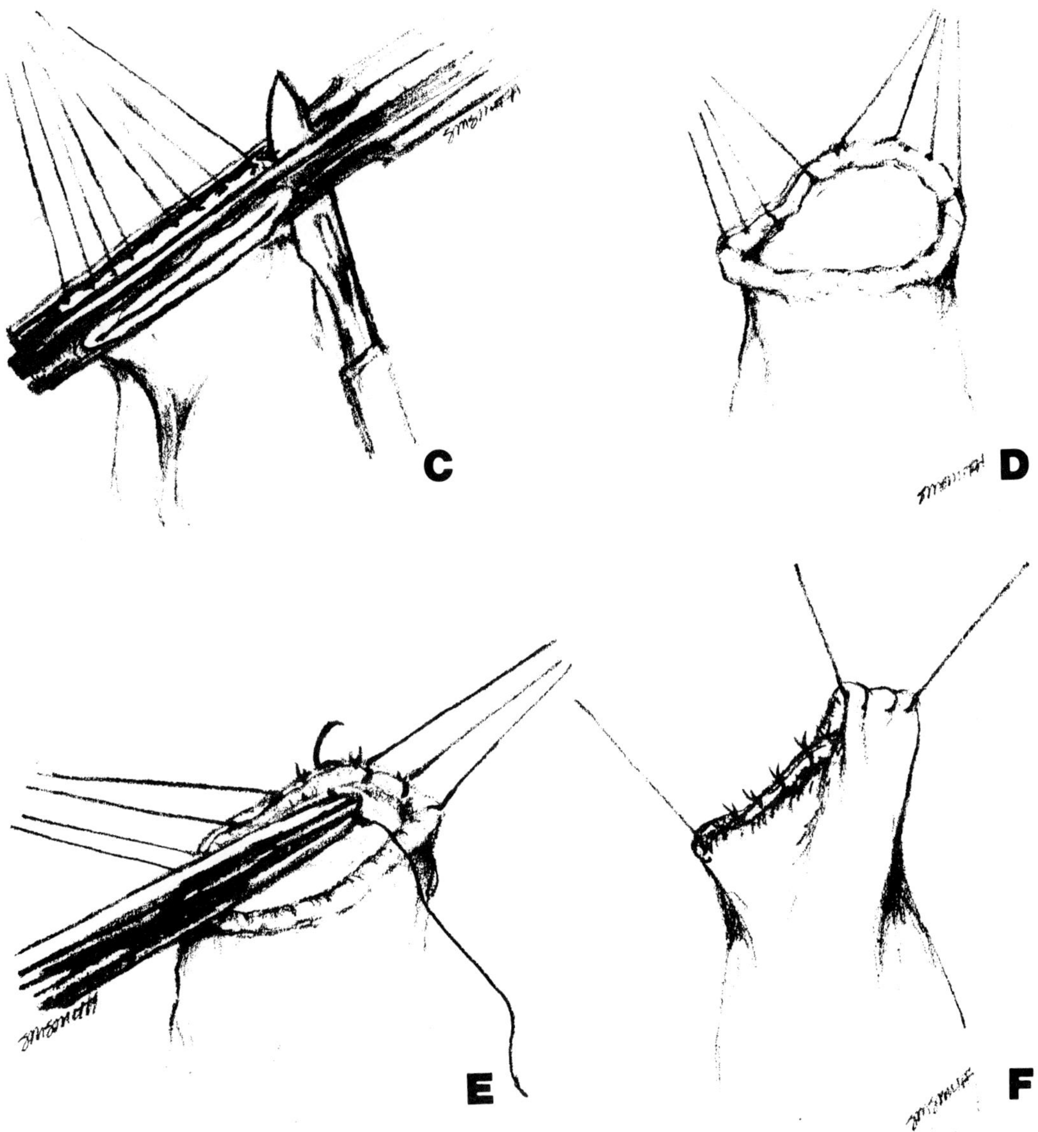

FIGURE 19.3 Continued

Reasons for an anastomotic leak include poor surgical technique and inadequate proximal decompression. Consequently, the intraoperative placement of a nasogastric tube is essential. Decompression with low suction should be continued until bowel function returns. This typically occurs within 2–3 days of the operation. The presence of persistent fever, abdominal rigidity, and diminished or absent bowel function should raise the clinical suspicion of a leaking anastomosis and merits additional evaluation.

INJURIES TO THE LARGE BOWEL

Fortunately, colonic or sigmoid injuries are exceptionally rare at the time of cesarean delivery even with concomitant cesarean hysterectomy. When such injuries are encountered, the bowel has usually not undergone mechanical preparation; thus, possible fecal spilling and infection are major considerations. As with small bowel injuries, recognition is usually not a major problem. The principal management decision is whether or not to divert the fecal stream. Regardless of the decision, consultation with a general surgeon appears prudent. Nonetheless, certain generalizations can be made. Small (<1 cm) injuries to the unprepared bowel should be treated with primary repair, using a double-layered closure as described for the small bowel.[32] Antibiotic therapy to cover gram-negative bacteria and aerobic organisms, such as clindamycin or gentamicin, should be initiated. Postoperative nasogastric suction should be considered, with feeding delayed until bowel function has returned to normal.

When an extensive bowel injury with fecal contamination is encountered, a temporary colostomy is indicated. Depending on the level of the injury, the colon may be mobilized and the injured portion exteriorized as a colostomy. Alternatively, with injuries in the rectosigmoid, repair of the injured site, with diversion of the fecal stream proximally via a transverse colostomy, is considered appropriate therapy. Antibiotic therapy, as discussed above, should also be started. After recovery and healing, the colon can safely undergo reanastomosis. Consultation with a general surgeon should be strongly considered for any but the simplest injuries.

SUMMARY

Even the most skillful and cautious obstetrician will occasionally encounter injury to the genitourinary and gastrointestinal tracts. Strict adherence to exacting surgical technique will minimize their occurrence. In general, obstetricians should be familiar with the following surgical situations: 1) bladder injury and repair, 2) evaluation of ureteral integrity, and 3) recognition and repair of small lacerations of the small bowel. However, the advice of urologic and general surgical consultants should be obtained.

The opinions expressed in this chapter are those of the authors and not necessarily those of the United States Navy or the Department of Defense.

REFERENCES

1. Higgins CC: Ureteral injuries during surgery. A review of 87 cases. *JAMA* 199:82, 1967.

2. Everett HS, Mattingly RF: Urinary tract injuries resulting from pelvic surgery. *Am J Obstet Gynecol* 71:502, 1956.
3. Mattingly RF, Borkowf HI: Lower urinary tract injuries in pregnancy, in Barber HK, Graber EA (eds): *Surgical Disease in Pregnancy.* Philadelphia, WB Saunders Co, 1974.
4. Nielsen TF, Hokegard K-H: Cesarean section and intraoperative surgical complications. *Acta Obstet Gynaecol Scand* 63:104, 1984.
5. Mattingly RF, Borkowf HI: Acute operative injury to the lower urinary tract. *Clin Obstet Gynecol* 5:123, 1978.
6. Buchsbaum HJ, Schmidt JD (eds): The urinary tract in clinical and surgical gynecology and obstetrics, in *Gynecologic and Obstetric Urology.* Philadelphia, WB Saunders Co, 1978.
7. Mickal A, Begneaud WP, Hawes TP Jr: Pitfalls and complications of cesarean section hysterectomy. *Clin Obstet Gynecol* 12:660, 1969.
8. Barclay DL: Cesarean hysterectomy. A thirty year experience. *Obstet Gynecol* 35:120, 1970.
9. McCausland AM, Cailloutte JC, Beunallack DA, et al: A comparative study of vesicovaginal fistulas following delivery. *Am J Obstet Gynecol* 79:1110, 1960.
10. Dunlop DL: Midforceps operations at the University of Alberta Hospital (1963–1967). *Am J Obstet Gynecol* 103:471, 1969.
11. Hassim AM: Uterine rupture with extrusion of the fetus into the bladder. *Int Surg* 49:130, 1968.
12. Raghaviah NV, Devi AI: Bladder injury associated with rupture of the uterus. *Obstet Gynecol* 46:573, 1975.
13. Eglinton GS, Phelan JP, Yeh S-Y, et al: Outcome of a trial of labor after prior cesarean delivery. *J Reprod Med* 29:3, 1984.
14. Eisenkop SM, Richman R, Platt LD, et al: Urinary tract injury during cesarean section. *Obstet Gynecol* 60:591, 1982.
15. Mattingly RF (ed): *TeLinde's Operative Gynecology,* ed 5. Philadelphia, JB Lippincott Co, 1977.
16. Williams TJ: Urologic Injuries, in Wynn RM (ed): *Obstetrics and Gynecology Annual.* New York, Appleton-Century-Crofts, 1975.
17. Harrow BR: Conservative and surgical management of bladder injuries following pelvic operations. *Obstet Gynecol* 33:852, 1969.
18. Vermesh M, Zbella EA, Menchaca A, et al. Vesical endometriosis following bladder injury. *Am J Obstet Gynecol* 153:894, 1985.
19. O'Leary JL, O'Leary JA: A simplified method of determining ureteral patency at operation. *Am J Obstet Gynecol* 101:271, 1966.
20. Beland G: Early treatment of ureteral injuries found after gynecologic surgery. *J Urol* 118:25, 1977.
21. Raney AM: Ureteral trauma: Effects of ureteral ligation with and without delegation—Experimental studies and case reports. *J Urol* 119:326, 1978.
22. Gurin JI, Garcia RL, Melman A, et al: Pathologic effect of ureteral ligation with clinical implications. *J Urol* 128:1404, 1982.
23. Kamholz JH, Reisman DD, Kantor HI: Treatment for the surgically ligated ureter. *Obstet Gynecol* 9:599, 1957.
24. Glenn JF (ed): *Urologic Surgery.* Hagerstown, Md, Harper & Row, Publishers, Inc, 1975.
25. Politano VA: Vesicouterine reflux, in: Glenn JF (ed): *Urologic Surgery,* ed 2. Hagerstown, Md, Harper & Row, 1975.
26. Prout GR, Koontz WW Jr: Partial vesical immobilization: An important adjunct in ureteroneocystostomy. *J Urol* 115:132, 1976.
27. Harrow BR: A neglected maneuver for uretero-vesical implantation following injury at gynecologic operations. *J Urol* 100:280, 1968.

28. Boari A, Casati E: Contributo Sperimentale alla plastica delluretere. *Attz dell 'Academia de le science Medicine e Natarali in Ferrara* 68:149, 1894.
29. Ockerblad NF: Reimplantation of the ureter into the bladder by a flap method. *J Urol* 57:845, 1947.
30. Shires GT: Trauma, in Schwartz SI (ed): *Principles of Surgery*. New York, McGraw-Hill BookCo,1984.
31. Paloyan D: Intestinal problems in gynecologic surgery, in Sciarra J (ed): *Gynecology*, Vol. 1. Philadelphia, Harper & Row, Publishers, Inc, 1982.
32. Carey LC, Catalano PW: The intestinal tract in relation to gynecology, in Mattingly RF (ed): *TeLinde's Operative Gynecology*. Philadelphia, JB Lippincott Co, 1977.
33. Wheeless CR Jr: The Gambee intestinal anastomosis in gynecologic surgery. *Obstet Gynecol* 46:448, 1975.

Chapter 20

Antibiotic Prophylaxis

Patrick Duff, MD

The most common complication associated with cesarean delivery is infection.[1] Figure 20.1 shows the frequency of postoperative infection in women undergoing abdominal delivery without benefit of prophylactic antibiotics.[2] In general, the highest incidence of infection occurs in young, indigent women having surgery after extended duration of labor and ruptured membranes. Conversely, the lowest incidence of infection occurs in women of the middle and upper socioeconomic classes having elective, scheduled cesarean delivery.

Many investigations have demonstrated that prophylactic antibiotics are of value in reducing the incidence of certain types of postcesarean infections. The purpose of this chapter is to examine the rationale for surgical prophylaxis and the mechanism of action of prophylactic antibiotics, and then to review the results of investigations designed to test the clinical utility of prophylaxis.

CRITERIA FOR USE OF PROPHYLACTIC ANTIBIOTICS

Three clinical criteria should be fulfilled to justify perioperative use of prophylactic antibiotics. The surgical procedure, by necessity, must be performed through a contaminated operative field. There must be a high incidence of postoperative infection, ie, exceeding 15%–20%, in the absence of prophylaxis. Finally, there must be serious sequelae that may result from the primary operative-site infection.

Unscheduled cesarean delivery clearly fulfills these criteria. The operation inevitably is associated with considerable bacterial contamination of the endometrial and peritoneal cavities. If some form of prophylaxis is not administered, the incidence of postcesarean endomyometritis is unacceptably high. In most patient populations, the incidence of this infec-

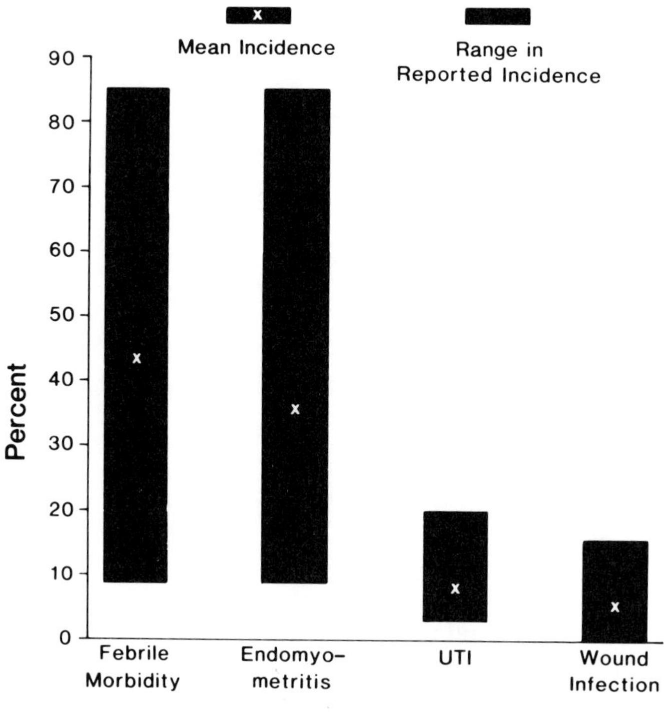

FIGURE 20.1 Frequency of postoperative infection in women undergoing cesarean delivery without benefit of prophylactic antibiotics.

tion averages 35%–40%.[2] In patients who develop endomyometritis, potentially life-threatening sequelae such as septic shock, pelvic abscess, and septic pelvic vein thrombophlebitis can occur.

MECHANISM OF ACTION OF PROPHYLACTIC ANTIBIOTICS

Prophylactic antibiotics appear to act in two principal ways. By destroying some bacteria and slowing the growth of others, they directly decrease the size of the bacterial inoculum present at the surgical site. They also alter the characteristics of the serosanguineous fluid that collects in the pelvic cavity after surgery, rendering it less suitable to support the growth of microorganisms. Other possible mechanisms of action include interference with the production of bacterial proteases and interference with attachment of bacterial to mucosal surfaces. In addition, antibiotics may, in a way that still is not completely understood, enhance the host's phagocytic capacity.[3]

Burke[3] has demonstrated that the timing of delivery of antibiotics to injured tissue is of critical importance in determining the efficacy of prophylaxis. The greatest therapeutic effect occurs when antibiotics are administered just before, or coincident with, the time when maximal bacterial contamination and tissue trauma occur. When antibiotic administration is delayed for more than 3 hours after the time of bacterial inoculation, the protective effect against infection is lost.

OBJECTIVES IN THE USE OF PROPHYLACTIC ANTIBIOTICS

One major objective in the use of prophylactic antibiotics is reduction of the incidence of endomyometritis. This infection causes the patient considerable discomfort and usually results in an increased duration and expense of hospitalization. Infected patients usually remain in the hospital 2 days longer than uninfected ones and incur additional hospital charges in the range of \$600 to \$1,000. In addition, endomyometritis is the usual precursor of such serious complications as pelvic abscess, septic shock, and septic pelvic vein thrombophlebitis.

A second objective in the use of prophylaxis is reduction of the incidence of major wound infections. Such disorders usually require a second surgical procedure to open and debride the incision. They may also result in dehiscence and evisceration. For these reasons, wound infection is even more likely than endomyometritis to result in marked prolongation of the patient's hospitalization.

The third objective in the use of prophylactic antibiotics is to decrease the duration and expense of hospitalization. The final objective is prevention of the rare, life-threatening complications of operative-site infection.

RESULTS OF CLINICAL TRIALS OF SYSTEMIC PROPHYLAXIS

Early Trials of Prophylaxis

The first formal investigations of antibiotic prophylaxis for cesarean delivery were published in the late 1960s and early 1970s.[4–9] These initial investigations all concluded that prophylaxis was of value in decreasing the incidence of infection-related morbidity after cesarean delivery.

There were significant weaknesses in the design of these initial investigations, however. Although prospective, the randomization scheme was not optimal in all studies. Most of the investigations were not double-blinded. With one exception,[4] the course of antibiotics was therapeutic ($\geq$3 days) rather than prophylactic. Several of the studies utilized two or three antibiotics for prophylaxis rather than one. Certain of the drugs selected for prophylaxis, eg, the aminoglycosides, would be considered suitable agents for specific treatment of established infections but not necessarily for prophylaxis.

The definitions of postoperative infections in these early clinical trials were not uniform. Specifically, most authors evaluated overall "febrile or

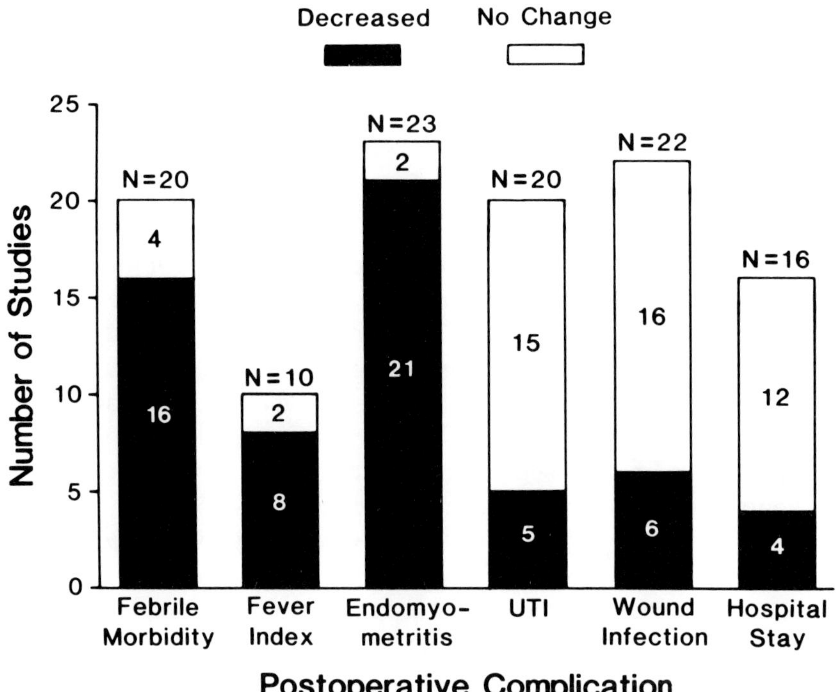

FIGURE 20.2 Clinical effects of systemic prophylactic antibiotics in women having cesarean delivery.

infectious morbidity" rather than the incidence of individual infections such as endomyometritis, urinary tract infection, or wound infection. Finally, few of the initial investigations provided detailed microbiologic study of the patients who became infected despite prophylaxis.

Despite these shortcomings, the early investigations served two important purposes. They focused the attention of obstetricians on the alarmingly high incidence of infection associated with cesarean delivery, and stimulated other investigators to conduct further clinical studies of prophylactic antibiotics.

Results of Recent Clinical Trials

Since the mid-1970s, more than 20 prospective, randomized, placebo-controlled trials of systemic prophylaxis for cesarean delivery have been published.[10–32] Figures 20.2 and 20.3 provide a graphic summary of the results of these investigations. Several of the findings of these studies merit special emphasis.

Virtually without exception, all studies have demonstrated a significant decrease in the frequency of endomyometritis in women having unscheduled abdominal delivery after extended duration of labor and rup-

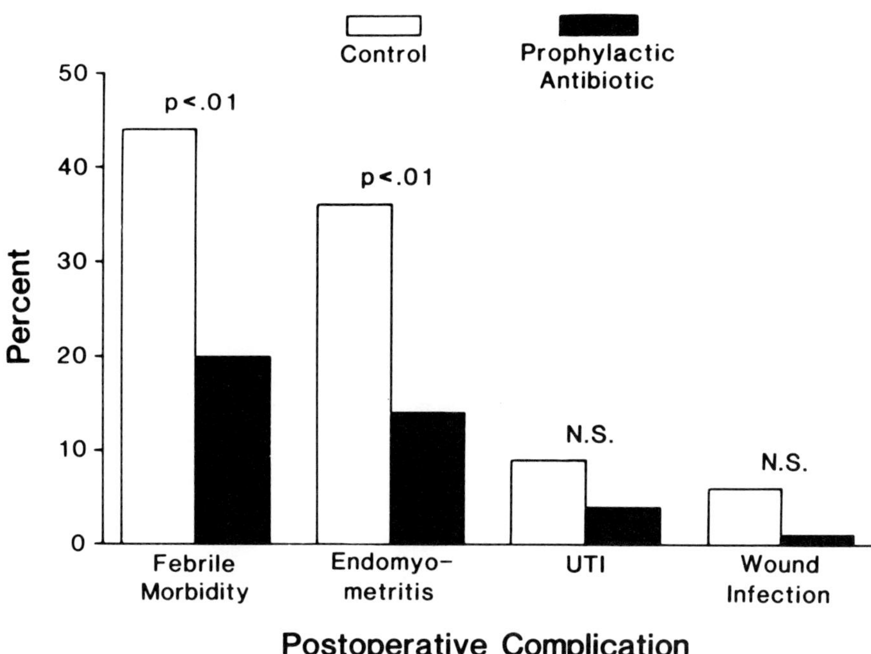

FIGURE 20.3 Reduction in frequency of postcesarean infection in women receiving systemic prophylactic antibiotics.

tured membranes. The reduction in the incidence of endomyometritis has averaged 50%–60% in most studies. These data are so convincing that it is probably not reasonable to utilize placebo controls in future studies of prophylaxis in these high-risk patients.

Most investigations have not shown a statistically significant decrease in endomyometritis in women undergoing elective, scheduled abdominal delivery. There may be some patient populations, however, in which the underlying frequency of infection is high enough so that, even in this situation, prophylaxis has a beneficial effect in reducing the incidence of postoperative morbidity and decreasing the expense of hospitalization.

The drugs most frequently used for prophylaxis have been the cephalosporins. Although it is widespread practice in the United States to utilize the newer extended-spectrum cephalosporins for prophylaxis, there is no evidence that these agents are better for this purpose than ampicillin or a first-generation cephalosporin. To date, four authors[33–36] have compared limited-spectrum agents to extended-spectrum antibiotics for prophylaxis. In these trials, 415 patients received an extended-spectrum agent and 476 received a more limited-spectrum agent (Table 20.1). None of the individual trials, or all considered collectively, have been able to show that the more expensive, extended-spectrum drugs are more effective in decreasing the incidence of postoperative endomyometritis.

TABLE 20.1 Limited versus Extended-Spectrum Agents as Prophylaxis for Cesarean Delivery

Author	No. of Patients	Drugs	Endometritis (%)
Louie et al[33]	70	Cefazolin	4.3
	60	Ampicillin	3.3
	58	Cefotaxime	6.9
Stiver et al[34]	119	Cefazolin	2.5
	124	Cefoxitin	4.0
Rayburn et al[35]	124	Cefazolin	3.2
	130	Moxalactam	7.7
Duff et al[36]	96	Cefazolin	19.8
	103	Cefonicid	12.6

Note: The first three investigations utilized 3 perioperative doses of antibiotic. The last used only a single dose.

Most investigators have utilized a 3-dose regimen for prophylaxis. There now are at least seven reports, however, demonstrating that a single dose of antibiotic is comparable in efficacy to multidose regimens.[37–43] The results of these investigations are summarized in Table 20.2.

Three investigators specifically sought to determine whether an extended course of antibiotics was more effective than limited perioperative prophylaxis in decreasing the incidence of postcesarean infection. Elliott and co-workers[20] demonstrated that a 3-day course of ampicillin was more effective than a 3-dose regimen in decreasing the incidence of febrile morbidity and endomyometritis and in shortening the duration of hospitalization. D'Angelo and Sokol,[17] however, were unable to confirm a signif-

TABLE 20.2 Results of Investigations Utilizing Single-Dose Prophylactic Regimens for Cesarean Delivery

			Incidence of Endometritis (%)		
Author	No. of Patients	Study Design	Single Dose	Comparison Group	*P*
Padilla et al[37]	71	Ampicillin (2 g) versus placebo	15	57	.05
Saltzman et al[38]	100	Ceftizoxime (2 g) versus placebo	6.0	24.5	.05
Ganesh et al[39]	57	Trimethoprim (240 mg) plus sulfamethoxazole (1,200 mg) versus placebo	21.0	46.0	.05
McGregor et al[40]	70	Cefotetan (2 g) versus cefoxitin (2 g × 3)	15.2	8.3	NS
Saltzman et al[41]	158	Mezlocillin (4 g) versus mezlocillin (4 g × 3) versus cefoxitin (2 g × 3)	5.9	4.0/4.0	NS
Gonik[42]	100	Cefotaxime (2 g) versus cefotaxime (2 g × 3)	10.0	14.0	NS
Varner et al[43]	36	Cefotetan (2 g) versus cefoxitin (2 g × 3)	10.0	0	NS

icant difference in the combined incidence of wound infection and endomyometritis when a 5-day course of treatment with cefazolin plus cephalexin was compared to a 4-dose course of cefazolin. DePalma et al[31] studied two drug regimens (cefamandole and penicillin plus gentamicin) and were unable to confirm an advantage for extended early therapy over limited perioperative prophylaxis. This latter study is noteworthy because the authors' patients were at exceptionally high risk of postcesarean infection as a result of their low socioeconomic status, and extended duration of labor and ruptured membranes.

At the present time, it is not possible to identify precisely that subset of women who are at such high risk of infection that they need early treatment with therapeutic antibiotics rather than simple prophylaxis.[44] Until a laboratory or clinical test with high sensitivity and predictive value is available, extended prophylactic or early-treatment regimens cannot be recommended.

For most surgical procedures, it is desirable to administer prophylactic antibiotics preoperatively, before tissue injury and bacterial contamination occur. If this policy were implemented for cesarean delivery, of course, the neonate would be exposed to antibiotic prior to birth. In theory, even this limited exposure might interfere with the ability of the pediatrician to evaluate the newborn for sepsis. Fortunately, multiple reports have now confirmed that delay in administration of antibiotics until after delivery of the fetus does not diminish the effectiveness of prophylaxis.

Most investigators have been unable to demonstrate that antibiotic prophylaxis decreases the incidence of abdominal wound infection. In the studies in which a positive effect was confirmed, the incidence of wound infection in the control population was high, ranging from 7.4% to 16.1%.[4,5,15,26,28,37] In the studies that demonstrated no reduction in wound infection, the incidence of infection in the control population was lower, ranging from 0% to 7%. With such a low frequency of infection in the control groups, many of the studies with negative findings may not have had a sufficient sample size to detect a beneficial treatment effect.

At present, no serious maternal side effects have occurred as a result of the use of antimicrobial prophylaxis for cesarean delivery. There are case reports, however, of at least two deaths from anaphylaxis in patients who received intraoperative injections of cephalothin during nonobstetric surgical procedures.[45] Therefore, the possibility of untoward side effects must always be considered when a decision is made to utilize prophylactic antibiotics.

Several recent investigations[46,47] have demonstrated that changes in the vaginal flora occur in women who receive prophylactic antibiotics at the time of cesarean delivery. The alterations in flora depend upon the specific drug selected for prophylaxis and the length of time it is administered.

The clinical significance of these changes in the flora of the lower genital tract is not entirely clear. No investigator has yet documented an increased incidence of more serious complications in women who become infected despite receiving prophylaxis. Of particular concern, however, is the increased isolation of enterococci in women who develop infections after receiving prophylactic cephalosporins. Many antibiotics used singly or in combination for the treatment of postcesarean infection do not provide effective coverage against enterococci. Therefore, if prophylactic antibiotics are to be used routinely on an obstetric service, careful surveillance must be maintained to detect unusual changes in antimicrobial susceptibilities.

There are three principal components of an effective surveillance system. First, genital tract and blood cultures should be performed in all patients who become infected despite receiving prophylaxis. The antibiotic susceptibility patterns of bacteria isolated from these patients should be evaluated to determine if selection of resistant microorganisms is occurring. Second, the clinical course of these women should be monitored to determine if they are experiencing a suboptimal response to the usual antibiotic regimens selected for therapy of postoperative infection. Finally, the hospital laboratory should conduct a periodic review of the susceptibility patterns of commonly isolated microorganisms to detect gradual changes in antimicrobial resistance throughout the hospital.

ALTERNATIVES TO SYSTEMIC PROPHYLAXIS

Extraperitoneal Cesarean Delivery

There is one prospective study[48] that directly compared the effects of extraperitoneal cesarean delivery versus systemic antibiotics on the frequency of postoperative endomyometritis. Wallace and co-workers assigned 127 women having unscheduled cesarean delivery to one of three treatment groups: transperitoneal cesarean delivery without systemic antibiotic prophylaxis ($n = 36$), extraperitoneal cesarean delivery without prophylaxis ($n = 75$), and extraperitoneal cesarean delivery with prophylaxis ($n = 16$). Compared to the former groups, only women in the last group experienced a statistically significant reduction in the incidence of endomyometritis. Although there are some weaknesses in the design of this study, the results suggest that extraperitoneal cesarean delivery is not as effective as systemic prophylactic antibiotics in preventing postcesarean endomyometritis.

Intraoperative Antibiotic Irrigation

Intraoperative irrigation is an alternative method of administering prophylactic antibiotics for cesarean delivery. This technique appears to exert its primary effect by delivering a high concentration of antibiotic directly to the site of maximum bacterial contamination and tissue injury.[49] Systemic absorption of antibiotic does occur, however, especially when both intrauterine and intraperitoneal irrigation are performed.[50] Serum levels of antibiotics, in fact, may exceed the minimal inhibitory concentrations for many genital tract pathogens.

Table 20.3 presents a summary of the published investigations of intraoperative irrigation.[51–63] Several of the findings of these studies merit special emphasis.

With only two exceptions,[53,54] all of the investigations have shown that antibiotic irrigation is superior to no treatment or to saline irrigation in reducing the incidence of endomyometritis.

Unlike the situation with systemic prophylaxis, not all antibiotics have been equally effective when administered by irrigation. For example, Conover and Moore[54] showed that whereas intravenous cefoxitin reduced the incidence of postcesarean endomyometritis, topical cefoxitin did not. Similarly, Dashow and co-workers[63] evaluated four different antibiotic solutions for topical irrigation (cefamandole, ampicillin, cephapirin, and moxalactam). Only patients who received cefamandole had a significant reduction in the incidence of postcesarean endomyometritis.

The observed differences in treatment effect appear to be due, at least in part, to differences in irrigation techniques. For example, there are differences between the volume of diluent, and hence the concentration of antibiotic, used in different studies. Some authors have irrigated both the uterine and peritoneal cavities; others have irrigated only the former. Some investigators have allowed the irrigant solution to remain in the uterus and/or peritoneal cavity, whereas others have immediately aspirated the solution. Differences in the pharmacokinetic properties of the drugs, particularly the half-life of the antibiotic in serum and tissue, may also be important in explaining the varied results of these studies. On the basis of the information presently available, cefamandole appears to be the agent with the most thoroughly documented evidence of efficacy.

Most of the studies that have compared intraoperative irrigation to systemic prophylaxis have utilized 3 doses for systemic administration and 1 dose for irrigation. In a comparison of this nature, there is a distinct cost advantage for irrigation over systemic administration. Recent reports,[37–43] however, have demonstrated that a single dose of systemic prophylaxis can be just as effective and economical as a single dose of drug administered by irrigation. Therefore, irrigation should be regarded as comparable, but not superior, to systemic administration of antibiotics.

In view of these latter findings, the principal argument in favor of irrigation is that it minimizes systemic absorption of antibiotic and, hopefully, reduces the risk of an untoward drug effect. Conversely, the major advantage of systemic prophylaxis is that it is a simpler and less time-consuming method of antibiotic administration.

TABLE 20.3 Clinical Trials of Intraoperative Antibiotic Irrigation

Author	No of Patients	Antibiotic	Study Design	Results
Long et al[51]	90	Cefamandole (2 g)	Prospective, randomized, blinded Two control groups: no irrigation and saline irrigation	Decreased fever index and decreased incidence of febrile morbidity and endomyometritis in antibiotic group
Rudd et al[52]	398	Cefamandole (2 g)	Treated patients were enrolled in a prospective manner. Study utilized historical controls who received no treatment	Decreased incidence of endomyometritis in treated patients
Levin et al[53]	128	Cefoxitin (2 g) Cephapirin (2 g)	Prospective, randomized, blinded Placebo controls	No significant difference in any measure of treatment effect
Conover et al[54]	124	Cefoxitin (2 g)	Prospective, randomized, blinded Placebo controls Compared irrigation to three doses of systemic antibiotics	Only systemic antibiotics were effective in decreasing the incidence of endomyometritis
Leveno et al[55]	103	Cefamandole (2 g)	Prospective, randomized, blinded Historical controls Compared irrigation to three doses of systemic antibiotics	Both regimens were of comparable effectiveness in decreasing incidence of endomyometritis
Boothby et al[56]	53	Cefoxitin (2 g)	Prospective, randomized, blinded No placebo or historical controls Compared irrigation to four doses of systemic antibiotics	No significant difference in incidence of endomyometritis in the two groups
Kellum et al[57]	262	Cefamandole (2 g)	Prospective, randomized. Two control groups: no irrigation and saline irrigation	Decreased incidence of endomyometritis in antibiotic group

Jensen et al[58]	200	Cefoxitin (2 g)	Treated patients were enrolled in a prospective manner Utilized historical controls who received no treatment	Decreased incidence of endomyometritis and decreased duration of hospitalization in the antibiotic group
Bourgeois et al[59]	223	Cefamandole (2 g)	Prospective, randomized. Two control groups: no irrigation and saline irrigation	Decreased incidence of endomyometritis in the antibiotic group
Saravolatz et al[60]	64	Ceforanide (2 g)	Prospective, randomized, blinded Compared irrigation to one dose of systemic antibiotics	No difference in treatment effect
Gonen et al[61]	208	Cefamandole (2 g)	Prospective, randomized, blinded Compared irrigation to six doses (1 g) of systemic antibiotics	No difference in treatment effect
Elliott and Flaherty[62]	158	Cefoxitin (2 g)	Prospective, randomized, blinded Controls received no treatment Compared irrigation to eight doses of systemic antibiotics and to a regimen that included irrigation and systemic administration	Decreased incidence of febrile morbidity and endomyometritis in the treated groups. The three treatment groups were of comparable effectiveness
Dashow et al[63]	360	Cefamandole (2 g) Cephapirin (2 g) Ampicillin (2 g) Moxalactam (2 g)	Prospective, randomized, blinded Placebo controls	Decreased incidence of febrile morbidity and endomyometritis in the cefamandole group

Use of systemic antibiotics in conjunction with intraoperative irrigation does not enhance the effectiveness of prophylaxis.[60–62] Therefore, there is no justification for combining both modalities.

CONCLUSIONS

The principal beneficial effect of prophylactic antibiotics is the reduction in the incidence of endomyometritis in women having unscheduled cesarean delivery. Utilization of prophylaxis in this group of patients is clearly cost effective.

The limited-spectrum (first-generation) cephalosporins or ampicillin should be considered the drugs of choice for prophylaxis. There is no evidence to date that the more expensive extended-spectrum cephalosporins or penicillins are more effective for prophylaxis.

There is no justification for administering more than 3 perioperative doses of antibiotic. In fact, in most patient populations, a single dose of antibiotic will provide a degree of prophylaxis comparable to that achieved with multidose regimens.

Intraoperative irrigation with an antibiotic solution is an acceptable, but not superior, alternative to systemic administration of antibiotics.

REFERENCES

1. Duff P: The pathophysiology of postcesarean endomyometritis. *Obstet Gynecol* 67:269, 1986.
2. Schwartz WH, Grolle K: The use of prophylactic antibiotics in cesarean section. A review of the literature. *J Reprod Med* 26:595, 1981.
3. Burke JF: Preventive antibiotic management in surgery. *Ann Rev Med* 24:289, 1973.
4. Gibbs RS, DeCherney AH, Schwarz RH: Prophylactic antibiotics in cesarean section: A double-blind study. *Am J Obstet Gynecol* 114:1048, 1972.
5. Gibbs RS, Hunt JE, Schwarz RH: A follow-up study on prophylactic antibiotics in cesarean section. *Am J Obstet Gynecol* 117:419, 1973.
6. Miller RD, Crichton D: Ampicillin prophylaxis in cesarean sections. *S Afr J Obstet Gynecol* 6:69, 1968.
7. Morrison JC, Coxwell WL, Kennedy BS, et al: The use of prophylactic antibiotics in patients undergoing cesarean section. *Surg Gynecol Obstet* 136:425, 1973.
8. Weissberg SM, Edwards NL, O'Leary JA: Prophylactic antibiotics in cesarean section. *Obstet Gynecol* 38:290, 1971.
9. Rothbard ML, Mayer W, Wystepek A, et al: Prophylactic antibiotics in cesarean section. *Obstet Gynecol* 45:421, 1975.
10. Wong R, Gee CL, Ledger WJ: Prophylactic use of cefazolin in monitored obstetric patients undergoing cesarean section. *Obstet Gynecol* 51:407, 1978.
11. Kreutner AK, Del Bene VE, Delamar D, et al: Perioperative antibiotic prophylaxis in cesarean section. *Obstet Gynecol* 52:279, 1978.
12. Kreutner AK, Del Bene VE, Delamar D, et al: Perioperative cephalosporin prophylaxis in cesarean section: Effect on endometritis in the high-risk patient. *Am J Obstet Gynecol* 134:925, 1979.
13. Phelan JP, Pruyn SC: Prophylactic antibiotics in cesarean section: A double-blind study of cefazolin. *Am J Obstet Gynecol* 133:474, 1979.

14. Gordon HR, Phelps D, Blanchard K: Prophylactic cesarean section antibiotics: Maternal and neonatal morbidity before or after cord clamping. *Obstet Gynecol* 53:151, 1979.
15. Gall SA: The efficacy of prophylactic antibiotics in cesarean section. *Am J Obstet Gynecol* 134:506, 1979.
16. Duff P, Park RC: Antibiotic prophylaxis for cesarean section in a military population. *Military Med* 145:377, 1980.
17. D'Angelo LJ, Sokol RJ: Short- versus long-course prophylactic antibiotic treatment in cesarean section. *Obstet Gynecol* 55:583, 1980.
18. Harger JH, English DH: Selection of patients for antibiotic prophylaxis in cesarean sections. *Am J Obstet Gynecol* 141:752, 1981.
19. Gibbs RS, St Clair PJ, Castillo MS, et al: Bacteriologic effects of antibiotic prophylaxis in high-risk cesarean section. *Obstet Gynecol* 57:277, 1981.
20. Elliott JP, Freeman RK, Dorchester W: Short versus long course of prophylactic antibiotics in cesarean section. *Am J Obstet Gynecol* 143:740, 1982.
21. Polk BF, Krache M, Phillippe M, et al: Randomized clinical trial of perioperative cefoxitin in preventing maternal infection after primary cesarean section. *Am J Obstet Gynecol* 142:983, 1982.
22. Apuzzio JJ, Reyelt C, Pelosi M, et al: Prophylactic antibiotics for cesarean section: Comparison of high- and low-risk patients for endomyometritis. *Obstet Gynecol* 59:693, 1982.
23. Duff P, Smith PN, Keiser JF: Antibiotic prophylaxis in low-risk cesarean section. *J Reprod Med* 27:133, 1982.
24. Padilla SL, Spence MR, Beauchamp PJ: Single-dose ampicillin for cesarean section prophylaxis. *Obstet Gynecol* 61:463, 1983.
25. Hawrylyshyn PA, Bernstein P, Papsin FR: Short-term antibiotic prophylaxis in high-risk patients following cesarean section. *Am J Obstet Gynecol* 145:285, 1983.
26. Green SL, Sarubbi FA, Bishop EH: Prophylactic antibiotics in high-risk cesarean section. *Obstet Gynecol* 51:569, 1978.
27. Wallace RL, Yonekura ML: The use of prophylactic antibiotics in patients undergoing emergency primary cesarean section. *Am J Obstet Gynecol* 147:533, 1983.
28. Young R, Platt L, Ledger W: Prophylactic cefoxitin in cesarean section. *Surg Gynecol Obstet* 157:11, 1983.
29. Hager WD, Williamson MM: Effects of antibiotic prophylaxis on women undergoing nonelective cesarean section in a community hospital. *J Reprod Med* 28:687, 1983.
30. Tully JL, Klapholz H, Baldini LM, et al: Perioperative use of cefoxitin in primary cesarean section. *J Reprod Med* 28:827, 1983.
31. DePalma RT, Leveno KJ, Cunningham FG, et al: Identification and management of women at high risk for pelvic infection following cesarean section. *Obstet Gynecol* 55(suppl):185, 1980.
32. DePalma RT, Cunningham FG, Leveno KG, et al: Continuing investigation of women at high risk for infection following cesarean delivery. *Obstet Gynecol* 60:53, 1982.
33. Louie TJ, Binns FAO, Baskett TF, et al: Cefotaxime, cefazolin, or ampicillin prophylaxis of febrile morbidity in emergency cesarean sections. *Clin Ther* 5:83, 1982.
34. Stiver HG, Forward KR, Livingstone RA, et al: Multicenter comparison of cefoxitin versus cefazolin for prevention of infectious morbidity after nonelective cesarean section. *Am J Obstet Gynecol* 45:158, 1983.
35. Rayburn W, Varner M, Galask R, et al: Comparison of moxalactam and cefazolin as prophylactic antibiotics during cesarean section. *Antimicrob Agents Chemother* 27:337, 1985.
36. Duff P, Robertson AW, Read JA: Prophylactic antibiotics for cesarean delivery: Single-dose cefazolin versus cefonicid. *Obstet Gynecol* 70:718, 1987.

37. Padilla SL, Spence MR, Beauchamp PJ: Single-dose ampicillin for cesarean section prophylaxis. *Obstet Gynecol* 61:463, 1983.
38. Saltzman DH, Eron LG, Kay HH, et al: Single-dose antibiotic prophylaxis in high-risk patients undergoing cesarean section. *Obstet Gynecol* 65:655, 1985.
39. Ganesh V, Apuzzio JJ, Dispenziere B, et al: Single-dose trimethoprimsulfamethoxazole prophylaxis for cesarean section. *Am J Obstet Gynecol* 154:1113, 1986.
40. McGregor JA, French JI, Makowski E: Single-dose cefotetan versus multidose cefoxitin for prophylaxis in cesarean section in high-risk patients. *Am J Obstet Gynecol* 154:955, 1986.
41. Saltzman DH, Eron LJ, Tuomala RE, et al: Single-dose antibiotic prophylaxis in high-risk patients undergoing cesarean section. *J Reprod Med* 31:709, 1986.
42. Gonik B: Single versus three-dose cefotaxime prophylaxis for cesarean section. *Obstet Gynecol* 65:189, 1985.
43. Varner MW, Weiner CP, Petzold CR, et al: Comparison of cefotetan and cefoxitin as prophylaxis in cesarean section. *Am J Obstet Gynecol* 154:951, 1986.
44. Duff P, Gibbs RS, St Clair PJ, et al: Correlation of laboratory and clinical criteria in the prediction of postcesarean endomyometritis. *Obstet Gynecol* 63:781, 1984.
45. Spruill FG, Minette LJ, Sturner WQ: Two surgical deaths associated with cephalothin. *JAMA* 229:440, 1974.
46. Gibbs RS, St Clair PJ, Castillo MS, et al: Bacteriologic effects of antibiotic prophylaxis in high-risk cesarean section. *Obstet Gynecol* 57:277, 1981.
47. Stiver HG, Tyrrell DL, Livingstone RA, et al: Comparative cervical microflora shifts after cefoxitin or cefazolin prophylaxis against infection following cesarean section. *Am J Obstet Gynecol* 149:718, 1984.
48. Wallace RL, Eglinton GS, Yonekura ML, et al: Extraperitoneal cesarean section: A surgical form of infection prophylaxis? *Am J Obstet Gynecol* 148:172, 1984.
49. Elliot JP, Flaherty JF: Comparison of lavage or intravenous antibiotics at cesarean section. *Obstet Gynecol* 67:29, 1986.
50. Duff P, Gibbs RS, Jorgensen JH, et al: The pharmacokinetics of prophylactic antibiotics administered by intraoperative irrigation at the time of cesarean section. *Obstet Gynecol* 60:409, 1982.
51. Long WH, Rudd EG, Dillon MB: Intrauterine irrigation with cefamandole naftate solution at cesarean section: A preliminary report. *Am J Obstet Gynecol* 138:755, 1980.
52. Rudd RG, Cobey EA, Long WA, et al: Prevention of endomyometritis using antibiotic irrigation during cesarean section. *Obstet Gynecol* 60:413, 1982.
53. Levin DK, Gorchels C, Andersen R: Reduction of post-cesarean infectious morbidity by means of antibiotic irrigation. *Am J Obstet Gynecol* 147:273, 1983.
54. Conover WB, Moore TR: Comparison of irrigation and intravenous antibiotic prophylaxis at cesarean section. *Obstet Gynecol* 63:787, 1984.
55. Leveno KJ, Quirk JG, Cunningham FG, et al: Perioperative antimicrobials at cesarean section: Lavage versus three intravenous doses. *Am J Obstet Gynecol* 149:463, 1984.
56. Boothby R, Benrubi G, Ferrell E: Comparison of intravenous cefoxitin prophylaxis with intraoperative cefoxitin irrigation for the prevention of post-cesarean section endometritis. *J Reprod Med* 29:830, 1984.
57. Kellum RB, Roberts WE, Harris JB, et al: Effect of intrauterine antibiotic lavage after cesarean birth on postoperative morbidity. *J Reprod Med* 30:527, 1985.
58. Jensen LP, Dobin AJ, O'Sullivan MJ, et al: Prevention of endomyometritis by local application of antibiotic solution during cesarean section. *Am J Obstet Gynecol* 152:565, 1985.
59. Bourgeois FJ, Pinkerton JA, Andersen W, et al: Antibiotic irrigation prophylaxis in the high-risk cesarean section patient. *Am J Obstet Gynecol* 153:197, 1985.
60. Saravolatz LD, Lee C, Drukker B: Comparison of intravenous administration with

intrauterine irrigation with ceforanide for nonelective cesarean section. *Obstet Gynecol* 66:513, 1985.

61. Gonen R, Sambert I, Levinski R, et al: Effect of irrigation or intravenous antibiotic prophylaxis on infectious morbidity at cesarean section. *Obstet Gynecol* 67:545, 1986.
62. Elliott JP, Flaherty JF: Comparison of lavage or intravenous antibiotics at cesarean section. *Obstet Gynecol* 67:29, 1986.
63. Dashow EE, Read JA, Coleman FH: Randomized comparison of five irrigation solutions at cesarean section. *Obstet Gynecol* 68:473, 1986.

Chapter 21

Blood Transfusion

David A. Sacks, MD

Acute massive blood loss is a known potential complication of pregnancy. It is thus not surprising that the first reported human-to-human blood transfusion was performed as a treatment for postpartum hemorrhage.[1] Hemorrhage remains one of the major causes of maternal mortality. It is second only to infection as a cause of postcesarean morbidity. Although only 1%–6% of all cesarean deliveries require blood transfusion,[2] the potential for unpredictable massive blood loss demands that the obstetrician be prepared for such a contingency. The purpose of this chapter is to discuss the indications for transfusion and to familiarize the reader with the basics of blood banking and component therapy. Potential complications of transfusion, as well as some of the ethical dilemmas related to transfusion, will also be discussed.

INDICATIONS FOR TRANSFUSION

Although much has been written about the use of blood in situations of acute blood loss, clear indications for blood replacement are lacking. A variety of indications for blood replacement including estimates of blood loss, hemoglobin level or hematocrit, and changes in vital signs have been proposed. Each of these will now be addressed.

Total blood volume in the nonpregnant woman varies from 64 to 80 mL/kg, or 4,480 to 5,600 mL for a 70-kg woman. Blood volume is most closely related to lean body mass and is proportionately decreased with obesity.[3] During pregnancy there is an expansion in plasma volume by 1,250–1,300 cc, peaking between 32 and 34 weeks. The plasma volume expansion of multiparas exceeds that of primigravidas by 200–250 cc. Plasma volume at term is proportional to the baby's birth weight. The plasma volume of mothers carrying twins exceeds that of singletons by

50%. The expansion in red cell mass is proportionately less than the expansion in plasma volume during pregnancy, equaling 250 cc in the unsupplemented woman and 450 cc in the iron-supplemented woman.[4]

The average blood loss at cesarean is 1,000 mL.[5,6] Both Brant[5] and Wilcox et al[6] showed that actual losses were approximately twice the surgeons' visual estimates. The former investigator also showed no relationship between actual blood loss and alterations in hemoglobin levels. Formulas based on intraoperative hematocrit changes have been devised to estimate the need for transfusion.[7] Schneider et al devised a nomogram based on physiologic parameters designed to aid in determining the number of units to be transfused.[8] However, formulas and nomograms are of little practical value during acute massive blood loss such as may be encountered during cesarean. Because of the protective effect of increased blood volume during pregnancy and the lack of a rapid, accurate means of assessing intraoperative blood loss, replacement at cesarean based exclusively upon estimates of blood loss seems unjustified.

Some authors have proposed arbitrary guidelines for transfusions based on hemoglobin concentration[9] or hematocrit.[10] The disproportionate expansion of plasma volume relative to red cell mass in normal pregnancy causes a fall in both of these values.[4] Furthermore, studies in both dogs and humans have shown tolerance of lowered hematocrits as long as normovolemia is maintained. As hematocrit declines, blood viscosity and resistance to flow both decrease. The resulting increased cardiac output serves to maintain tissue oxygenation in the face of declining red cell mass. Working with splenectomized dogs, Messmer et al showed that at hematocrits as low as 20%, the microcirculatory flow was adequate to keep tissue oxygen content at or close to normal levels in skeletal muscle, the liver, pancreas, small intestine, and kidney.[11] Singler and Furman[12] studied children who underwent surgery, using normovolemic hemodilution. Maintenance of low peripheral vascular resistance was associated with adequate cellular oxygenation with intraoperative hematocrits as low as 14%.[12] Czer and Shoemaker[13] suggested that raising the hematocrit above 33% in patients undergoing major surgery may not be beneficial. There was no improvement in oxygen delivery following transfusion if the pretransfusion hematocrit was above 33%. Survival was greatest in the group whose pretransfusion hematocrit was between 27% and 33%.

The dramatic hemodynamic changes that take place at the time of operative delivery may be affected by the choice of anesthetic. Regional anesthesia may produce a transient hypotensive effect. The immediate postdelivery increase in cardiac output may be modified by epidural anesthesia.[14] Halothane in concentrations of up to 1% does not increase blood loss.[15]

From the foregoing, it becomes apparent that a rational decision to replace blood lost at cesarean should be based on consideration of not only the volume of the vascular system and the oxygen-carrying capacity, but also the dynamics of circulation. The ultimate consequence of severe hemorrhage is irreversible hypoxic organ damage.[3,16] Because that diagnosis may be made only in retrospect, it seems reasonable to initiate transfusion upon the appearance of early signs of hemodynamic decompensation. These include hypotension, narrowed pulse pressure, tachycardia, cool skin, and oliguria. Central hemodynamic monitoring, particularly in a patient with underlying cardiovascular disease, hypertensive disorder, or coagulopathy, may be a useful adjunct.[17]

TYPE AND SCREEN VERSUS TYPE AND CROSSMATCH

A number of publications[18–27] have suggested the potential benefit of typing and screening rather than crossmatching blood in anticipation of major surgery. When a *type and screen* is ordered, the ABO and Rh of the potential recipient's blood are determined. Her serum is then mixed with specially selected O-positive reagent red blood cells, which by law must contain antigens that will react with all of the common clinically significant antibodies.[28] An antibody enhancement solution, such as bovine serum albumin, may be added at this point. The addition of albumin facilitates the detection of incomplete antibodies or of antibodies that are capable of attaching to a specific antigen but are unable to cause agglutination in a saline suspension of erythrocytes. Following incubation at 37°C the cell–serum mixture is washed with isotonic saline. After being decanted, the sedimented cells are mixed with antihuman globulin. The presence of agglutination indicates the presence of antibodies in the potential recipient's serum to at least one of the antigens on the surface of the test red cells.[19] A *crossmatch* follows the same steps as detailed above, except that the donor cells are tested against recipient serum.

A patient who has a negative antibody screen and who receives type-specific, uncrossmatched blood will exhibit an antibody-mediated transfusion reaction only if her serum has antibodies to a rare antigen on donor red cells. The likelihood of this is remote. Heisto[29] found 16 antibodies in the sera of 23,857 (0.07%) patients that had escaped detection during typing and screening. Boral et al[30] found 5 such antibodies among 17,483 specimens (0.03%).

Friedman[18] reviewed transfusion practices in over 10,000 patients undergoing cesarean delivery; 8.5% of low cervical and 12.8% of other cesarean patients required transfusion. The mean number of units transfused per patient was 2.0. Similar data were reported by Penney et al.[22] Both Reisner[23] and Hill and Lavin[24] transfused 3% of their patients requiring cesarean delivery, whereas Chestnut[25] transfused only 1.9% of 213 patients. Cesarean birth thus appears to be an operative procedure in which blood transfusion is infrequently required.

There are potential benefits to be derived from a policy of typing and screening blood. Significant cost savings may be realized from avoiding

TABLE 21.1 Blood Ordering for Cesarean Delivery

Type and crossmatch 2 or more units
Active vaginal bleeding
Placenta previa
Coagulopathy
Positive antibody screen
Type and screen 2 units
All others

unnecessary crossmatches.[19,21,23,26] The shelf life of whole blood or packed cells in anticoagulant citrate-phosphate-dextrose-adenine-1 (CPD-A-1) is 35 days and in sodium chloride-adenine-glucose-mannitol (SAGM) preservative 42 days. Blood that has been crossmatched is usually held for a single potential recipient for no more than 1 or 2 days. In contrast, type-specific units may be "double-tagged" for two or more potential recipients who have been found to have no antibodies on screening. Therefore, by increasing the number of patients who may be covered by a limited blood bank inventory, typing and screening serves to decrease wastage of banked blood.

Should blood be required during cesarean delivery for a patient for whom only a type and screen has been performed, a crossmatch may be undertaken. If the need is urgent, a "quick spin" crossmatch in which donor red cells are mixed with patient serum may be performed. The absence of agglutination or hemolysis following brief centrifugation indicates compatibility. If the intraoperative need for blood is extremely urgent, a unit of O-negative blood may be transfused while awaiting completion of crossmatching.

Based on the foregoing, a rational blood-ordering policy for cesarean may be suggested (Table 21.1). Patients with positive antibody screens, as well as those at increased risk for hemorrhage, should have crossmatched blood available. The majority of patients—who are at low risk for transfusion—may be safely managed with blood that has been typed and screened.

AUTOLOGOUS BLOOD DONATION AND TRANSFUSION

The storage of blood for transfusion back to the donor at a later time has been employed for general surgery[31] as well as cesarean deliveries.[31–35] Advantages include the avoidance of hemolytic transfusion reactions, isoimmunization, and blood-borne infections.

In addition, unused blood may be utilized for homologous transfusion.

An indication for autologous blood unique to obstetrics is the management of pregnancies complicated by alloantibodies to high-incidence ("public") antigens.[32,36,37] Obtaining compatible blood for either maternal or neonatal transfusion for these patients is extremely difficult. Autologous blood may be kept in standard preservatives or may be frozen and stored for up to 3 years.[38] Sandler et al[33] reported on a patient with an anti-Lu^b antibody who did not require the use of her frozen cells during either of two term pregnancies. One year thereafter, that blood was available for emergency surgery for an ectopic pregnancy.

The drop in hemoglobin concentration following donation during pregnancy has been reported to be as high as 1.5 g/dL.[34] Although most authors[32–34] have not encountered major complications of blood donations during pregnancy, Davis[35] reported a patient who, near term, developed hypotension and fetal bradycardia during phlebotomy. It thus seems prudent to monitor both maternal vital signs and fetal heart rate during phlebotomy of a pregnant woman beyond the mid-trimester.

TRANSFUSION OF WHOLE BLOOD AND BLOOD COMPONENTS

Donor Blood

Testing of donor blood includes determination of ABO and Rh types. Testing for unexpected antibodies is done routinely for donors who have been pregnant previously, or who have themselves been blood recipients, or when otherwise indicated. Those units containing clinically significant antibodies should be processed into components containing minimal amounts of plasma.[38] All donor blood has also been screened and found to be negative for hepatitis B surface antigen, hepatitis B core antibody, syphilis, and human immunodeficiency virus (HIV) antibody.[39] A normal value of alanine aminotransferase is now also required as presumptive evidence of the absence of non-A, non-B hepatitis.

Blood Administration

Normal saline (0.9% USP) is most commonly recommended as the only fluid to be administered with blood transfusion.[40–43] Hypotonic solutions (eg, 5% dextrose in water) have been shown to cause in vitro hemolysis. Calcium-containing solutions (eg, lactated Ringer's) may cause clot formation of blood stored in citrate.[44]

Medications should never be added to blood. The pH of the medication may be high enough to cause hemolysis. Determining whether blood or the medication is the cause of a reaction is difficult when the two are administered simultaneously. Furthermore, if a unit of blood containing medication is discontinued, the patient will have received an incomplete dose.

Patients receiving rapid transfusion and those receiving blood during surgery may benefit from having the transfused blood warmed. Administration of 3,000 mL or more of cold banked blood at rates in excess of 50 cc/min has been associated with ventricular arrhythmias and cardiac arrest.[45] Because a patient undergoing a cesarean may have a decrease in body temperature, the administration of even 1 or 2 units of cold banked blood may further decrease the core temperature. A decrease of as little as 0.5°–1°C may cause severe postoperative shivering, which in turn may increase oxygen consumption by as much as 400%.[42] Caution should be exercised in using microwave blood warmers, as uneven or excessive heating may cause hemolysis.[46]

Although there is no minimum time over which a unit of blood must be transfused, there is a theoretical risk of bacterial contamination the longer blood is kept at room temperature. Therefore, the administration of a unit of blood should be completed within 4 hours. Blood requiring a longer infusion time should be divided into aliquots. A unit of blood that has been warmed above 10°C but has not been used may not be returned to the blood bank for reissue.[40]

Platelet aggregates develop after 2–4 days of storage. The larger fibrin–white blood cell–platelet aggregates do not form until 10 days of storage. To prevent transfusion of these macroaggregates, blood filters with a pore size of 170 μm should be used routinely. Whether the use of micropore (20- to 40-μm) filters prevents adult respiratory distress syndrome is not clear at present. The routine use of such filters is not recommended.[40,42,43]

Emergency Transfusion

Resuscitation following acute massive blood loss is a two-step process. First, normovolemia is restored, using crystalloid or colloid.[47] Second, blood is transfused to restore the oxygen-carrying capacity. The patient's blood type may be rapidly established in most blood banks. In an emergency, the administration of type-specific blood is preferable to O-negative (universal donor) blood for a variety of reasons. Type-specific blood, even in the absence of an antibody screen, will be compatible over 99% of the time.[48] O-negative whole blood and packed cells may contain anti-A and anti-B IgG and IgM antibodies in sufficient quantity to cause hemolysis of recipient cells. Because these antibodies may also hemolyze donor red cells, it is best not to switch back to the patient's own type-specific cells once therapy has been initiated with O-negative blood. Finally, O-negative is one of the least common blood groups and should therefore be saved for recipients of the same type.

Blood Storage

Most banked blood is stored in citrate-phosphate-dextrose (CPD), citrate-phosphate-dextrose-adenine (CPD-A), or sodium chloride-adenine-glucose-mannitol (SAGM) anticoagulant-preservative. The average unit of whole blood contains 450 cc of blood.[49] The citrate ion binds calcium,

TABLE 21.2 Metabolic Changes in Whole Blood Stored in CPDA-1

	Storage	Time	Days
	0	14	35
Whole blood lactate (mg/dL)	19	91	202
Whole blood pH	7.16	6.93	6.73
Plasma dextrose (mg/dL)	432	357	282
Plasma sodium (mEq/L)	169	159	153
Plasma potassium (mEq/L)	3.3	17.6	17.2
Plasma chloride (mEq/L)	84	79	79
Plasma bicarbonate (mEq/L)	12	12.5	8.0
Whole blood ammonia (μg/dL)	82	423	703
Hematocrit (%)	35	35	36
Plasma hemoglobin (mg/dL)	0.5	24.7	45.6
WBC ($\times 10^3$)	7.2	3.0	2.9
2,3-DPG (μmol/g hemoglobin)[52]	13.2	—	0.7

Source: Latham JT, Bove JR, Weirich FL: Chemical and hematologic changes in stored CPDA-1 blood. *Transfusion* 22:158, 1982.

thus preventing coagulation. Dextrose enables the erythrocytes to continue anaerobic glycolysis, thereby continuing the production of adenosine triphosphate (ATP). ATP maintains cell viability by preserving membrane function, the sodium-potassium pump, and cell shape and deformability.[48] The addition of adenine to the anticoagulant-preservative (CPD-A) prolongs the permissible storage time from 21 to 35 days. Adenine increases erythrocyte survival by allowing the red cells to resynthesize ATP.[42] Mannitol prevents hemolysis of erythrocytes. The addition of SAGM preservative to red cells anticoagulated in CPD further extends the storage time to 42 days.[50] Storage of blood at 1°–6°C slows the rate of glycolysis approximately 40 times in comparison with the rate at body temperature.[42] U.S. federal government regulations require that at least 70% of transfused erythrocytes remain in circulation for 24 hours after transfusion. This requirement is exceeded by holding the shelf lives of blood stored in CPD to 28 days, in CPD-A to 35 days, and in SAGM to 42 days.

Stored blood undergoes many metabolic changes with time[51,52] (Table 21.2). Stored erythrocytes metabolize glucose to lactate. With falling pH, alterations in red cell function and shape occur. Some stored red cells become spherocytic, which renders them rigid and incapable of passing through the microcirculation.[48] Storage temperatures of 1°–6°C stimulate the sodium-potassium pump, causing red cells to lose potassium and gain sodium. With an increase in osmotic fragility, red cells lyse and plasma hemoglobin increases. Granulocyte function and viability decrease markedly after 24–48 hours. After 24 hours of storage at 1°–6°C, only 10%–25% of platelets remain viable. All clotting factors except labile factors V and VIII remain stable up to 35 days of storage. At 35 days, factor VIII levels have been reported to fall to 20% and factor V levels to 10%.[53] Loss of 2,3-diphosphoglycerate (2,3-DPG) results in greater erythrocyte in vitro oxygen affinity.

Although heparin is an anticoagulant, it is not a preservative, because it lacks glucose. Further, the anticoagulant effect of heparin may be neutralized during storage by thromboplastic substances released by cellular elements in blood. For these two reasons, heparinized whole blood must be used within 48 hours of collection.[42] Heparinized blood has been used in open-heart surgery to avoid cardiac abnormalities that may be associated with depressed calcium levels due to the presence of citrate. Except in the rare patient with a potentially life-threatening arrhythmia, heparinized whole blood is inappropriate for cesarean delivery.

Blood Components

Whole Blood

Whole blood is indicated for those patients in whom acute massive bleeding has resulted in hemorrhagic shock.[40] Whole blood restores the oxygen-carrying capacity, intravascular volume, coagulation factors, and colloid osmotic pressure while exposing the patient to the fewest number of donors.[41,48] The hematocrit of a typical unit varies from 36% to 40%,[40] depending on the actual value of the unit and the donor's hematocrit. A unit of whole blood will raise the hematocrit approximately 3%–4%. Both during and after storage, water shifts out of erythrocytes. In the massively transfused patient, that shift could occur in vivo, resulting in a drop in hematocrit, which might be incorrectly interpreted as continuing blood loss.[49]

Red Blood Cells

Centrifugation or sedimentation of whole blood results in its separation into red cells and plasma. Red cells stored in CPD-A have a hematocrit of 70%–80% and those stored in SAGM, 55%–60%.[50] Red blood cells are indicated for patients in whom normovolemia has been restored but whose oxygen-carrying capacity is below normal. A unit of packed cells will raise the hematocrit approximately 3%–4%. The contents of a unit of red blood cells vary, depending upon the time of separation.

If separation is done within 6 hours of collection, as when harvesting platelets, much of the buffy coat (the layer containing platelets and leukocytes) is removed. If, however, a unit of stored whole blood is separated later, it is likely that the resultant packed cells will contain some lysed and/or aggregated leukocyte and platelet fragments.

There is some debate over the use of packed erythrocytes in the face of hypovolemia.[41,42,48,49,54] In reporting on patients undergoing major cardiovascular surgery, Shackford et al[55] demonstrated significantly lower colloid osmotic pressure in patients receiving packed cells compared with those transfused with whole blood. However, there were no significant differences in either cardiac index or intrapulmonary shunts between both groups.

Because of the increased hematocrit of cells stored in CPD-A, packed red cells have increased viscosity, which may impede the rate of flow. This problem may be obviated by mixing the cells at the time of administration with isotonic saline. This does not, however, appear to be a problem for cells stored in SAGM.[50]

Patients who have had several pregnancies, as well as those who have had multiple transfusions, may develop antibodies to leukocyte antigens and/or plasma protein. Leukocytes are responsible for the majority of febrile transfusion reactions, whereas plasma antigens are responsible for the majority of urticarial allergic reactions. Leukocytes may be removed from erythrocytes by inverted centrifugation, by microfiltration, or by washing cells with saline. Batch washing will remove not only 90% of the leukocytes but also almost all of the plasma.[56] Washed cells have certain disadvantages, however. Because saline contains no nutrients for cell metabolism, washed erythrocytes must be used within 24 hours. The limited shelf life of washed cells is also related to the fact that washing takes place in an open system, which increases the risk of bacterial contamination.[40] Finally, washing removes up to 30% of erythrocytes, along with leukocytes and plasma. To give the same oxygen-carrying capacity found in a unit of unwashed cells, a greater number of units must be transfused. This potentially exposes the patient to a greater number of donors. Because anesthetized patients rarely manifest febrile or urticarial reactions, washed cells are rarely indicated for intraoperative use.[49] Most patients who have one febrile reaction are unlikely to have a second.[57] Because of the problems involved, it seems best to reserve washed cells for those patients who have had two or more documented transfusion reactions.

Frozen red blood cells are prepared by adding glycerol, a cryoprotective agent, to cells that are less than 5 days old. The cells are then frozen to −80° to −200°C. The glycerol does not prevent some freezing from occurring, but it does prevent puncture of the erythrocytes by ice crystals. Cells frozen in glycerol may be stored for up to 3 years. If, upon thawing, the cells containing glycerol are transfused, they will lyse because water will enter the cells more rapidly than the glycerol will leave. For that reason, the glycerol is removed by exposure to solutions of progressively decreasing concentration. This process is both time-consuming and expensive.

The use of frozen-thawed-deglycerolized cells is recommended primarily for those patients who have repeated transfusion reactions with washed red cells. Another indication, mentioned previously, is autotransfusion of rare donor cells.

Platelets

Random donor platelets are prepared by slow centrifugation of fresh whole blood. Platelets so obtained may be stored at 20°–24°C, with constant agitation for 72 hours, or at 1°–6°C for 48 hours.[40] Hypoxic conditions within the storage bag result in increased lactate production, which, over 72 hours, produces a fall in the pH of the suspending plasma to 6.0. Below pH 6.0, platelet viability is severely impaired. Newer types of plastic bags are permeable to oxygen and permit storage of platelets for up to 5 days at 22°C.[58]

Although compatibility testing is not required, the use of incompatible units may result in isoimmunization, in that red cells and their fragments may be present in platelet-rich plasma. During and following cesarean section, the most likely indication for platelet transfusion is thrombocytopenia (usually defined as less than 50,000/μL). The average dose is 6–10 units.

The failure to demonstrate an increase in platelet count 1 hour after transfusion suggests the presence of recipient isoantibodies to human leukocyte A (HLA) antigens. This may be overcome by the use of single-donor, HLA-matched platelets.[59] The latter are prepared by a 2- to 3-hour apheresis. In this procedure, platelets from a single donor are sequentially harvested from 3–4 L of blood passed through a rotating in-line centrifuge. A unit of single-donor platelets contains 3 × 10-inch platelets, equivalent to 6–8 units of random-donor platelets. The plasma volume of a unit is 200–300 mL. One unit of single-donor platelets will raise the adult platelet count by 30,000–60,000/μL.

Fresh Frozen Plasma

Plasma is that portion of blood in which the particulate components are suspended. It consists mainly of water, with 7% being protein and 2% carbohydrate and lipid. Fresh frozen plasma (FFP) is prepared by centrifuging whole blood within 6 hours of phlebotomy. The plasma may be stored at −18°C or less for up to 1 year. A thawed unit must be used within 24 hours. The volume of a unit is 200–250 mL. It contains all of the coagulation factors, including labile factors V and VIII. Although compatibility testing is not required, transfused units should be ABO-compatible with recipients' red cells.

A variety of indications for FFP have been suggested, including coagulation deficiencies seen with liver disease and therapeutic plasma exchange in thrombotic thrombocytopenic purpura and immunodeficiencies. However, only its use in the face of massive transfusion, such as might be encountered at cesarean delivery, will be discussed here. There is little to support the routine use of FFP to replace diluted coagulation factors in patients receiving several units of stored blood.[60,61] In patients receiving massive transfusions, most procoagulants are present in concentrations in excess of 30%, a level adequate, in most instances, to maintain hemostasis.[49] Furthermore, thrombocytopenia is a more frequent cause of bleeding than depletion of coagulation factors in massively transfused patients.[60] As with any blood product, FFP may transmit bloodborne diseases. For all these reasons, the prophylactic use of FFP in patients receiving multiple transfusions is not indicated.[62] It would seem reasonable, however, to consider FFP for the massively transfused patient who continues to bleed but is not thrombocytopenic. Serial partial thromboplastin and prothrombin tests should be followed to determine the dose and effectiveness of FFP.

Other Blood Components

There are other blood components (eg, cryoprecipitate, plasma protein fraction) that are not routinely used when cesarean is performed for obstetric indications. A discussion of their use is beyond the scope of this chapter. The interested reader is referred to the appropriate textbooks.[39,40,63]

COMPLICATIONS OF TRANSFUSIONS

Metabolic Changes

Oxygen Affinity

Because of the decline in 2,3-DPG, blood stored in CPD or CPD-A increases its oxygen affinity over time. This is reflected in a left shift of the oxygen–hemoglobin dissociation curve. The magnitude of this shift depends upon the volume of cells transfused and the duration of storage. This shift is corrected within 24 hours of transfusion.[64] The increased oxygen affinity causes blood passing through the lungs to become saturated at a lower pO_2. In other body tissues, increased oxygen affinity may theoretically result in impaired oxygen delivery, in that oxygen may not be released until the tissue pO_2 is in the hypoxic range. However, clinical studies have not confirmed specific organ hypoxia in the face of transfusion with stored erythrocytes. Bowen and Fleming[65] suggested as a reason for this a compensatory increase in capillary blood flow.

Citrate Toxicity

Citrate toxicity is not a direct consequence of the infusion of citrate, but rather the result of calcium binding by the citrate ion. Transfusion of citrated blood at a rate in excess of 1 unit/5 min will depress ionic calcium by nearly 50%.[66] On completion of transfusion, the calcium level rapidly returns toward normal in the patient with adequate perfusion. This rapid return is probably related to both the rapid metabolism of citrate by the liver and the rapid mobilization of calcium from endogenous stores. Thus, in the absence of persistent hypoperfusion or severe liver disease, citrate intoxication is rare. Indeed, cardiac arrhythmias are more likely to be precipitated by calcium ion infusion than by citrate toxicity.[39] Because measurement of ionic calcium is not readily performed in many institutions, electrocardiographic changes with or without associated muscle tremors may be the only manifestations of citrate intoxication. The administration of calcium chloride or calcium gluconate (0.5–1 mL of 10% solution per 100 cc of transfused blood) may be cautiously undertaken in such patients.

Acid–Base Changes

Blood stored in CPD becomes progressively more acidotic with time (Table 21.2). However, the transfusion of large volumes of stored blood to combat casualties was associated with a correction of metabolic acidosis in those patients in whom blood pressure was restored.[16] It thus seems that restoration of perfusion facilitates correction of metabolic acidosis, regardless of the pH of transfused blood. Furthermore, the transfused citrate is rapidly metabolized to pyruvate and bicarbonate, which may, in turn, result in metabolic alkalosis.

Hyperkalemia

Hyperkalemia may occur after massive transfusion of 2 or more blood volumes (roughly equivalent to 20 or more units of whole blood). It is always associated with citrate-induced metabolic alkalosis, although it may be masked by respiratory or metabolic acidosis. Although it is usually self-limited, hyperkalemia may result in cardiac arrhythmias or seizures.[39]

Transfusion Reactions

Up to 5% of recipients of blood products suffer immediate reactions, and 7% develop delayed reactions.[40] Febrile and allergic reactions are seen more frequently than the more serious hemolytic transfusion reactions. A large proportion of fatal transfusion reactions are due to clerical error[46,67] and are therefore potentially avoidable.

Hemolytic Reactions

Hemolytic transfusion reactions are categorized as acute or delayed. The former are further identified depending on whether the site of hemolysis is intravascular or extravascular.

Acute intravascular hemolytic reactions are almost always due to the transfusion of ABO-incompatible erythrocytes. Naturally occurring anti-A and anti-B IgM antibodies bind complement efficiently. In the process

TABLE 21.3 Signs and Symptoms of Acute Intravascular Hemolytic Transfusion

1. Hypotension[a]
2. Fever with or without chills
3. Chest or back pain
4. Dyspnea
5. Nausea, vomiting
6. Flushing, urticaria
7. Excessive bleeding, DIC[a]
8. Hemoglobinemia
9. Hemoglobinuria[a]
10. Oliguria/renal failure[a]
11. Jaundice

[a] May be found under general anesthesia.

of complement activation, C3a and C5a fragments are cleaved from the larger C3 and C5 molecules, respectively. These basic peptides release histamine from mast cells, causing increased capillary permeability, as well as edema and contraction of smooth muscles. Subsequent hypotension and shock may be aggravated by kinin-like activity of C2 fragments and by non-histamine-dependent kinin activity of C3a.[68]

The common signs and symptoms of acute hemolytic reactions are listed in Table 21.3. Of these, hypotension, uncontrollable bleeding, and hemoglobinuria may be the only signs when the reaction takes place intraoperatively. Disseminated intravascular coagulation (DIC) may result from either the release of thromboplastic substances from erythrocyte stroma or from the antibody–antigen reaction, activating Hageman factor, platelets, and leukocytes.[68] Acute renal failure may be due to tubular deposition of acid hematin and/or to deposition of fibrin subsequent to DIC. Alternatively, renal tubular ischemia may be secondary to complement- and/or kinin-mediated vasomotor changes.

Acute extravascular hemolysis is usually due to IgG-mediated hemolysis seen with such antibodies as Rh, Kell, and Duffy. Signs and symptoms are similar to those listed for intravascular hemolysis (Table 21.3). Vasomotor symptoms are, however, rare, because of the lack of complement activation.

The management of an acute hemolytic transfusion reaction is both diagnostic and supportive (Table 21.4). Alkalinizing urine to prevent deposition of acid hematin is of questionable value, but is likely harmless.[42]

Delayed hemolytic reactions are due to antibodies whose concentration is too low for detection at the time of transfusion. Symptoms occur after a variable time period of up to 21 days and may include a fall in hemoglobin, fever, malaise, hemoglobinemia, or hyperbilirubinemia. Although monitoring of the hematocrit as well as the renal and coagulation status is prudent, no active intervention is usually indicated.

Nonimmune causes of hemolysis that may be seen at the time of transfusion include infusion of hypotonic solutions (eg, 5% dextrose in water), overheated or frozen cells, and contaminated blood. Differentiat-

TABLE 21.4 Management of Hemolytic Transfusion Reactions

1. Discontinue transfusion
2. Keep IV line open with normal saline
3. Support blood pressure and respiration
4. Treat DIC
5. Maintain urine output; consider diuretics
6. Alkalinize urine
7. Check blood bag label, patient identification for clerical errors
8. Return blood container, transfusion set, and intravenous solutions
9. Inspect postreaction serum or plasma for hemolysis and compare with prereaction sample
10. Perform direct antiglobulin test in postreaction sample and compare with prereaction sample
11. Depending on results of steps 3–6, other tests may include:
    a. Determination of ABO and Rh on prereaction and postreaction samples from patient and donor blood
    b. Repeat tests for antibodies in donor or recipient and repeat crossmatching using prereaction and postreaction blood specimens from patient and donor blood
    c. Gram stain and culture of blood container
    d. Bilirubin 5–7 hours after transfusion
    e. Postreaction urine for hemoglobin
    f. Coagulation studies

ing these from an acute hemolytic reaction may be extremely difficult. When suspected, the source of nonimmune hemolysis should be vigorously pursued and eliminated.

Febrile Reactions

Fever as an independent sign occurring with blood transfusion is most likely due to antileukocyte antibodies. These are found most often in either multigravidas or patients who have received multiple transfusions. Temperature elevations rarely exceed 38°C. Management of a febrile transfusion reaction usually entails only slowing the rate of transfusion and administering an antipyretic.[68] Indications for the use of washed or frozen-thawed erythrocytes were included in the discussion of blood components. The fevers seen with acute hemolytic reactions and with transfusion of infected blood are usually higher than those seen with febrile reactions. Associated clinical findings (Table 21.3) may help to identify the source of the fever. When the findings are unclear, initiation of care for a hemolytic reaction (Table 21.4) seems appropriate.

Allergic Reactions

Allergic reactions are due to antibodies to transfused plasma proteins. Rarely, an IgA-deficient recipient may develop IgG anti-IgA antibodies. Findings vary from urticaria of the arms and trunk to severe anaphylactic reactions. Although the former is more common, the latter may be life-threatening. Treatment of a mild reaction includes slowing of transfusion and subcutaneous administration of epinephrine and antihistamines. Severe reactions require stopping the transfusion and administering intravenous hydrocortisone and vasopressors.[69] Patients who have a history of previous mild allergic transfusion reactions should receive an antihistamine prior to transfusion. Washed or frozen-thawed red cells or cells from an IgA-deficient donor should be considered for those with a history of severe allergic transfusion reactions.

Depletion of Coagulation Proteins and Platelets

Massive transfusion is defined as the replacement of 1 or more total blood volumes (approximately 5,000 mL or 10 units of whole blood) within 24 hours.[40] There is an inverse relationship between the volume of blood replaced and the platelet count.[70–72] It is not clear whether the apparent depletion of platelets and coagulation proteins is due to dilution, consumption of coagulation factors precipitated by shock and tissue damage, or both. What is clear is that there is no apparent correlation between the volume of blood transfused and the frequency of pathologic bleeding.[71–73] Therefore, the *routine* administration of platelets or FFP after a given number of units of blood have been transfused is likely not beneficial. It would seem reasonable, however, to perform serial coagulation tests for the massively transfused patient and to replace platelets and/or plasma in the presence of clinical bleeding and laboratory evidence of clotting factor deficiencies.

Infections

Hepatitis

Posttransfusion hepatitis (PTH) remains the most frequent cause of death following transfusion.[43] Approximately 10% of blood recipients will develop PTH.[74] Of these, the majority are anicteric.[42,43,74] There is an increased risk with an increasing number of units transfused.[75]

Despite the disqualification of prospective donors who are positive for hepatitis B surface antigen (HBsAg),[31] hepatitis B remains the cause of 10% of PTH. One explanation for this is the possibility that the virus may be present in the donor in concentrations too low to be detected by third-generation tests. Alternatively, donor screening may be done during the temporal "window" between the disappearance of HBsAg and the appearance of anti-HBs antibody. The recent addition of screening donors for hepatitis B core antibody (HBcAb), which is present concurrently within that window, may further decrease the number of cases of PTH caused by hepatitis B.

Non-A, non-B hepatitis (NANB) is responsible for the majority of PTH. It is characterized by the presence of liver enzyme changes consistent with viral hepatitis and the absence of serologic markers for either hepatitis A or B. The time from exposure to enzyme elevation for NANB is usually 7–8 weeks (versus 12 weeks for hepatitis B). Approximately 20%–30%

of patients become icteric. The disease is usually mild, although fatal cases have been reported. Diagnosis of anicteric NANB is made by the observation, within 14–180 days of transfusion, of two elevations of alanine aminotransferase (ALT) in tests done at least 5 days apart.[42] From 10% to 60% of patients with NANB will develop chronic hepatitis, defined by persistent elevations of ALT after 1 year.

Because of the lack of a serologic marker for NANB, screening of donors for elevated ALT has been initiated by the Red Cross. However, ALT values vary with age, sex, and use of alcohol. An elevated ALT, therefore, is not specific for NANB. Further, NANB has been reported in recipients of blood from donors whose ALT was normal.[74] Clearly, the development of a virus-specific test for NANB is desperately needed.

Acquired Immune Deficiency Syndrome (AIDS)

AIDS is a lethal disease transmitted by human immunodeficiency viruses (HIV). As of January 4, 1988, 1,243 cases of AIDS whose likely source was a transfused blood product had been reported.[76] These blood products include whole blood, red cells, platelets, and plasma. Antibody to HIV has also been found in patients transfused with washed or frozen red cells.[77] Although over 3 million people receive transfusions each year, the risk of acquiring AIDS from blood components is apparently low. Federal guidelines[78] require the disqualification of donors from high-risk groups, as well as serologic screening. Since the institution of screening of prospective donors for serologic evidence of HIV in March 1985, 1,115 cases of transfusion-associated AIDS have been reported.[76] The apparent persistence of blood-borne transmission of AIDS despite serologic screening of prospective donors may be explained, in part, by the latency between exposure to the virus and the development of antibodies.[79]

The practice of designating donors is opposed by the three national blood bank organizations.[80] The assumption that a family member or friend is not a carrier of AIDS may not be valid. Further, large-scale use of designated donors may cause regular donors to delay donating until blood is needed by a family member or friend, thus jeopardizing the nation's blood supply.

Cytomegalovirus (CMV)

CMV is a DNA virus found in the leukocytes of 10% of asymptomatic individuals. Fifty percent of adults have antibody to CMV.[43] However, the virus may persist despite the presence of antibody. Posttransfusion CMV is acquired in about 30% of recipients. These infections occur with equal frequency in seropositive and seronegative individuals.[81] Over 90% of infected immunocompetent individuals exhibit no symptoms. The remainder usually have a mild, heterophile-negative mononucleosis-like syndrome. Preterm infants weighing less than 1,250 g delivered from CMV antibody–negative mothers are at increased risk for life-threatening infection.

There are no reports of congenitally acquired CMV infection secondary to transfusion to a seronegative mother. However, disease transmission in such patients remains a theoretical risk, particularly those in whom delivery remote from term is a possibility (eg, placenta previa). These patients may benefit from transfusion with either blood from seronegative donors or frozen deglycerolized red cells.[81]

Malaria

Current American Association of Blood Banks policy allows individuals who have visited endemic areas but who reside in nonendemic areas to donate blood 6 months after returning from the endemic area. However, those who have received antimalarial prophylaxis may not donate blood for 3 years following cessation of treatment. Those who have had active disease may not donate blood until 3 years after cessation of treatment or after becoming asymptomatic.[38] Despite these precautions, an occasional case of posttransfusion malaria is reported.[74] This is probably related to the lack of a sensitive, inexpensive laboratory test for this disease.

Syphilis

Transmission of syphilis by stored blood is extremely rare, because the spirochete cannot survive refrigeration at 4°C. Because spirochetes may circulate before the test becomes reactive, a negative serologic test for syphilis in a donor does not preclude the possibility of infection. A case of transfusion-associated syphilis in a patient given 25 units of seronegative platelet concentrates and 6 units of packed red blood cells has been reported.[82]

Posttransfusion Purpura

Posttransfusion purpura is a rare but potentially fatal delayed complication of blood transfusion. The majority of reported cases have occurred in women with previous sensitizing pregnancies and/or transfusions.[83] The disease is characterized by the appearance, within 5–12 days of transfusion, of thrombocytopenia associated with petechiae and bleeding from mucosal surfaces. Clinical findings may include epistaxis, melena, hematuria, and menorrhagia.

The postulated mechanism of this disease is the development of an isoantibody to the Pl^{A1} platelet antigen. Following transfusion of Pl^{A1}-positive platelets to a Pl^{A1}-negative recipient, antibody–antigen complexes form and remain in circulation. The latter adsorb onto the patient's own

Pl^{A1}-deficient platelets, which are then destroyed by her own antiplatelet antibodies. The rarity of this complication may be explained, in part, by the fact that only 2% of the population is deficient in the Pl^{A1} antigen. Although the disease is usually self-limited, successful treatment with plasma exchange has been reported.[83,84]

REFUSAL OF TRANSFUSION

The pregnant woman who, for personal or religious reasons, refuses blood transfusion places her obstetrician squarely on the horns of a dilemma. Conflicting responsibilities to the maternal and fetal patient raise a number of difficult ethical and legal issues.[85]

Alternatives to transfusion include intraoperative extracorporeal hemodilution[86,87] and the use of plasma volume expanders. The former ensures maintenance of peripheral perfusion despite a decrease in red cell mass. However, a hemorrhagic death despite restoration of normovolemia has been reported.[88] Among the plasma volume expanders, only the perfluorochemicals (PFCs) have the capacity to carry oxygen, and then only in solution. This may require prolonged patient exposure to high inspired oxygen tensions until endogenous hemoglobin is restored.[89] Side effects of PFCs include chest discomfort and pulmonary and systemic hypotension. These are complement mediated and are usually averted by the use of prophylactic corticosteroids.[90] No PFC is currently licensed in the United States.

It is thus apparent that only blood will be lifesaving in some instances of acute massive hemorrhage. Such hemorrhage may be encountered during cesarean delivery. The physician who decides to transfuse the unconsenting patient does so at the risk of legal scrutiny. A body of case law has emerged that makes the mother's right of refusal subordinate to the viable fetus's right to live.[85] However, transfusing a patient despite her refusal may expose the physician and the hospital to civil liability. The obstetrician is therefore advised to become familiar with the manner in which the local court will conduct a telephone hearing in dealing with emergencies. Obtaining legal counsel early in the course of prenatal care is preferable to retrospective legal scrutiny.

CONCLUSION

The need for blood transfusion may arise in caring for the patient who requires a cesarean. The obstetrician should be familiar with the indications for component therapy and should be prepared to manage potential complications. As with any other therapeutic modality, the risks and benefits of transfusion should be carefully and knowledgeably weighed prior to administration of blood and blood products.

REFERENCES

1. Blundell J: A successful case of transfusion. *Lancet* 1:431, 1829.
2. Petitti DB: Maternal mortality and morbidity in cesarean section. *Clin Obstet Gynecol* 28:763, 1985.
3. Mattox KL: Disorders of surgical bleeding and blood transfusion problems, in Hardy JD (ed): *Hardy's Textbook of Surgery.* Philadelphia, JB Lippincott Co, 1983, pp 73–81.
4. Martin C: Physiologic changes during pregnancy: The mother, in Quilligan EJ, Kretchmer N (eds): *Fetal and Maternal Medicine.* New York, John Wiley & Sons, Inc, 1980, pp 140–180.
5. Brant HA: Blood loss at cesarean section. *J Obstet Gynaecol Br Commonwealth* 73:456, 1966.
6. Wilcox CF, Hunt AB, Owen CA: The measurement of blood lost during cesarean section. *Am J Obstet Gynecol* 77:772, 1959.
7. Gross JB: Estimating allowable blood loss: Corrected for dilution. *Anesthesiology* 58:277, 1983.
8. Schneider AJ, Stockman JA, Oski FA: Transfusion nomogram: An application of physiology to clinical decisions regarding the use of blood. *Crit Care Med* 9:469, 1981.
9. Gibbs CE, Misenhimer HR: The use of blood transfusions in obstetrics. *Am J Obstet Gynecol* 93:26, 1965.
10. Stoelting RK, Miller RD: *Basics of Anesthesia.* New York, Churchill Livingstone, 1984, pp 248–249.
11. Messmer K, Gornandt L, Jesch F, et al: Oxygen transport and tissue oxygenation during hemodilution with dextran. *Adv Exp Med Biol* 37:669, 1976.
12. Singler RC, Furman EB: Hemodilution: How low a minimum hematocrit? *Anesthesiology* 53:572, 1980.
13. Czer LSC, Shoemaker WC: Optimal hematocrit value in critically ill postoperative patients. *Surg Gynecol Obstet* 147:363, 1978.
14. Ueland K, Metcalfe J: Heart disease in pregnancy. *Clin Perinatol* 1:349, 1974.
15. Skovsted P, Misfeldt BB, Viby Mogensen J, et al: The effects of anesthesia on blood loss at cesarean section. *Acta Anaesthesiol Scand* 17:153, 1973.
16. Collins JA: The pathophysiology of hemorrhagic shock. *Prog Clin Biol Res* 108:5, 1982.
17. Clark SL, Horenstein JM, Phelan JP, et al: Experience with the pulmonary artery catheter in obstetrics and gynecology. *Am J Obstet Gynecol* 152:374, 1985.
18. Friedman BA: An analysis of surgical blood use in United States hospitals with application to the maximum surgical blood order schedule. *Transfusion* 19:268, 1979.
19. Lee K, Lachance V: Type and screen for elective surgery. *Transfusion* 20:324, 1980.
20. Mintz PD, Henry JB, Boral LI: The type and antibody screen. *Clin Lab Med* 2:169, 1982.
21. Ness PM, Rosche ME, Barrasso C, et al: The efficacy of type and screen to reduce unnecessary cross matches for obstetric patients. *Am J Obstet Gynecol* 140:661, 1981.
22. Penney GC, Moores HM, Boulton FE: Development of a rational blood-ordering policy for obstetrics and gynaecology. *Br J Obstet Gynaecol* 89:100, 1982.
23. Reisner LS: Type and screen for cesarean section: A prudent alternative. *Anesthesiology* 58:476, 1983.
24. Hill ST, Lavin JP: Blood ordering in obstetrics and gynecology: Recommendations for the type and screen. *Obstet Gynecol* 62:236, 1983.
25. Chestnut DH: Blood replacement for repeat cesarean section: "Type and screen" preferable to cross matching. *NC Med J* 46:139, 1985.
26. Parker RT: Blood replacement for repeat cesarean section. *NC Med J* 46:141, 1985.

27. Nakamura Y, Takano A, Shinagawa S: Type and screen system for elective surgery in obstetrics and gynecology. *Acta Obstet Gynaecol Jpn* 37:141, 1985.
28. Code of Federal Regulations. Title 21. Vol 6, Parts 660.6–660.36. Washington, DC, US Government Printing Office, 1981.
29. Heisto H: Pretransfusion blood group serology. *Transfusion* 19:761, 1979.
30. Boral LI, Hill SS, Apollon CJ, et al: The type and antibody screen, revisited. *Am J Clin Pathol* 71:578, 1979.
31. Rebulla P, Giovanetti AM, Petrini G, et al: Autologous blood predeposit for elective surgery: A program for better use and conservation of blood. *Surgery* 97:463, 1985.
32. Milles G, Browne WH, Barrick RG: Autologous transfusions for elective cesarean section. *Am J Obstet Gynecol* 103:1166, 1969.
33. Sandler SG, Beyth Y, Laufer N, et al: Autologous blood transfusions and pregnancy. *Obstet Gynecol* 53:625, 1979.
34. Katz AR, Walker WA, Ross PJ, et al: Autologous transfusion in obstetrics and gynecology. *Int J Gynaecol Obstet* 16:345, 1979.
35. Davis R: Banked autologous blood for caesarean section. *Anaesth Intensive Care* 7:358, 1979.
36. Sacks DA, Johnson CS, Platt LD: Isoimmunization in pregnancy to Gerbich antigen. *Am J Perinatol* 2:208, 1985.
37. Sacks DA, Johnson CS: Yt^a isoimmunization in pregnancy. *J Reprod Med* 28:407, 1983.
38. American Association of Blood Banks: *Standards for Blood Banks and Transfusion Services,* ed 11. Arlington, Va, American Association of Blood Banks, 1984.
39. American Association of Blood Banks, American Red Cross, Council of Community Blood Centers: Circular of information for the use of human blood and blood components, 1984.
40. Snyder EL (ed): *Blood Transfusion Therapy.* Arlington, Va, American Association of Blood Banks, 1983.
41. Wallas CH: Selected topics in blood component therapy. *Prog Clin Pathol* 9:47, 1984.
42. Miller RD, Brzica SM: Blood, blood component, colloid, and autotransfusion therapy, in Miller RD (ed): *Anesthesia,* vol 2. New York, Churchill Livingstone, 1981, pp 885–922.
43. Dahlke MB: Red blood cell transfusion therapy. *Med Clin North Am* 68:639, 1984.
44. Ryden SE, Oberman HA: Compatibility of common intravenous solutions with CPD blood. *Transfusion* 115:250, 1975.
45. Boyan CP, Howland WS: Cardiac arrest and temperature of bank blood. *JAMA* 183:58, 1963.
46. Pineda AA, Brzica SM, Taswell HF: Hemolytic transfusion reaction—recent experience in a large blood bank. *Mayo Clin Proc* 53:378, 1978.
47. Shoemaker WC: Evaluation of colloids, crystalloids, whole blood, and red cell therapy in the critically ill patient. *Clin Lab Med* 2:35, 1982.
48. Isbister JP: Haemotherapy for acute haemorrhage. *Anaesth Intensive Care* 12:217, 1984.
49. Schmidt PJ: Component therapy. *Int Anaesthsiol Clin* 20:23, 1982.
50. Högman CF, Akerblom O, Hedlund K, et al: Red cell suspensions in SAGM medium. *Vox Sang* 45:217, 1983.
51. Latham JT, Bove JR, Weirich FL: Chemical and hematologic changes in stored CPDA-1 blood. *Transfusion* 22:158, 1982.
52. Moore GL, Peck CC, Sohmer PR, et al: Some properties of blood stored in anticoagulant CPDA-1 solution. A brief summary. *Transfusion* 21:135, 1981.
53. Bowie EJW, Thompson JH, Owen CA: The stability of antihemophilic globulin and labile factor in human blood. *Mayo Clin Proc* 39:144, 1964.

54. Gould SA, Rice CL, Moss GS: The physiologic basis of the use of blood and blood products. *Surg Ann* 16:13, 1984.
55. Shackford SR, Virgilio RW, Peters RM: Whole blood versus packed-cell transfusions. *Ann Surg* 193:337, 1981.
56. Meryman HT, Bross J, Lebovitz R: The preparation of leukocyte-poor red blood cells: A comparative study. *Transfusion* 20:285, 1980.
57. Menitove JE, McElligott MC, Aster RH: Febrile transfusion reaction: What component should be given next? *Vox Sang* 42:318, 1982.
58. Murphy S, Kahn RA, Holme S, et al: Improved storage of platelets for transfusion in a new container. *Blood* 60:194, 1982.
59. Daly PA, Schiffer CA, Aisner J, et al: Platelet transfusion therapy. One-hour post-transfusion increments are valuable in predicting the need for HLA-matched preparations. *JAMA* 243:435, 1980.
60. Braunstein AH, Oberman HA: Transfusion of plasma components. *Transfusion* 24:281, 1984.
61. Martin DJ, Lucas CE, Ledgerwood AM, et al: Fresh frozen plasma supplement to massive red blood cell transfusion. *Ann Surg* 202:505, 1985.
62. Consensus Conference: Fresh-frozen plasma. *JAMA* 253:551, 1985.
63. Mollison PL: *Blood Transfusion in Clinical Medicine,* ed 7. Oxford, Blackwell Scientific Publications, 1983.
64. Valtis DJ, Kennedy AC: Defective gas-transport function of stored blood red cells. *Lancet* 1:119, 1954.
65. Bowen JC, Fleming WH: Increased oxyhemoglobin affinity after transfusion of stored blood: Evidence for circulatory compensation. *Ann Surg* 180:760, 1974.
66. Denlinger JK, Narhwold ML, Gibbs PS, et al: Hypocalcemia during rapid blood transfusion in anaesthetized man. *Br J Anaesth* 48:995, 1976.
67. Myhre BA: Fatalities from blood transfusion. *JAMA* 244:1333, 1980.
68. Webster BH: Clinical presentation of haemolytic transfusion reactions. *Anaesth Intensive Care* 8:115, 1980.
69. Rush B, Lee NLY: Clinical presentation of nonhaemolytic transfusion reactions. *Anaesth Intensive Care* 8:125, 1980.
70. Lucas CE, Ledgerwood AM: Clinical significance of altered coagulation tests after massive transfusion for trauma. *Am Surg* 47:125, 1981.
71. Mannucci PM, Federici AB, Sirchia G: Hemostasis testing during massive blood replacement. *Vox Sang* 42:113, 1982.
72. Sohmer PR, Scott RL: Massive transfusion. *Clin Lab Med* 2:21, 1982.
73. Harrigan C, Lucas CE, Ledgerwood AM, et al: Serial changes in primary hemostasis after massive transfusion. *Surgery* 98:836, 1985.
74. Kahn RA: Diseases transmitted by blood transfusion. *Hum Pathol* 14:241, 1983.
75. Conrad ME, Knodell RG, Bradley EL, et al: Risk factors in transmission of non-A, non-B post-transfusion hepatitis. *Transfusion* 17:579, 1977.
76. Word J (CDC): Personal communication.
77. AIDS-Hemophelia French Study Group: Immunologic and virologic status of multitransfused patients: Role of type and origin of blood products. *Blood* 66:896, 1985.
78. CDC: Update: Revised Public Health Service definition of persons who should refrain from donating blood and plasma—United States. *MMWR* 34:547, 1985.
79. Perkins HA, Samson S, Garner J, et al: Risks of AIDS for recipients of blood components from donors who subsequently develop AIDS. *Blood* 70:1604, 1987.
80. Perkins HA: Transfusion-associated AIDS. *Am J Hematol* 19:307, 1985.
81. International Forum: Transfusion-transmitted CMV infections. *Vox Sang* 46:387, 1984.
82. Chambers RW, Foley HT, Schmidt PJ: Transmission of syphilis by fresh blood components. *Transfusion* 9:32, 1969.

83. Budd JL, Wiegers SE, O'Hara JM: Relapsing post-transfusion purpura. *Am J Med* 78:361, 1985.
84. Rank BH, Gay C, Burke L, et al: Post-transfusion purpura as a gynecologic complication. *Obstet Gynecol* 55:725, 1980.
85. Sacks DA, Koppes RH: Blood transfusion and Jehovah's Witnesses: Medical and legal issues in obstetrics and gynecology. *Am J Obstet Gynecol* 154:483, 1986.
86. Khine HH, Naidu R, Cowell H, et al: A method of blood conservation in Jehovah's Witnesses: Incirculation diversion and refusion. *Anesth Analg* 57:279, 1978.
87. Lichtiger B, Dupuis JF, Seski J: Hemotherapy during surgery for Jehovah's Witnesses: A new method. *Anesth Analg* 61:618, 1982.
88. Harris TJB, Parikh NR, Rao YK, et al: Exsanguination in a Jehovah's Witness. *Anaesthesia* 38:989, 1983.
89. Tremper KK, Levine E, Friedman A, et al: The preoperative treatment of severely anemic patients with a perfluorochemical blood substitute, Fluosol-DA 20%. *Anaesthesiology* 55:A9, 1981.
90. Karn KE, Ogburn PL, Julian T, et al: Use of a whole blood substitute, Fluosol-DA 20%, after massive postpartum hemorrhage. *Obstet Gynecol* 65:127, 1985.

Chapter 22

Resuscitation of the Newborn Infant

Stephen D. Minton, MD

Cesarean delivery is indicated in any situation in which delivery of the fetus must be accomplished and in which induction of labor, additional labor, or vaginal delivery of the fetus per se is deemed to be of greater risk to the mother or the fetus than abdominal delivery.[1,2] As has been shown in other chapters of this book, there are both maternal (toxemia, maternal cardiovascular disease, etc), fetal (breech presentation, maternal genital herpes, etc), and combined (placenta previa, etc) indications for cesarean delivery. Regardless of the indication, the physiologic adjustments necessary immediately after birth often require some degree of neonatal resuscitation.

It has been shown that skillful resuscitation of the asphyxiated newborn can prevent brain damage and minimize subsequent neonatal morbidity.[3] Because an important part of resuscitation is anticipation and preparation, it is important to inform the pediatrician and/or nursery personnel of the impending compromised neonate as early as possible. Special equipment, drugs, and blood products may need to be assembled. If communication between the delivering physician and the physician caring for the infant occurs early enough, more appropriate resuscitation can be applied to the child and the neonatal outcome may be improved.

TRANSITIONAL PHYSIOLOGY

At birth, dynamic, complex changes occur during the transition from intrauterine to extrauterine life. This process encompasses not only changes in the function of specific organ systems such as the pulmonary and cardiovascular systems, but also a reorganization of metabolic processes to achieve a new steady state for the newborn infant. For most infants, the transition is very smooth and occurs in a coordinated fashion. However, for some, the transition is delayed or complicated, and for a small percentage of infants it never occurs. To apply appropriate resuscitative procedures, one must have a good understanding of the development of each of the critical systems and the transition that normally occurs from intrauterine to extrauterine life. If we are to reduce neonatal morbidity and mortality, we must be able to detect those infants whose transition does not proceed appropriately. Because the most critical physiologic changes occur in the pulmonary and cardiovascular systems at birth, we will discuss those systems first.

Pulmonary System

The lungs are initially seen in the embryo at approximately 21 days of gestation as an outgrowth from the laryngotracheal groove. This outgrowth divides into two parts, one of which becomes the larynx and trachea and the other the forerunners of the primary bronchi and lungs. At approximately the fourth gestational month, one can see changes in the epithelial lining of the bronchi from cuboidal to pseudocuboidal cells. By 18 weeks gestation, alveolization is beginning. Lining the alveoli are type II pneumocytes, which become distinguishable around 20–24 weeks gestation.[4] These cells produce surfactant, which can be detected in the amniotic fluid of fetuses between 25 and 30 weeks.[5,6] As gestation progresses, the absolute quantity of surfactant increases in both the lung and the amniotic fluid. By 33–36 weeks, adequate quantities of surfactant for alveolar stability are usually present.[5,6] During this period, the qualitative composition of amniotic fluid surfactant also changes. By 37 weeks, phosphatidylglycerol is found in the amniotic fluid of most fetuses. This is the major component of surfactant upon which alveolar stability is based and can be used as an indicator of pulmonary maturity.[7,8] It is also important to remember that, in utero, the alveoli are open at nearly normal neonatal lung volume and filled with fluid.[9]

Capillary invasion around the developing alveolar sacs begins at approximately 18 weeks.[10] The pulmonary and bronchial circulations are well developed by the 25th week of gestation, with multiple, mutual connections at the alveolar level.[9]

The neuromuscular system as it relates to respiration is well defined even in the very-low-birth-weight infant.[9] The fetus initiates some respiratory movement in utero, which increases in frequency as it approaches term.[11,12] These breathing maneuvers are often associated with rapid eye movement (REM) sleep.[13] Usually these efforts are rapid, discoordinate motions of the chest and abdominal walls. During these fetal breathing maneuvers, amniotic fluid moves in and out of the lungs. In the full-term fetus, as much as 600 mL of amniotic fluid per day can be breathed in and out.[14]

During vaginal delivery, the fetal thoracic cage is compressed by the birth canal, with pressures of 30–160 cm/H_2O.[15] This can forcibly eject from the airways as much as 30 mL of tracheal/lung fluid.[16] Subsequent recoil of the neonatal chest wall after vaginal delivery usually produces inspiration of air, resulting in an air–liquid interface in the larger airways. The precise mechanism of the first extrauterine inspiration remains somewhat obscure but probably relates to the multiple unfamiliar stimuli that the infant faces.[17] These include cold, air, light, noise, gravity, and pain, as well as chemical factors such as hypercapnia, respiratory acidosis, and hypoxia. A great deal of pressure is required initially to open a normal alveolus, but once this has been accomplished, the alveoli may be fully inflated with only a small increase in pressure.[9] This is due to the decrease in surface tension caused by the surfactant.

In cesarean birth, the chest wall is not compressed as extensively as it is during vaginal birth, and the expulsion of tracheal fluid through the airways is therefore not accomplished as successfully. As the infant begins to breathe, there are great increases in blood and lymph flow through the lungs.[9] When the lung fluid is ejected from the airways by breathing, hydrostatic alveolar pressure on the pulmonary capillaries decreases, resulting in increased blood flow into the lungs. This causes capillary fluid to transudate into the interstitium. Alveolar fluid may be directly absorbed into the interstitial spaces at the alveolar corners. The dramatic increase in lung fluid absorption usually begins to subside by 6 hours of age.[18] It is of clinical interest to note that immature rabbit and lamb fetuses delivered by section are both slow to clear their lung fluid.[9] The clinical condition of increased fluid in the lungs is referred to as "transient tachypnea of the newborn."

The very premature newborn may not have enough surfactant to keep the alveoli open, resulting in delayed excretion and reabsorption of fluid. In addition, such an infant may require assisted mechanical ventilation, which will often maintain pulmonary vascular resistance at a higher level for a prolonged period of time.

Cardiovascular System

Fetal circulation differs markedly from that of the neonate.[19] In the fetus, the placenta rather than the lung is the organ of oxygen uptake and CO_2 elimination. In the fetus, blood flowing to the placenta by way of the umbilical arteries has a partial pressure of oxygen in the range of 20 torr and a partial pressure of carbon dioxide in the range of 45 torr.[20] Oxygenated blood, with a partial pressure of approximately 35 torr of oxygen and 40 torr of carbon dioxide, returns to the fetus from the placenta via the umbilical vein. A portion of this blood goes directly into the inferior vena cava via the ductus venosus, and the remainder flows through the liver before entering the inferior vena cava. As blood passes from the inferior vena cava into the right atrium, the major portion is shunted directly through the foramen ovale into the left atrium and then into the left ventricle and out of the aorta. Thus oxygenated blood is preferentially delivered to the heart, head, and upper extremities. Blood returning from the superior vena cava and blood coming from the inferior vena cava that does not cross the foramen ovale is directed into the right ventricle and flows out of the pulmonary artery toward the lungs. However, most of the blood coming out of the pulmonary artery is shunted across the ductus arteriosus into the descending aorta, where it mixes with blood coming from the left ventricle.

This particular cardiovascular arrangement represents essentially two circuits in parallel. The pulmonary circulation has a high resistance because the pulmonary arteries are tightly constricted in response to a low PO_2, a mild metabolic acidosis, and increased tension of alveoli filled with fetal lung fluid.[19,20] Pulmonary blood flow in the fetus is therefore low and represents only 10%–20% of the right ventricular output.[20] On the other hand, a major portion of the systemic circulation is in the low-resistance vascular bed of the placenta, which receives 40% of the combined output of the two ventricles.[19] This system in utero allows the majority of blood to bypass the pulmonary circulation. The tissues receiving their blood supply from the ascending aorta (the heart and the brain) are perfused with more highly oxygenated blood than those supplied by the descending aorta below the ductus, for example, the kidneys and intestine.

Factors determining the rate of exchange at the placenta include surface area, the diffusion coefficient of gases through a membrane, and concentration gradients across the membrane.[21] Uterine blood flow is 500–750 mL/min. The fetus must maintain an umbilical blood flow of 250–350 mL/min to maintain a normal fetal/maternal PO_2 relationship. During labor, uterine and placental blood flow is diminished or transiently halted with uterine contractions.

With the delivery of the infant and the initiation of the first breath, there is a series of important and dramatic changes in the neonatal cardiovascular system.[19] As the lungs begin to expand, the partial pressure of oxygen rises and results in a fall in pulmonary vascular resistance. This fall in pulmonary vascular resistance is followed by a fall in the pressures in the pulmonary artery and, subsequently, in the right ventricle and right atrium. As fluid is absorbed out of the alveolar sacs, pulmonary blood flow further increases, as does pulmonary venous return to the left atrium. As the umbilical cord is clamped, the systemic vascular resistance increases due to the removal of the low-vascular-resistance placenta. As a result, aortic, left ventricular, and left atrial blood pressures rise. When left atrial pressure exceeds right atrial pressure, the foramen ovale closes, stopping right-to-left blood flow. When systemic vascular pressure in the aorta exceeds pulmonary vascular pressure, flow through the ductus arteriosus reverses. Perfusion with oxygenated blood causes constriction of the ductus arteriosus. It is likely that one or more vasoactive substances, including arachidonic acid metabolites, also play a role in this constriction.[19,22–26] However, even when newborn infants are well oxygenated, complete closure does not occur immediately.[19,27] Persistence of the ductus arteriosus is particularly common in premature infants because of a diminished constriction response of the ductus to a rise in PaO_2 and other stimuli.[19,27] With these alterations in vascular resistance and flow, the course of neonatal circulation becomes similar to that of the adult, with two circuits in series rather than in parallel.

Temperature Control

Fetal thermal homeostasis is provided entirely by the uterine environment. A 0.5°–1.0°C gradient between the fetus and the mother exists to dissipate heat from the fetus.[28–30] Although the initial exposure to a colder environment at the time of birth may be helpful in establishing adequate ventilation, it has been shown that stresses from extreme heat and cold diminish the likelihood of survival.[31]

After birth, the infant's core temperature may drop rapidly, due mainly to evaporation from its moist body.[32,33] This drop in temperature is exacerbated by the often cold delivery rooms, resulting in large temperature gradients and convective heat loss from the neonate. In the very-low-birth-weight infant with a small amount of subcutaneous tissue and relatively large surface area per mass ratio, such heat loss is even more significant.[33] In the cold-stressed infant, significant metabolic acidosis may develop due to free fatty acids and glycerol produced from the compensatory heat-producing metabolism of brown fat.[34]

In an attempt to compensate for potential cold stress, the neonate is usually placed under a radiant warmer to minimize heat loss. If the temperature is not servo-controlled, the infant may in fact become too hot or heat stressed. Such infants compensate by vasodilating the peripheral circulation in an effort to dissipate the excessive heat. This protective mechanism, however, may reduce the effective circulating blood volume, resulting in potential relative hypovolemia. If the infant is already relatively hypovolemic from another cause (ie, nuchal cord, placenta abruptio), such changes may be especially detrimental.

PATHOPHYSIOLOGY OF ASPHYXIA

Appropriate resuscitation mandates an understanding of birth asphyxia. Tissues can be deprived of oxygen by two major pathogenic mechanisms, ie, *hypoxemia,* which is a diminished amount of oxygen in the blood supply, or *ischemia,* which is a diminished amount of blood perfusing the tissues. In most instances during the perinatal period, hypoxemia or ischemia occur as a result of *asphyxia,* which refers to an impairment or

TABLE 22.1 Major Biochemical Effects of Hypoxemia on Carbohydrate and Energy Metabolism

↑ Glucose influx to brain
↑ Glycogenolysis
↑ Glycolysis
↓ Brain glucose Glucose utilization > glucose influx
↑ Lactate (and H^+) production and tissue acidosis
↓ Phosphocreatine
↓ Oxidative phosphorylation
↓ ATP

Source: Adapted from Volpe JJ: Hyponic-ischemic encephalopathy, in Volpe JJ (ed): *Neurology of the Newborn.* Philadelphia, WB Saunders Co, 1987, p 148.

failure in the exchange of the respiratory gases, ie, oxygen and carbon dioxide. When asphyxia occurs, there is a rise in $PaCO_2$ and a fall in the pH and PaO_2.

Under aerobic conditions, the concerted actions of glycolysis, the citric acid cycle, and the electron transport system result in the formation of 38 molecules of adenosine triphosphate (ATP), with its high-energy phosphate bonds, for each molecule of glucose oxidized.[35]

Aerobic Conditions

$$\text{Glucose} + 2\ \text{NAD}^+ + 2\ \text{ADP} + 2\ \text{P}_i \rightarrow 2\ \text{pyruvate} + 2\ \text{NADH} + 2\ \text{ATP}$$

$$2\ \text{Pyruvate} + 2\ \text{NADH} + 36\ \text{ADP} + 36\ \text{P}_i + 6\ \text{O}_2 \rightarrow 2\ \text{NAD}^+ + 6\ \text{CO}_2 + 44\ \text{H}_2\text{O} + 36\ \text{ATP}$$

Sum:

$$\text{Glucose} + 38\ \text{ADP} + 38\ \text{P}_i + 6\ \text{O}_2 \rightarrow 6\ \text{CO}_2 + 44\ \text{H}_2\text{O} + \boxed{38\ \text{ATP}}$$

Hypoxemia is accompanied by a number of major biochemical changes in carbohydrate and energy metabolism (Table 22.1).[35,36] The earliest significant changes are a decrease in brain glycogen, an elevation in lactate, and a decrease in phosphocreatinine.[35] These are followed by a decrease in brain glucose and, finally, ATP. The changes appear to reflect principally the impaired production of high-energy phosphate, secondary to failure of the coupled mitochondrial system of the citric acid cycle and the electron transport chain, in turn a consequence of the lack of the ultimate electron acceptor, oxygen. Glycolysis becomes the sole source of ATP production, and because lactate is the principal product of anaerobic glycolysis, only two molecules of ATP are generated for each molecule of glucose metabolized.

Anaerobic Conditions

$$\text{Glucose} + 2\ \text{ADP} + 2\ \text{P}_i \rightarrow 2\ \text{lactate}^- + 2\text{H}^+ + \boxed{2\ \text{ATP}}$$

The accumulation of lactate and associated hydrogen ions is initially beneficial because it signifies the adaptive response of the individual to oxygen deprivation.[35] However, if persistent, this can become a serious deleterious factor.

An understanding of the pathophysiology of asphyxia is extremely important when determining the approach to resuscitation of an asphyxiated newborn infant. Much of our current information regarding asphyxia has been derived from animal experiments; however, one must be very cautious in extrapolating this information to the human neonate, because there is great variability in the response of different species to asphyxia.[37]

The sequence of events described with asphyxia in the rhesus monkey fetus is probably closely analogous to that of the human fetus. Dawes[37] and Adamsons et al[38] delivered rhesus monkey fetuses by cesarean section in which, prior to delivery, catheters were placed in fetal vessels and the head was covered with a saline-filled rubber bag to prevent air breathing. The monkeys were asphyxiated by tying the umbilical cords at birth. Figure 22.1 illustrates the changes in three physiological variables (respiratory rate, heart rate, and blood pressure) during 10 minutes of *total* asphyxia and subsequent resuscitation. As can be seen from the figure, the monkey had rapid gasps occurring shortly after the onset of asphyxia. This was accompanied by thrashing movements of the extremities. This ceased after 1–2 minutes and was followed by primary apnea. During primary apnea, the heart rate dropped to approximately 100 bpm (normal is 180–220 bpm in the infant monkey). Blood pressure, however, was maintained. During primary apnea, spontaneous respirations could be induced by appropriate sensory stimuli. Primary apnea lasted for approximately 1 minute, followed by a series of spontaneous gasps for 4 or 5 minutes. These respiratory gasps gradually became weaker and terminated at the last gasp after approximately 8 minutes of total asphyxia. The apnea occurring at this point is termed "secondary apnea." During secondary apnea, the heart rate falls lower and the blood pressure is *not* maintained. During secondary apnea, spontaneous respirations cannot be induced by external sensory stimuli. Death occurs if secondary apnea is not reversed within several minutes.

Resuscitation of the monkey was performed by positive-pressure ventilation. The longer the delay in initiating adequate resuscitative measures

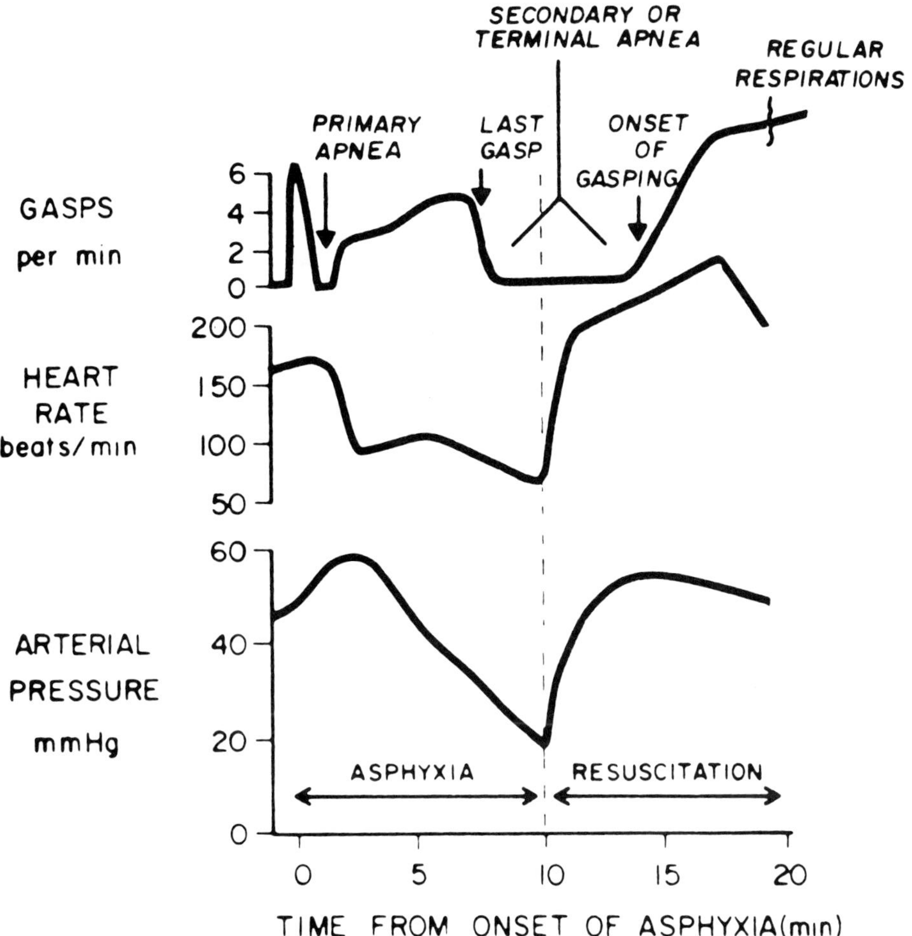

FIGURE 22.1 Changes in physiologic parameters during asphyxiation and resuscitation of the rhesus monkey fetus at birth. (Adapted from Dawes CA: *Foetal and Neonatal Physiology [Year Book]*. Chicago, Year Book Publishers, 1968; and Adamson K Jr, Behrman R, Dawes G, et al: *J Pediatr* 65:807, 1964, with permission.)

after the last gasp, the longer the time to the first gasp after resuscitation. It has been stated that for every 1-minute delay in resuscitation during secondary apnea, there is a 2-minute delay until a gasp is noted and a 4-minute delay in rhythmic breathing.[38,39]

Circulatory Changes during Asphyxia

As demonstrated in Figure 22.1, as asphyxia progresses, the monkey initially has a falling heart rate, with a subsequent fall in blood pressure. This results in a decrease in cardiac output.[37] Concomitant with this decrease in cardiac output is a redistribution of available cardiac output in an attempt to provide increased oxygenated blood to the vital organs—

brain, heart, and adrenal glands.[40,41] Decreased blood flow is seen in the kidneys, spleen, lungs, and carcass.[40,41] During asphyxia, the mechanism by which this redistribution is accomplished requires a larger contribution of the oxygenated blood returning from the placenta through the ductus venosus and inferior vena cava into the right atrium to be shunted across the foramen ovale into the left atrium and subsequently to the heart and brain.[42] This will temporarily maintain the absolute volume of blood perfusing the heart and brain on a per gram of tissue basis in the face of falling cardiac output.[42] If, however, cardiac output decreases by 80%, the percentage of cardiac output going to the heart, adrenal glands, and paleoencephalon, although increased significantly, will not be sufficient to preserve adequate flow to these organs.[42]

Diving Seal Reflex

Reflex circulatory adjustments occur in diving sea mammals. These adjustments include a profound bradycardia, a decrease in oxygen consumption and body temperature, and an accumulation of lactic acid in muscle, but not in blood.[43] With these changes, the seal is able to maintain central arterial blood pressure and oxygenation during prolonged periods under the water. When the seal resurfaces, the circulatory system reverts to the predive state, and after air breathing starts, the lactic acid is extracted from the muscle by the bloodstream and delivered to the liver for metabolism. It has been postulated that such circulatory adjustments may occur in the human newborn to protect vital organs from hypoxia occurring at the time of delivery. This hypothesis is based in part on the observation that blood lactate levels in the newborn increase shortly after the onset of respiration, with higher levels noted in the severely depressed newborn. However, careful calculations reveal that this reflex plays only a small part in fetal/newborn resistance to hypoxia.

During fetal asphyxia, the placenta tends to vasodilate in order to allow more blood in the placenta for gas exchange. This reduces effective circulating blood volume in the neonate. If the fetus is born during this period of redistribution of blood volume between the fetus and placenta, the total effective blood volume in the newborn will be reduced.

A falling PaO_2 and pH and a rising $PaCO_2$ will cause vasoconstriction of the pulmonary blood vessels, increasing right-to-left shunting at both the foramen ovale and ductus arteriosus levels. In utero this protective mechanism results in increased blood return to the placenta for oxygen uptake and is beneficial. However, with removal of the placenta, the neonatal lung becomes the organ of gas exchange and these shunts are harmful. Thus, such "protective mechanisms" may potentiate rather than relieve asphyxia.

Biochemical Changes during Asphyxia

During total asphyxia of the rhesus monkey, dramatic changes in acid-base parameters occur (Figure 22.1). The pH drops from 7.3 to 6.8 after

10 minutes of total asphyxia.[37,38] In addition, blood lactate levels rise rapidly, resulting in metabolic acidosis. If asphyxia is severe, the development of lactate exceeds the buffering capacity of the blood as well as the ability of the neonatal liver to oxidate the lactate. In addition to the severe metabolic acidosis, there is an immediate rapid elevation in the $PaCO_2$ from 45 to 150 torr at 10 minutes.[37,38] The rising $PaCO_2$ (respiratory acidosis) and rising lactate (metabolic acidosis) cause a profound drop in the pH. In the monkey, PaO_2 fell from 25 torr prior to total asphyxia to virtually zero at 10 minutes.[37,38] In addition, in response to either hypoxia or hyperthermia, there is a rise in free fatty acids and glycerol, both products of neutral fat hydrolysis. These acids further potentiate the metabolic acidosis.

Glucose oxidation is the main source of fuel for the newborn and essentially the only source of fuel to the brain. It has been postulated that in utero there may be a decrease in the transfer of glucose across the placenta secondary to hypoxia.[44] This decreased transfer of glucose to the fetus may result in the release of fetal catecholamines, which will mobilize free fatty acids and glycerol.[44] Because glucose is the main source of fuel to the brain, hypoglycemia results in mobilization of hepatic glycogen immediately after birth to provide a continuing source of glucose.[42] If there has been a redistribution of cardiac output secondary to asphyxia, there may be decreased blood flow to the liver and a decrease in the ability of the newborn to mobilize hepatic glycogen. Thus hypoglycemia can play a significant role in the subsequent outcome of asphyxia. On the other hand, the administration of excessive glucose during asphyxia can also be dangerous, causing an increase in the production of lactic acid, which worsens the acidosis, as well as contributing to cerebral edema during acidosis. During the buffering process, potassium is displaced from its binding site, leaves the red cell and enters the plasma. Thus, plasma potassium rises during asphyxia and can have significant cardiogenic effects.[20] However, as renal excretion of potassium continues, total body potassium may be depleted. Upon relief of asphyxia, these buffering processes are reversed. Potassium leaves the plasma and enters the red cell, binding to hemoglobin, resulting in plasma hypokalemia. This plasma hypokalemia combined with total body hypokalemia can also have profound effects on the heart and the gastrointestinal system.

Hypocalcemia develops during asphyxia and may lead to myocardial failure.[20] The mechanism of this change is unknown.

Several studies suggest that the brain tissue can utilize glycerol, ketone bodies, and lactate as metabolic substrates.[45–50] However, efficient utilization of these substrates requires high oxygen concentrations. Thus, it is unlikely that these pathways are actually utilized under conditions of hypoxia and glycogen depletion.[42]

It may be that the human fetus at term is relatively less mature and tolerates greater amounts of asphyxia than the rhesus monkey without developing brain damage, and that the time to the last gasp is longer than in the rhesus monkey.[37] The human infant may also have a marked prolongation of primary apnea and/or time to the last gasp.[42] Thus, in any individual newborn, the actual time course of asphyxic damage and the possibility of subsequent neurologic dysfunction cannot be easily estimated.

When an apneic newborn is encountered in the delivery room, it is extremely difficult to determine whether primary or secondary apnea is present. The latter must be assumed if the infant does not immediately respond to external stimuli and resuscitative efforts. Retrospectively, on the basis of the infant's response, it may be possible to estimate the severity of the asphyxial episode.

RISKS OF CESAREAN BIRTH FOR THE INFANT

Although a cursory review of the available evidence suggests that the safest, most atraumatic method of delivery for an infant is invariably cesarean, abdominal delivery is, in fact, not without potential risks to the infant.[1,2] Such risks must always be considered in the risk/benefit formula of decision making.

Uteroplacental hypoperfusion is one of the more common complications of abdominal delivery. It may result from placing the mother in the supine position, with resultant compression of the major maternal blood vessels.[1,2,51] Uteroplacental blood flow is also dependent on adequate maternal cardiac output and perfusion pressure. Anesthetic techniques that interfere with maternal cardiovascular integrity can produce fetal depression.[52] This can be provoked by (1) decreasing maternal cardiac output secondary to decreased venous return, (2) decreasing maternal cardiac output secondary to maternal myocardial depression (usually produced by an overdose of a potent inhalation anesthetic or local anesthetic drug), or (3) decreased maternal systemic blood pressure caused by sympathectomy of high spinal or epidural anesthesia.[1,52]

Anesthetic agents have additional risks for the neonate. Inhalation agents can cross the placenta rapidly because they are usually nonionized, highly lipid-soluble substances of low molecular weight.[52] The concentration of these agents in the fetus is directly dependent on the concentration and duration of the anesthetic in the mother. If excessive concentrations of anesthetic are given to the mother for inordinately long periods of time, the incidence of fetal depression is markedly increased.[53,54] For example, with general anesthesia, if the induction to delivery time is greater than 20 minutes,[55] neonatal neurological depression, evidenced by flaccidity, cardiorespiratory depression, and decreased muscle tone, should be anticipated. This can result in insufficient respiratory effort in the newborn, with resultant hypoventilation and possible hypoxemia.[20,33,56]

Cesarean delivery has also long been recognized to be associated with an increase in neonatal respiratory morbidity at all gestational ages.[57,58] However, despite the effort to define the frequency of this complication and its specific pathophysiology, there still remains a great deal of dispute concerning this phenomenon. This syndrome, often referred to as "transient tachypnea of the newborn (TTN)" or "neonatal wet lung syndrome," may be due to a number of different problems. Additional respiratory morbidity may be due to iatrogenic prematurity, in which inaccurate gestational date estimation results *unexpectedly* in a premature infant. Work done by Boon and associates[59] in 1981 demonstrated a reduced air volume in the lungs of neonates delivered by cesarean compared with those delivered vaginally. These pulmonary findings, in combination with the frequently seen chest x-ray pattern of increased fluid in the lungs of many newborns following cesarean delivery, suggest that the TTN may be an incomplete adaptation of the fetal lung to extrauterine life. Some have suggested that the physiologic and mechanical events of labor and delivery are necessary for complete pulmonary adaptation. Another observation suggesting the importance of labor in lung maturation is the higher incidence of respiratory morbidity following section without a trial of labor than in section with a trial of labor.[60] These observations imply that labor may be a physiologic stimulus to prepare the fetus for extrauterine pulmonary life.

When reviewing complications of cesarean delivery, accidental lacerations to the fetus during the surgical procedure must be included.[1,61] The frequency of these accidents appears to be related to the experience of the surgeon. The most common situation leading to laceration occurs with a well-thinned-out lower uterine segment in a patient who has ruptured membranes. In these cases, the uterus at the incision site may be only 2 or 3 mm thick. The incidence of neonatal laceration is unknown, but this should be an uncommon occurrence. The major importance of inadvertent scalpel lacerations is usually only cosmetic.

Cesarean delivery also accounts for the added risk to infants of future pregnancies. These dangers include a higher than usual incidence of placenta previa,[62] fetal death due to antepartum rupture of vertical uterine incisions,[1] and neonatal respiratory disease associated with subsequent elective cesarean delivery.[58]

AN APPROACH TO DELIVERY ROOM MANAGEMENT OF THE NEWBORN

The extent of the resuscitative measures needed by the newborn after cesarean can be determined only after the infant's condition is evaluated by an individual with considerable clinical experience. There is no substitute for adequate training and periodic review of the techniques used by the resuscitators. In addition, anticipation is the key to successful resuscitation. The physician responsible for the resuscitation should arrive

TABLE 22.2 Apgar Scoring Chart

Sign	Score 0	1	2
Heart rate	Absent	Below 100 bpm	Over 100 bpm
Respiratory effort	Absent	Weak, irregular (hypoventilation)	Good cry
Muscle tone	Limp or flaccid	Some flexion or extremities	Well flexed, active motion
Reflex irritability (place catheter in nose or slap sole of foot)	No response	Grimace	Cry, cough, or sneeze
Color	Cyanotic, pallid	Acrocyanotic	Pink

Source: Adapted from data of Apgar V: A proposal for a new method of evaluation of the newborn infant. *Anesth Analg* 32:260, 1953.

early enough to set out the necessary equipment and see that it is functioning properly. This procedure is facilitated when the appropriate supplies have been identified and organized in a prearranged manner on a resuscitation cart or attached to a wall board.[63] Another major advantage of arriving before the delivery is that information obtained from the obstetrician concerning the pregnancy and labor makes it possible to anticipate some problems that may be present at birth. Transmitting this information to personnel in the nursery will enable special preparations to be made for anticipated problems. The pediatrician who arrives after the delivery is obviously at a disadvantage with respect to organizing equipment and obtaining the relevant history. In addition, it may be difficult to assess accurately the time and the sequence of events that have occurred following the delivery of the infant. The current approach to resuscitation of the newborn infant closely follows the guidelines recommended by the American Heart Association.[64]

Apgar Scoring

The severity of depression of the newborn infant must be evaluated to determine the course of immediate management. The most practical guideline, as well as the one almost universally utilized, is based on the Apgar scoring chart[65] (Table 22.2). Five variables (heart rate, respiratory effort, muscle tone, reflex irritability, and color) are evaluated. Each of these variables is given a score of 0 to 2, with 0 indicating no response and 2 being the best score. The total score is calculated and recorded at 1 minute and 5 minutes following delivery. Because this score is the basis for the resuscitative effort, a review of the mechanism of Apgar scores seems appropriate.

Heart Rate

Normal newborns have a heart rate varying between 100 and 170 bpm. The term infant usually has a heart rate closer to 120 bpm. The preterm infant generally has a higher heart rate—approximately 140–160 bpm at 28–30 weeks. The best method for obtaining an accurate heart rate is by listening with a stethoscope. Another method is by palpation of either the umbilical cord or an appropriate artery (usually femoral, brachial, or carotid). Severe asphyxia and decreased cardiac output are often associated with bradycardia. However, as previously mentioned, the diving seal reflex can produce bradycardia without hypoxia. It must be noted that maternal drugs, hyperthermia, or moderate asphyxia may result in tachycardia rather than bradycardia.

Respiratory Efforts

Respirations are usually initiated in the first 30 seconds of life and are normally regular in rhythm by 90 seconds of age. Maternal drugs, severe asphyxia, hypovolemia, or central nervous system damage may be associated with apnea. It should be noted that the longer the patient hypoventilates, the more difficult it will be to correct the acidosis.

Muscle Tone

Muscle tone is evaluated by observation of the neonate. Decreased muscle tone may be due to maternal drugs, asphyxia, central nervous system damage, severe prematurity (<1,000 g), or, in rare instances, diseases such as congenital myasthenia gravis. The premature infant's muscle tone is less developed than the term infant's and must be taken into account when giving an Apgar score.

Reflex Irritability

This response is elicited by stimulating the infant in either of two ways. First, the child may have the soles of the feet slapped or stimulated. Second, a catheter may be inserted into the nose in an attempt to elicit a cry. A grimace scores only 1, and no response scores 0.

Color

Color is the least important yet most obvious variable. Many normal neonates continue to have cyanotic hands and feet (acrocyanosis) well after initial Apgar scores are obtained. If central cyanosis persists beyond the first few minutes, low cardiac output or pulmonary disease must be considered. This is especially true if the infant remains cyanotic while being ventilated with oxygen.

The Apgar score is principally used to determine the need for resuscitation, as well as the response of the newborn to the resuscitation. Such evaluation should continue from birth until the newborn has gone through its transition and no longer requires resuscitative efforts. If the Apgar score is less than 7 at 5 minutes, it is recommended that additional scores be obtained every 5 minutes for up to 20 minutes unless two successive scores are 8 or greater.

Based on this scoring system, three groups of newborns have been identified. An Apgar score of 7–10 indicates that the newborn is normal. An Apgar score between 4 and 6 indicates moderate depression. An Apgar score between 0 to 3 is associated with severe depression. The course of management of each of the three groups is described below.

Apgar Score of 7–10

Any newborn requiring resuscitation should be placed in a servo-controlled neutral thermal environment. It is the author's opinion that at the present time an overhead radiant heat source is most effective and should be used in every delivery room for neonatal resuscitation. Hypothermia of the newborn should be avoided. It has been demonstrated that a naked, wet, term neonate placed on an open table in the delivery room with an ambient temperature of 25°C will lose 4°C in skin temperature in 5 minutes and 2°C in core temperature in 20 minutes.[32] A dried infant under a radiant heat source loses almost no heat over the same time. Therefore, the skin should be dried with a warm towel and the infant should be placed immediately under the radiant warmer.

If the neonate is allowed to become cold stressed, it will attempt to compensate. The major response will be via chemical thermogenesis.[33,66] Brown fat stored in the dorsum of the neck, between the scapulae, and in the perinephric area will be biochemically degraded to free fatty acids and glycerol by brown fat lipase. This oxidation will produce large quantities of heat but will also result in metabolic acidosis.

The infant with an Apgar score of 7–10 will rarely need any resuscitative effort unless the Apgar score suddenly falls after birth.

The infant's oropharynx and nostrils should be suctioned with a soft rubber bulb syringe immediately after delivery of the head. This is best accomplished by the obstetrician before the rest of the child is delivered. The pharynx should be aspirated first, then the nose. It is best to avoid nasopharyngeal stimulation with a catheter, because reflex bradycardia, apnea, and/or laryngospasm may occur.[67] If the stomach needs to be suctioned, as can be the case in some infants born by section, one should wait until the infant is stable and pink before passing the DeLee catheter.

Some neonates require external stimuli to initiate breathing. This is especially true if the infant has primary apnea. Such stimulation may include gentle intermittent spanking of the feet or buttocks or stimulation of the lumbar spinal region.

Supplemental oxygen applied by cannula may be required for brief periods as the child goes through the transition from intrauterine to extrauterine circulation.

This infant may be sent to the admit nursery or kept in the delivery room as appropriate.

Apgar Score of 4–6

The newborn with an Apgar score of 4–6 probably has mild to moderate depression. The initial resuscitative response is the same as that of the neonate with an Apgar score of 7–10. This includes drying, placement under a radiant warmer for temperature support, external stimulation, and attention to establishing a clear airway. Many of these infants will respond almost immediately.

If apnea is present, it is usually primary apnea. Give 5–10 breaths with a positive-pressure mask and 100% supplemental oxygen, and hand ventilate using just enough positive pressure to obtain a moderate chest rise. This will usually result in rapid improvement.

If the child does not respond to the above regimen or becomes worse over several minutes, with an Apgar score dropping to 0–3, management should proceed as for severe depression (Apgar score of 0–3).

Apgar Score of 0–3

The infant with an Apgar score of 0–3 is considered severely depressed and probably asphyxiated until proven otherwise. He or she is usually apneic, with a heart rate of less than 100 bpm, obtunded, and cyanotic. This is a medical emergency. Again, the child is quickly dried and placed under a radiant warmer. The airway is cleared. If the heart rate is over 100 bpm or if the resuscitator feels that the infant may have primary apnea, a 30- to 45-second attempt to resuscitate, using an adequately sealed face mask and positive-pressure oxygen by bag, can be utilized. Adequate ventilation with oxygen usually requires a rate of approximately 40–60 breaths per minute. Approximately 20–25 cm H_2O pressure is needed to inflate the lungs of a normal newborn, but pressure twice that high may be needed initially.[68–70] The inspiratory phase should be slightly less than half the time of the ventilation cycle. Adequate ventilation is best determined by chest wall movement and auscultation of breath sounds with the stethoscope. Preparation for immediate intubation should be made while the bag and mask ventilation is being tried. Bag and mask ventilation pressures may not be sufficient in newborns delivered by cesarean section to expand the alveoli. Frothy fluid extruding from the trachea may partially fill the posterior pharynx. If there is a rise in the Apgar score, the bag and mask ventilation can be continued. If there is no response (as indicated by an increase in heart rate and color, increased gasping, and some spontaneous movement), endotracheal intubation should be performed.

Endotracheal intubation should be performed under direct laryngoscopic visualization. The head of the newborn should be placed in a straight position without hyperextending the neck. The Miller laryngoscope No. 0 or 1 straight blade is held in the left hand and inserted near the midline along the right index finger, which has been inserted into the mouth. The laryngoscope blade is advanced along the tongue until the epiglottis is visualized. The blade should be advanced into the area between the base of the tongue and the base of the epiglottis. As the blade is gently raised, the epiglottis swings anteriorly, revealing the larynx. If secretions or meconium are noted, gentle suctioning should be done before insertion of the endotracheal tube. The endotracheal tube is placed in the mouth, on the right side, and gently advanced through the vocal cords into the trachea. After intubation, the laryngoscope blade is carefully withdrawn while the position of the tube is maintained by the right hand on the infant's face. The ventilation bag is attached. Air entry into the chest is then checked with a stethoscope. A straight endotracheal tube is preferred. For preterm infants, tubes between 2.5 and 3.0 mm may be used. For term infants, 3.0- to 4.0-mm tubes are usually required. Be sure to determine if breath sounds are equal, chest rise is adequate, ventilation rate is 40–60 bpm, and the endotracheal tube is in the trachea. For infants whose hearts do not respond within 30 seconds to effective ventilation (by reaching a heart rate of over 80 bpm), external cardiac compression should be started. This is best performed by placing the hands around the neonate's chest with both thumbs over the sternum at the junction of the upper two-thirds and lower one-third.[71] Do not place the thumbs over the xiphoid process. The fingers are used to support the back. The sternum is compressed at a rate of 100–120 times/min. It is very important to compress the chest adequately. This often requires compression of one-half the anteroposterior diameter of the chest. One should frequently evaluate the effectiveness of cardiac massage by checking any available peripheral pulse. Attach an electrocardiographic monitor to the infant as soon as possible.

If the heart rate does not improve or deteriorates, and adequate ventilation and oxygenation are being provided, one must assume that significant metabolic acidosis is present. This will decrease myocardial contractility and increase right-to-left shunting of blood around the lungs. Administration of 2–3 mEq/kg of 0.5 mEq/mL sodium bicarbonate over 2–3 minutes may partially correct the acidosis. Sodium bicarbonate should be given only when there is adequate ventilation, because it is metabolized to carbon dioxide, which may exacerbate the ongoing acidosis.[20,72] Epinephrine, 0.1 mg/kg, in a ratio of 1:10,000, can be administered by an umbilical vessel catheter or by the endotracheal route.[73] Epinephrine improves myocardial contractility, muscle tone, and peripheral perfusion. It stimulates spontaneous myocardial contractions (in asystole) and the response to electrical countershock. It is less effective in the presence of severe metabolic acidosis and may need to be repeated at 5-minute intervals because of the short duration of action. Intracardiac epinephrine (0.1 mg/kg) should be utilized only as a last resort. If the heart rate does not go above 100 bpm with the aforementioned regimen, one must assume severe asphyxia and proceed with advanced cardiopulmonary resuscitation. Place an umbilical arterial catheter[74] and obtain an arterial blood gas determination. If acidosis is still present, give 2–3 Eq sodium bicarbonate (0.5 mEq/cc) per kilogram over 2–3 minutes and repeat as needed.

Hypovolemia associated with problems such as nuchal cord, placenta previa, and abruptio placenta may increase the likelihood of persistent fetal circulation and delay in the physiologic adaptations after birth. Therefore, assess the blood volume status with blood pressure, physical examination (capillary refill normally <3 seconds), and central venous pressure (umbilical venous catheter placed above the diaphragm) if needed. Central venous pressures can be very helpful in differentiating hypovolemic from cardiogenic shock.[75] If hypovolemia is present, volume expanders such as albumin or blood may be indicated. We give 10–15 cc/kg via slow intravenous push over 5 minutes. Do not give volume expansion for a "low blood pressure" if the infant is pink and/or well perfused.

If respiratory depression due to maternal narcotic analgesics is possible, the narcotic antagonist naloxone (0.01 mg/kg) can be administered either intramuscularly or intravenously. Usually the infant's tone and respiratory effort will improve dramatically. If naloxone is effective, assess the infant closely; repeat doses may be needed, because the narcotic has a longer half-life than the naloxone.

Hypoglycemia is a common complication of perinatal distress. Because glucose is the main source of fuel for the newborn and essentially the only source of fuel for the brain, it is mandatory to evaluate continually for hypoglycemia and provide infusions of glucose as needed. If glucose is indicated, give 2 mL/kg of D10 water IV push over 2 minutes.

If the infant has not responded to the above regimen, it will be necessary to repeat arterial blood gas administration. Usually the bicarbonate and epinephrine will need to be repeated. If the heart rate is still less than 100 bpm, give calcium gluconate 10% (100 mg/mL) in a dose of 100–200 mg/kg through the umbilical artery catheter over 1–2 minutes. Calcium gluconate increases myocardial contractility and may enhance ventricular excitability (in asystole) or conduction velocities (in electromechanical dissociation). However, it can produce severe sinus bradycardia or asystole if given too fast or through an umbilical venous catheter. It may be repeated every 10 minutes to a maximum dose of 2 g.

If the heart rate is still less than 100 bpm, give atropine (0.1 mg/1.0 mL), 0.10–0.40 mL/kg intravenously, over 1 minute. Atropine reduces vagal tone, with a resultant increase in sinoatrial node discharge and atrioventricular node conduction (increases the heart rate). It is useful for bradycardia resulting in hypotension, ventricular ectopy, myocardial ischemia, and temporary treatment of second- and third-degree heart block. It may precipitate tachyarrhythmias or, in insufficient doses, cause a paradoxical bradycardia. The minimum dose is 0.10 mg; the maximum dose is 0.40 mg.

If the heart rate is still less than 100 bpm, reassess ventilation again. The value of continued resuscitation needs to be considered at this point.

SPECIAL PROBLEMS

Very-Low-Birth-Weight Neonates

The preterm infant is faced with the task of adapting to an extrauterine environment with organ systems that are physiologically immature. Many of the normal neonatal transitions that occur within a short period of time after birth in the term infant take longer to occur in the very-low-birth-weight infant, and, in fact, some may not occur for weeks. Therefore, it becomes imperative that the resuscitator apply prompt, effective resuscitation but avoid any unnecessary manipulation or overcompensation for the neonate's effort during this transitional period.

A special dilemma presented by the very-low-birth-weight infant is Apgar scoring. Because the Apgar score was based on term neonates, when rigidly applied, it is very easy to overestimate the degree of neonatal depression by underestimating reflex activity and muscle tone, which are less well developed in the very-low-birth-weight infant. Because Apgar scoring is used as the guideline in resuscitation, this underestimation may lead to overaggressive resuscitation. Therefore one must avoid unnecessary resuscitation, which may delay the very-low-birth-weight infant's normal progress through transition.

Respiratory distress syndrome (RDS) continues to be one of the most common clinical problems encountered by preterm infants. Many of these neonates will have tachypnea, nasal flaring, expiratory grunting, chest retractions, decreased chest compliance, and decreased breath sounds. If an initial resuscitation is required, it is imperative to respond promptly and effectively to avoid unnecessary hypoxia. This may be accomplished with an appropriately sized premature mask and bag or may require endotracheal intubation and hand ventilation. An optimal system will provide continuous positive airway pressure (CPAP). Spontaneous respiratory effort, when effective and sustained, is probably more effective in increasing tidal volume and establishing functional residual capacity than mechanical ventilation of the lung. It is extremely important not to overventilate these infants. By overventilation, one can increase right-to-left shunting through the foramen ovale and the ductus arteriosus. In addition, one can cause barotrauma to the pulmonary parenchyma, which may subsequently lead to pulmonary interstitial emphysema and air leaks. Therefore, it becomes imperative to have an experienced, skilled resuscitator evaluate the clinical stability of the infant, anticipate his or her future respiratory needs, and weigh the findings against the risk of the resuscitative efforts.

The second problem to anticipate in the resuscitation of very-low-birth-weight infants born by cesarean is vascular hypovolemia and/or hypotension. These neonates can have rapid changes in intravascular volume, and they are predisposed to intracranial hemorrhage and right-to-left pulmonary shunting, both associated with hypovolemia. In addition, there may be loss of autoregulation of cerebral blood flow in the presence of moderate or severe asphyxia. It is, therefore, important to identify the hypovolemia or hypotension quickly in these babies and to give an appropriate amount of fluids if indicated. It is just as important not to give too much volume, again because of the possibility of producing systemic hypertension and increasing the risk of cerebral capillary blood vessel rupture.[21,76] We commonly employ central venous lines to assist in determining blood volume status.

The very low birth weight appropriate for the gestational age infant is often accompanied by impaired glucose homeostasis immediately after birth.[77] These infants may have functionally immature gluconeogenic and glycogenolytic enzyme systems in addition to poor glycogen stores. They have relatively large brains (13% of the body mass in the newborn versus 2% in the adult). This may lead to greater glucose consumption when oral and parenteral intake is low. Therefore, following initial resuscitation, an intravenous glucose infusion of approximately 5–7 mg/kg/min should be started to minimize the risk of hypoglycemia.

Intrauterine infection plays a significant role in extreme prematurity. Chorioamnionitis is a frequent finding. One must always be alert to its association and diligent in evaluating for its presence. Evaluation of the complete blood count, appropriately obtained cultures, and urine directogen are often helpful in determining the etiology and treatment.

Hypovolemia

It has been clearly demonstrated that certain conditions in the fetus may lead to major abnormalities in the distribution of total blood volume. These include:

1. Nuchal cord or compression of the umbilical cord, which may selectively obstruct venous flow more than arterial flow, thereby trapping a large volume of blood in the placenta
2. Placenta previa
3. Abruptio placenta
4. Vellamentous insertion of the cord
5. Fetal asphyxia at delivery

Initially, it may be difficult to determine whether or not the blood volume is adequate in an asphyxiated child. In severe asphyxia, the infant may shunt blood away from the skin in order to protect the brain, heart, and adrenals. For this reason, there may be decreased capillary refill in the periphery, which may be interpreted as a reduction in blood volume. Asphyxia may also cause an abnormal heart rate, metabolic acidosis, and poor peripheral perfusion, manifested by pallor, slow capillary refill, and a large difference between core and skin temperatures. Blood pressures may or may not be helpful in distinguishing asphyxia from hypovolemia. In these difficult cases, central venous pressures assessed through umbilical venous catheters placed above the diaphragm are very useful. If a child is born pale and/or chalky white and has a history of one of the above-mentioned conditions, it may be necessary to expand the circulating blood volume quickly. We have found that expansion with either a 5% albumin solution or plasmanate often rapidly returns the infant to a normal condition.

Meconium Aspiration

The care of the newborn delivered by cesarean with meconium-stained amniotic fluid should be the same as that of a vaginally delivered child. The obstetrician should carefully suction the hypopharynx before delivery of the shoulders. This may be the single most important factor in preventing severe meconium aspiration syndrome.[78,79] If this material is not removed during delivery, the infant may aspirate it into the lower airways during spontaneous breathing, or it may be pushed in by mask and bag ventilation. The previously mentioned obstetrical care should clear the upper airway in more than 90% of infants.[78] However, approximately 10% of infants will still have meconium left in the trachea just below the vocal cords. Direct visualization of the larynx should be done by a skilled observer as quickly as possible. This should be done even if respirations have been initiated, because tenacious meconium may still be removable. If meconium is present on the vocal cords, intubation should be accomplished, and the airways should be suctioned with the largest suction catheter that can be passed.[78] An alternative is direct DeLee suctioning of the trachea by laryngoscopy. This process may need to be repeated several times. It has been suggested that no positive pressure be applied to the airway until the first cleansing is completed. However, remember that the major underlying cause of the passage of meconium is hypoxemia. One does not want to potentiate any possible nervous system damage. Therefore, one must try to return the oxygen and heart rate to the normal range as quickly as possible. This type of suctioning and treatment significantly reduces the incidence of morbidity and mortality due to meconium aspiration syndrome.[78,79]

Drug-Depressed Infants

Infants born by cesarean may be exposed to narcotic analgesics during labor or delivery.[56] Meperidine is one of the most commonly used drugs. If it is given intramuscularly within 1.5–2.0 hours before delivery, the drug concentration will be at its maximum in the serum of the mother and fetus at the time of birth. Often these children will have a *falling* Apgar score, because the first Apgar score is the most reflective of intrauterine conditions and the second Apgar of extrauterine life. There are two approaches to the care of these neonates. One is to establish an airway for providing adequate ventilation until the effect of the drug has passed. The other is to treat the narcotic depression with naloxone, 0.01 mg/kg, administered either intramuscularly or intravenously.[23,33] Typically, the infant's tone or respiratory effort, if depressed due to narcotic analgesics, should improve dramatically. Because narcotic-induced respiratory depression has been reported to last for up to 5 hours,[80] the infant should be carefully observed; later, doses of naloxone should be administered if renarcotization occurs. However, the narcotic antagonist may create acute drug withdrawal in infants whose mothers have used narcotics frequently during pregnancy.[33]

Intrauterine Growth Retardation

The growth-retarded fetus is at higher risk for perinatal morbidity and mortality, the risk rising with the severity of the growth retardation.[81–84] Because much of the literature has not separated symmetrically from asymmetrically growth-retarded infants, it is difficult to interpret all of the current findings.

As many as 65% of growth-retarded infants are likely to present in the delivery room with one or more severe and often life-threatening problems.[85] Neonatal asphyxia is more common in small-for-dates infants.[85–87] Most do not enjoy adequate placental nutritional support. Therefore, their glycogen reserves are low. In addition, they may be marginally oxygenated. These infants can develop hypoxemia and acidosis rapidly. At birth, resuscitation must be prompt and vigorous.

The respiratory difficulties that these children face at birth are usually due to aspiration of amniotic fluid from asphyxia.[88] If meconium has been passed, meconium aspiration may occur. The severity of the condition is related to the quantity of material aspirated.

The premature growth-retarded infant may experience accelerated pulmonary maturity secondary to the intrauterine stress. However, very premature growth retarded infants can have RDS, just as their preterm AGA counterparts do.

Some growth-retarded infants have persistent fetal circulation as a component of their lung disease.[88] This may occur due to chronic intrauterine hypoxia. One must be sure that congenital cardiac anomalies are not coexistent.

Thermal regulation is also a problem in these children, who have poor fat insulation, decreased carbohydrate stores,[89] a lack of response to glycogenic amino acids,[90] and decreased brown fat stores.[91] Hypoglycemia is seen most frequently in those infants whose growth retardation is most severe. It is most likely to occur during the first 12 hours of age but may appear during the first 48 hours of life. Hypoglycemia in these infants occurs because of the low glycogen stores combined with the high metabolic rate. Gluconeogenesis also appears to be impaired in these children compared to the AGA infant.

Polycythemia occurs in 15%–39% of growth-retarded infants near term[92,93] and is associated with elevated erythropoietin levels.[94] Intrauterine hypoxemia is postulated to be an important factor in polycythemia.[95]

Falling Apgar Score

In an infant with a 5-minute Apgar score that is less than the 1-minute Apgar score despite appropriate resuscitative management, prompt and accurate diagnosis is essential. Two possible diagnoses have been mentioned: drug depression and hypovolemia. Infants with central nervous system disease may also have a falling Apgar score.[96] Another possibility is tension pneumothorax.[42,97] One should listen for breath sounds and check the point of maximum intensity of the heart to determine if there has been a shift. A child with diaphragmatic hernia may also have decreased breath sounds and a shift of the heart, as well as a scaphoid abdomen. Infants with the above-mentioned conditions can rapidly deteriorate. Under rare conditions, bilateral choanal atresia or severe micrognathia may also lead to a falling Apgar score. Additional diagnostic modalities include transillumination of the chest and chest x-ray.

An infrequently seen but important disease is Potter's syndrome. Infants with this disease often have the characteristic facies and extremities of uterine constraint. There is usually a history of oligohydramnios, either on the basis of renal agenesis, or, if early enough in gestation, on the basis of premature rupture of membranes and amniotic fluid leaks. These infants have very poor lung compliance, often with severe pulmonary hypoplasia. Despite high ventilatory pressures through a bag and mask or an endotracheal tube, there is very little chest expansion and markedly decreased breath sounds bilaterally. Chest x-rays show very small, hypoplastic lung fields. These neonates are very difficult to manage, and the vast majority of them die. Recent research on the use of high-frequency jet ventilation or high-frequency oscillation in pulmonary hypoplasia has shown some promising early results.[98]

HYPOXIC-ISCHEMIC ENCEPHALOPATHY FOLLOWING ASPHYXIA AND RESUSCITATION

The goal of resuscitation is to provide appropriate intervention and adequate resuscitation in order to prevent or minimize brain damage. "Neonatal hypoxic-ischemic encephalopathy (HIE)" is the term used most frequently to designate the clinical and neuropathologic changes that are thought to occur in the fetal/neonatal brain following either intrapartum or neonatal asphyxia. In both the premature and the full-term infant, this injury is the single most important perinatal cause of neurological morbidity. The subsequent neurological defects of concern are principally a variety of motor deficits often grouped together as cerebral palsy with or without mental retardation and/or seizures. Much of the theory of HIE is based either on animal data or on clinical postmortem correlations in human studies.

The primary disturbance in neural tissue is a deficit in oxygen supply. The effects of hypoxemia on brain carbohydrate and energy metabolism are the same as previously mentioned in discussing the pathophysiology of asphyxia (Table 22.1). Glycolysis is accelerated, and an attempt to increase glucose concentrations in the brain is made by increased glycogenolysis and by increased net uptake of glucose from the blood.[99] Despite this acceleration, brain energy demands cannot be met, and ATP levels begin to fall after 2 minutes and decrease by 30% after 6 minutes.

Regional changes in glucose metabolism have been examined in newborn dogs subjected to acute hypoxemia and studied by autoradiographic 2-[^{14}C]deoxyglucose technique.[100] The authors found increased glucose utilization in most gray matter structures and every white matter structure. There was an accumulation of lactate in the brain in both gray and white matter. However, only in white matter did a decline in energy state occur. Thus, it appears that anaerobic glycolysis, with its accelerated glucose utilization, was capable of preserving the energy state in gray but not in white matter. Because glucose levels declined drastically in white compared to gray matter, it appeared that glucose influx could not meet the increased demands for glucose in white matter. The rate of glucose metabolism appears limited by glucose influx from blood, because local cerebral blood flow is increased insignificantly to white matter but dramatically to gray matter.[101] This imbalance between glucose needs and glucose delivery may contribute to the propensity of neonatal cerebral white matter to hypoxic injury.

The progression of lactate formation leads to tissue acidosis. Several deleterious effects then ensue. First is the impairment of cerebral vascular autoregulation. The brain loses its ability to fine-tune autoregulation of blood flow to areas with increased needs. The potential for ischemic brain injury increases when cerebral perfusion pressure falls. Second, phosphofructokinase activity is inhibited by low pH; thus, the brain's remaining source of ATP, ie, glycolysis, will be eliminated. Third, advanced tissue acidosis will lead directly to cellular injury and ultimately to necrosis.

It has become increasingly apparent that alterations in cerebral blood flow are of prime importance in understanding the neuropathological and neurological consequences of all varieties of perinatal asphyxia. Tight coupling of cerebral function, metabolism, and blood flow has been well established and can be demonstrated by a variety of correlative physiological, biochemical, and clinical studies.[102–104] Both total and regional cerebral blood flow change significantly with maturation. In general, cerebral blood flow increases with postnatal age.[105,106] This correlates with increases in cerebral metabolic rates and energy demands.

There are impressive regional differences in cerebral blood flow. Blood flows are highest in cerebral gray matter, nuclear structures of the brain stem, and diencephalon, and lowest in cerebral white matter. Blood flow to the cerebral cortex is approximately five- to tenfold that of subcortical white matter.[35] Studies of blood flow to various regions of the primate cerebrum indicate that the parasagittal areas, especially the posterior ones, have significantly lower flow than other cerebral regions.[107]

Cerebral blood flow has clearly been shown to be regulated by the following major factors:

1. *Autoregulation* appears to be operative over a broad range of arterial blood pressure in both preterm and term lambs and neonatal dogs.[108–112] The autoregulatory range in the preterm newborn is slightly narrower. With decreasing gestational age, resting mean arterial blood pressure values approach the lower limit of the autoregulatory curve. Therefore, the margin for safety in the preterm fetus is small at the lower end of the autoregulatory curve, suggesting increased vulnerability to ischemic brain injury with modest hypotension.
2. *Alterations in arterial* $PaCO_2$ have a marked effect on cerebral blood flow in perinatal animals.[101,113] In general, there is a limited vasodilatory response in cerebral white matter, which may have implications for the vulnerability of this region to HIE.[101]
3. *Alterations in arterial* PaO_2 can also cause distinct changes in cerebral blood flow.[101] Decreases in oxygen tension result in increases in flow, and vice versa. Cerebral white matter has limited vasodilatory capacity.
4. *Acidemia* can cause a sharp increase in cerebral blood flow, whether produced by hypoxemia or lactate infusion.

Neuropathology of HIE

The neuropathological features of neonatal HIE vary considerably with the gestational age of the infant, nature of the insult, type of intervention, and so forth. The major neurological groups are shown in Table 22.3.

TABLE 22.3 Major Neuropathological Groups of Neonatal HIE

Variety of Lesion	Site of Injury	Regional Sites	Pathogenesis	Gestational Age
Selective neuronal necrosis	Neurons	Cerebral cortex, diencephalon, basal ganglion, midbrain, pons, medulla, cerebellum	Oxygen deprivation	Both term and preterm
Status marmoratus	Neurons, gliosis, hypermyelination	Basal ganglia, thalamus	Probable oxygen deprivation	Term > preterm
Parasagittal cerebral injury	Neurons	Cerebral cortex and subcortical white matter in parasagittal superomedial aspects of cerebral convexities (watershed areas)	Principally ischemic	Term > preterm
Periventricular leukomalacia	White matter	Occipital radiation at the trigone of the lateral ventricles and in white matter around foramen of Monroe (watershed areas)	Principally ischemic	Preterm > term
Focal (and multifocal) ischemic brain necrosis	Gray and white matter	Lesions within the distribution of major cerebral vessels	Principally ischemic	Sixth month of gestation to the first postnatal weeks or months

Selective neuronal necrosis is the most common variety of injury observed in neonatal HIE. There is necrosis of neurons in a characteristic though often widespread distribution.[114] Oxygen deprivation plays a dominant role in the pathogenesis of this condition.[115] Neuronal necrosis often coexists with other varieties of injury.

Status marmoratus is a striking lesion involving the basal ganglia and thalamus, and is the least common variety of HIE.[116] The lesion is not seen in its complete form until the latter part of the first year of life, although it may represent a perinatal injury. The major features are neuronal loss, gliosis, and hypermyelination. The pathogenesis is unclear but appears to be often related to oxygen deprivation.[35,116]

Parasagittal cerebral injury refers to a lesion of the cerebral cortex and subcortical white matter with a characteristic distribution, ie, the parasagittal, supermedial aspects of the cerebral convexities.[35] The injury is usually bilateral. The pathogenesis is principally an ischemic lesion in the full-term infant. The areas of necrosis are in the border zones between the end fields of the major cerebral arteries (ie, anterior, middle, and posterior cerebral arteries). Hypotension and loss of autoregulation of cerebral blood flow may play an important role in the pathogenesis of this lesion.[35]

Periventricular leukomalacia refers to necrosis of white matter in a characteristic distribution, usually adjacent to the external angles of the lateral ventricles.[35] It is principally an ischemic lesion affecting premature infants more often than term infants. Hemorrhage is not an uncommon secondary complication.

Focal and multifocal ischemic brain necrosis usually occurs within the distribution of major cerebral vessels, generally from approximately the sixth month of gestation to the first postnatal weeks or months.[35] Areas of immature brain have a propensity to undergo dissolution because of their high water content, relative paucity of myelinated fibers, and deficient astroglial response.[117] Often a cavity will form (ie, porencephaly, hydranencephaly, and multicystic encephalomalacia).[118]

Ability of the Newborn to Survive Asphyxia

It has been clearly shown in several mammalian species, including the human, that newborns survive asphyxia much better than adults.[119] The biochemical and physiological bases for this relative resistance are not entirely understood, but animal experiments indicate several factors to be of major importance. Younger animals survive longer because their cerebral rate of utilization of high-energy compounds is significantly less than the rate of adult animals.[120–123] The lower cerebral rate of energy utilization in young animals is considered to be secondary to the anatomical and electrophysiological immaturity of the perinatal brain.[121] Another major factor is the availability of substrate for anaerobic degradation. The substrate may be stored locally, as with myocardial glycogen, or mobilized from the liver glycogen to supply the brain.

The cardiovascular system also plays a role in the fetus/infant's ability to survive hypoxic-ischemic insult. There is a relative resistance of the myocardium of young animals to asphyxia due to their greater stores of myocardial glycogen and the greater aerobic capacity of their mitochondria in election transport and oxidative phosphorylation.[37] If the circulation remains intact, there can be a redistribution of lactate and hydrogen ion to tissues still being profused, and thus a means of buffering brain cells during asphyxia.[124] However, this tolerance to hypoxic-ischemic insult not only leads to increased survival capabilities but also increases susceptibility to permanent brain damage following asphyxia.[119]

Prognosis in HIE

The outcome of infants sustaining HIE is influenced by several factors. These include the duration and severity of the insult, gestational age, presence of seizures, associated infections, and metabolic and traumatic derangements.[125] Because there are many factors that determine the final outcome, it is often difficult to form a prognosis for any single infant. However, certain associations have been identified.

Gestational age is an important predictor of mortality in asphyxiated newborns. Nelson and Ellenberg[126] found a higher mortality rate in premature asphyxiated infants. Conversely, they found an increased risk of cerebral palsy in term survivors. Sarnat and Sarnat[127] studied a group of infants who were either stillborn or born without spontaneous, sustained breathing for a minimum of 20 minutes. Seventy percent of the term infants survived, compared to 32% of the preterm infants. The long-term morbidity was 36% for the term infants and 11% for the preterm infants.

The Apgar score has been implicated in long-term neurological follow-up studies. A low Apgar score indicates an abnormal condition but does not necessarily imply any specific etiology. Infants who have an Apgar score of 0–3 at 5 minutes do have higher mortality and greater central nervous system morbidity than infants who have an Apgar score of 4–6 or 7–10. The longer the score is low, the greater its significance. An infant with a 0–3 Apgar score at 20 minutes has a 53% mortality. In full-term surviving neonates with an Apgar score of 0–3 at 5 minutes, the incidence of cerebral palsy is approximately 1%. If the score is 0–3 at 15 minutes, 9% of the survivors will have cerebral palsy; if it is 0–3 at 20 minutes, 57% of the infants will have cerebral palsy.

Although the Apgar score does not allow one to time precisely the duration of the asphyxic episode, one can obtain a time estimate by evaluating both the Apgar score and the return of Apgar score function. For example, an infant tends to lose function in the following order: color, respiration, tone, reflexes, and heart rate. Following effective resuscitation, these functions tend to reappear in the following order: heart rate, reflexes, color, respiration, and tone. The time required for tone and respirations to return may indicate the severity or duration of the asphyxic insult to the central nervous system. Mulligan et al[128] found a 19% immediate mortality and an 18% morbidity among 39 surviving term infants who did not have spontaneous respirations for more than 1 minute after birth. De Souza et al[129] followed 15 term infants who survived apnea for 10 minutes or more after birth. Two had severe neurological deficits and five

TABLE 22.4 Clinical Staging of Posthypoxic Encephalopathy

Factor	Stage I	Stage II	Stage III
Level of consciousness	Alert	Lethargy	Coma
Muscle tone	Normal	Hypotonia	Flaccidity
Tendon reflexes	Increased	Increased	Depressed or absent
Myoclonus	Present	Present	Absent
Complex reflexes			
Sucking	Active	Weak	Absent
Moro response	Exaggerated	Incomplete	Absent
Grasping	Normal to exaggerated	Exaggerated	Absent
Oculocephalic (doll's eyes)	Normal	Overreactive	Reduced or absent
Autonomic function			
Pupils	Dilated	Constricted	Variable or fixed
Respiration	Regular	Variations in rate and depth, periodic	Ataxia, apnea
Heart rate	Normal or tachycardia	Bradycardia	Bradycardia
Seizures	None	Common	Uncommon
Electroencephalogram	Normal	Low voltage, periodic and/or paroxysmal	Periodic or isoelectric

Source: Adapted from Sarnat HB, Sarnat MS: Neonatal encephalopathy following fetal distress. *Arch Neurol* 33:696, 1975.

had delayed language development. A delay of greater than 30 minutes to spontaneous respiration in term infants has indicated universally damaged infants.[130]

Neurological examination in the immediate neonatal period provides a useful index for predicting later neurological outcome. Brown et al[131] found a significant risk of cerebral palsy to be associated with certain behavioral and neurological signs (feeding difficulties, cyanotic spells, apnea, apathy) following the occurrence of perinatal asphyxia. Sarnat and Sarnat,[127] using their Clinical Staging of Posthypoxic Encephalopathy (Table 22.4), demonstrated that stage I newborn infants who are alert or even hyperalert, have normal muscle tone with increased reflexes, and so on, invariably recover without neurological deficits. Infants in stage II, who are lethargic and have diffuse muscular hypotonia, later develop normally if clinical and electroencephalographic abnormalities are fully reversed by 5 days of age. Stage III encephalopathy in comatose, flaccid, and unresponsive neonates is associated with high mortality (50%) and universal morbidity among the survivors.

Neonatal seizures are frequently associated with intrapartum asphyxia. Seizures per se are not associated exclusively with late neurological sequelae. However, seizure occurrence within the first 12 hours, the appearance of status or serial seizures, or a persistently abnormal electroencephalogram with burst suppression or low-voltage background are signs of significant neonatal neurological dysfunction. Infants with hypoxic ischemic encephalopathy who have seizures are described as having a poorer long-term neurological prognosis.[125,128,132]

The presence of hypodensities on computed tomography scan in full-term infants is correlated with a less than optimal motor and mental outcome.[133,134] Technetium brain scanning can provide valuable information concerning the site and extent of injury. O'Brien et al[135] studied 85 full-term infants with HIE related to intrauterine asphyxia. They found increased uptake of the radionucleide on delayed images in areas of tissue injury.

Long-term sequelae of the major neurological injuries include the following:[35]

Selective neuronal necroses: mental retardation, spastic quadriparesis, seizure disorder, ataxia, bulbar and pseudobulbar palsy, hyperactivity, and impaired attention

Status marmoratus: choreoathetosis, mental retardation, spastic quadriparesis

Parasagittal cerebral injury: spastic quadriparesis, intellectual deficits

Periventricular leukomalacia: spastic diplegia, intellectual deficits

Focal (and multifocal) necrosis: spastic hemiparesis and quadriparesis, mental retardation, seizure disorder

COUNSELING PARENTS

It is extremely important to remember that resuscitation is a major disruption of contact between mother, father, and baby at the time of birth. If possible, it is extremely helpful for the person in charge of resuscitation to explain to the parents before the cesarean what therapeutic maneuvers may be needed and why. In some cases, when a cesarean is being planned and time permits, it is useful to give the father and mother a tour of the newborn intensive care unit ahead of time.

At delivery, it is important to take at least a few seconds to show the mother her baby after resuscitation before taking the child to the newborn intensive care unit. Again, if at all possible, face-to-face interaction between baby and mother can be rewarding. Even in the most complicated cases, this can usually be done. Such efforts also begin the rapport between physician and parents that is vital for later effective communication.

REFERENCES

1. Creasy AK, Resnick R: *Maternal-Fetal Medicine Principles and Practice.* Philadelphia, WB Saunders Co, 1984, pp 472–478.
2. Dunn LJ: Cesarean section and other obstetrical operations, in Danforth DN (ed):

Obstetrics and Gynecology, ed 4. Philadelphia, Harper & Row, Publishers, Inc, 1982, pp 769–778.

3. Behrman RE, James LS, Klaus M, et al: Treatment of the asphyxiated newborn infant. *J Pediatr* 74:981, 1969.
4. Kikkawa Y: Morphology and morphologic development of the lung, in Scarpelli EM (ed): *Pulmonary Physiology of the Fetus, Newborn and Child.* Philadelphia, Lea & Febiger, 1975, pp 37–60.
5. Bleasdale JE, Wallis P, MacDonald PC, et al: Characterization of the forward and reverse reactions catalyzed by CDP-diacylglycerol: Inositol transferase in rabbit lung tissue. *Biochem Biophys Acta* 575:135, 1979.
6. Kulovich MV, Gluck L: The lung profile II. Complicated pregnancy. *Am J Obstet Gynecol* 135:64, 1979.
7. Hallman M, Gluck L: Phosphatidylglycerol in lung surfactant function. III. Possible modifier of surfactant function. *J Lipid Res* 17:257, 1976.
8. Suzuki Y: Effect of protein, cholesterol and phosphatidylglycerol on the surface activity of the lipid–protein complex reconstituted from pig pulmonary surfactant. *J Lipid Res* 23:62, 1982.
9. Nelson NM: The onset of respiration, in Avery GB (ed): *Pathophysiology and Management of the Newborn.* Philadelphia, JB Lippincott Co, 1987, pp 176–197.
10. Tooley WH: Evaluation of fetal maturity development of the fetal lung, in Creasy RK, Resnik R (eds): *Maternal-Fetal Medicine: Principles and Practice.* Philadelphia, WB Saunders Co, 1984, pp 369–376.
11. Patrick J, Natale R, Richardson B: Patterns of human fetal breathing activity at 34 to 35 weeks gestational age. *Am J Obstet Gynecol* 132:507, 1978.
12. Boddy K, Mantell CD: Observations of fetal breathing movements transmitted through maternal abdominal wall. *Lancet* 2:1219, 1972.
13. Dawes GS, Fox HE, Laduc BM, et al: Respiratory movements and rapid-eye-movement sleep in the foetal lamb. *J Physiol* 220:119, 1972.
14. Duenhoelter JH, Pritchard JA: Fetal respiration: Quantitative measurements of amniotic fluid inspired near term by human and rhesus fetuses. *Am J Obstet Gynecol* 125:306, 1976.
15. Nelson NM: Respiration after birth, in Smith CA, Nelson NM (eds): *Physiology of the Newborn Infant,* ed 4. Springfield, Ill, Charles C Thomas, 1976.
16. Saunders RA, Milner AD: Pulmonary pressure/volume relationships during the last phase of delivery and the first postnatal breaths in human subjects. *J Pediatr* 93:667, 1978.
17. Burns BP: The central control of respiratory movements. *Br Med Bull* 19:7, 1963.
18. Egan EA, Olver RE, Strang LB: Changes in non-electrolyte permeability of alveoli and the absorption of lung liquid at the start of breathing in the lamb. *J Physiol* 244:161, 1975.
19. Adams FH: Fetal and neonatal circulations, in Adams FH, Emmanowlides GC (eds): *Heart Disease in Infants, Children, and Adolescents,* ed 3. Baltimore, Williams & Wilkins Co, pp 11–17.
20. Phibbs RH: Delivery room management of the newborn, in Avery GB (ed): *Pathophysiology and Management of the Newborn.* Philadelphia, JB Lippincott Co, 1987, pp 212–231.
21. Kaiser IH: Fertilization and physiology and development of fetus and placenta, in Danforth DN (ed): *Obstetrics and Gynecology,* ed 4. Philadelphia, Harper & Row, Publishers, Inc, 1982, pp 294–325.
22. Clyman RI, Heymann MA: Pharmacology of the ductus arteriosus. *Pediatr Clin North Am* 28:77, 1981.
23. Clyman RI, Campbell D, Heymann MA, et al: Persistent responsiveness of the neonatal ductus arteriosus in immature lambs. *Circulation* 71:141, 1985.

24. Levin DL, Mills LJ, Weinberg AG: Hemodynamic, pulmonary, vascular, and myocardial abnormalities secondary to pharmacologic constriction of the fetal ductus arteriosus. *Circulation* 60:360, 1979.
25. Printz MP, Skidgel RA, Friedman WF: Studies of pulmonary prostaglandin biosynthetic and catabolic enzymes as factors in ductus arteriosus patency and closure. *Pediatr Res* 18:19, 1984.
26. Stenmark KR, James SL, Voelkel NF, et al: Leukotriene C_4 and D_4 in neonates with hypoxemia and pulmonary hypertension. *N Engl J Med* 309:77, 1983.
27. Perloff JK: Patent ductus arteriosus, in Perloff JK (ed): *The Clinical Recognition of Congenital Heart Disease,* ed 3. Philadelphia, WB Saunders Co, 1987, pp 467–489.
28. Adamsons K Jr, Towell ME: Thermal hoemeostasis in the fetus and newborn. *Anesthesiology* 26:531, 1965.
29. Wood C, Beard RW: Temperature of human fetus. *J Obstet Gynaecol Br Commonwealth* 71:768, 1964.
30. Mann TP: Observations on temperatures of mothers and babies in the perinatal period. *J Obstet Gynaecol Br Commonwealth* 75:316, 1968.
31. Silverman W, Fertig J, Berger A: The influence of the thermal environment upon the survival of newly born premature infants. *Pediatrics* 22:876, 1958.
32. Dahm L, James L: Newborn temperature and calculated heat loss in the delivery room. *Pediatrics* 49:504, 1972.
33. Sills J, Coen RW: The neonate, in Creasy RK, Resnik R (eds): *Maternal-Fetal Medicine: Principles and Practice.* Philadelphia, WB Saunders Co, 1984, pp 1093–1111.
34. Adamsons K Jr, Grandy G, James L: The influence of thermal factors upon oxygen consumption of the newborn human infant. *J Pediatr* 66:495, 1965.
35. Volpe JJ: Hypoxic-ischemic encephalopathy, in Volpe JJ (ed): *Neurology of the Newborn.* Philadelphia, WB Saunders Co, 1987, pp 160–279.
36. Siesjo BK, Plum F: Pathophysiology of anoxic brain damage, in Gaull GE (ed): *Biology of Brain Dysfunction.* New York, Plenum Press, 1973, p 319.
37. Dawes CS: *Foetal and Neonatal Physiology (Year Book).* Chicago, Year Book Publishers, 1968.
38. Adamsons K Jr, Behrman R, Dawes G, et al: Resuscitation by positive pressure ventilation and tris-hydroxy-methyl-aminomethane of rhesus monkeys asphyxiated at birth. *J Pediatr* 65:807, 1964.
39. James L: Onset of breathing and resuscitation. *J Pediatr* 65:807, 1964.
40. Behrman R, Lees M, Peterson E, et al: Distribution of the circulation in the normal and asphyxiated fetal primate. *Am J Obstet Gynecol* 108:956, 1970.
41. Fisher DJ: Increased regional myocardial blood flows and oxygen deliveries during hypoxemia in lambs. *Pediatr Res* 18:602, 1984.
42. Fisher DE, Paton JB: Resuscitation of the newborn infant, in Klaus MH, Fanaroff AA (eds): *Care of the High Risk Neonate.* Philadelphia, WB Saunders Co, 1986, pp 31–50.
43. Scholander P: The master switch of life. *Sci Am* 209:92, 1963.
44. Stave U, Wolf H: Metabolic effects of hypoxia neonatorum, in Stave U (ed): *Physiology of the Perinatal Period.* New York, Appleton-Century-Crofts, 1970.
45. Daniel P, Love E, Moorehouse L, et al: Factors influencing utilization of ketone-bodies by brain in normal rats and rats with ketoacidosis. *Lancet* 2:637, 1971.
46. Gardiner R: The effects of hypoglycemia on cerebral blood flow and metabolism in the newborn calf. *J Physiol* 298:37, 1980.
47. Hawkins R, Williamson D, Krebs H: Ketone-body utilization by adult and suckling rat brain in vivo. *Biochem J* 122:13, 1971.
48. Hellmann J, Vannucci R, Nardis E: Blood-brain barrier permeability to lactic acid in the newborn dog: Lactate as a cerebral metabolic fuel. *Pediatr Res* 16:40, 1982.
49. Shambaugh G, Mrozak S, Freinkel N: Fetal fuels I. Utilization of ketones by isolated

tissues at various stages of maturation and maternal nutrition during late gestation. *Metabolism* 26:623, 1977.

50. Sloviter H, Shimkin P, Suhara K: Glycerol as a substrate for brain metabolism. *Nature* 210:1334, 1966.
51. Goodlin RC: Aortocaval compression during cesarean section. *Obstet Gynecol* 37:702, 1971.
52. Naulty JS: Obstetric anesthesia, in Avery GB (ed): *Neonatology, Pathophysiology and Management of the Newborn,* ed 3. Philadelphia, JB Lippincott Co, 1987, pp 159–175.
53. Moya F: Volatile inhalation agents and muscle relaxants in obstetrics. *Acta Anesthesiol Scand* 25(suppl):368, 1966.
54. Fox FS, Smith JB, Namba Y, et al: Anesthesia for cesarean section. *Am J Obstet Gynecol* 133:15, 1979.
55. Marx GF, Joshi CW, Orkin LR: Placental transmission of nitrous oxide. *Anesthesiology* 32:429, 1970.
56. Morishima HO: Obstetric analgesia and anesthesia, in Danforth DN (ed): *Obstetrics and Gynecology,* ed 4. Philadelphia, Harper & Row Publishers, Inc, 1982, pp 663–679.
57. Clifford SH: A consideration of the obstetrical management of premature labor. *N Engl J Med* 210:570, 1934.
58. Usher R, McLean F, Maughan GB: Respiratory distress syndrome in infants delivered by cesarean section. *Am J Obstet Gynecol* 88:806, 1964.
59. Boon AW, Milner AD, Hopkin IE: Lung volumes and lung mechanics in babies born vaginally and by elective and emergency lower segmental cesarean section. *J Pediatr* 98:812, 1981.
60. Bowers SK, MacDonald HM, Shapiro ED: Prevention of iatrogenic neonatal respiratory distress syndrome: Elective repeat cesarean section and spontaneous labor. *Am J Obstet Gynecol* 143:186, 1982.
61. Gerber AH: Accidental incision of the fetus during cesarean delivery. *Int J Gynaecol Obstet* 12:46, 1974.
62. Singh PM, Rodrigues C, Gupta AN: Placenta previa and previous cesarean section. *Acta Obstet Gynecol* 60:367, 1981.
63. Clark J, Brown Z, Jung A: Resuscitation equipment board for nurseries and delivery rooms. *JAMA* 236:2427, 1976.
64. Standards and guidelines for cardiopulmonary resuscitation (CPR) and emergency cardiac care (ECC). V. Advanced cardiac life support for neonates. *JAMA* 244:453, 1980.
65. Apgar V: A proposal for a new method of evaluation of the newborn infant. *Anesth Analg* 32:260, 1953.
66. Hey E, Scopes JW: Thermoregulation in the newborn, in Avery GB (ed): *Pathophysiology and Management of the Newborn.* Philadelphia, JB Lippincott Co, 1987, pp 201–211.
67. Cordero L Jr, Hon E: Neonatal bradycardia following nasopharyngeal stimulation. *J Pediatr* 78:441, 1971.
68. Karlberg P, Chery R, Escardo F, et al: Pulmonary ventilation and mechanics of breathing in the first minutes of life, including the onset of respiration. *Acta Paediatr Scand* 51:121, 1962.
69. Milner A, Vyas H: Lung expansion at birth. *J Pediatr* 101:879, 1982.
70. Boon AW, Milner AD, Hopkin IE: Lung expansion, tidal exchange and formation of the functional residual capacity during resuscitation of asphyxiated neonates. *J Pediatr* 95:1031, 1979.
71. Todres I, Rogers M: Methods of external cardiac massage in the newborn infant. *J Pediatr* 86:781, 1975.

72. Murray JF: *The Normal Lung. The Basis for Diagnosis and Treatment of Pulmonary Disease.* Philadelphia, WB Saunders Co, 1976, pp 199–222.
73. Lindemann R: Resuscitation of the newborn with endotracheal administration of epinephrine. *Acta Paediatr Scand* 73:210, 1984.
74. Kitterman JA, Phibbs RH, Tooley WH: Catheterization of umbilical vessels in newborn infants. *Pediatr Clin North Am* 17:895, 1970.
75. Cabal LA, Devaskar U, Siassi B, et al: Cardiogenic shock associated with perinatal asphyxia in preterm infants. *J Pediatr* 96:705, 1980.
76. Goldberg R, Chung D, Goldman S, et al: The association of rapid volume expansion and intraventricular hemorrhage in the preterm infant. *J Pediatr* 96:1060, 1980.
77. Fluge G: Clinical aspects of neonatal hypoglycemia. *Acta Paediatr Scand* 63:82, 1974.
78. Carson BS, Losey RW, Bowes WA Jr, et al: Combined obstetric and pediatric approach to prevent meconium aspiration syndrome. *Am J Obstet Gynecol* 126:712, 1976.
79. Gregory GA, Gooding CA, Phibbs RH, et al: Meconium aspiration in infants: A prospective study. *J Pediatr* 85:807, 1974.
80. Koch G, Wandel H: Effects of pethidine on the postnatal adjustment of respiration and acid-base balance. *Acta Obstet Gynecol Scand* 47:27, 1968.
81. Drillen C: The small-for-dates infant: Etiology and prognosis. *Pediatr Clin North Am* 17:9, 1970.
82. Fitzhardinge P, Steven E: The small-for-dates infant. II. Neurologic and intellectual sequelae. *Pediatrics* 50:50, 1972.
83. Gruenwald P: Infants of low birth weight among 5,000 deliveries. *Pediatrics* 34:157, 1964.
84. Low J, Galbraith R: Pregnancy characteristics of intrauterine growth retardation. *Obstet Gynecol* 44:122, 1974.
85. Ownsted M, Moar V, Scott WA: Perinatal morbidity and mortality in small-for-dates babies: The relative importance of some maternal factors. *Early Hum Dev* 5:367, 1981.
86. Len CC, Moawad AH, Rosenow PJ, et al: Acid-base characteristics of fetuses with intrauterine growth retardation during labor and delivery. *Am J Obstet Gynecol* 137:553, 1980.
87. Low J, Boston R, Pancham S: Fetal asphyxia during the intrapartum period in intrauterine growth retarded infants. *Am J Obstet Gynecol* 113:352, 1972.
88. Klaus MH, Fanaroff AA: *Care of the High-Risk Neonate.* Philadelphia, WB Saunders Co, 1986, pp 80–88.
89. Shelley H: Carbohydrate reserves in the newborn infant. *Br Med J* 1:273, 1964.
90. Williams P, Fisher R Jr, Sperling M, et al: Effects of oral alanine on blood glucose and insulin concentrations in small-for-gestational age infants. *N Engl J Med* 292:612, 1975.
91. Aherne W, Hull D: Brown adipose tissue and heat production in the newborn infant. *J Pathol Bacteriol* 223:91, 1966.
92. Haworth J, Dilling L, Younsoszai M: Relation of blood glucose to hematocrit, birth weight, and other body measurements in normal and growth retarded infants. *Lancet* 2:901, 1967.
93. Humbert JR, Abelson H, Hathway WE, et al: Polycythemia in small for gestational age infants. *J Pediatr* 75:812, 1969.
94. Finne P: Erythropoietin levels in cord blood as an indicator of intrauterine hypoxia. *Acta Paediatr Scand* 55:478, 1966.
95. Gruenwald P: Chronic fetal distress and placental insufficiency. *Biol Neonate* 5:215, 1963.

96. Volpe JJ, Hill A: Neurologic disorders, in Avery GB (ed): *Pathophysiology and Management of the Newborn*. Philadelphia, JB Lippincott Co, 1987, pp 1073–1132.
97. Martin RJ, Klaus MH, Fanaroff AA: Respiratory problems, in Klaus MH, Fanaroff AA (eds): *Care of the High Risk Neonate*. Philadelphia, WB Saunders Co, 1986, pp 171–201.
98. Wetzel RC, Gioia FR: High frequency ventilation. *Pediatr Clin North Am* 34:15, 1987.
99. Holowach-Thurston J, Haubart RE, Jones EM, et al: Decrease in brain glucose in anoxia in spite of elevated plasma glucose levels. *Pediatr Res* 7:691, 1973.
100. Duffy TE, Cavazzutti M, Cruz NF, et al: Local cerebral glucose metabolism in newborn dogs: Effects of hypoxia and halothane anesthesia. *Ann Neurol* 11:233, 1982.
101. Cavazzutti M, Duffy TE: Regulation of local cerebral blood flow in normal and hypoxic newborn dogs. *Ann Neurol* 11:247, 1982.
102. Kuschinsky W, Wahl M: Local chemical and neurogenic regulation of cerebral vascular resistance. *Physiol Res* 58:656, 1978.
103. Busija DW, Heistad DD: Factors involved in the physiological regulation of the cerebral circulation. *Rev Physiol Biochem Pharmacol* 101:162, 1984.
104. Siesjo BK: Cerebral circulation and metabolism. *J Neurosurg* 60:883, 1984.
105. Vannucci RC, Plum F: Pathophysiology of perinatal hypoxic-ischemic brain damage, in Gaull GE (ed): *Biology of Brain Dysfunction*. New York, Plenum Press, 1975, p 1.
106. Rudolph AM, Heymann MA: The circulation of the fetus in utero. *Circ Res* 21:163, 1967.
107. Resvich M, Brann AW Jr, Shapiro HM, et al: Regional cerebral blood flow during prolonged partial asphyxia, in Meyer JS, Resvich M, Lechner H, et al (eds): *Research on the Cerebral Circulation*. Springfield, Ill, Charles C Thomas, 1972, p 216.
108. Camp D, Kotagal UR, Kleinman LI: Preservation of cerebral autoregulation in the unanesthetized hypoxemic newborn dog. *Brain Res* 241:207, 1982.
109. Lou HC, Lassen NA, Friis-Hansen B: Impaired autoregulation of cerebral blood flow in the distressed newborn infant. *J Pediatr* 94:118, 1979.
110. Hernandez MJ, Brennan RW, Bowman GS, et al: Autoregulation of cerebral blood flow in the newborn dog. *Ann Neurol* 6:177, 1979.
111. Papile LA, Rudolph AM, Heymann MA: Autoregulation of cerebral blood flow in the preterm fetal lamb. *Pediatr Res* 19:159, 1985.
112. Tweed WA, Cote J, Pash M, et al: Arterial oxygenation determines autoregulation of cerebral blood flow in the fetal lamb. *Pediatr Res* 17:246, 1983.
113. Purves MJ, James IM: Observations on the control of cerebral blood flow in the sheep fetus and newborn lambs. *Circ Res* 25:651, 1969.
114. Norman MG: Perinatal brain damage. *Perspect Pediatr Pathol* 4:41, 1978.
115. Larroche JCL: *Developmental Pathology of the Neonate*. Amsterdam, Elsevier North-Holland, 1977.
116. Malamud N: Status marmoratus: A form of cerebral palsy following either birth injury or inflammation of the central nervous system. *J Pediatr* 37:610, 1950.
117. Raybaud C: Destructive lesions of the brain. *Neuroradiology* 25:265, 1983.
118. Schmitt HP: Multicystic encephalopathy, a polyetiologic condition in early infancy: Morphologic, pathogenetic and clinical aspects. *Brain Dev* 1:1, 1984.
119. Vannucci RC, Voorhies TM: Resistance of the immature to hypoxia-ischemia, in Sarnat HB (ed): *Topics in Neonatal Neurology*. New York, Grune & Stratton, 1984, pp 48–55.
120. Duffy TE, Kohle SJ, Vannucci RC: Carbohydrate and energy metabolism in perinatal rat brain: Relation to survival in anoxia. *J Neurochem* 24:271, 1975.
121. Holowach-Thurston J, McDougal DB Jr: Effect of ischemia on metabolism of the brain of the newborn mouse. *Am J Physiol* 216:348, 1969.

122. Vannucci RC, Vasta F, Vannucci SJ: Glucose supplementation does not accentuate hypoxic-ischemic brain damage in immature rats: Biochemical mechanisms. *Pediatr Res* 19:396, 1985.
123. Lowry OH, Passonneau JV, Hasselberger FX, et al: Effect of ischemia on known substrates and cofactors of the glycolytic pathway in brain. *J Biol Chem* 239:18, 1964.
124. Adamsons K Jr: Brain damage in the fetus and newborn from hypoxia or asphyxia, in James L, Myers R, Gaull G (eds): *Report of the 57th Ross Conference on Pediatric Research*. Columbus, Ohio: Ross Laboratories, 1967, p 75.
125. Vannucci RC, Voorhies TM: Resistance of the immature to hypoxia-ischemia, in Sarnat HB (ed): *Topics in Neonatal Neurology*. New York, Grune & Stratton, 1984, pp 76–78.
126. Nelson KB, Ellenberg JH: Apgar scores as predictors of chronic neurologic disability. *Pediatrics* 68:36, 1981.
127. Sarnat HB, Sarnat MS: Neonatal encephalopathy following fetal distress. *Arch Neurol* 33:696, 1975.
128. Mulligan JC, Painter MJ, O'Donoghue PW, et al: Neonatal asphyxia. II. Neonatal mortality and long-term sequelae. *J Pediatr* 96:903, 1980.
129. DeSouza SW, McCartney E, Nolan M, et al: Hearing, speech, and language in survivors of severe perinatal asphyxia. *Arch Dis Child* 56:245, 1981.
130. Steiner H, Neligan G: Perinatal cardiac arrest. *Arch Dis Child* 50:692, 1975.
131. Brown JK, Purvis RJ, Forfar JO, et al: Neurological aspects of perinatal asphyxia. *Dev Med Child Neurol* 16:567, 1974.
132. Rose RL, Lombrosco CT: Neonatal seizure states. *Pediatrics* 45:404, 1970.
133. Fitzhardinge PM, Flodmark O, Fitz CR, et al: The prognostic value of computed tomography and autopsy in premature and fullterm neonates that have suffered perinatal asphyxia. *Radiology* 137:93, 1980.
134. Magilner AD, Wertheimer IS: Preliminary results of a computed tomography study of neonatal brain hypoxic-ischemic encephalopathy. *J Comput Assist Tomogr* 4:457, 1980.
135. O'Brien MJ, Ash JM, Gilday DL: Radionuclide brain scanning in perinatal hypoxia/ ischemia. *Dev Med Child Neurol* 21:161, 1979.

Postoperative Complications

Chapter 23

Routine Postcesarean Care and Management of Common Complications

Susan E. Rutherford, MD, and
Jeffrey P. Phelan, MD

Successful and timely recovery after cesarean delivery begins with preoperative and intraoperative anticipation of possible complications. Preparation for surgery and preexisting problems such as chorioamnionitis, the need for prophylactic antibiotics, and the impact of specific types of anesthesia are discussed in other chapters.

Although the development of routine procedures is a safeguard against inadvertent error, all guidelines must ultimately be adapted to individual patients. The purpose of this chapter is to review basic principles of postoperative care and the rationale behind them. This includes discussions of normal postoperative recovery, such as fluid management, analgesia, ambulation, and nutrition, as well as problems specific to individual organ systems.

INITIAL RECOVERY

As the patient begins to recover from anesthesia, she must be observed carefully for changes in cardiovascular or respiratory status. Vital signs are usually monitored at least every 15 minutes in the recovery room. When the patient is awake and alert after general anesthesia, or has experienced significant return of sensory and motor function after regional anesthesia, and has stable vital signs, she may be transferred to the ward. Routine ward policies for monitoring of vital signs and initial care may be utilized in uncomplicated patients. For example, vital signs may be obtained every 30 minutes for the first 2 hours and less frequently thereafter. Observation of vaginal bleeding, uterine consistency, incisional bleeding, and urine output should accompany the recording of vital signs.

FLUID AND ELECTROLYTES

Intraoperative fluid administration and blood loss are key determinants of immediate postoperative therapy, particularly if either has been excessive. In addition to blood loss, hypovolemia may be caused by a transfer of extracellular fluid into interstitial spaces, including the peritoneal cavity and bowel lumen, especially in the presence of peritonitis. Such fluid extravasation occurs to a lesser degree due to irritation of the peritoneal surface during any abdominal surgery (so-called third spacing).

Water constitutes 50%–70% of body weight (the lower proportion in obese patients). Two-thirds of body water (roughly 40% of body weight) is in the intracellular space and one-third (20% of body weight) in the extracellular (interstitial and intravascular) space. An infusion of 5% dextrose in water will be distributed evenly throughout all of the water-containing spaces in order to maintain balanced osmolarity. In contrast, normal saline remains principally as extracellular fluid; 25% remains intravascular. Thus, correction of hypovolemia, using crystalloid solutions, requires at least the equivalent of normal saline. The role of hypertonic saline is not yet clearly defined. Hypovolemia associated with a low intravascular colloid osmotic pressure may be better corrected when the administration of serum albumin is included to prevent loss of additional water into the interstitial space.

Postoperative oliguria (less than 400 mL per 24 hr) or anuria (less than 50 mL per 24 hr) should prompt consideration of hypovolemia. Loss of the ability to concentrate urine may indicate acute renal failure. In the presence of severe hypovolemia, replacement of fluids may be monitored with a central venous pressure line to prevent fluid overload and pulmonary edema. Patients with severe preeclampsia or septic shock may not have normal cardiac function and may require a pulmonary artery catheter for adequate monitoring. Patients with renal failure, septic shock, or a nasogastric tube are especially likely to develop electrolyte imbalances.

ANALGESIA

Adequate pain relief is that which provides satisfactory patient comfort without obtundation or respiratory depression. Both respiratory and gastrointestinal complications can be worsened by excessive quantities of pain medication. An adequate frequency of administration obviates the need for high individual doses and prevents wide swings in blood levels with alternating pain and obtundation. Selected medications and doses for the immediate postoperative period and when the patient can tolerate oral medications are listed in Table 23.1.

In therapeutic doses, none of the commonly used narcotic analgesics have a significant effect on lactation or the nursing infant. For example, meperidine is found in only trace amounts in breast milk.[2,3] On the other

TABLE 23.1 Selected Medications and Suggested Doses for Postcesarean Analgesia

Parenteral medications		
Morphine sulfate	8–15 mg SC	Every 3–4 hours
Meperidine	75–100 mg IM	Every 3–4 hours
Hydromorphone	2 mg IM	Every 4–6 hours
Meperidine with promethazine	50–75 mg meperidine 25 mg promethazine IM	Every 3–4 hours
Oral medications		
Hydromorphone	2 mg PO	Every 4–6 hours
Oxycodone	5 mg PO	Every 6 hours
Acetaminophen (300 mg) with codeine phosphate (30 mg)	1–2 tablets PO	Every 4 hours
Acetaminophen (300 mg) with codeine phosphate (60 mg)	1 tablet PO	Every 4 hours

Source: Goodman LS, Gilman A (eds): *The Pharmacological Basis of Therapeutics*, ed 5. New York, Macmillan Publishing Co, 1975.

hand, salicylates may affect infant platelet function, although only 0.5% of the daily dose appears in breast milk.[2]

Recent reports describe the efficacy of intrathecal or epidural opiate administration for postoperative analgesia. With such analgesia, sensory fibers appear to be selectively blocked. In one study, analgesia from morphine administered epidurally lasted 29.3 ± 3.5 hours after cesarean delivery.[4]

AMBULATION

Historically, surgical patients were kept in bed for what now seems prolonged periods of time. One concern was abdominal wound dehiscence. Inferior suture materials contributed to this complication. The first article advocating early ambulation (in vaginal celiotomy patients on the first to third day) was published in 1899. In 1915, the recommendations of a major surgical textbook were: "Fowler's position . . . may hasten involution and favors drainage; it should, however, not be begun until the patient has recovered from the shock of the operation. The baby may begin to nurse at the breast in 12 hours, if the mother's condition is satisfactory. Throughout the first week the bowels are moved by enemata, the first clyster being given on the third or fourth day. The diet is limited to fluids until the bowels have been moved. If the convalescence is uncomplicated, the patient is allowed to sit up in bed on the ninth, and to get up on the twelfth or fourteenth day."[5]

After the turn of the century, a few practitioners began to allow and finally to encourage early ambulation. The initially observed benefits were the same as those seen today: lower mortality, more rapid return of spontaneous bowel activity without catharsis, fewer pulmonary complications, less liability to "circulatory disturbances"—specifically, venous thrombosis and pulmonary embolism—less overall weakening, and a faster, more complete recovery.[6] Observations of laboratory animals about 1940 showed that those allowed to move around at will experienced more rapid wound healing. However, not until the 1940s did early ambulation become popular in the United States.

The upright position encourages reinflation of the dependent alveoli and prevents pulmonary complications. The ability to ambulate to the bathroom makes removal of the urinary catheter more convenient. Removal of the catheter promotes return of bladder tone and decreases the risk of nosocomial infection. Bowel motility is also enhanced by ambulation, with a concurrent decrease in the incidence of nausea, vomiting, and abdominal distention.

A reasonable approach in the uncomplicated patient might be to allow sitting and, if possible, ambulation with assistance by 8–12 hours postoperatively, regardless of the type of anesthesia. Success with this approach is clearly related to the motivation of the individual patient and attention from the nursing staff. The majority of patients ambulate by 24 hours postoperatively. In those patients who are too ill to ambulate, more individualized care, such as helping to turn in bed and changes of bed position, may be necessary.

LABORATORY STUDIES

Routines vary widely with individual physician preference. Consideration of a patient's physiologic status should guide the selection and timing of routine laboratory tests. Determination of hematocrit or hemoglobin is useful in discovering unsuspected blood loss, particularly following equilibration of fluids. This is usually performed on the first postoperative day and repeated as necessary. Measurements of blood volume 1 hour postpartum have shown decreases of 600 mL in women delivered vaginally and 1,000 mL in those undergoing cesarean delivery.[7] The hematocrit changes by approximately 2% during the first few postpartum days; an increase is seen after normal vaginal delivery and a decrease after cesarean delivery.[7]

Routine urine cultures with discontinuance of an indwelling catheter will help determine bateriuria but may not reflect clinically significant infection. Abnormal clinical findings such as tachycardia, hypotension, oliguria, bleeding, and fever may require additional laboratory tests to assist in diagnosis or monitoring of therapy.

Fetal-maternal hemorrhage is greater in patients undergoing cesarean than vaginal birth.[8,9] Unsensitized Rh-negative patients require an estimate of the degree of fetal-maternal bleeding, such as with the use of the Kleihauer-Betke acid elution technique for detection of fetal erythrocytes. Maternal hematocrit and estimation of blood volume are necessary to calculate the amount of bleeding that has occurred. A dose of 300 μg of

Rh immune globulin will, in all but exceptional cases, protect the mother against sensitization. The administration of sufficient Rh immune globulin is manifested by a positive antibody titer during the postoperative period.

POSTOPERATIVE NUTRITION

The optimal way to provide nutrition for a postoperative patient is via the gastrointestinal tract if it is functional. Well-nourished, healthy patients can tolerate the trauma of a surgical procedure and the perioperative deprivation of nutrients with little difficulty provided they receive adequate intravenous water, electrolytes, and calories in the form of dextrose. The dextrose prevents some of the protein catabolism that would otherwise be needed for gluconeogenesis. The enteral route is the safest for providing additional protein, amino acids, and fats, except for extreme cases wherein the gastrointestinal tract is nonfunctional. Once oral feeding has begun, it is important that the patient have adequate intake of calories, protein, minerals, trace elements, and vitamins.

Nonobstetric adult patients who do not eat have been found to lose, on the average, 0.5–1 lb of weight per day of hospitalization. Under these circumstances, energy is provided by catabolism of body fat stores as well as metabolically active protein (largely skeletal muscle).[10]

Those patients with complications, such as a large blood loss, retroperitoneal hematoma, or sepsis, have a more extreme catabolic response and usually a more significant partial starvation during convalescence. Their available fat and protein reserves will be exhausted in 2–4 weeks.[10] Those patients who do not receive oral feeding within 1 week should be considered for enteral or parenteral nutrition.

A solid food diet should, as much as possible, approximate the patient's normal eating habits. Regular hospital diets are based on the Recommended Daily Dietary Allowances of the Food and Nutrition Board, National Academy of Sciences–National Research Council. However, because most individuals' protein intake is usually higher, most hospital diets contain more protein. In prescribing diets, care should be taken to avoid foods that the patient cannot tolerate, such as milk products in those with lactose intolerance.

There are a variety of liquid food diets, including mixed processed foods and elemental defined-formula diets. Such diets vary in osmolality, digestibility, caloric density, lactose content, viscosity, fat content, taste, and expense.[11] These are useful in the patient who cannot be fed with solid food but has adequate gastrointestinal function for a liquid diet. Complications can include discomfort or erosions from a feeding tube, aspiration, vomiting, cramping, diarrhea, rapid expansion of the extracellular fluid compartment, and metabolic disturbances.

The most common nutritional deficit in the surgical population is protein-calorie undernutrition.[12] All but the eight essential amino acids can be synthesized endogenously. Patients undergoing simple surgery experience metabolic and endocrine events similar to those of simple starvation. For approximately 2 days during reduced oral intake, liver glycogenolysis can maintain serum glucose. After that, protein catabolism yields amino acids, which are converted to glucose. If feeding is resumed within a week, liver and muscle glycogen, as well as catabolized muscle protein, will be replaced.[12] Severely injured patients or those undergoing extensive surgery also experience a hypermetabolic state. Patients in an adequate nutritional state prior to surgery experience faster wound healing, fewer infections, and more rapid recovery.[13] Minor surgery results in a 4%–8% postoperative weight loss and major surgery in a 15%–25% weight loss.[14]

RESPIRATORY COMPLICATIONS

Respiratory complications are the most common source of morbidity after major surgical procedures. The majority are the result of changes in the ventilatory pattern associated with abdominal surgery, secondary to postoperative pain. Monotonous, shallow breathing without spontaneous deep breaths leads to decreases in functional residual capacity, residual volume, vital capacity, expiratory flow rates, and compliance, as well as increased work of breathing.[15] The initial effect is atelectasis.

Atelectasis consists of collapsed, airless alveoli and comprises 90% of postoperative pulmonary complications.[16,17] It is most often platelike and subsegmental, although entire segments, lobes, or a lung may collapse. Of patients having abdominal surgery, 83% develop pulmonary function changes[18] and 4%–20% have clinical evidence of atelectasis.[16,17] Patients with lower abdominal or transverse incisions are less likely to develop atelectasis.

The absence of periodic deep breaths, sighing, or yawning is the primary cause of atelectasis. Alveolar-capillary units are normally recruited by deep inspiration every 5–10 minutes.[19] Closure of small (less than 1 mm) airways occurs in portions of the lung that are ventilated little more than their residual volume. Failure to reexpand the lung causes an increasing number of alveoli to become poorly ventilated. After collapse of the small airways, the distally trapped gas is absorbed and the alveoli collapse, resulting in atelectasis. If collapse occurs in an entire segment, there is no longer movement of air in the bronchus and secretions easily accumulate, forming a mucous plug. The tendency toward airway closure increases with age due to lower lung elastic recoil. Postoperative pain, analgesics, smoking, supine body position, obesity, and increased abdominal girth such as that associated with ileus favor premature airway closure and atelectasis.

During expiration, airway closure occurs first in the dependent or compressed portions of the lung. Due to compression of the lung above them, these parts of the lung are most subject to atelectasis. With abdominal distention and splinting, the diaphragm is slightly elevated and the lobes adjacent to the diaphragm are also at greater risk of atelectasis.

Lack of intermittent lung expansion also leads to changes in regional pulmonary blood flow and decreased surfactant levels at the alveolar surfaces. This contributes to the reduction in functional residual capacity and to early airway closure.

Depression of mucociliary activity, the duration of anesthesia, and the patient's general physical and mental condition also affect the incidence of atelectasis. During anesthesia a mixture of gases low in nitrogen and high in oxygen favors more rapid absorption of trapped air and alveolar collapse. Aspiration may also lead to atelectasis and/or pneumonia. Patients with chronic lung disease such as smokers or those with asthma, bronchitis, or emphysema are at greater risk for the development of atelectasis. Such patients have a greater volume of secretions, and their mucociliary clearance mechanisms are also impaired.

Atelectasis usually appears within the first 24 hours and rarely later than 48 hours after an operation. Inspiratory insufficiency initially leads to the development of small, diffuse atelectatic lesions that easily reverse with intermittent deep breathing or inspiration greater than the tidal volume range. From this point, most postoperative atelectasis spontaneously improves. Atelectasis that persists or progresses becomes clinically significant when it is associated with some discomfort or distress on the part of the patient.[20]

Signs of established atelectasis include basilar rales, diminished breath sounds, dullness to percussion of the chest, bronchial breathing, tachypnea, and fever or tachycardia. Atelectasis is rarely severe enough to compromise oxygenation. If this occurs, an arterial blood gas determination will show decreased PO_2 and normal or decreased PCO_2 consistent with pulmonary shunting. The respiratory rate may be normal or increased. The dyspnea and cyanosis of atelectasis may resemble pneumonia. Its persistence provides a site for the development of pneumonia.

Radiologic findings vary according to the type of atelectasis. Plate-like atelectasis appears as linear horizontal densities, usually in the basilar lung segments. Segmental (sublobar) uninflated areas most often also occur basally. Collapse of a lobe or an entire lung may appear as a relative opacity (Figure 23.1) or yield lateralizing signs, including shift of the mediastinum on chest x-ray. Miliary atelectasis may appear as a diffuse reticular pattern or generally increased opacification due to overall volume loss (Figure 23.2). The different findings and degrees of atelectasis should be considered as part of a continuous clinical spectrum.

When pneumonia follows atelectasis, it most often occurs between the 4th and 10th postoperative days. It does not inevitably follow atelec-

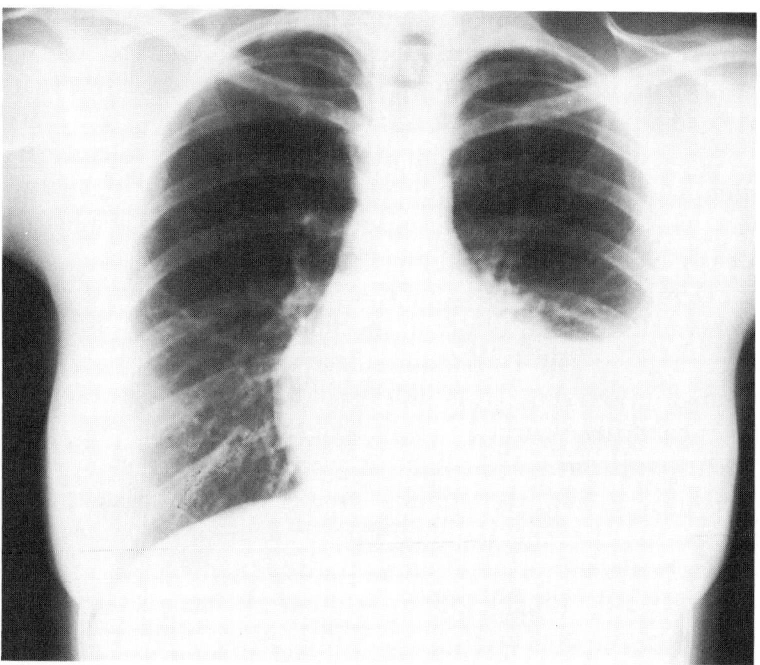

FIGURE 23.1 Segmental atelectasis.

tasis, as most patients recover without developing pneumonia. Systemic factors such as peritonitis or postsurgical impairment of the immune system render the patient more susceptible to pneumonia.[21]

The criteria that will aid in the diagnosis of pneumonia are illustrated in Table 23.2. In addition, a sputum culture will aid in identifying the organisms found on Gram stain and establish sensitivities ensuring administration of the proper antibiotics.

Prevention of respiratory complications begins with an adequate history and a physical examination. Abstinence from smoking and refraining from elective surgery in the presence of a respiratory infection will avoid many postoperative respiratory complications. Postoperative atelectasis is four times more common in patients who smoke more than 20 cigarettes per day than in nonsmokers.[22] It is also helpful to teach deep-breathing exercises or incentive spirometry preoperatively. The only mechanical advantage to incentive spirometry is measurement of respiratory parameters. Encouragement by hospital staff and patient compliance appear to be the most important factors in effective use of spirometers.

Blow gloves and blow bottles, by virtue of the inspiratory effort required for proper use, can also be effective. The usefulness of chest percussion and postural drainage varies, depending on the clinical circumstances.

Postoperatively, hyperinflation by sighing or deep breathing is essen-

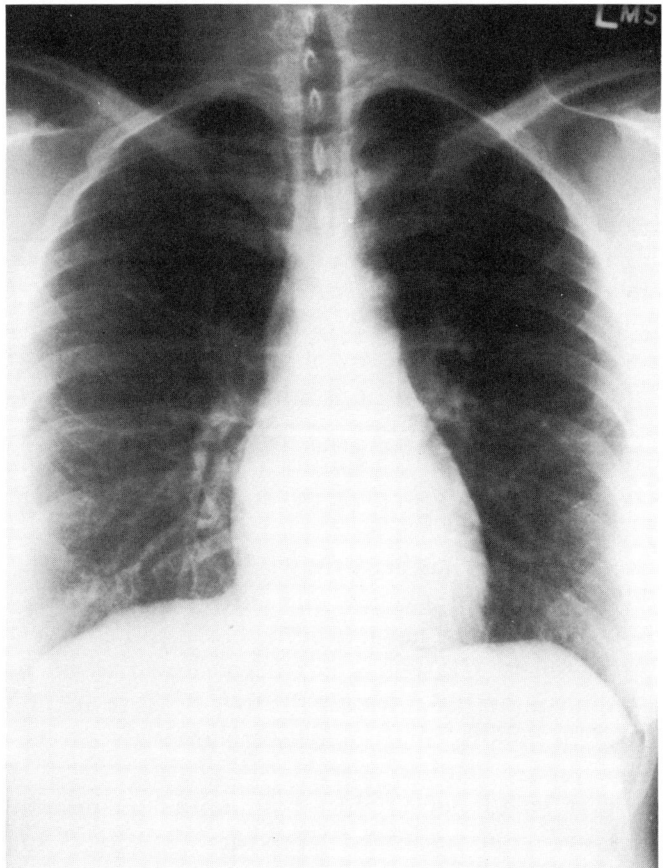

FIGURE 23.2 Miliary (diffuse alveolar) atelectasis.

tial. The resultant alveolar distention also stimulates coughing. Coughing, in turn, helps to loosen secretions and dislodge mucous plugs. Endotracheal suction and the instillation of 1–2 mL of saline may be necessary to stimulate these actions in a few patients. Rarely, bronchoscopy may be needed.

Frequent change of body position prevents the same areas of lung from remaining dependent. Medication to relieve incisional pain without de-

TABLE 23.2 Clinical Findings Consistent with Postcesarean Pneumonia

Temperature elevation greater than 101°F
Leukocytosis
A new radiologic infiltrate on chest x-ray
Production of purulent sputum
Granulocytes and a single bacterial species on Gram-stained sputum smear

pressing respiration and early ambulation will also help prevent atelectasis. Most postcesarean patients should be able to sit up and many will be able to ambulate by 8–12 hours postoperatively.

Incentive spirometry requires the patient to sustain maximal inspiration to achieve alveolar inflation.[15] It is the most widely used modality for the prevention and treatment of postoperative atelectasis in the United States and is employed in approximately 95% of hospitals.[23] In 57% of the hospitals surveyed, more than three-fourths of the patients with postoperative atelectasis were treated with incentive spirometry. Chest physiotherapy, intermittent positive pressure breathing (IPPB), continuous positive airway pressure (CPAP) by mask, and blow bottles were found to be used much less frequently for prophylaxis. For treatment, chest physiotherapy and IPPB were used in approximately 80% of hospitals, but in fewer patients than incentive spirometry.[23] Measuring inspired lung volumes may be useful in prescribing the appropriate treatment and monitoring progress.

Incentive spirometry has been shown in controlled studies to be superior to IPPB in both effectiveness and cost.[24,25] IPPB with bronchodilators or bronchodetergents has not been shown to be of benefit in prophylaxis or treatment. CPAP has not been shown to be necessary in patients who can voluntarily take deep breaths. Because humidity less than 70% in inhaled air inhibits ciliary activity and dries secretions, mucolytics and humidified air are helpful.

Oxygen may be administered to maintain adequate arterial oxygen tension. Excessive concentrations of oxygen, however, may lead to increased gas absorption in obstructed airways and lower surfactant levels, which will worsen atelectasis and increase ventilation-perfusion mismatching.[22]

The same conservative measures employed in the treatment of atelectasis should also be used in the patient with pneumonia. In addition, antibiotics appropriate to the offending organism should be given and adjusted according to the culture and sensitivity results.

Intubation and ventilation are rarely necessary in the postcesarean population. Extremely small vital capacities (less than 10–12 mL per kilogram of body weight), tachypnea (more than 35–40 bpm), respiratory acidosis, and hypoxia unresponsive to conservative measures will usually require ventilatory assistance. Intubation and CPAP or positive end-expiratory pressure (PEEP) without mechanical ventilation may be adequate.[21]

ADULT RESPIRATORY DISTRESS SYNDROME (ARDS)

ARDS may result from shock, sepsis, or trauma; hypovolemia and infection are the usual etiologies in an obstetrical population. In comparison to atelectasis or pneumonia alone, the clinical symptoms and signs are more severe: tachypnea, dyspnea, bronchoconstriction, increased work of breathing, ventilation-perfusion mismatch, increased pulmonary shunting and dead space, and hypoxia. Pathologically, there is loss of the pulmonary microvascular membrane integrity with edema, hemorrhage, and the deposition of proteinaceous intra-alveolar hyaline membranes. Early changes are completely reversible, but after 4–5 days, inflammation and tissue destruction may result in pulmonary fibrosis and may lead to death. ARDS mandates intensive respiratory care and careful management of cardiac function, fluid balance, and electrolytes.

PULMONARY EDEMA

Pulmonary edema is caused by any one or a combination of left ventricular failure, decreased colloid osmotic pressure, or alveolar-capillary disruption. It may be provoked by fluid overload or may be secondary to other processes such as preeclampsia, sepsis, or cardiac disease. Administration of blood, colloid, crystalloid, or absorption of irrigation fluid may contribute to fluid overload. Anesthetics, narcotics, hypnotic agents, and arrhythmias decrease myocardial contractility and may lead to incomplete cardiac emptying. Noxious agents (gases or vapors) or aspiration of gastric contents may cause injury to the alveolar membrane. The underlying cause of the pulmonary edema must be treated if possible. Usual management includes the administration of diuretics and, if necessary, invasive hemodynamic monitoring. A pulmonary artery catheter will provide information needed to follow the response to diuresis or to provide inotropic or vasoactive drugs.

DEEP VENOUS THROMBOSIS AND PULMONARY EMBOLISM

These topics are covered in Chapter 28.

POSTOPERATIVE BOWEL COMPLICATIONS

Gastrointestinal dysfunction may be due to postoperative ileus, secondary to intra-abdominal sepsis, bleeding into the gastrointestinal tract, gastrointestinal fistulas, or a large variety of intestinal and metabolic conditions. Anesthesia, wound pain, and the medications required for the treatment of pain may also contribute to ileus and may prevent oral intake in the immediate postoperative period. Abdominal surgery delays oral feeding due to a slower return of bowel peristalsis, particularly among those patients undergoing upper abdominal or retroperitoneal surgery. The stomach and sigmoid colon are the last to resume peristalsis, taking up to 3–4 days. In contrast, the small bowel rapidly regains its function and can absorb water, electrolytes, glucose, and amino acids within 1–2 days.

TABLE 23.3 Clinical Findings Consistent with Postcesarean Ileus

Nausea and/or vomiting
Abdominal distention
Absent flatus
Minimal or absent bowel sounds
Distended loops of bowel on abdominal x-ray

In primates, electromechanical evidence of normal small bowel contractile activity has been found within 5–10 hours of an abdominal operation.[26] Although transit time is delayed, gas usually does not accumulate in the small intestine. The type of operation, duration, or extent of manipulation of the intestine do not affect the duration of reduced motility.[27] The sigmoid colon appears to be the slowest to recover normal motility postoperatively, taking approximately 2–3 days.[28] As with the small intestine, the duration of operation and the extent of handling of the colon do not appear to affect the reduction of bowel motility.[26,27]

Postoperative nausea is usually mild and transient, though it may last as long as 24 hours. This varies with the anesthetic agent used and with postoperative analgesia. Commonly, return of colonic function is awaited and oral nutrition is begun when bowel sounds are auscultated and flatus is passed. Normal bowel sounds from the small intestine may be heard prior to adequate stomach and colonic activity. Passage of flatus signals significant return of colonic activity, and a bowel movement indicates return of normal function. Rather than wait for the presence of active bowel sounds, some feel that oral clear liquids may be begun as soon as the nausea has subsided. It is not clear whether there is any benefit to cold versus hot liquids. Ice chips help to relieve a dry mouth with only a small amount of liquid. However, it has been suggested that ice chips enhance swallowing of air, leading to discomfort from gastric distention.

A limited volume of clear liquids has historically been followed by a full liquid diet including milk and, subsequently, solid foods.[10] However, in patients without evidence of ileus, a regular diet as tolerated may be begun 24–72 hours postoperatively.[12] A regular diet will usually be tolerated by the third postoperative day. Early feeding of solids may actually enhance early return of bowel function by stimulating the gastrocolic reflex.

The occurrence of nausea, vomiting, or abdominal distention indicates reduced intestinal activity and possibly ileus (Table 23.3). Other signs include minimal or absent evidence of peristalsis and absence of flatus. Radiologic evidence includes gas-filled, distended loops of bowel, with or without air-fluid levels (Figure 23.3). Withholding oral intake and observation are usually adequate treatment. If ileus is persistent, nasogastric suction may be required. Rarely, placement of a long tube such as a Miller-

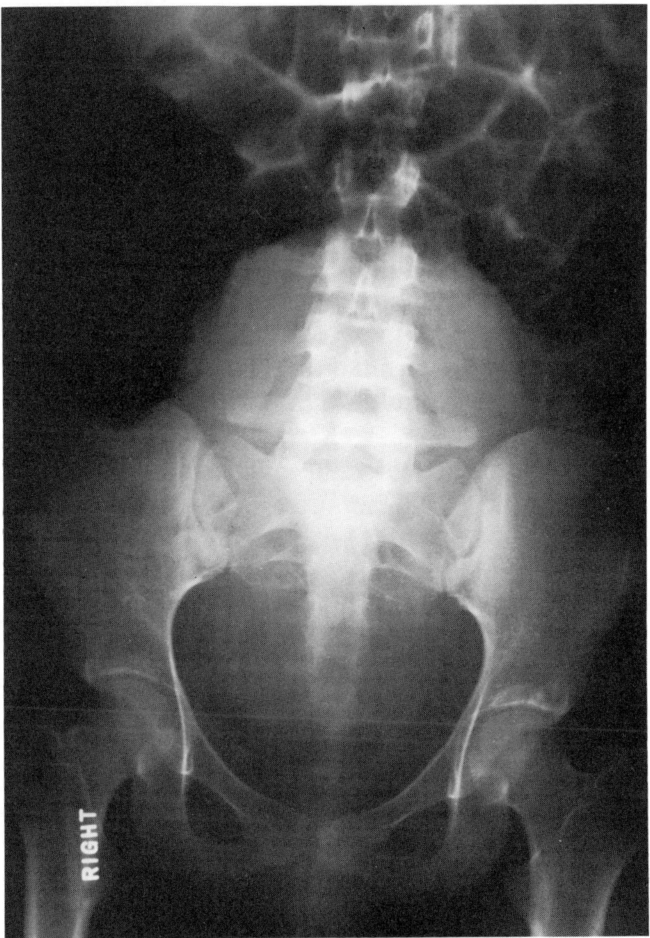

FIGURE 23.3 Postoperative adynamic ileus cephalad to the postpartum uterus.

Abbot tube into the small intestine may be necessary. Ensuring normal fluid and electrolyte status is essential to facilitate return of normal bowel function. Administration of water-soluble radiocontrast material has been reported as useful in differentiating ileus from mechanical small bowel obstruction. Colonic pseudo-obstruction, in which physical and radiologic findings suggest mechanical obstruction of the large bowel, is rare. A specific pathologic entity is absent, and the etiology is thought to be a neurostimulatory imbalance. Early administration of a water-soluble enema is the therapy of choice.[29]

Severe colicky pains, sometimes referred to as "gas pains," frequently occur on the second or third postoperative day. They may be accompanied by signs of ileus such as distention and tympany. The depression of intestinal function by analgesic agents augments this reaction. Palliative measures may include a hot water bottle, heating pad, or rectal tube. Enemas will help to stimulate bowel motility, but should be used only if return of bowel function is imminent and avoided if obstruction is suspected.

Mechanical bowel obstruction may appear as an ileus or as expected postoperative bowel inactivity in the early stages. Peristaltic rushes with high-pitched sounds signal bowel obstruction and occur in addition to symptoms of nausea, vomiting, and abdominal distention. Conservative management consists of restricting oral intake and placement of a nasogastric tube or possibly a long tube. Maintenance of normal fluid status, electrolytes, hematocrit, and serum proteins is essential. Failure to respond to conservative therapy necessitates surgical consultation and possible abdominal exploration.

Immediate postoperative enteral feeding has been combined with esophagogastric aspiration to aliment successfully a variety of surgical patients. The main disadvantage of such therapy is the requirement of a nasogastric-duodenal tube or gastrostomy. An elemental diet is also required to prevent clogging of the tube. Advantages include a much more rapid recovery of bowel function with avoidance of paralytic ileus, a shorter hospital stay, and possibly a lower incidence of sepsis and wound complications. The resultant positive nitrogen and energy balances may explain the finding of increased wound strength. The patient can also drink water freely. This procedure has been applied most frequently in patients undergoing bowel surgery or cholecystectomy, but has also been used in gynecologic patients.[30]

COMMON POSTOPERATIVE URINARY TRACT COMPLICATIONS

Urinary tract infection is the second most common cause of postcesarean febrile morbidity, with a reported incidence of 2%–16%.[31] In one study >7.3% of postoperative clean catch urine specimens had more than 10^5 bacteria per milliliter in culture.[32] One percent of patients had both endometritis and bacteriuria.[32]

The most common etiology of nosocomial urinary tract infections among hospitalized patients in general is urethral catheterization (80%), particularly with indwelling catheters.[33] The incidence of infection increases with the duration of an indwelling catheter at a rate of 4%–7.5% per day during the first 10 days.[33] Critically ill patients and diabetics are more likely to develop bacteriuria. Women are at greater risk than men, as approximately 80% of women may harbor urethral bacteria.[33]

A variety of techniques have been utilized to attempt to reduce the incidence of catheter-related infections. These include systemic antibiotics and eradication of bacteria in drainage bags with antiseptic solutions. With proper insertion technique and the advent of closed system drainage, the incidence of infection has decreased. The supplemental benefit of antibiotic coverage and drainage bag irrigation is small, if significant at all.[33]

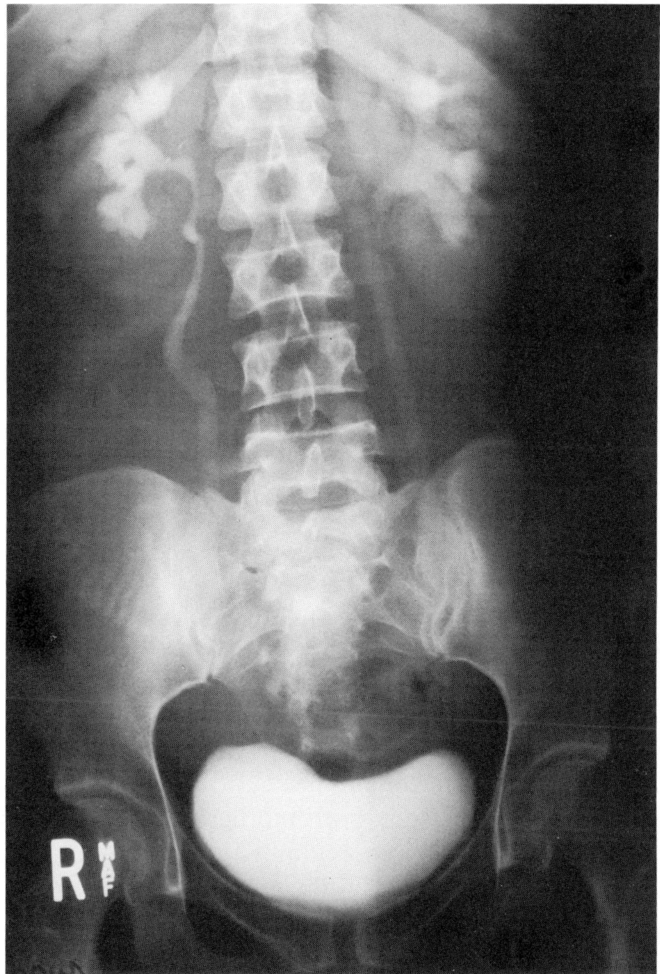

FIGURE 23.4 Intravenous pyelogram showing left pelvic brim ureterolithiasis.

Urinary tract infection must be considered in postoperative cesarean patients with fever. Catheter-related infections are primarily asymptomatic but can lead to bacteremia in 1% of cases.[33] Gram-negative bacilli and enterococci are common offenders. A persistent fever in these postoperative patients may be due to infection, but the differential diagnosis also includes obstruction due to surgical complications or urolithiasis. A radiograph of the abdomen and an intravenous pyelogram will be helpful in determining the etiology (Figure 23.4) if the clinical picture suggests obstruction.

BREAST-FEEDING IN THE POSTCESAREAN PATIENT

Women who have experienced a cesarean delivery, especially if unanticipated, will often need reassurance that their role as a mother to their newborn is no different than that of someone who has delivered vaginally.

Sensitivity and encouragement are especially important for those mothers who may feel that they have failed because a cesarean delivery was necessary. In addition, cesarean mothers may need practical physical assistance in their efforts to breast-feed during the initial postoperative period.

Breast-feeding must be individualized to the condition of the mother and infant. For example, a cesarean delivery is more likely for a preterm than a term infant, and the preterm infant may not be able to breast-feed initially. The importance of producing breast milk manually or mechanically for the preterm infant should be stressed and the mother encouraged in her efforts. Pooled term breast milk may not provide the concentration of nutrients needed by a very preterm infant (eg, 32 weeks or less). Recent studies have shown higher nitrogen (protein), fat, energy, sodium, and chloride contents in preterm compared to term milk.[34,35] The mother herself may be very ill and unable to move easily enough to handle her newborn on her own for breast-feeding. Conversely, if a regional anesthetic has been used, with help a mother may be able to breast-feed in the recovery room.

The techniques used for breast-feeding are virtually the same for vaginally delivered and cesarean mothers. Those with the discomfort of cesarean incisions may initially prefer positions that minimize pressure on the maternal abdomen, such as the lateral Sim's position. If the mother is sitting or reclining in a semi-Fowler's position, additional pillows may be necessary to support her arm and head and the baby on her abdomen.

Pain medication may affect both mother and infant, though rarely does it interfere with lactation. Commonly used analgesics, such as morphine, meperidine, codeine, acetaminophen, and ibuprofen in therapeutic doses, have no reported adverse effects.[36] However, administration of pain medication immediately after a feeding will allow drug levels to peak prior to the next feeding (most medications given orally or parenterally peak in less than 90 minutes), minimizing drowsiness in the mother and the amount of drug potentially transferred to the infant.

The choice of drugs administered to the mother should be affected by her desire for lactation (Table 23.4). Some necessary diagnostic or therapeutic agents such as radiopharmaceuticals require temporary interruption of lactation. Others, such as tetracycline and chloramphenicol, may be avoided entirely in preference to other agents. Antibiotic therapy is commonly needed in postoperative cesarean patients. The transfer of antibiotics to maternal milk is extremely small. Penicillins and cephalosporins are transferred in only trace amounts. Except for tetracyclines, chloramphenicol, and macrolides (eg, erythromycin), the concentration of other antibiotics such as aminoglycosides remains below 1 μg/mL in breast milk.[37]

The differential diagnosis in a postoperative cesarean patient with a fever includes breast engorgement and mastitis. Breast engorgement is associated with obstructed excretory ducts and, at most, a low-grade fever.

TABLE 23.4 Selected Drugs and Their Levels in Breast Milk

Drug	Levels in Breast Milk and Effect
Contraindicated during Breast-Feeding	
Antineoplastic agents	Possible immune suppression, growth abnormality
Bromocriptine	Suppresses lactation
Cimetidine	Concentrated in breast milk; inhibition of drug metabolism, CNS stimulation in infant
Ergotamine	Vomiting, diarrhea, convulsions
Gold salts	Rash, renal and hepatic inflammation
Methimazole, thiouracil	Interference with thyroid function Propylthiouracil may be used
Phenindione	Hemorrhage
Discontinue Breast-Feeding Temporarily	
Chloramphenicol	1.3% of dose, levels 50% of serum level or more; no reported effect, possible blood dyscrasia
Metronidazole	Levels similar to serum level; decreased appetite, vomiting, possible blood dyscrasia
Radiopharmaceuticals	Significant levels for hours to weeks, varying with substance
Sulfa	0.12% of dose; interferes with conjugation of bilirubin; never use with G6PD deficiency
Tetracyclines	0.03% of dose; levels 60% of serum level or more

Source: Vorherr H: Drug excretion in breast milk. *Postgrad Med* 56:97, 1974; Lepage G, Collet S, Bougle D, et al: The composition of preterm milk in relation to the degree of prematurity. *Am J Clin Nutr* 40:1042, 1984; Committee on Drugs, American Academy of Pediatrics: The transfer of drugs and other chemicals into human breast milk. *Pediatrics* 72:375, 1983.

Nursing by the baby, manual expression, or mechanical pumping will relieve the obstruction. Mastitis usually begins as a cellulitis from cracks in the nipple rather than as an intraductal process. Flu-like symptoms, chills, and myalgias may herald its onset, frequently accompanied by a temperature of 102°F (39°C). Local erythema and tenderness also occur.

Nonepidemic puerperal mastitis occurs in approximately 1%–10% of nursing mothers, of whom up to 10% may develop an abscess.[38,39] From one-third to one-half of these infections are found to have *Staphylococcus aureus* in cultures of breast milk.[38,40] Many infants are found to have similarly positive nasopharyngeal cultures.

Diagnosis may be aided by laboratory examination of the breast milk. Leukocyte counts $<10^6$/mL are associated with $<10^3$ bacteria per milliliter and probable milk stasis. Their outcome is good without treatment. In contrast, $>10^6$ leukocytes and $>10^3$ bacteria per milliliter suggest infectious mastitis, in which only 15% may have a good result without treatment and 11% develop abscesses.[41,42]

As many as half of the patients with puerperal mastitis may be resistant to penicillin in vitro, but much fewer fail to respond clinically.[38,40] The most useful oral antibiotics are penicillinase-resistant penicillins or erythromycin, for those allergic to penicillin, in doses of 500 mg four times a day (Table 23.5). Clindamycin may be indicated in cases of serious breast infections or for those suspected of having a mixed flora.[43]

TABLE 23.5 Antibiotics Found to Be Effective in the Treatment of Puerperal Mastitis

Penicillinase-resistant penicillins
Oxacillin
Nafcillin
Cloxacillin
Dicloxacillin
For penicillin-allergic patients
Erythromycin
Other medications
Clindamycin

For both breast engorgement and mastitis, continuation of nursing is therapeutic and is the most effective way of draining an obstructed area. Local hot, wet compresses may help dilate mammary ducts in those with breast engorgement. Because engorgement may contribute to breast abscess formation in patients with mastitis, continued nursing or emptying of the breasts is crucial. There are no adverse effects on infants who continue to nurse. Treatment with antibiotics in the early stage of cellulitis is also extremely important in preventing abscess formation.

CONCLUSION

Attention to detail in the postoperative management of cesarean patients will avert many complications. Practices such as early ambulation have helped to foster an attitude of recovery and health. The benefits of rapid recovery are not only physical but also emotional and financial. Effort on the part of the entire health care team is required to accomplish these goals.

The opinions expressed in this chapter are those of the authors and not necessarily those of the United States Navy or the Department of Defense.

REFERENCES

1. Goodman LS, Gilman A (eds): *The Pharmacological Basis of Therapeutics,* ed 5. New York, Macmillan Publishing Co, 1975.
2. Vorherr H: Drug excretion in breast milk. *Postgrad Med* 56:97, 1974.
3. Townsend RJ, Benedetti TJ, Erickson SH, et al: Excretion of ibuprofen into breast milk. *Am J Obstet Gynecol* 149:184, 1984.
4. Rosen MA, Hughes SC, Shnider SM: Epidural morphine for the relief of postoperative pain after cesarean delivery. *Anesth Analg* 62:666, 1983.
5. Frank RT: Obstetrical surgery, in Johnson AB (ed): *Operative Therapeusis.* New York, D Appleton and Co, 1915, pp 513–514.
6. Leithauser DJ: *Early Ambulation and Related Procedures in Surgical Management.* Springfield, Ill, Charles C Thomas, 1946, pp 10–26.

7. Metcalfe J, Ueland K: Maternal cardiovascular adjustments to pregnancy. *Prog Cardiovasc Dis* 16:363, 1974.
8. Zipursky A, Pollock J, Neelands P, et al: The transplacental passage of foetal red blood-cells and the pathogenesis of Rh immunisation during pregnancy. *Lancet* 2:489, 1963.
9. Fear FE, Queenan JT: Factors affecting the trans-placental passage of fetal erythrocytes. *Obstet Gynecol* 29:444, 1967.
10. Randall HT: Enteral nutrition, in *Manual of Preoperative and Postoperative Care.* Committee on Pre and Postoperative Care, American College of Surgeons. Philadelphia, WB Saunders Co, 1983, pp 68–85.
11. Heymsfield SB, Horowitz J, Lawson DH: Enteral hyperalimentation, in Berk JE (ed): *Developments in Digestive Diseases,* vol 3. Philadelphia, Lea & Febiger, 1980, pp 59–83.
12. Horowitz J, Smith J, Lawson DH, et al: Nutritional management of the surgical patient, in Lubin MF, Walker HK, Smith RB III (eds): *Medical Management of the Surgical Patient.* Boston, Butterworths, 1982, pp 3–60.
13. Vogel CM, Kingsbury RJ, Baue A: Intravenous hyperalimentation: A review of two and one-half years' experience. *Arch Surg* 105:414, 1972.
14. Kinney JM, Long CL, Gump FE, et al: Tissue composition of weight loss in surgical patients. I. Elective operation. *Ann Surg* 168:459, 1968.
15. Bartlett RH, Brennan ML, Gazzaniga AB, et al: Studies on the pathogenesis and prevention of postoperative pulmonary complications. *Surg Gynecol Obstet* 137:925, 1973.
16. Schwartz SI: Complications, in Schwartz SI (ed): *Principles of Surgery,* ed 2. New York, McGraw-Hill Book Co, 1974, pp 461–490.
17. Ward RJ, Danziger F, Bonica JJ, et al: An evaluation of postoperative respiratory maneuvers. *Surg Gynecol Obstet* 123:51, 1966.
18. Beecher HK: Measured effect of laparotomy on respiration. *J Clin Invest* 12:639, 1933.
19. Van De Water JM: Preoperative and postoperative techniques in the prevention of pulmonary complications. *Surg Clin North Am* 60:1339, 1980.
20. O'Donohue WJ: Prevention and treatment of postoperative atelectasis: Can it and will it be adequately studied? *Chest* 87:1, 1985.
21. Lewis FR: Management of atelectasis and pneumonia. *Surg Clin North Am* 60:1391, 1980.
22. Wellman JJ: Respiratory care in the surgical patient, in Lubin MF, Walker HK, Smith RB III (eds): *Medical Management of the Surgical Patient.* Boston, Butterworths, 1982, pp 281–330.
23. O'Donohue WJ: National survey of the usage of lung expansion modalities for the prevention and treatment of postoperative atelectasis following abdominal and thoracic surgery. *Chest* 87:76, 1985.
24. Van de Water JM, Watring WG, Linton LA, et al: Prevention of postoperative pulmonary complications. *Surg Gynecol Obstet* 135:229, 1972.
25. Dohi S, Gold MI: Comparison of two methods of postoperative respiratory care. *Chest* 73:592, 1978.
26. Wilson JP: Post-operative motility of the large intestine in man. *Gut* 16:689, 1975.
27. Graber JN, Schulte WJ, Condon RE, et al: Relationship of duration of postoperative ileus to extent and site of operative dissection. *Surgery* 92:87, 1982.
28. Woods JH, Erickson LW, Condon RE, et al: Postoperative ileus: A colonic problem? *Surgery* 84:527, 1978.
29. Spira IA, Wolff WI: Colonic pseudo-obstruction following termination of pregnancy and uterine operation. *Am J Obstet Gynecol* 126:7, 1976.

30. Moss G: Early enteral feeding after abdominal surgery, in Deitel M (ed): *Nutrition in Clinical Surgery,* ed 2. Baltimore, Williams & Wilkins Co, 1985, pp 220–231.
31. Farrell SJ, Andersen HF, Work BA Jr: Cesarean section: Indications and postoperative morbidity. *Obstet Gynecol* 56:696, 1980.
32. Rehu M, Nilsson CG: Risk factors for febrile morbidity associated with cesarean section. *Obstet Gynecol* 56:269, 1980.
33. Fowler JE Jr, Marshall V: Nosocomial catheter-associated urinary tract infection. *Infect Surg* 2:43, 1983.
34. Gross SJ, David RJ, Bauman L, et al: Nutritional composition of milk produced by mothers delivering preterm. *J Pediatr* 96:641, 1980.
35. Lepage G, Collet S, Bougle D, et al: The composition of preterm milk in relation to the degree of prematurity. *Am J Clin Nutr* 40:1042, 1984.
36. Committee on Drugs, American Academy of Pediatrics: The transfer of drugs and other chemicals into human breast milk. *Pediatrics* 72:375, 1983.
37. Matsuda S: Transfer of antibiotics into maternal milk. *Biol Res Preg* 5:57, 1984.
38. Marshall BR, Hepper JK, Zirbel CC: Sporadic puerperal mastitis: An infection that need not interrupt lactation. *JAMA* 233:1377, 1975.
39. Neifert MR, Seacat JM: Contemporary breast-feeding management. *Clin Perinatol* 12:319, 1985.
40. Niebyl JR, Spence MR, Parmley TH: Sporadic (nonepidemic) puerperal mastitis. *J Reprod Med* 20:97, 1978.
41. Thomsen AC, Espersen T, Maigaard S: Course and treatment of milk stasis, noninfectious inflammation of the breast, and infectious mastitis in nursing women. *Am J Obstet Gynecol* 149:492, 1984.
42. Thomsen AC, Hansen KB, Moller BR: Leukocyte counts and microbiologic cultivation in the diagnosis of puerperal mastitis. *Am J Obstet Gynecol* 146:938, 1983.
43. Wong MK, Smith CV, Phelan JP: Antepartum mastitis. *J Reprod Med* 31:511, 1986.

Chapter 24

The Role of Ultrasonography in the Management of the Postcesarean Patient

Harbinder S. Brar, MD

Sonography during pregnancy is an established and valuable tool to aid in the diagnosis of a variety of obstetric disorders. The use of postpartum sonography is now being used increasingly to assess the uterine cavity for retained products of conception and endometritis. In postcesarean patients, the common complications include hemorrhage, endomyometritis, and thromboembolism.[1] Ultrasound is a useful adjunctive diagnostic tool in the differential diagnosis of these complications and in evaluation of the abdominal wall and pelvis for hematomas and abscesses. Retained products of conception within the uterus are also easily visualized with ultrasound, although this diagnosis will rarely be entertained in postoperative cesarean patients. Thromboembolic episodes are frequent during puerperium, especially in postcesarean patients, and are attributed to the hypercoagulable state of pregnancy and vascular stasis.[2,3] Noninvasive impedance phlebography is a valuable tool to diagnose deep venous thrombosis in the lower extremities. Pearson and Creasman[4] reported an overall 95.6% diagnostic accuracy rate using this method, although it is of limited value when thrombosis involves the pelvic veins. Under these circumstances, one must resort to phlebography if confirmation of the diagnosis is needed.

SONOGRAPHIC ANATOMY OF THE POSTPARTUM PELVIS

The female pelvis undergoes drastic biochemical, physiological, and anatomical changes during pregnancy. During the postpartum period, the uterus gradually returns to the nonpregnant state in 6 weeks. This is due to the disappearance of both the hormonal and mechanical effects of pregnancy. On the first postpartum day, the uterine fundus is at or below the level of the umbilicus and the uterus is slightly dextroverted ("physiologic

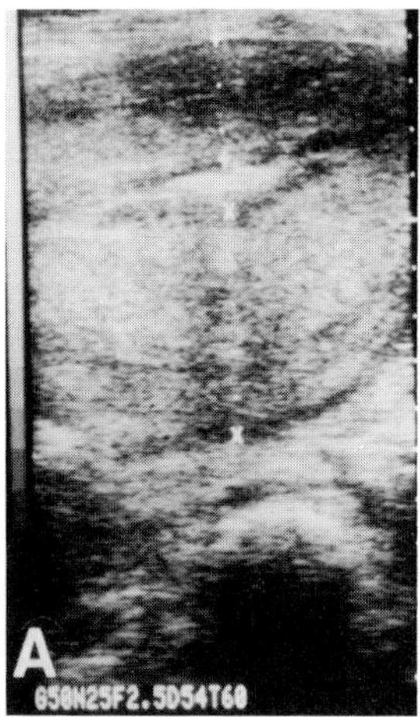

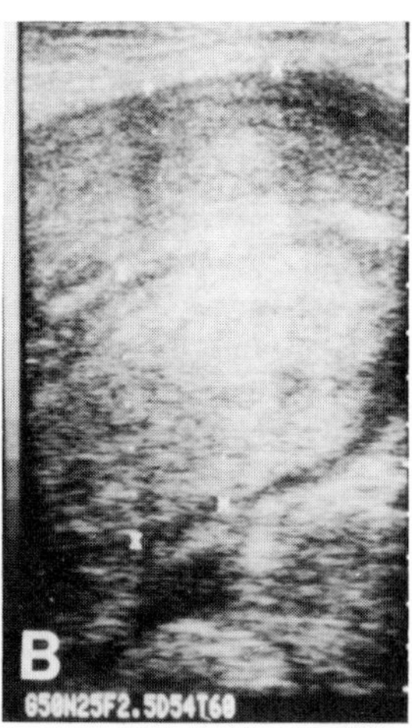

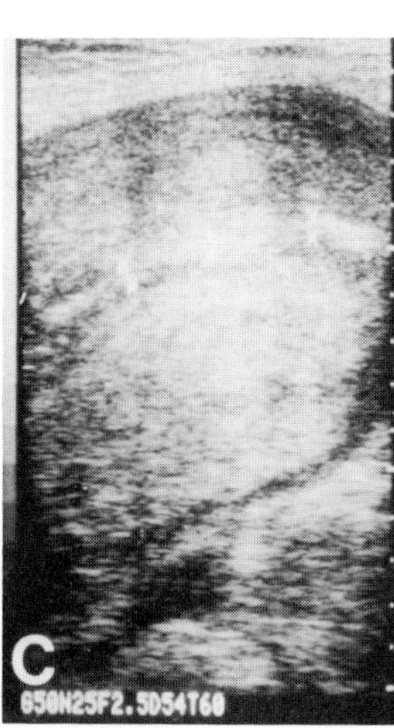

FIGURE 24.1 Ultrasound evaluation of a postpartum uterus. (A) The transverse uterine wall thickness. It measures 2.6 cm anteriorly and 4.8 cm posteriorly from the uterine cavity. (B) A longitudinal section of the uterus. The uterine wall thickness measures 3.3–3.4 cm anteriorly and 5.6–5.8 cm posteriorly from the uterine cavity. (C) A postpartum uterine cavity. It measures 0.4–0.6 cm in thickness. Please note the white band indicative of an empty uterine cavity.

right torsion of the uterus").[5] In a study of 25 normal postpartum patients, uterine wall thickness varied from 3 to 6.5 cm.[6] The walls are slightly thicker in multiparas compared to primiparas. On ultrasound (Figure 24.1), the walls of the uterus appear homogeneous, although subtle irregularities of the contour may be seen after cesarean.[7] The endometrial cavity is usually seen as a slit, the anteroposterior (AP) thickness varying from 0.5 to 1.3 cm.[6] A full bladder is advisable when performing an ultrasound examination in the postpartum period, as it provides an acoustic window and pushes the antiflexed puerperal uterus posteriorly, thus positioning the endometrial cavity at right angles to the sound waves and improving visualization.[8] Additionally, it pushes gas-filled loops of bowel away from the pelvis, which usually hinder visualization of the cul-de-sac, adnexa, and uterus.

The broad ligaments contain loose areolar tissue, uterine artery and veins, fallopian tubes, and round ligaments. They are not prominent in the nonpregnant patient, and therefore are not well visualized on ultrasound. By contrast, they are seen relatively easily in the pregnant and postpartum period because of the large and tortuous uterine vessels (Figure 24.2).

The ovaries are difficult to visualize postpartum because gas-filled loops of bowel obscure their depiction from their extrapelvic position, where they are usually displaced by the large uterus. The cul-de-sac and the abdominal cavity, however, can be visualized for the presence of free fluid and ascites or hemoperitoneum.[9]

Postpartum uterine involution can also be assessed with ultrasound.

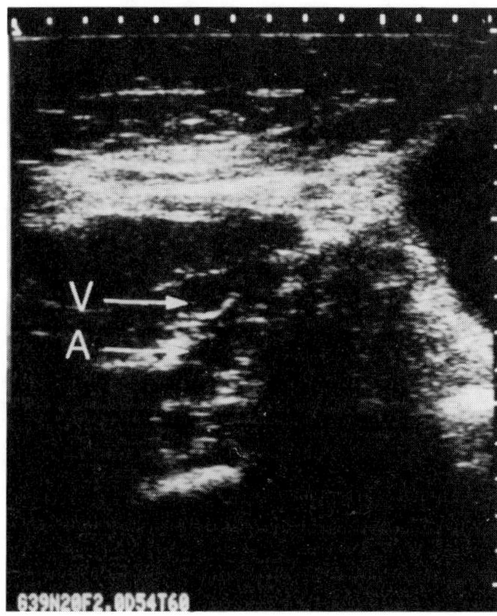

FIGURE 24.2 The uterine artery (A) and uterine vein (V) in the broad ligament of a postpartum gravida.

Van Ness et al determined that the uterine area decreased 31% in the first week, 48% in the second and third weeks, and 18% after the 21st day.[10] Although involution can be judged clinically with relative ease, ultrasound may play a complementary role in those patients in whom an adequate clinical pelvic examination is not technically feasible due to pain, surgery, or obesity.

POSTOPERATIVE PUERPERAL INFECTION

Puerperal endomyometritis is suspected when the postoperative patient experiences temperature of 100.4°C or more on 2 consecutive days, not including the first day of fever.[1] The incidence of endomyometritis in postcesarean patients varies from 13% to 70%.[1] The diagnosis is usually made clinically by a process of exclusion, and patients generally respond rapidly to antibiotics. Therefore, the value of sonography is limited and may be unnecessary in the majority of cases. Occasionally the infection can spread outside the uterine cavity, leading to parametritis, septic pelvic thrombophlebitis, and peritonitis. Sonographic findings of endometritis are variable and include a dilated uterine cavity with fluid and/or gas, fluid in the cul-de-sac, and, often, a normal sonogram. Endometritis can result from both retained products of conception and contamination of the uterine cavity by microorganisms from the vagina.

Sonographic findings of retained products of conception may mimic those of endometritis. Retained products of conception are relatively easy to identify because their echo pattern differs so markedly from that of the myometrium. A sonographically "empty" uterus (Figure 24.1) indicates with virtual certainty that no retained products of conception are present, but an abnormal scan may represent blood, fluid, infection, or retained

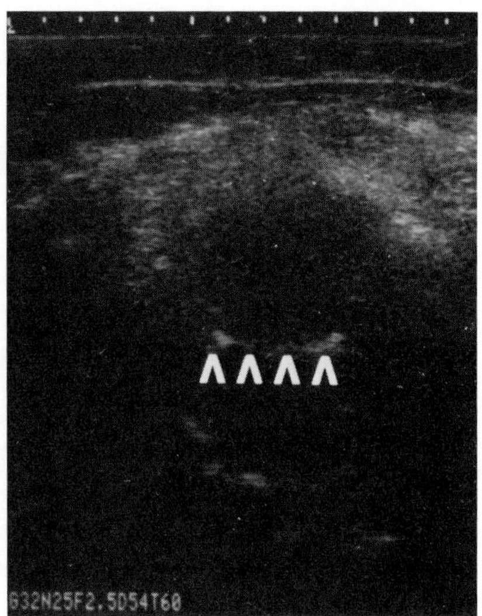

FIGURE 24.3 Ultrasound evaluation of a post-cesarean patient at the level of the uterine incision. Note the echoes generated by the suture material.

products of conception.[11,12] Milder forms of endometritis usually result in normal sonograms. As the disease advances, exudation into the uterine cavity becomes visible sonographically. Gas-forming organisms, including *Escherichia coli* and *Clostridium perfringens,* are frequently present in endometritis, and the gas is easily detectable on the sonogram. Because air can also be introduced into the uterus during surgical manipulations, it is important to perform sonograms prior to dilatation and curettage.

Infections and abscesses may also develop in the uterine incision and abdominal wall, and ultrasound plays an adjunctive role in their diagnosis. Burger et al[13] reported a variable sonographic appearance of the uterine incision after cesarean delivery. Usually the uterine incision contains strong echoes generated from the suture material used (Figure 24.3). Small seromas and hematomas (in the uterine incision, broad ligament, and under the bladder flap) may develop and are visible on ultrasound during the first postoperative week. Any fluid-filled collection seen with ultrasound around the uterine incision in a febrile patient is strongly suggestive of abscess formation. Occasionally abscesses may develop, with characteristic fluid and gas collections, shaggy walls, and internal echoes, and free cul-de-sac fluid may indicate peritonitis. If a patient is hemodynamically unstable, blood may be present. In such a case, ultrasound-directed paracentesis may clarify the situation (Figure 24.4).[9] It is usually impossible to distinguish with certainty between an infected and an uninfected fluid collection, but irregularity of the wall, internal echoes, or the appearance of numerous bright echoes increase the probability of infection. The diagnostic approach to a postsurgical pelvic abscess includes several modalities. Computed tomography may be preferable, as it permits thorough assessment of the entire peritoneal cavity and may identify gas or fresh hemorrhage within a fluid collection. On the other hand, sonography

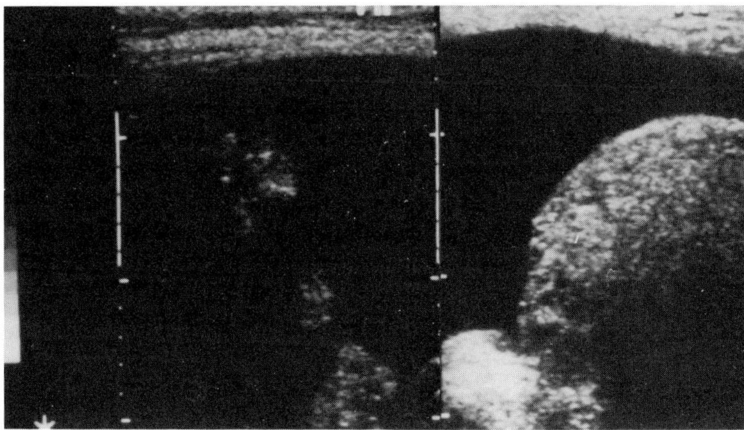

FIGURE 24.4 Postpartum patient with sonographic evidence of intra-abdominal fluid. Paracentesis demonstrated ascitic fluid.

may be difficult due to the presence of ileus, wounds, and bandages, but it has the advantage of identifying peristalsis in fluid-filled structures (bowel) and of allowing percutaneous aspirations using sonographic guidance with real-time instruments.[14]

Abdominal wall disorders, even though superficial, are difficult to detect clinically due to tenderness to palpation. The abdominal wall and rectus sheath can be studied in detail with a 5- or 7-mHz short internal focus transducer. Seromas, hematomas, and abscesses in the anterior abdominal wall are easily visualized with ultrasound and have similar sonographic findings. They usually resolve slowly but should be drained in a febrile patient. Ultrasound guidance may be helpful under these circumstances.

PUERPERAL THROMBOPHLEBITIS

An increased incidence of thrombophlebitis and thromboembolic episodes during pregnancy, puerperium, and the postcesarean period is known to occur secondary to the hypercoagulable state, venous stasis, and puerperal infection.[15] Impedance phlebography is useful in the diagnosis of deep vein thrombosis of the calf and thighs.[4] Although pelvic and ovarian thrombophlebitis is difficult to diagnose using this technique, computed tomography and sonography may aid in the diagnosis of ovarian vein thrombophlebitis in a limited number of cases.[16] This condition, which complicates 0.18% of patients,[2] is usually diagnosed on the basis of clinical findings. For instance, these patients frequently present with lower abdominal pain, nausea, vomiting, and fever unresponsive to traditional antibiotics. Examination may reveal a ropelike mass (thrombosed ovarian vein), more commonly on the right side. The differential diagnosis includes broad ligament hematoma, pelvic abscess, ovarian torsion, appendicitis, and volvulus of bowel. Although no cases diagnosed by ultrasonography have been reported, ultrasound may aid in making or excluding other diagnoses, such as broad ligament hematoma, pelvic abscess, or ovarian torsion. Shaffer et al reported a case of ovarian vein thrombophlebitis diagnosed by computed tomography.[17]

POSTPARTUM HEMORRHAGE

Postpartum hemorrhage in a postcesarean patient is usually due to uterine atony, placenta accreta, or bleeding from the uterine incision. Uterine atony may be visualized as a large uterus on ultrasound, with the endometrial cavity enlarged by echo-free space that represents blood. Bleeding from the uterine incision into the broad ligament or under the bladder flap is also seen easily as echo-free collections on ultrasound. If bleeding occurs freely into the abdominal cavity, fluid is seen on ultrasound and paracentesis under ultrasound guidance can confirm the diagnosis. Retained products of conception as a cause of hemorrhage are rare in this group. Rarely, postpartum hemorrhage may be due to retained products of conception in a postcesarean patient. Sonography may be helpful in these rare situations. Delayed postpartum hemorrhage secondary to placental polyp or subinvolution of the uterus can also be readily visualized.

OTHER POSTOPERATIVE COMPLICATIONS

Urinary Tract Complications

The proximity of the bladder and ureter to the operative field makes the urinary tract vulnerable to infection, surgical trauma, and mechanical compression from adjacent hematomas, abscesses, and seromas. Infection of the urinary tract is easily diagnosed with urinalysis and culture. Acute renal failure is an uncommon postoperative complication of cesarean delivery. Once the diagnosis of acute renal failure has been established and a prerenal cause has been excluded, an ultrasound examination should be performed as the primary screening procedure to differentiate between urinary tract outflow obstruction and parenchymal disease. Postrenal acute renal failure is potentially correctable; furthermore, prompt diagnosis and intervention are necessary to prevent secondary renal parenchymal loss. Obstruction must be bilateral in order to cause acute renal failure. Acute urinary bladder retention is not uncommon postoperatively and is easily seen on ultrasound as a distended bladder. An indwelling catheter usually resolves the problem (Figure 24.5).

The collecting system is normally dilated in pregnancy, but excessive dilatation with acute renal failure in a patient with intraoperatively par-

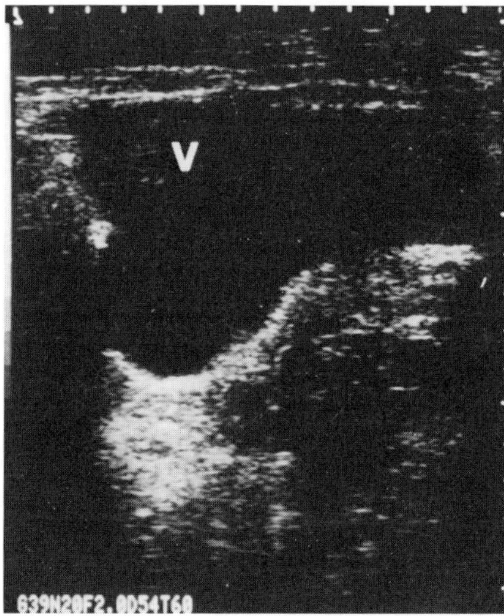

FIGURE 24.5 Acute urinary retention in a postpartum patient.

ametrial extensions or postoperatively pelvic hematomas and abscesses is highly suspicious of bilateral ureteral obstruction. If bilateral dilatation is detected, the scanning procedure should be continued to determine the level and etiology of the obstructing lesion. A dilated ureter proximal to the site of obstruction can often be demonstrated. Scanning the pelvis with the urinary bladder distended is required to identify obstructing masses of pelvic origin. Further diagnostic procedures such as antegrade or retrograde pyelography should be performed once obstruction is suspected on ultrasound examination.

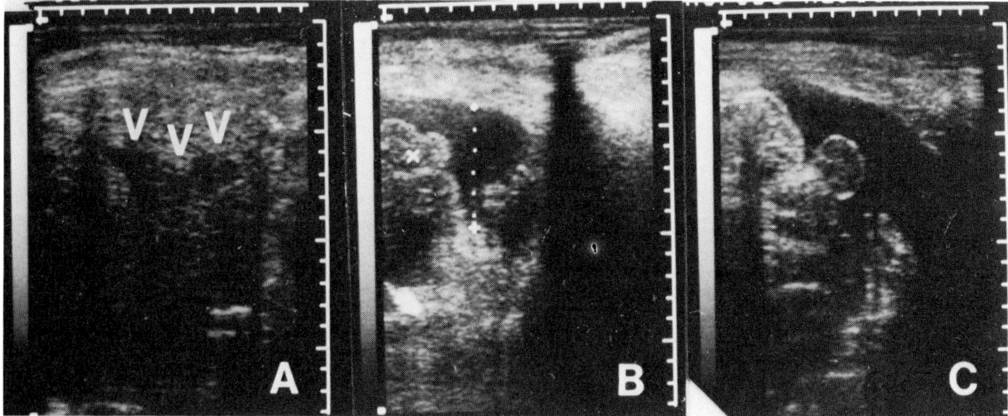

FIGURE 24.6 Ultrasound evaluation of a postcesarean preeclamptic patient demonstrates the following: (A) subcapsular hematomas of the liver (V), (B) intra-abdominal fluid with floating bowel (X), and (C) intra-abdominal fluid accumulation determined to be blood by paracentesis.

Intra-abdominal Complications

A postcesarean patient who continues to be febrile, despite the use of adequate antibiotics, should be thoroughly evaluated for conditions such as septic thrombophlebitis, pelvic and abdominal wall hematomas, and abscesses. Abdominal ultrasonography may be helpful in the management and diagnosis of these complications. Abscesses present most often as complex, predominantly cystic masses with occasional fluid levels. Subphrenic abscesses can be seen on ultrasound but are more difficult to visualize, and scanning needs to be done with the patient in different positions for adequate visualization of the subphrenic space. Additionally, pleural effusion should not be mistaken for subdiaphragmatic fluid collections. Infrequently, a hepatic subcapsular hematoma may also be seen on ultrasound in a patient with preeclampsia (Figure 24.6).

REFERENCES

1. Vorherr H: Puerperal genitourinary infection, in Sciarra J (ed): *Gynecology and Obstetrics,* vol 2. Philadelphia, Harper & Row, Publishers, Inc, 1982, chap 91, pp 1–29.
2. Brown TK, Mannick RA: Puerperal ovarian vein thrombophlebitis—A syndrome. *Am J Obstet Gynecol* 109:263, 1971.
3. Montalto NJ, Bloch E, Malfetano JH, et al: Postpartum thrombophlebitis of the ovarian vein. *Obstet Gynecol* 34:867, 1969.
4. Pearson DLC, Creasman WT: Diagnosis of deep venous thrombosis in obstetrics and gynecology by impedance phlebography. *Obstet Gynecol* 58:52, 1981.
5. Vorherr H: Puerperium: Maternal involutional changes—Management of puerperal problems and complications, in Sciarra J (ed): *Gynecology and Obstetrics,* vol 2. Philadelphia, Harper & Row, Publishers, Inc, chap 90, pp 30–44.
6. Lee CY, Madrazo BL, Drukker BH: Ultrasonic evaluation of the postpartum uterus in the management of postpartum bleeding. *Obstet Gynecol* 58:227, 1981.
7. Gross BH, Callen PW: Ultrasound of the uterus, in Callen PW (ed): *Ultrasonography in Obstetrics and Gynecology.* Philadelphia, WB Saunders, Co, 1982, p 227.
8. Madrazo BL: Postpartum sonography, in Sanders RC, Jones E (eds): *Ultrasonography in Obstetrics and Gynecology,* ed 3. New York, Appleton-Century-Crofts Medical, 1986, p 449.
9. Rodriguez MH, Smith J, Clark SL, Phelan JP: Ultrasound-guided paracentesis in complicated postpartum patients. *J Reprod Med* (in press).
10. Van Rees D, Bernstine RL, Crawford W: Involution of the postpartum uterus: An ultrasonic study. *J Clin Ultrasound* 9:55, 1981.
11. Malvern J, Campbell S, May P: Ultrasonic scanning of the puerperal uterus following secondary postpartum haemorrhage. *Br J Obstet Gynaecol* 80:320, 1973.
12. Robinson HP: Sonar in the puerperium. *Scott Med J* 14:234, 1972.
13. Burger NF, Dararas B, Boes EGM: An echographic evaluation during the early puerperium of the uterine wound after cesarean section. *J Clin Ultrasound* 10:271, 1982.
14. Gerzof SG, Robbins AH, Johnson WC, et al: Percutaneous catheter drainage of abdominal abscesses. A five year experience. *N Engl J Med* 305:653, 1981.

15. Villasanta U: Thromboembolic disease in pregnancy. *Am J Obstet Gynecol* 93:142, 1965.
16. Wilson PC, Lerner RM: Diagnosis of ovarian vein thrombophlebitis by ultrasonography. *J Ultrasound Med* 2:187, 1983.
17. Shaffer PB, Johnson JC, Bryan D, et al: Diagnosis of ovarian vein thrombophlebitis by computed tomography. *J Comp Assist Tomogr* 5:436, 1981.

Chapter 25

Diagnosis and Management of Postcesarean Wound Complications

Stanley A. Gall, Jr, MD, and
Stanley A. Gall, MD

"Little thought is given to the fact that every open wound, surgical or accidental, receives bacterial organisms and that the term 'infection' is applied only in those instances in which the process of wound healing is impaired by this contamination."[1] The healing of the celiotomy and uterotomy incisions of cesarean delivery are, on occasion, afflicted by an imbalance between host defense systems and unavoidable bacterial contamination.

This chapter will deal with the process of healing of surgical wounds, with particular emphasis on cesarean delivery–associated infectious morbidity. The complications of uterine and urinary tract infections occurring in conjunction with cesarean delivery are dealt with elsewhere (Chapters 22 and 26). This discussion will focus on wound healing, microbial contamination, conduct of surgery, operating techniques, and patient characteristics influencing wound infection. The chapter will conclude with a discussion of the diagnostic and therapeutic considerations of postcesarean wound infection.

Wound infections complicate different procedures to a degree commensurate with the species and concentration of bacteria introduced into the wound, the condition of the tissues of the wound after surgical manipulation, and the general condition of the larger support system, the host. Stratification of surgical wounds in regard to their probable bacterial inoculum was achieved by the categories of the National Research Council established in 1964 (Table 25.1). By this classification system, cesarean delivery is considered clean refined in elective repeat cases with intact membranes and clean contaminated otherwise.

Infection rates vary according to these classifications and increase dramatically with increasing wound soilage. Clean refined cases are reported to have infection rates of 1.3%–4.7%, whereas infection in con-

TABLE 25.1 Classification of Wounds

Clean
No inflammation
No break in technique
Neither gastrointestinal nor respiratory tract entered, but transection of appendix or cystic duct considered clean in absence of acute inflammation
Entrance of genitourinary or biliary tract considered clean in absence of infected urine or bile
Subdivided into refined-clean (elective, not drained, and primarily closed) and other clean (clean cases other than refined-clean)
Clean-Contaminated
Entrance of gastrointestinal or respiratory tract without significant spillage
Minor break in technique
Entrance of genitourinary tract or biliary tract in the presence of infected urine or bile
Contaminated
Major break in technique
Acute bacterial inflammation with pus
Spillage from gastrointestinal tract
Traumatic wound, fresh, from relatively clean source
Dirty
Presence of pus
Perforated viscus
Traumatic wound, old, or from dirty source

Source: National Academy of Sciences–National Research Council, Division of Medical Sciences, Ad Hoc Committee of the Committee on Trauma: Postoperative wound infections: The influence of ultraviolet irradiation of the operating room and of various other factors. *Ann Surg* 160(suppl 12):1, 1964.

taminated cases may range as high as 48.7%.[2,3] Wound infection rates for cesarean delivery are variable, ranging from 1% to 7%.[4–9]

The cesarean delivery rate has spiraled upward in recent years for a variety of reasons. Because the complications of cesarean delivery exceed those of vaginal delivery, overall infectious morbidity has also increased. Cesarean delivery rates in 1970 were only 5.5%, increasing to 15.2% in 1978 and 22% in 1986. Maternal infectious morbidity results in increased discomfort and pain, as well as increased expense due to longer hospital stays. It has been estimated that a wound infection prolongs the average hospital stay about 6 days and increase the cost to the patient from $775 to $1,302.[10] More importantly, infection is one of the major causes of maternal mortality from cesarean delivery.[11]

HISTORICAL ASPECTS

The historical foundations of antisepsis stem from the treatment of non-surgical wounds and begin with the first recorded surgical history of 48 cases in the Edwin Smith papyrus of 3,000 B.C.[12,13] The Egyptian treatment of wounds was notable for gentleness in the handling of tissues and for suture and bandage approximation of soft tissue wounds. Expectant management was a notable part of their practice, particularly in infected wounds.

Hippocrates, the great teacher and first father of medicine from the fifth century B.C., advocated avoiding treatment of wounds with dressing, ointments, oils, or grease. He felt that wounds should be dried with no bandage, except for the application of cataplasm.

Galen of Pergamum, writing in the second century A.D. and the dominant influence on medicine for the next 1400 years, recognized the importance of incision and drainage of abscesses, albeit to allow better balance of the humors causing the disease.

The first strong attacks on the dogma of Galenic thought came from Paracelsus (1493–1541). Although his theories were not an improvement, he began the process of questioning the humoral theories. In 1545 Ambrose Pare published his story of turning away from the use of boiling oil in the treatment of gunshot wounds in the Battle of Metz. This rediscovery of improved healing with gentle treatment of traumatic wounds was the beginning of modern wound treatment. Pare advocated turpentine, rose oil, egg yolk, and aqua vitae for wounds, popularized the use of ligature in amputation, and introduced podalic version.

In 1840, hypochlorite was promulgated by Semmelweiss for washing the hands and instruments. This seminal contribution to the attack on puerperal sepsis was the first cogent work concerning surgical asepsis. In 1843 Oliver Wendell Holmes published on "The Contagiousness of Puerperal Sepsis" in the United States, wherein he recommended washing hands, changing clothing and washing after postmortems, and avoiding delivery after contact with cases of sepsis.[14]

Lister first used carbolic acid on compound fractures in 1865 and Reyher introduced phenol to Germany in 1874, utilizing the antiseptic as an immediate treatment on the battlefield. He developed the concept of primary debridement and secondary closure, with a success unsurpassed until the application of antibiosis in World War II.

WOUND INFECTION

The balance of the factors of wound healing, bacterial inoculum, local wound conditions, and the patient's systemic support of the wound determine the ultimate result. Wounds with even small inoculums may become infected because of poor surgical technique, and even perfect wound handling does not prevent infection in cases of gross contamination. Direct contamination by the air or breaks in sterile technique are most easily understood; however, the final common pathway for organisms to the wound from the multitude of other sources is unknown.

The sources of bacteria are broadly divided into the patient herself; the operator and the surgical team; the surgical instruments, solutions, drapings, and dressings; and the air and surrounding environment. Preventive measures to reduce the patient's endogenous flora begin upon admission. Remote sites of infection must be treated, if possible, prior to elective surgery. The presence of a remote infection was found to be an independent determinant of wound infection, increasing the overall rate from 6.7% to 18.4%.[3] Elimination of the source is preferable to merely attempting to block its access to the wound. Reduction of the patient's gross cutaneous flora is accomplished by preoperative showers. Using hexachlorophene, Cruse and Foord were able to reduce the infection rate from 2.3% to 1.3%.[2] Removal of hair from the operative site is required to allow the adhesion of dressings, but any method of hair removal is associated with an increased infection rate, likely damaging the skin in some fashion and providing breaks for bacterial entry. If shaving is required, it should be done in the operating room. Alexander et al showed that clipping hair on the morning of surgery resulted in significantly lower infection rates than clipping hair the evening prior to surgery or shaving at any time.[15] Cruse and Foord examined clean cases and noted a decrease in the infection rate from 2.5% in a shaved group, to 1.7% in a group where the pubic hair was clipped, to 1.4% when an electric clipper was used, and to 0.9% when no clipping or shaving was done.[2] Infection rates of clean-contaminated and clean cases of tubal ligation and total abdominal hysterectomy were not affected by any method of hair removal, with no data available for cesarean delivery.[3]

Preparation of the patient's skin in the operating room is a combination of mechanical cleansing of dirt and debris, removal of bacteria, and the application of a bactericidal solution. Bacteria, notably *Staphylococcus aureus,* are resident in the hair follicles, and can be appreciably reduced but not totally eliminated. The antiseptic agents most commonly used for preparation of the patient's skin and the surgeon's hands include iodophors, chlorhexidine, and hexachlorophene. Iodophors and chlorhexidine are bactericidal on contact and have a wide range of antimicrobial activity. Hexachlorophene has been abandoned by some because of its slower onset of activity, predominance of gram-positive activity, pH and solvent dependence, and the demonstration of systemic absorbance.[16]

Preparation of the patient should be accomplished with sterile supplies and the wearing of sterile gloves after scrubbing. The popular use of plastic skin drapes offers no advantage over cloth drapes, as the fluids encountered during surgery cause loosening at the edges and destroy the protective effect. Plastic drapes are useful for covering and isolating sources of infection such as fistulas or ostomies. Wound drapes, on the other hand, have been found to be nearly 100% successful in reducing the introduction of endogenous and exogenous bacteria into abdominal wounds.[17]

Cesarean delivery involves the transmission of vaginal and uterine contents to the peritoneum and wound. In a study of 65 premenopausal women, vaginal cultures revealed an average of 9.1 different organisms, 3.9 species of aerobic bacteria, 0.5 species of microaerophilic bacteria, and 4.7 species of anaerobic bacteria, with predominance of lactobacilli,

TABLE 25.2 Aerobic and Anaerobic Bacteria Commonly Present in Amniotic Fluid with Ruptured and Intact Membranes

Bacteria	Ruptured Membranes	Intact Membranes
Anaerobic	*Bacteroides vicius*	*Fusobacterium nucleatum*
	Peptostreptococcus anaerobius	*Bacteroides corrodens*
	Peptococcus asaccharolyticus	*Bacteroides ochraceus*
	Bacteroides species	*Peptostreptococcus micros*
Aerobic	Group B streptococci	*Staphylococcus epidermidis*
	Diphtheroids	Nonhemolytic streptococci
	Escherichia coli	*Hemophilus influenzae*
	Enterococcus	*Listeria monocytogenes*
	Klebsiella pneumoniae	*Pseudomonas aeruginosa*
	Corynebacterium vaginale	*Klebsiella pneumoniae*
	Staphylococcus epidermidis	Group B streptococci

Source: Gall SA: Infections in the female genital tract. *Comp Ther* 9:34, 1983.

peptococci, peptostreptococci, and bacteroid species.[18] During pregnancy, however, the number of species and proportion of anaerobes decreases, while those of lactobacilli, diphtheroids, and *Candida albicans* increase markedly. *Escherichia coli* is present in 30% of women, whereas group B streptococci, anaerobic species, and staphylococci are found in less than 10%. Group A streptococci are rare.[19]

Factors predisposing the patient to increased bacterial concentration in the uterus and/or vagina prior to delivery result in an increased infection rate. The celiotomy wound in cesarean delivery was believed by Sweet et al to be contaminated similarly to abdominal trauma or gunshot wounds.[20] As demonstrated by Gall,[18] rupture of membranes results in a change in the flora of the amniotic cavity as vaginal bacterial colonize the amniotic fluid (Table 25.2). In a study of amniotic fluid cultures done at the time of primary cesarean delivery, 66/88 (75%) of patients were culture positive, with an average of 3.5 organisms, with 44% being highly virulent bacteria.[21] It is important to note that patients with unrecognized chorioamnionitis and premature labor may have pathogens consistent with bowel flora even in the absence of rupture of membranes.[18] Compared with elective cases, Nielsen and Hokegard found an increase in infectious morbidity in patients undergoing cesarean following labor with ruptured membranes. This was particularly evident in emergent cases (Table 25.3). Gibbs found that the use of internal fetal monitoring was relatively unimportant as a determinant of infection compared to the duration of labor, the presence of ruptured membranes, and multiple vaginal examinations.[22] Other studies consistently reported a significant increase in infectious morbidity with increasing length of ruptured membranes, longer labor, and greater number of vaginal exams,[4–6,11,23] although the independent contribution of any of one of these factors is unclear.

The flora isolated from the postcesarean delivery wound infection parallel the amniotic flora and are similar to those of postpartum endo-

TABLE 25.3 Wound Infection Rates in Cesarean Delivery

Case Status	Wound Infection Rate (%)
Rupture of membranes, no uterine contractions	29.7
All emergent cases	24.2
Uterine contractions, membranes intact	16.9
Emergent, membranes intact, no contractions	7.8
Elective	4.7

Source: Nielsen TF, Hokegard KH: Postoperative cesarean section morbidity: A prospective study. *Am J Obstet Gynecol* 146:911, 1983.

metritis, with a mixed anaerobic and aerobic character. *Staphylococcus aureus, E. coli, Proteus mirabilis, Bacteroides* species, and beta-hemolytic streptococci are frequently isolated. Clostridial species are more rarely found.[20] This mixed nature of the infection creates a synergistic system between the aerobes and anaerobes that may follow a particularly fulminant course. Thus, bacterial contamination of cesarean wounds involves large microbial doses of relatively virulent organisms. This level of inoculum is especially relevant because the minimal infecting dose of bacteria under optimal conditions is only 1×10^5 per gram of tissue.

Other sources of bacterial wound contamination were examined by Howe and Marston in their 1962 study of lengthy abdominal operations. Elaborate sampling and cultures of the air, operating theater, nasopharynx of patients, operating team, ward staff, blood, and wounds correlated 10 of 18 infected cases with a human source of *Staphylococcus aureus*.[24] The authors documented that the majority of serious wound infections arose from seeding in the operating room and came from surgical personnel or the patient. One case of possible blood-borne infection was also documented. No incident of contamination in 330 cases implicated the surgeon's gloves. Surgical instruments are easily and completely sterilized, as are disposable sutures and other operative paraphernalia, but these may become contaminated by other sources and thus serve as a final pathway to the patient's wound. The use of impervious, nonwettable gowns and drapes is as important as the use of masks. Eliminating superfluous operating room personnel and traffic further limits the human sources. Extremely efficient air filtering systems with positive-pressure rooms and laminar flow have rendered the use of ultraviolet lights unimportant in the majority of cases.[25]

In addition to sterile technique, other factors are important in the prevention of wound infection. These include adequate hemostasis, debridement of devitalized and dead tissue, approximation of tissue in the absence of tension, and obliteration of dead space. Each of these basic procedures contributes significantly to proper healing.

Restoration of adequate tissue oxygen partial pressure (PO_2) is also essential for healing. Tissue oxygenation assumes a critical role in bacterial phagocytosis and intracellular killing.[26] Neutrophil chemotaxis is unchanged over a wide range of tissue PO_2, but the ability to carry out intracellular killing, particularly against *Staphylococcus* and gram-negative organisms such as *E. coli, Serratia marcescens, Klebsiella pneumoniae,* and *Proteus* species is markedly reduced in hypoxic environments. Intracellular killing is a result of markedly increased phagocytic cell oxygen consumption and reduction to form superoxides, hydroxyl radicals, hydrogen peroxide, and singlet oxygen. These very active substances are lethal antimicrobial agents.[27] Postoperative hypotension and anemia also contribute to infection by limiting oxygen and phagocyte delivery to the tissue.[2,5,6,23]

WOUND HEALING

The initial period of hypoxia and the trauma of surgical manipulation cause a brief vasoconstriction and then a prolonged period of capillary dilatation. Precapillary sphincters relax, increasing blood flow per gram of tissue. Endothelial junctions become less closely adherent, allowing exudation of serum from the postcapillary venules under the influence of prostaglandins, histamine, and kinins. With this hyperemia and hemoconcentration, capillary stasis ensues. Products from the activated complement and coagulation systems aid in phagocyte chemotaxis. The fibrin clot establishes the earliest structure within the wound and forms a seal against microbial contamination at the wound surface.

Phagocytic cells from the blood marginate and then egress into the wound, initially in a proportion similar to their ratio in the blood. The polymorphonuclear leukocytes, with a shorter life span, die, leaving behind additional digestive enzymes; mononuclear cells predominate after 1–2 days. At this time, fibroblasts have extended from the capillary adventitia. Aided by the fibrinolytic activity of the proliferating network of capillary endothelium, these cells create the initial collagen fiber networks that will form the basis for the healed wound's scar. Wound strength is markedly increased by the deposition of collagen in the wound and its organization by the fibroblasts.[28]

This rich interplay between phagocytic cells, capillary endothelium, and fibroblasts serves to eliminate debris, including bacteria, to revascularize the wound, and then to rebuild the damaged tissue. Poor surgical technique hinders this process. Dead and devitalized tissues become additional debris to be removed. Regions that are underperfused have low oxygen tension and rapidly dropping oxidation-reduction potential. This hinders the penetration and function of phagocytes. These regions become a rich medium free of host defenses. These bacterial strongholds allow continued wound inflammation, tissue edema, and delayed healing. Additionally, fibroblasts are unable to function at low oxygen tensions, delaying restoration of wound integrity. The cesarean delivery wound is often contaminated with foreign material, particularly debris from the products of conception. Careful irrigation of the uterus and the wound helps to decrease this insult.

A balance must be reached in surgical technique between hemostasis and devitalization. Overly enthusiastic hemostasis with electrocautery or ligatures, which include extraneous tissue or are too tightly tied, both unnecessarily create areas of dead tissue. Delicate technique in using fine transfixion ligatures, for hemostasis as advocated by Halsted,[29] and avoiding electrocautery as much as possible by taking time to compress small bleeders gently, are rewarded by improved tissue viability. Gentle irrigation is used to remove debris and dilute bacterial contamination. Cruse and Foord found that any use of electrocautery doubled wound infection rates across all categories.[2] This detrimental effect was eliminated when the finer McEndoe cautery was substituted for the Bovie at Foothills Hospital.[30]

Seromas and hematomas produce effects similar to those of devitalized tissue in that oxygen tension is very low and phagocytic penetration is poor. Hematomas provide an additional barrier to healing, as fibroblasts have no fibrinolytic capability. Further collagen construction must wait for the fibrinolytic activity of the capillary endothelium, humoral factors, or macrophages. These fluid collections mechanically prevent tissue apposition, compromise circulation to surrounding tissue by compression, and provide a rich nidus for bacterial activity. Wound tissue placed under tension will similarly experience decreased circulation and the creation of dead space by bridging effects.

Surgical drains are indicated in cases where the collection of blood, serum, or infected fluid is anticipated. The removal of such materials prevents their mechanical disruption of the wound and the development of bacterial reservoirs. The presence of such a path from the outside merits careful consideration. Penrose drains are always culture positive at their deep end upon removal; however, the closed wound suction system remains sterile as long as flow continues. Drains should always be brought out of the body through a stab wound separate from the surgical incision and removed when they are no longer productive. The closed suction system allows simple collection of all drainage, facilitating its disposal and reducing its potential as an infective source to other patients on the ward. An additional advantage of the closed suction drain is its ability to aid in closure of dead space and to promote early adherence of tissue. This is especially relevant in the obese patient who has a large amount of relatively avascular tissue. Tissue tension should be primarily relieved by approximation of the strong fascial layer, but retention sutures in the massively obese patient may be required.

Sutures, despite their positive effects, represent foreign bodies in a wound and increase the likelihood of infection. The surgeon's choice and use of sutures is important. A simple piece of silk placed in a wound provides a nidus for infection and decreases the minimal inoculum of bacteria required for infection by a factor of 10,000. Increasing diameter and braided strands increase infection rates, as they provide a greater area for bacterial lodgement. Suture should be chosen on the basis of strength and the period of time during which that suture strength will be required. Ideally, the smallest-diameter suture that provides adequate strength should be used.

Chromic gut lasts for only 2–3 weeks and is inadequate as a fascial suture, but is appropriate for the repair of the uterine incision. Polyglycolic acid (PGA) suture has a linear decrease to zero strength over 4 weeks; PDS suture may remain for 6 months; and Dacron, cotton, silk, nylon, and polypropylene are not absorbed. A review of abdominal wound closure techniques concluded that monofilament running suture placed at least 1.5 cm from the cut edge provides the most preferable fascial closure, and when properly performed, obviates the need for retention sutures.[28] Polypropylene or PGA sutures are excellent choices for fascial approximation in cesarean delivery. Importantly, polypropylene will retain its strength in the event of an infection, preserving the integrity of the fascial layer.[28]

THE OBESE PATIENT

The poorly vascularized fatty tissue of the obese patient presents particular problems in avoiding wound tension, closing dead space, and ensuring adequate tissue PO_2. Fatty tissue tolerates contamination less well than better-perfused tissues. Green and Sarubbi identified obesity as one of four factors significantly associated with febrile morbidity after cesarean delivery.[5] Nielsen and Hokegard's 1983 prospective study corroborated these findings.[6] Their definition of obesity (weight at delivery = desirable pregravid weight + 30 lb) was particularly stringent. Obesity is a strong independent factor in wound infection regardless of the degree of contamination and despite an association with increased age and longer procedures.[31] Gallup recommends a midline incision, a superficial Hemovac drain, nonabsorbable monofilament fascial closure with a Smead-Jones stitch, and avoidance of subcutaneous suture[32] (see also Chapter 12). Other authors recommend a periumbilical transverse incision, thereby avoiding both operating through a large panniculus and placing an incision under a large, moist skinfold.[33] In the obese patient, subcutaneous suture only provides extra foreign material in a wound already predisposed to infection. Fragile adipose tissue tends to heal relatively poorly and requires particular attention to gentle technique.

OTHER HOST FACTORS

Changes in the immune system secondary to pregnancy are also important considerations in wound infection. Tolerance to survival of the fetal allograft implies an adaption in the maternal immune system. Humoral and cellular immune responses are blunted, natural killer activity is decreased, and thymus-dependent leukocyte reactivity is reduced.[19] Pregnant women are more susceptible to infections from several different bacteria and have a greatly increased incidence of candidiasis. Other systemic factors increasing wound infection rates include the use of steroids, poor nutritional status, diabetes, and blood transfusions. Approximately 2%–4% of Americans have documented diabetes and an additional 2%–4% have abnormal glucose metabolism. Prevalence increases with age, involving 40%–60% of those in the ninth decade of life.[34] Pregnancy is a diabetogenic state in which abnormal carbohydrate metabolism is frequent. However, incidence figures during pregnancy are difficult to obtain. High glucose levels and ketosis provide an enriched culture medium and adversely affect the ability of cells to phagocytose bacteria. Diabetes was found to be a significant risk factor for wound infection by Cruse.[9] However, in the National Research Council study, the increase in the wound infection rate from 7.4% to 10.4% was explained entirely by the advanced age of the diabetic population studied. Hjortrup et al. found a 25% increase in complications in a diabetic population undergoing major vascular, abdominal, or femoral neck fracture surgery.[35] These data suggest that close monitoring of blood glucose levels during the peripartum period is important in decreasing susceptibility to infection. Diabetic patients also have an increased nasopharyngeal staphylococcus carriage rate and tend to be more obese than nondiabetic patients. Other significant factors affecting the diabetic during pregnancy are an increased risk of preeclampsia, an increased birth weight, and an increased frequency of labor dystocia, all of which predispose to an increased cesarean delivery rate in this population.[36]

Exogenous corticosteroid administration has been shown to affect wound healing and host antimicrobial activity. The National Research Council found an increase in infection rate from 7.1% to 16% in patients receiving steroids. Although these patients were somewhat older and had longer preoperative stays the difference was felt to be significant. Cruse and Foord were not able to demonstrate a difference in infection rates in patients receiving steroids.[2] Steroid administration causes an increase in circulating neutrophils, and leukocyte and monocyte numbers are decreased. This acute change is due primarily to a redistribution phenomenon and occurs with long-term administration as well. Monocytes have a demonstrably impaired ability to effect intracellular killing in these patients; however, no primary effect on the humoral or cell-mediated response to infection is noted after steroid administration. Host defenses may be affected secondarily, as all phases of the inflammatory process are inhibited. Capillary dilatation and resulting local edema, fibrin deposition, and prostaglandin production are severely reduced, and leukocyte migration, macrophage phagocytosis, and plasminogen activator production are inhibited. Because capillary and fibroblast proliferation is reduced, collagen deposition is adversely affected. This ultimately delays the development of wound strength.[37]

Urgency of operation also contributes to the rate of wound infection in cesarean delivery. Hawrylyshyn noted an increase in wound infection from 3.7% in nonemergent primary cesarean delivery to 15.4% in emergency cases. This rate is comparable to the 3.2% rate in elective repeat abdominal delivery.[4] Green and Sarrubi found urgency (elective versus emergent) to be a significant independent factor in the overall infection rate.[5] Nielsen and Hokegard found that infection from all sources rose significantly from 4.7% in elective cases to 24.2% in emergent procedures.[6] These increases may be due to inadequate patient preparation, derangements in circulation stability associated with emergent cases, or unknown factors.

Another factor, the time of day when the operation was performed, was not found to be significant in the National Research Council study.[3] Procedures performed from midnight to 8 A.M. were associated with a doubling in infection rate,[30] but factors such as case mix were not considered. When these factors were taken into account, the time of day differences were insignificant.[2]

Finally, prophylactic antibiotics have been shown to decrease cesarean delivery infection rates. For more details, see Chapter 20.

DIAGNOSIS AND TREATMENT OF WOUND INFECTION

Timely diagnosis and treatment is essential in the care of a wound infection. Locally, the infected wound is marked by the cardinal signs of inflammation and often drainage of purulent material. Note should also be made of the presence of subcutaneous emphysema, usually indicating clostridial or other anaerobic infection. The patient may also display leukocytosis and fever. Any wound displaying inflammation that separates at the skin edges should be considered infected. Any infected wound should be opened to the fascia along the affected portion, and a Gram stain and aerobic and anaerobic blood cultures obtained. The success of anaerobic cultures may be enhanced by the inclusion of small pieces of tissue debrided from the wound. These must be placed in appropriate anaerobic transport media to ensure an adequate laboratory specimen. All positive cultures should have sensitivities determined. Endometrial cultures may also be indicated if foul-smelling lochia and uterine tenderness are present. These cultures must also be transported in anaerobic media.

Treatment of the wound site must follow the principles of wound healing.[1] First, inadequate nutrition, anemia, and hypovolemia must be corrected. Collections of purulent matter should be incised and drained; simple aspiration is inadequate. Sharp debridement of dead and devitalized tissue may be followed by enzymatic debridement or chemical debridement with hydrogen peroxide or Dakin's solution. All antiseptic solutions are cytotoxic, and saline lavage should follow their use. Once granulation tissue begins to form, these solutions must be avoided unless gross infection remains. It is incorrect to destroy granulation tissue by making the wound bleed with each dressing change. This vascularized tissue is a prerequisite to eventual secondary closure or epithelialization of the wound surface. Wet-to-dry dressings should be discontinued and replaced with dry or wet-to-wet dressings once granulation tissue appears. This rich vascular carpet affords an excellent surface that, when approximated, will quickly continue the healing process. If the wound is to be left open for closure by secondary intention, a sterile scab should be allowed to form under which epithelialization may most efficiently take place. If the wound is too large to epithelialize from the skin edges, split thickness skin grafts may be applied to this surface.

Systemic antibiotics are generally not indicated for simple wound infections because drainage is sufficient. *Staphylococcus* is the most frequent isolate, particularly in the more superficial areas of the wound.[18] However, wound infections frequently have mixed flora, with *Bacteroides* species and *Enterobacter* being the most frequent anaerobic isolates. *Chlamydia* and *Ureaplasma* may prove to be important organisms as culture techniques for these species improve. An argument for avoiding systemic antibiotics is that resolution of one component of such a mixed infection often cures the problem.[38] Should systemic therapy be required, initial coverage should be governed by consideration of susceptibility to the isolates most frequently found in these wounds in the hospital in question. Broadly speaking, aerobic gram-positive organisms such as *Staphylococcus* will require penicillinase-resistant compounds, nafcillin, or methicillin, whereas *Streptococcus* remains susceptible to penicillin. *Enterococcus* requires either ampicillin, semisynthetic penicillin, or vancomycin in addition to an aminoglycoside. Aerobic gram-negative species are generally covered by aminoglycosides. Anaerobic gram-negative species require clindamycin, metronidazole, or chloramphenicol. Gram-positive anaerobes are sensitive to penicillin but may be missed with newer cephalosporins.[20] Once susceptibilities on positive cultures are completed, the most appropriate drug combination should be employed.

NECROTIZING FASCIITIS

The most serious complication of wound infection is necrotizing fasciitis. This condition requires extensive surgical debridement. Necrotizing infections of the abdominal wall may be due to clostridial organisms (clostridial myonecrosis) or to single or multiple nonclostridial organisms acting synergistically (necrotizing fasciitis). The spectrum of clostridial infection ranges from simple contamination to myonecrosis. Localized clostridial cellulitis requires local debridement, whereas spreading cellulitis may be rapidly fatal secondary to septic shock and disseminated intravascular coagulation.

With clostridial myonecrosis, the muscle has been rendered susceptible by ischemic injury. Contiguous viable muscle tissue is invaded by clostridial exotoxins, causing the muscle to become pale and edematous. Later it does not contract when incised, and looks beefy red and nonviable. There may be associated cutaneous changes, with the formation of fluid-filled bullae and frank gangrene. These findings may be difficult to distinguish from nonclostridial necrotizing fasciitis.

Necrotizing fasciitis is usually a synergistic infection that destroys subcutaneous tissues. About 80% of the cases reported are associated with minor trauma or surgery. The level of involvement, ie, superficial or deep, is related principally to the portal of entry of the organisms. The process extends from the source of devitalized fascia, with undermining of skin and progressive necrosis of the subcutaneous tissues. Gangrene of the skin occurs, with thrombosis of nutrient vessels in the subcutaneous tissue. The presence of crepitus suggests gas formation. This is caused by bacterial metabolism in an anaerobic environment and is seen more often in infection caused by facultative bacteria.

A high index of suspicion and an aggressive attitude are essential to the treatment of necrotizing fasciitis, and early diagnosis is critical. Debridement must be performed promptly and must include excision of all devitalized tissue. Such debridement may have to be repeated on multiple occasions. Adjuncts to treatment include high dose penicillin, an aminoglycoside, and either clindamycin or metronidazole as antibiotics along with hyperharic oxygen.

FASCIAL DEHISCENCE

Fascial dehiscence is an infrequent condition, occurring in 4.7% of wound infections.[23] This is a troublesome complication, greatly increasing morbidity and requiring a return to the operating theater. The presence of a large serosanguineous discharge from the wound heralds a fascial dehiscence. It is preferable to inspect and open the wound under sterile conditions in the operating room. The wound needs to be investigated, cleaned, debrided, and closed with Smead-Jones or retention sutures. Occasionally, loops of small bowel may protrude through an incision. This is a surgical emergency. The small bowel should be covered with wet sterile dressing and definitive closure performed in an operating room.

SUMMARY

Increased cesarean delivery rates and the greater infectious morbidity associated with this procedure mandate surveillance of factors involved in wound infections. Efforts to reduce bacterial contamination include timely delivery—avoiding emergency operations, treatment of concurrent remote infections, appropriate patient preparation—clipping hair instead of shaving, and reducing operating room personnel. Surgical technique should emphasize the principles of wound healing such as hemostasis, approximation of tissues, gentle handling to avoid unnecessary tissue devitalization, and avoidance of suture and dead space. Drains should be of the closed suction type and exteriorized through a separate stab incision. Perioperative management must be concerned with adequate volume and hematocrit support, tight control of serum glucose levels, and avoidance of corticosteroids if possible as well as the use of prophylactic antibiotics.

Postoperatively, frequent and regular inspection and palpation of every wound leads to early diagnosis and treatment of infections that do occur. Incision and drainage, appropriate debridement and dressings, cultures, and systemic antibiotics are integral parts of postoperative wound care. As the wound infection is eliminated, decisions on whether to perform secondary closure or allow healing by secondary intention must be made.

REFERENCES

1. Reid MR: Some considerations of the problems of wound healing. *N Engl J Med* 215:753, 1936.
2. Cruse PJE, Foord R: A five-year prospective study of 23,649 surgical wounds. *Arch Surg* 107:206, 1973.
3. National Academy of Sciences–National Research Council, Division of Medical Sciences, Ad Hoc Committee of the Committee on Trauma: Postoperative wound infections: The influence of ultraviolet irradiation of the operating room and of various other factors. *Ann Surg* 160(suppl 12):1, 1964.
4. Hawrylyshyn PA, Bernstein P, Papsin FR: Risk factors associated with infection following cesarean section. *Am J Obstet Gynecol* 139:294, 1981.
5. Green SL, Sarubbi FA: Risk factors associated with postcesarean section febrile morbidity. *Obstet Gynecol* 49:686, 1977.
6. Nielsen TF, Hokegard KH: Postoperative cesarean section morbidity: A prospective study. *Am J Obstet Gynecol* 146:911, 1983.
7. Levin DK, Gorchels C, Andersen R: Reduction of post-cesarean section infectious morbidity by means of antibiotic irrigation. *Am J Obstet Gynecol* 147:273, 1983.
8. Farrell SJ, Andersen HF, Work BA: Cesarean section: Indications and postoperative morbidity. *Obstet Gynecol* 56:696, 1980.
9. Cruse P: Infection surveillance: Identifying the problems and the high-risk patient. *South Med J* 70 (suppl 1):4, 1977.
10. Green JW, Wenzel RP: Postoperative wound infection: A controlled study of the increased duration of hospital stay and direct cost of hospitalization. *Ann Surg* 185:264, 1977.
11. Petitti DB: Maternal mortality and morbidity in cesarean section. *Clin Obstet Gynecol* 28:763, 1985.
12. Wangensteen OH, Wangensteen SD, Klinger CF: Some pre-listerian and post-listerian antiseptic wound practices and the emergency of asepsis. *Surg Obstet Gynecol* 137:677, 1973.
13. Zimmerman LM, Veith I: *Great Ideas in the History of Surgery*. New York, Dover Publications, 1967.

14. Lister J: On the antiseptic principle in the practice of surgery. *Lancet* 2:353, 1867.
15. Alexander JW, Fischer JE, Boyajian M, et al: The influence of hair-removal methods on wound infections. *Arch Surg* 118:347, 1983.
16. Altemeier WA, Burke JF, Pruitt BA, et al: *Manual on Control of Infections in Surgical Patients,* ed 2. Philadelphia, JB Lippincott Co, 1984.
17. Raahave D: Effect of plastic skin and wound drapes on the density of bacteria in operation wounds. *Br J Surg* 63:421, 1976.
18. Gall SA: Infections in the female genital tract. *Comp Ther* 9:34, 1983.
19. Ho JL, Barza M: An approach to infectious disease, in Gleicher N (ed): *Principles of Medical Therapy in Pregnancy.* New York, Plenum Press, 1985.
20. Sweet RL, Yonekura ML, Hill G, et al: Appropriate use of antibiotics in serious obstetric and gynecologic infections. *Am J Obstet Gynecol* 136:719, 1983.
21. Gall SA, Hill GB: Single versus multiple dose piperacillin in primary cesarean operation. In press.
22. Gibbs RS, Jones PM, Wilder CJY: Internal fetal monitoring and maternal infection following cesarean section. *Obstet Gynecol* 52:193, 1978.
23. Gibbs RS, Blanco JD, St Clair PJ: A case-control study of wound abscess after cesarean delivery. *Obstet Gynecol* 62:498, 1983.
24. Howe CW, Marston AT: A study on sources of postoperative staphylococcal infection. *Surg Gynecol Obstet* 115:266, 1962.
25. Sanderson MC, Bentley G: Assessment of wound contamination during surgery: A preliminary report comparing vertical laminar flow and conventional theatre systems. *Br J Surg* 63:431, 1976.
26. Kuhn HH, Ullman U, Kuhn FW: New aspects on the pathophysiology of wound infection and wound healing—the problem of lowered oxygen pressure in the tissue. *Infection* 13:52, 1985.
27. Knighton DR, Halliday B, Hunt TK: Oxygen as an antibiotic. *Arch Surg* 119:199, 1984.
28. Poole GV: Mechanical factors in abdominal wound closure: The prevention of fascial dehiscence. *Surgery* 97:631, 1985.
29. Halsted WS: Ligature and suture material. *JAMA* 60:1119, 1913.
30. Cruse PJE, Foord R: The epidemiology of wound infection. *Surg Clin North Am* 60:27, 1980.
31. Polk HC: Operating room acquired infection: A review of pathogenesis. *Am Surg* 45:349, 1979.
32. Gallup DG: Modifications of celiotomy techniques to decrease morbidity in obese gynecologic patients. *Am J Obstet Gynecol* 150:171, 1984.
33. Krebs HB, Helmkamp BF: Transverse periumbilical incision in the massively obese patient. *Obstet Gynecol* 63:241, 1984.
34. Cahill GF: Diabetes mellitus, in Wyngaarden JB, Smith LH (eds): *Cecil Textbook of Medicine,* ed 16. Philadelphia, WB Saunders Co, 1982, p 1053.
35. Hjortrup A, Sorensen C, Dyremose E, et al: Influence of diabetes mellitus on operative risk. *Br J Surg* 72:783, 1985.
36. Pritchard JA, MacDonald PC, Gant NF: *Williams Obstetrics,* ed 17. Norwalk, Conn, Appleton-Century-Crofts, 1985, pp 598–604.
37. Gilman AG, Goodman LS, Gilman AC: *The Pharmacological Basis of Therapeutics,* ed 6. New York, Macmillan Co, 1980, p 1478.
38. Hirsch HA, Decker K: The therapy of anaerobic infections in obstetrics and gynecology. *Infection* 8(suppl 2):S195, 1980.

Chapter 26

Diagnosis and Management of Postcesarean Endomyometritis

Patrick Duff, MD

The incidence of cesarean delivery now exceeds 20% in many medical centers in the United States. As increasing numbers of abdominal deliveries have been performed, infection has become recognized as the most frequent complication associated with this surgical procedure. This chapter will review the pathophysiology, microbiology, and diagnosis of postcesarean endomyometritis and present appropriate measures for the treatment of this common infection.

INCIDENCE

If prophylactic antibiotics are not used, the incidence of postcesarean endomyometritis varies from a low of 5% to a high of approximately 85%, with a mean of 35% to 40% in most series.[1] In general, the lowest incidence of infection occurs in middle- and upper-income women undergoing scheduled abdominal delivery. Conversely, the highest incidence of infection occurs in young, indigent patients having surgery after extended duration of labor and ruptured membranes. Consistent use of prophylactic antibiotics at the time of abdominal delivery reduces the number of postoperative infections by approximately 50% to 60%.[2,3]

In women who develop postcesarean endomyometritis, the frequency of concurrent bacteremia varies from zero to 25%, with a mean of approximately 10%.[1,2] The incidence of life-threatening sequelae of endomyometritis such as pelvic abscess, septic shock, and septic pelvic thrombophlebitis is now less than 2%. Before the introduction of newer antibiotics with an expanded spectrum of activity against aerobic and anaerobic gram-negative bacilli, the incidence of serious complications of endomyometritis was as high as 4% to 5%.[2,3]

RISK FACTORS

The principal risk factors for postcesarean infection are young age, low socioeconomic status, extended duration of labor and ruptured membranes, and multiple vaginal examinations. The age and socioeconomic status of the patient appear to influence the incidence of infection because of their relationship to the general health and immunocompetence of the host. The number of vaginal examinations, length of labor, and duration of ruptured membranes are of importance in determining the size of the bacterial inoculum present in the uterus at the time of surgery. The duration of internal fetal monitoring, length of surgery, type of anesthesia, preoperative hematocrit, intraoperative blood loss, and experience of the surgeon are relatively weak risk factors for infection when corrections are made for duration of labor and ruptured membranes.[4–6]

MICROBIOLOGY

Postcesarean endomyometritis is a polymicrobial infection caused almost exclusively by bacteria normally present in the lower genital tract. The principal pathogens may be divided into four major groups: aerobic streptococci, anaerobic gram-positive cocci, and aerobic and anaerobic gram-negative bacilli.[1]

Of the aerobic streptococci, the most common pathogens are group B and group D streptococci. Peptococci and Peptostreptococci are the most frequently isolated anaerobic gram-positive cocci. *Escherichia coli* is the predominant aerobic gram-negative bacillus recovered from infected patients, although *Klebsiella pneumoniae* and *Proteus* species are occasional pathogens. The most common anaerobic gram-negative bacilli are *Bacteroides bivius, B. disiens, B. melaninogenicus, B. fragilis,* and *Gardnerella vaginalis.* In addition to these organisms, there now are limited data indicating that, in some instances, *Mycoplasma hominis* and *Chlamydia trachomatis* may cause intrauterine infection.[7] The role of *Ureaplasma urealyticum* in the pathogenesis of upper genitourinary tract infection has not been defined precisely at the present time, although it does not appear to be an important pathogen.

The microorganisms most frequently recovered from patients with bacteremia are *E. coli,* group B streptococci, *Bacteroides* species, anaerobic gram-positive cocci, and *G. vaginalis. M. hominis* has also been isolated from blood cultures in a small number of patients. Although most episodes of bacteremia are caused by a single pathogen, polymicrobial bacteremia has been described in association with postcesarean infection.[8–12]

PATHOPHYSIOLOGY

The development of any infection is dependent upon a complex balance between host defense mechanisms and bacterial virulence factors. Cesarean delivery alters this balance in such a way as to predispose the patient to intrauterine infection.[13] During labor and the ensuing abdominal delivery, the endometrial and peritoneal cavities invariably are contaminated with large numbers of bacteria. The size of the bacterial inoculum is especially high when surgery is performed after multiple vaginal examinations and extended duration of labor and ruptured membranes. The serosanguineous fluid that collects in the pelvic cavity after surgery provides an excellent culture medium for microorganisms, particularly anaerobes. Standard techniques for uterine closure, specifically the double layer of interlocking sutures, create a distinct zone of ischemia and necrosis in myometrial tissue that facilitates the growth of facultative and obligate anaerobes in the lower uterine segment.

The microorganisms inoculated into the pelvic and uterine cavities interact with one another in an intricate manner to produce infection. Aerobic gram-negative bacilli and group B streptococci frequently are associated with early onset of endomyometritis, peritonitis, and bacteremia. The aerobic streptococci, in particular, are capable of rapid dissemination through soft tissue planes. They may cause sufficient inflammatory injury in the operative site that conditions become optimal for accelerated growth of anaerobic bacteria. Anaerobic organisms, especially *Bacteroides* species, are the pathogens most likely to cause abscess formation.[14]

DIAGNOSIS

Clinical Manifestations

Symptoms and signs of endomyometritis usually develop 24 to 48 hours after surgery. The principal clinical manifestations are fever, tachycardia, lower abdominal pain, uterine and adnexal tenderness, and pelvic peritoneal irritation. Some patients will have induration or phlegmon formation in the broad ligament.

In the initial evaluation of the febrile postoperative patient, the major disorders that should be considered in the differential diagnosis are atelectasis, pneumonia, viral syndrome, appendicitis, and acute pyelonephritis. Lower urinary tract infections usually do not cause temperature elevation and systemic symptoms. In patients who fail to respond appropriately to antibiotic therapy, the differential diagnosis must be broadened to include undetected wound infection, mastitis, pelvic abscess, venous thromboembolism, collagen vascular disease, drug fever, factitious fever, and septic pelvic vein thrombophlebitis.[1]

Laboratory Evaluation

The initial laboratory evaluation should include hematocrit, differential white blood cell count, aerobic and anaerobic blood cultures, and aerobic

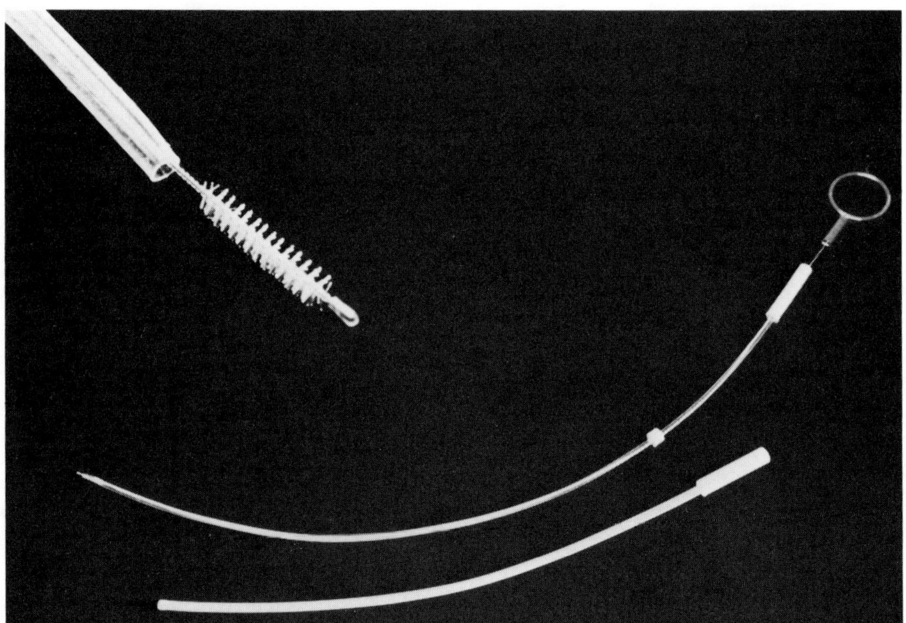

FIGURE 26.1 Uterine sampling device. To use this device, cleanse the cervix with an antiseptic solution. Insert the catheter transcervically. Push forward on the thumb screw to dislodge the ethylene glycol plug from the tip of the outer catheter and advance the biopsy brush into the upper uterine cavity. Rotate the brush through a 360° arc to obtain the uterine culture. Withdraw the brush into the inner catheter and then remove the latter. Cut off the brush and place it in an anaerobic transport medium. The specimen then may be cultured for both aerobes and anaerobes.

and anaerobic endometrial cultures. The best instrument presently available for obtaining endometrial cultures is a double-lumen catheter (Meditech, Watertown, Mass.) that contains a small biopsy brush (Figure 26.1).[15] This instrument, although more expensive than a standard culture device, offers distinct advantages in decreasing the contamination of endometrial cultures by the bacteria that colonize the endocervical canal and upper vagina.

A chest x-ray should be obtained only if there is clinical suspicion of extensive atelectasis, pneumonia, or pulmonary venous thromboembolism. Urine culture is indicated if the patient has physical findings suggestive of an upper tract infection. Pelvic ultrasound or computed tomographic scan of the pelvis may be of value in the unusual situation where a pelvic abscess or ovarian vein thrombosis is suspected.

TREATMENT

Results of Clinical Trials

Table 26.1 summarizes the dosage and spectrum of activity of the principal antibiotics that have been used in the treatment of postcesarean endo-

TABLE 26.1 Antibacterial Activity of Antibiotics Used to Treat Postcesarean Endomyometritis

		Spectrum of Activity				
Drug	**Dosage**	Groups A and B Streptococci	Group D Streptococci	Aerobic Gram-Negative Bacilli	Anaerobic Streptococci	Anaerobic Gram-Negative Bacilli
Penicillins						
Ampicillin	1–2 g, q6h	4+	4+	2–3+	3–4+	2+
Penicillin	5 million units, q6h	4+	0	0	3–4+	2+
Ticarcillin-clavulanic acid	3 g/0.1 g, q4–6h	3+	1+	3+	3–4	3+
Ampicillin-sulbactam	2g/1g, q6h	4+	4+	3+	3–4+	3+
Ureidopenicillins	3–4 g, q6h	3+	3–4+	3+	3–4+	3+
Cephalosporins						
Cefamandole	2 g, q4–6h	3+	0	3+	3–4+	2–3+
Cefazolin	2 g, q8h	3–4+	0	2–3+	3–4+	2+
Cefonicid	1–2 g, q12–24h	3+	0	3+	3–4+	2–3+
Cefoperazone	2–4 g, q12h	3+	0	3+	3–4+	2–3+
Ceforanide	1–2 g, q12h	3+	0	3+	3–4+	2–3+
Cefotaxime	2 g, q6–8h	3+	0	3+	3–4+	2–3+
Cefotetan	1–3 g, q12h	3+	0	3+	3–4+	3+
Cefoxitin	2 g, q6h	3+	0	3+	3–4+	3+
Ceftriaxone	1–2 g, q12–24h	3+	0	3+	3–4+	2–3+
Moxalactam	2 g, q8h	3+	0	3+	3–4+	3+
Carbapenems						
Imipenem-cilastatin	0.5 g, q6h	4+	2+	3–4+	3–4+	3–4+
Drugs Used in Combination Regimens						
Aminoglycosides	Variable	0	0	4+	0	0
Aztreonam	2 g, q8h	0	0	4+	0	0
Clindamycin	0.9 g, q8h	2–3+	0	0	4+	4+
Metronidazole	0.5 g, q6h	0	0	0	4+	4+

Source: Reprinted with permission from *Contemporary OB/GYN* March, 1987. The information presented in this table is based upon data from references 1, 16, and 17.

0, poor activity; 4+, excellent activity.

TABLE 26.2 Results of Combination Antibiotic Therapy for Postcesarean Endomyometritis

Antibiotic	No. of Patients	Incidence of Cure	
		Range (%)	Mean (%)
Penicillin + aminoglycoside[18–22]	373	61–78	75
Clindamycin + aminoglycoside[18,23–31]	521	86–100	92
Clindamycin + aztreonam[25,32]	72	86–91	90

myometritis.[1,16,17] Tables 26.2 and 26.3 present the cumulative results of over 30 investigations that have evaluated different combination and single-agent regimens for treatment of this infection. The following points deserve special emphasis.

The combination of penicillin-aminoglycoside is an inferior treatment modality.[18–22] When compared directly with any other treatment regimen except single-agent therapy with cefamandole or cefoperazone, penicillin-gentamicin produces significantly fewer cures. Moreover, approximately one-third of the patients who fail to respond to this regimen develop serious sequelae of their primary infection.

The combination of metronidazole plus aminoglycoside has not been tested extensively as initial therapy for postcesarean endomyometritis. Because metronidazole lacks activity against aerobic gram-positive cocci, it should be used in combination with both penicillin and an aminoglycoside in order to provide broad-spectrum coverage against genital tract pathogens.

The regimen that has been tested most extensively is clindamycin-aminoglycoside.[18,23–31,44,49,51] Treatment with this combination consistently cures over 90% of patients. Less than 0.5% of women receiving this therapy develop pelvic abscess, septic shock, or septic pelvic vein

TABLE 26.3 Results of Single-Agent Antibiotic Therapy for Postcesarean Endomyometritis

Antibiotic	No. of Patients	Incidence of Cure	
		Range (%)	Mean (%)
Cefamandole[23,33–36]	294	73–90	85
Cefoperazone[37]	107	Multicenter study	84
Cefotaxime[31]	143	Single study	97
Cefotetan[38]	59	Multicenter study	100
Cefoxitin[19,29,39–44]	224	50–100	85
Imipenem-cilastatin[45]	43	Multicenter study	98
Moxalactam[46–49]	278	86–91	89
Ticarcillin-clavulanic acid[50,51]	23	Single study	91
Ureidopenicillins[27,43,52–54]	108	91–100	92

thrombophlebitis. Approximately half of the observed treatment failures observed with this regimen are due to the presence of microorganisms, usually enterococci, that are resistant to both clindamycin and gentamicin. Most of the remaining failures are actually side-effect failures secondary to drug-induced diarrhea.

In otherwise healthy obstetric patients, nephrotoxicity or ototoxicity due to aminoglycosides is extremely rare. In fact, underdosing is the more common problem when aminoglycosides are utilized in obstetric patients.[55] In this regard, the development of a new monobactam antibiotic, aztreonam, is of special interest. This agent has essentially the same spectrum of activity as the aminoglycosides but does not cause serious side effects. The limited experience with this agent in combination with clindamycin for treatment of endomyometritis has been favorable.[25,32]

Cefamandole should not be used as a single agent for the treatment of postcesarean endomyometritis. Its major weakness is its relatively limited activity against *Bacteroides* species. Several of the newer cephalosporins (ceforanide, cefoperazone, ceftriaxone, and cefonicid) have this same limitation in coverage, and thus have no advantage over cefamandole despite their more favorable pharmacokinetic properties.

Of the extended-spectrum cephalosporins and carbapenems, the agents with the best in vitro activity against genital tract pathogens are cefoxitin, moxalactam, cefotetan, and imipenem-cilastatin. In selected clinical trials, both moxalactam and cefoxitin have produced cure rates comparable to those achieved with the combination regimen of clindamycin-aminoglycoside.

The experience to date with cefotetan and imipenem-cilastatin, although limited, has been favorable.[38,45] The former agent has two features that make it particularly attractive. It is relatively inexpensive compared to the other cephalosporins. In addition, it has an extended half-life, thus permitting twice-daily dosing. The superior spectrum of activity of imipenem-cilastatin, combined with its minimal toxicity but relatively high cost, justify restriction of its use to the treatment of seriously ill individuals who have life-threatening nosocomial infections.

Although cefotaxime has less in vitro activity against anaerobes than the agents noted above, the drug showed great efficacy in one recent clinical trial.[31] The results of this investigation are particularly notable because the patients being treated were indigent women with a high risk of developing serious complications of their primary infection.

The most common side effect associated with use of the newer cephalosporins and carbapenems is diarrhea. Approximately 2% to 3% of patients will require discontinuation of therapy because of this troublesome problem. Less common adverse reactions include neutropenia, thrombocytopenia, transaminase enzyme elevation, and pain at the site of injection. Although certain of these agents, notably moxalactam, cefoperazone, and cefamandole, have caused serious bleeding disorders in

TABLE 26.4 Pharmacy Charges for Antibiotic Therapy

Item	Range	Mean
Markup (over wholesale price)	10–961%	135%
Dispensing fee (per day)	\$0.79–\$14.65	\$5.47
Preparation fee (per dose)	\$0.80–\$31.50	\$9.09

Source: Figures in this table are based upon data presented in McCue JD, Hansen C, Gal P: Hospital charges for antibiotics, *Rev Infect Dis* 7:643, 1985.

some individuals, this complication is rarely observed in obstetric patients.[56]

In preliminary investigations, the new extended-spectrum penicillins—azlocillin, piperacillin, mezlocillin, and ticarcillin-clavulanic acid—have cured approximately 90% of infected patients.[27,43,50–54] In small comparative trials, these cure rates have not differed significantly from those achieved by the use of combination therapy with clindamycin-aminoglycoside.

Patients who have failed to respond to extended-spectrum single agents have not developed more serious complications than those treated initially with combination therapy. In addition, there is no evidence to date indicating that the use of these drugs in obstetric patients has resulted in superinfections with resistant organisms. Nevertheless, selection of resistant microorganisms, specifically enterococci, and induction of beta-lactamases in other microorganisms are serious theoretical concerns.

If only the direct cost of the antibiotic is considered, and if recommended doses of drugs are administered, the costs of the ureidopenicillins, ticarcillin-clavulanic acid, cefotetan, cefotaxime, and clindamycin-gentamicin are approximately the same. The combination of metronidazole-penicillin-gentamicin is about two-thirds as expensive as the preceding regimens. The cost of cefoxitin, moxalactam, and imipenem-cilastatin is about 33% to 50% more than that of the regimens described above. These cost estimates do not include indirect charges such as the expense of infusion sets, nursing and pharmacy fees, or the cost of laboratory tests performed to monitor patients for drug toxicity. Table 26.4 shows the results of a recent survey of hospital pharmacists who were asked to indicate the added charges imposed by their hospital for administration of antibiotic solutions.[57] Both the direct cost of the drug and the indirect charges associated with preparation of the drug by the pharmacy must be considered when selecting antibiotic therapy for postcesarean infection.

TREATMENT RECOMMENDATIONS

Once the diagnosis of endomyometritis is established, antibiotic therapy should be initiated with one of the following regimens.

Clindamycin plus aminoglycoside (or aztreonam)

TABLE 26.5 Differential Diagnosis of Refractory Puerperal Fever

Possible Cause	Diagnostic Study	Treatment
Resistant microorganism	Culture and sensitivity of endometrium and blood specimens	Modify antibiotic therapy
Wound infection	Physical examination Aspiration of wound	Incision and drainage of wound
Pelvic abscess	Physical examination Ultrasound CT scan	Continue antibiotics Surgical drainage
Septic pelvic vein thrombophlebitis	Physical examination CT scan Venogram	Continue antibiotics Anticoagulation
Viral syndrome	Differential white cell count to detect lymphocytosis or atypical lymphocytes Mononucleosis serology	Symptomatic treatment Discontinue antibiotics
Venous thromboembolism	Physical examination Venogram Ventilation-perfusion scan of lung	Anticoagulation
Collagen vascular disease	Fluorescent antinuclear antibody	Rheumatology consultation Discontinue antibiotics
Drug fever	Observation of temperature curve Differential white cell count to detect eosinophilia	Discontinue antibiotics
Factitious fever	Observation of patient	Discontinue antibiotics

Extended-spectrum cephalosporin (moxalactam, cefotaxime, cefoxitin, or cefotetan)

Extended-spectrum penicillin

Metronidazole-penicillin-aminoglycoside

In seriously ill patients, the combination of clindamycin plus gentamicin or aztreonam is the preferred regimen. In mildly to moderately ill women, either combination therapy or an extended-spectrum cephalosporin or penicillin is acceptable treatment. If the patient has received a cephalosporin for prophylaxis, treatment with a penicillin may be the better choice because of the possibility that enterococci may be one of the predominant organisms.

Most patients will show a clear response to treatment within 72 hours. The two most common causes of apparent treatment failure are concurrent wound infection and resistant microorganisms. If a wound infection develops, incision and drainage is indicated, but a change in antibiotics usually is not necessary. The principal microorganisms likely to be resistant to initial treatment regimens are aerobic gram-negative bacilli, enterococci, and *Bacteroides* species. If a resistant organism is thought to be present, antibiotic therapy should be modified. In patients receiving clindamycin plus an aminoglycoside or aztreonam, penicillin should be added to the treatment regimen to provide coverage against

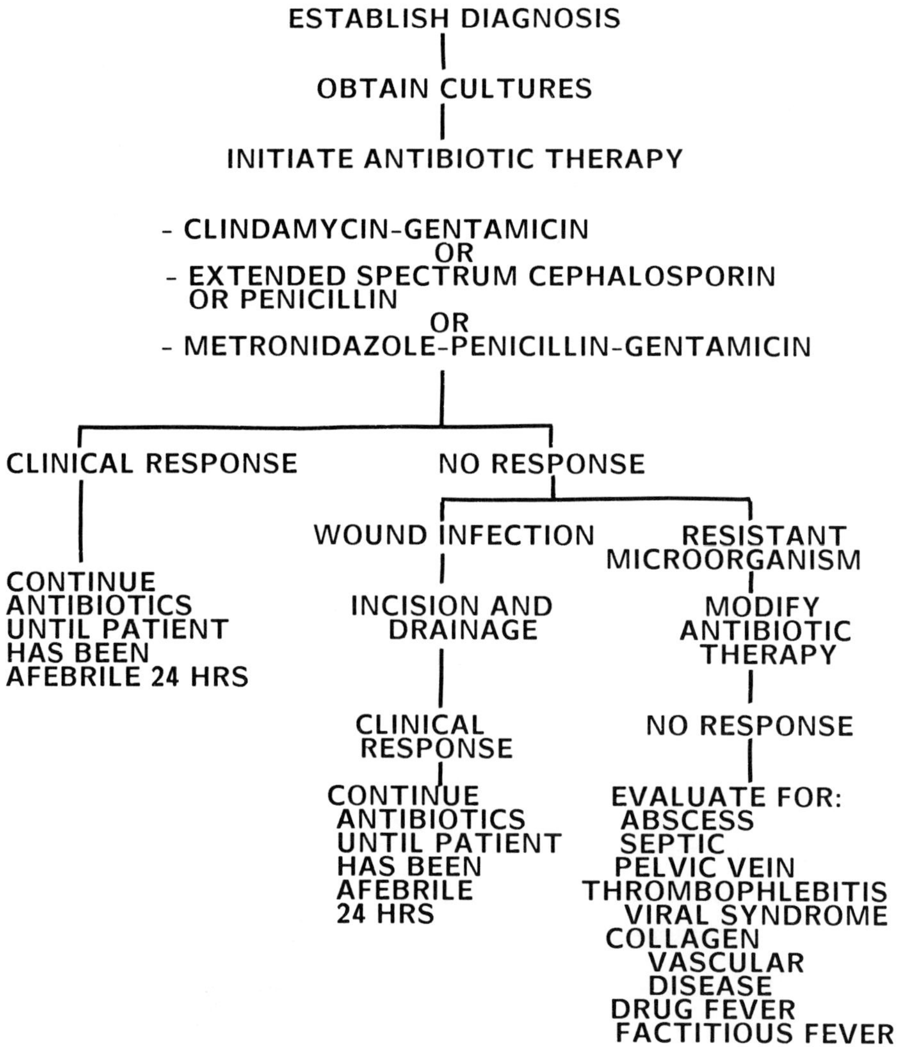

FIGURE 26.2 Treatment protocol for postcesarean endomyometritis.

enterococci. In patients receiving single-agent therapy, one alternative is to change the treatment to clindamycin plus penicillin plus an aminoglycoside. Another alternative would be to add an aminoglycoside if enhanced coverage of aerobic gram-negative bacilli is needed or to administer clindamycin or metronidazole if improved coverage of anaerobes is desired.

Parenteral therapy should be continued for a minimum of 24 hours after the patient becomes afebrile and asymptomatic. At this point, therapy may be discontinued. Patients do not need to be maintained on oral antibiotics after discharge from the hospital. Extended therapy of this nature adds to the patient's expense and increases the risk of side effects without providing any measurable therapeutic benefit. These treatment recommendations are summarized in Figure 26.2.

In patients who fail to improve after a change in antibiotic therapy, another detailed examination should be performed to detect a wound infection or pelvic abscess. Other possible causes of poor treatment response include viral syndrome, venous thrombophlebitis, factitious fever, and drug fever. Table 26.5 summarizes the differential diagnosis and management of refractory puerperal fever. If the treatment guidelines outlined above are followed, less than 1% of patients should present such a diagnostic dilemma for the clinician.

REFERENCES

1. Duff P: Pathophysiology and management of postcesarean endomyometritis. *Obstet Gynecol* 67:269, 1986.
2. Swartz WH, Grolle K: The use of prophylactic antibiotics in cesarean section. A review of the literature. *J Reprod Med* 26:595, 1981.
3. Cartwright PS, Pittaway DE, Jones HW, et al: The use of prophylactic antibiotics in obstetrics and gynecology: A review. *Obstet Gynecol Surv* 39:537, 1984.
4. Gibbs RS: Clinical risk factors for puerperal infection. *Obstet Gynecol* 55:178S, 1980.
5. Repke JT, Spence MR, Calhoun S: Risk factors in the development of cesarean section infection. *Surg Gynecol Obstet* 158:112, 1984.
6. Hagglund L, Christensen KV, Christensen P, et al: Risk factors in cesarean section infection. *Obstet Gynecol* 62:145, 1983.
7. Hoyme UB, Kiviat N, Eschenbach DA: Microbiology and treatment of late postpartum endometritis. *Obstet Gynecol* 68:226, 1986.
8. diZerega GS, Yonekura ML, Keegan K, et al: Bacteremia in post-cesarean section endomyometritis: Differential response to therapy. *Obstet Gynecol* 55:587, 1980.
9. Blanco JD, Gibbs RS, Castaneda YS: Bacteremia in obstetrics: Clinical course. *Obstet Gynecol* 58:621, 1981.
10. Bryan CS, Reynolds KL, More EE: Bacteremia in obstetrics and gynecology. *Obstet Gynecol* 64:155, 1984.
11. Reimer LG, Reller LB: *Gardnerella vaginalis* bacteremia: A review of thirty cases. *Obstet Gynecol* 64:170, 1984.
12. Monif GRG, Baer H: Polymicrobial bacteremia in obstetric patients. *Obstet Gynecol* 48:167, 1976.
13. Gilstrap LC, Cunningham FG: The bacterial pathogenesis of infection following cesarean section. *Obstet Gynecol* 53:545, 1979.
14. Weinstein WM, Onderdonk AB, Bartlett JG, et al: Experimental intra-abdominal abscesses in rats: Development of an experimental model. *Infect Immunol* 10:1250, 1974.
15. Duff P, Gibbs RS, Blanco JD, et al: Endometrial culture techniques in puerperal patients. *Obstet Gynecol* 61:217, 1983.
16. Tally FP, Cuchural GJ, Jacobus NV, et al: Susceptibility of the *Bacteroides fragilis* group in the United States in 1981. *Antimicrob Agents Chemother* 23:536, 1983.
17. Sutter BL, Finegold SM: Susceptibility of anaerobic bacteria to 23 antimicrobial agents. *Antimicrob Agents Chemother* 10:736, 1976.
18. DiZerega G, Yonekura L, Roy S, et al: A comparison of clindamycin-gentamicin and penicillin-gentamicin in the treatment of post-cesarean section endomyometritis. *Am J Obstet Gynecol* 134:238, 1979.
19. Duff P, Keiser JF, Strong SL: A comparative study of two antibiotic regimens for the treatment of operative site infections. *Am J Obstet Gynecol* 142:996, 1978.

20. Gibbs RS, Jones PM, Wilder CJ: Antibiotic therapy of endometritis following cesarean section. Treatment successes and failures. *Obstet Gynecol* 52:31, 1978.
21. Monif GRG, Hempling RE: Antibiotic therapy for the bacteroidaceae in post-cesarean section infections. *Obstet Gynecol* 57:177, 1981.
22. Cunningham FG, Hauth JC, Strong JD, et al: Infectious morbidity following cesarean section. Comparison of two treatment regimens. *Obstet Gynecol* 52:657, 1978.
23. Gibbs RS, Blanco JD, Castaneda YS, et al: A double-blind, randomized comparison of clindamycin-gentamicin versus cefamandole for treatment of post-cesarean section endomyometritis. *Am J Obstet Gynecol* 144:261, 1982.
24. Gibbs RS, Blanco JD, Duff P, et al: A double-blind, randomized comparison of moxalactam versus clindamycin-gentamicin in treatment of endomyometritis after cesarean section delivery. *Am J Obstet Gynecol* 146:769, 1983.
25. Gibbs RS, Blanco JD, Lipscomb KA, et al: Aztreonam versus gentamicin, each with clindamycin, in the treatment of endometritis. *Obstet Gynecol* 65:825, 1985.
26. Gall SA, Kohan AP, Ayers OM, et al: Intravenous metronidazole or clindamycin with tobramycin for pelvic infections. *Obstet Gynecol* 57:51, 1981.
27. Gilstrap LC, Maier RC, Gibbs RS, et al: Piperacillin versus clindamycin plus gentamicin for pelvic infections. *Obstet Gynecol* 64:762, 1984.
28. Sen P, Apuzzio J, Reyclt C, et al: Prospective evaluation of combinations of antimicrobial agents for endometritis after cesarean section. *Surg Gynecol Obstet* 151:89, 1980.
29. Drusano GL, Warren JW, Saah AJ, et al: A prospective randomized controlled trial of cefoxitin versus clindamycin-aminoglycoside in mixed anaerobic-aerobic infections. *Surg Gynecol Obstet* 154:715, 1982.
30. Blanco JD, Gibbs RS, Duff P, et al: Randomized comparison of ceftazidime versus clindamycin-gentamicin in the treatment of obstetrical and gynecologic infections. *Antimicrob Agents Chemother* 24:500, 1983.
31. Hemsell DL, Cunningham FG, DePalma RT, et al: Cefotaxime sodium therapy for endomyometritis following cesarean section: Dose-finding and comparative studies. *Obstet Gynecol* 62:489, 1983.
32. Pastorek JG, Cole C, Aldridge KE, et al: Aztreonam plus clindamycin as therapy for pelvic infections in women. *Am J Med* 78:47, 1985.
33. Cunningham FG, Gilstrap LC, Kappus SS: Cefamandole for treatment of obstetrical and gynecologic infections. *Scand J Infect Dis* 25:75S, 1980.
34. Gall SA, Hill GB: High-dose cefamandole therapy in obstetric and gynecologic infections. *Am J Obstet Gynecol* 137:914, 1980.
35. Gibbs RS, Huff RW: Cefamandole therapy of endomyometritis following cesarean section. *Am J Obstet Gynecol* 133:32, 1980.
36. Cunningham FG, Gilstrap LC, Kappus SS, et al: Treatment of obstetric and gynecologic infections with cefamandole. *Am J Obstet Gynecol* 133:602, 1979.
37. Ling FW, McNeeley SG, Anderson GD, et al: Clinical efficacy of cefoperazone in obstetric and gynecologic infections. *Clin Ther* 6:669, 1984.
38. Poindexter AN, Sweet R, Ritter M: Cefotetan in the treatment of obstetric and gynecologic infections. *Am J Obstet Gynecol* 154:946, 1986.
39. Gonzalez-Enders R, Yi A, Calderon J, et al: Treatment of postpartum endometritis with cefoxitin sodium. *J Antimicrob Chemother* 4:245S, 1978.
40. Hager WD, McDaniel PS: Treatment of serious obstetric and gynecologic infections with cefoxitin. *J Reprod Med* 28:337, 1983.
41. Sweet RL, Ledger WJ: Cefoxitin: Single-agent treatment of mixed aerobic-anaerobic pelvic infections. *Obstet Gynecol* 54:193, 1979.
42. Galask RP, Ohm M: Intravenous cefoxitin sodium for the treatment of infections in obstetric and gynaecological patients. *J Antimicrob Chemother* 4:241S, 1979.
43. Sweet RL, Robbie MO, Ohm-Smith M, et al: Comparative study of piperacillin versus

cefoxitin in the treatment of obstetric and gynecologic infections. *Am J Obstet Gynecol* 145:342, 1983.
44. Herman G, Cohen AW, Talbot GH, et al: Cefoxitin versus clindamycin and gentamicin in the treatment of postcesarean section infections. *Obstet Gynecol* 67:371, 1986.
45. Sweet RL: Imipenem-cilastatin in the treatment of obstetric and gynecologic infections: A review of worldwide experience. *Rev Infect Dis* 7:S522, 1985.
46. Gibbs RS, Blanco JD, Castaneda YS, et al: Therapy of obstetric infections with moxalactam. *Antimicrob Agents Chemother* 17:1004, 1980.
47. Gall SA, Addison WA, Hill GB: Moxalactam therapy for obstetric and gynecologic infections. *Rev Infect Dis* 4:S701, 1982.
48. Cunningham FG, Gibbs RS, Hemsell DL: Moxalactam for treatment of pelvic infections after cesarean delivery. *Rev Infect Dis* 4:S696, 1982.
49. Sweet RL, Ohm-Smith M, Landers DV, et al: Moxalactam versus clindamycin plus tobramycin in the treatment of obstetric and gynecologic infections. *Am J Obstet Gynecol* 152:808, 1985.
50. Pastorek JG, Aldridge KE, Cunningham GL, et al: Comparison of ticarcillin plus clavulanic acid with cefoxitin in the treatment of female pelvic infection. *Am J Med* 79(suppl 5B):161, 1985.
51. Apuzzio JJ, Kaminski Z, Gamesh V, et al: Comparative clinical evaluation of ticarcillin plus clavulanic acid versus clindamycin plus gentamicin in treatment of post-cesarean endomyometritis. *Am J Med* 79(suppl 5B):161, 1985.
52. Le Frock JL, Molaui A, Rolston K, et al: Mezlocillin versus cefoxitin in pelvic and intraabdominal infections. *Infect Surg* 1984.
53. Sorrell TC, Marshall JR, Yoshimari R, et al: Antimicrobial therapy of postpartum endomyometritis II. Prospective, randomized trial of mezlocillin versus ampicillin. *Am J Obstet Gynecol* 141:246, 1981.
54. Marshall JR, Chow AW, Shorrell TC: Effectiveness of mezlocillin in female genital tract infections. *J Antimicrob Chemother* 9:149, 1982.
55. Duff P, Jorgensen JG, Gibbs RS, et al: Serum gentamicin levels in patients with postcesarean endomyometritis. *Obstet Gynecol* 61:723, 1983.
56. Agnelli G, DelFavero A, Praise P, et al: Cephalosporin-induced hypoprothrombinemia: Is the *N*-methylthiotetrazole side chain the culprit? *Antimicrob Agents Chemother* 29:1108, 1986.
57. McCue JD, Hansen C, Gal P: Hospital charges for antibiotics. *Rev Infect Dis* 7:643, 1985.

Chapter 27

Postoperative Anesthetic Complications

Gary D. V. Hankins, MD, and
Larry C. Gilstrap III, MD

Postoperative anesthetic complications range in severity from the merely annoying spinal headache to the potentially lethal aspiration pneumonitis. The prevention of these complications has been discussed in previous chapters. This chapter will cover primarily therapeutic modalities once the complication has occurred.

General anesthesia is associated with less frequent but more severe complications than occur with conduction anesthesia. Aspiration of gastric contents presents as an immediate complication of general anesthesia, whereas hepatitis from the inhalational agents is a delayed complication. Spinal headaches, urinary retention, and cord hematomas are immediate complications of conduction anesthesia, whereas infection and arachnoiditis are generally delayed.

GASTRIC ASPIRATION

Anesthesia-related deaths account for 10% to 15% of all maternal deaths in the United States, the gastric aspiration syndrome representing the single most common cause of anesthetic fatality.[1–3] Krantz and Edwards reported that the aspiration syndrome complicated 1 in 11,000 vaginal deliveries and 1 in 430 cesarean deliveries, accounting for 1 maternal death in every 3,000 cesarean sections or every 30,000 to 40,000 vaginal deliveries.[4] A higher incidence of aspiration (0.89%) in the United Kingdom resulted in even more frequent deaths, with 1 in 5,000 to 6,000 pregnant women dying from this complication.[5] With the increasing cesarean delivery rate in this country, which has occurred largely since the above reports were published, we may anticipate even more fatalities from anesthetic-related aspiration.

Curtis Mendelson, the obstetrician who first called attention to the

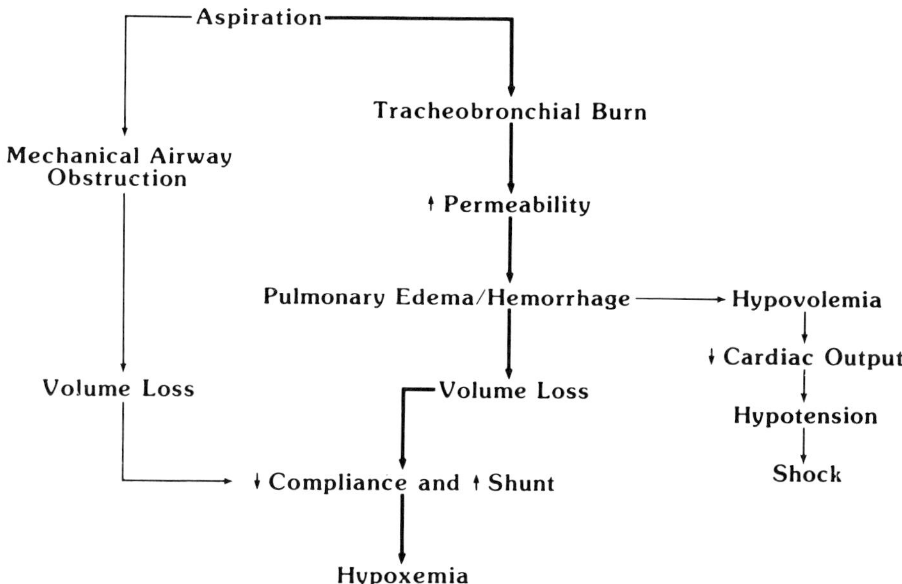

FIGURE 27.1 Pathophysiology of gastric aspiration syndrome.

gastric aspiration syndrome in 1946, astutely described the clinical characteristics of this condition.[6] He noted that some women aspirated copious amounts of solid debris and developed massive acute airway obstruction and suffocated. The majority, however, aspirated liquid material and promptly developed dyspnea, wheezing, cyanosis, and arterial hypoxemia. Accordingly, the injury was felt to be mediated principally by acidic gastric contents. Moreover, similar physiologic and pathologic lesions could be created in animal models by infusion of acidic fluid (pH <2.5) into the lungs. Indeed, the diagnosis of Mendelson's syndrome includes a lung injury produced by aspiration of gastric contents with a pH of <2.5. Subsequent animal data by Awe and associates, however, demonstrated that the aspiration of material with a pH of 5.5 produced hypoxemia equivalent to that seen after acid aspiration (pH = 1), but with much worse hypercapnia.[7] Other investigators also confirmed that pulmonary injury is produced by aspiration of either acidic or alkaline gastric contents.[8] They also emphasized that the addition of particulate matter, irrespective of the pH, increased the mortality rate in animal models.[8] Clinically, this observation had already been made in pregnant women, with severe lung injuries reported even after antacid use and with a gastric content pH of 6.4.[9]

The pathophysiology of the injuries produced by gastric aspiration is shown schematically in Figure 27.1. The gastric contents produce a chemical burn upon contact and initiate a cascade of events, central to which is increased pulmonary alveolar capillary membrane permeability.

TABLE 27.1 Signs and Symptoms of Aspiration Pneumonitis

Tachypnea
Bronchospasm
Wheezing
Rhonchi
Cyanosis
Hypoxia
Tachycardia
Hypotension

Water and plasma proteins, and in severe injuries red blood cells, flood the alveolus. This dilutes alveolar surfactant, much of which may have already been destroyed by the initial aspirate, and leads to further alveolar collapse and loss of lung volume. This alveolar collapse results in dramatic intrapulmonary shunts and in arterial hypoxemia that is refractory to supplemental oxygen therapy.[10] The fluid-filled lungs will also be stiff, and respirations will be labored if spontaneous, or may require high pressures if the patient is mechanically ventilated. The rapid flux of fluid and blood from the intravascular compartment into the pulmonary interstitium and alveoli may also result in hypovolemia, falling cardiac output, and systemic hypotension. The signs and symptoms of aspiration are summarized in Table 27.1. Not surprisingly, in the general population the mortality from gastric aspiration has shown a strong correlation with the magnitude of the original insult. When only one lung showed evidence of involvement, 41% of patients died compared to 90% when both lungs were involved.[11]

With prompt diagnosis and aggressive treatment, the outlook of the pregnant woman with aspiration pneumonitis should be far better than that of the general population, which often includes severely debilitated individuals with chronic disease. The pregnant woman is usually healthy prior to the aspiration, and by securing her airway, further aspiration and pulmonary insults are avoidable.

Aggressive treatment of the woman who is suspected or known to have aspirated is mandatory. Endotracheal intubation not only secures the airway but also allows suctioning and clearing of debris from the upper trachea and bronchi. Suctioning may also stimulate coughing and clearance of debris from the lower airways. Assisted mechanical ventilation can be instituted and continued until a chest radiograph and arterial blood gas studies have been obtained. If they are normal, the woman can be safely extubated. If they are abnormal, this aggressive approach may also prevent further deterioration in maternal status.

Positive-pressure ventilation and supplemental oxygen are the cornerstones of therapy for gastric aspiration.[10] Cameron et al, in an animal model, demonstrated increased survival when positive-pressure ventilation was instituted immediately, but no effect if it was delayed for 24 hours.[12]

The addition of positive end-expiratory pressure (PEEP) results in dramatic improvement in cases of fulminant pulmonary edema. Actual edema fluid formation, as well as arterial oxygenation, improve rapidly. The continuous positive intrapulmonary pressure will result in airway recruitment and pulmonary reinflation, which will, in turn, decrease the intrapulmonary shunt. Actual extravasation of fluid into the alveoli may also be diminished by PEEP. Levels of PEEP of 15 cm of water pressure or less are usually sufficient. At these pressures, we have not encountered deleterious effects of PEEP on venous return or cardiac output. These women may, however, be significantly volume depleted from the loss of both fluid and blood into the lung, and may tolerate PEEP poorly. If hypotension occurs and is not corrected by 500 mL of normal saline or lactated Ringer's solution, invasive hemodynamic monitoring is indicated to assist fluid management. Similarly, levels of PEEP greater than 15 cm of water, because of the potential adverse effect on venous return, may require a pulmonary artery catheter for safe monitoring. Because a capillary leak is present in the lungs, the lowest pulmonary capillary wedge pressure (PCWP) that will sustain adequate cardiac output and urine flow should be sought. If possible, the PCWP should be maintained at 12–15 mm Hg or less.

Supplemental oxygen will be required if a significant pulmonary injury has occurred. The goal of oxygen therapy is to maintain adequate tissue oxygenation while limiting exposure of the injured lung to the lowest possible inspired oxygen concentration. A hemoglobin saturation of 90%, corresponding to an arterial PO_2 of 60 mm Hg under usual circumstances, should serve both purposes. As demonstrated in Figure 27.2, hemoglobin saturations above 90% provide little additional oxygen-carrying capabilities. Moreover, attempts to attain a higher hemoglobin saturation can lead to deleterious effects on the lungs from oxygen toxicity. An arterial line may be necessary in such women to facilitate frequent blood gas sampling. Such an approach will decrease the patient's discomfort while ensuring that an arterial specimen is reliably available for blood gas analysis.

Bronchoscopy is indicated only if a major airway is obstructed by large particulate debris. Lavage is never indicated, as it is much more apt to worsen than to alleviate the injury. Other therapies that were once controversial, include the use of steroids and prophylactic antibiotics. Both Downs and Chapman and their colleagues, using animal models, found no beneficial effects of steroids on arterial oxygenation, cardiac output, and pulmonary artery pressure.[13,14] Other investigators found less lung water in steroid-treated patients at 48 hours postinsult but no beneficial effect on any other physiologic parameter.[15] Moreover, no one has shown improved survival with steroid therapy for the aspiration syndrome.[1] Although steroids are good in theory, there is insufficient evidence to support their use clinically.

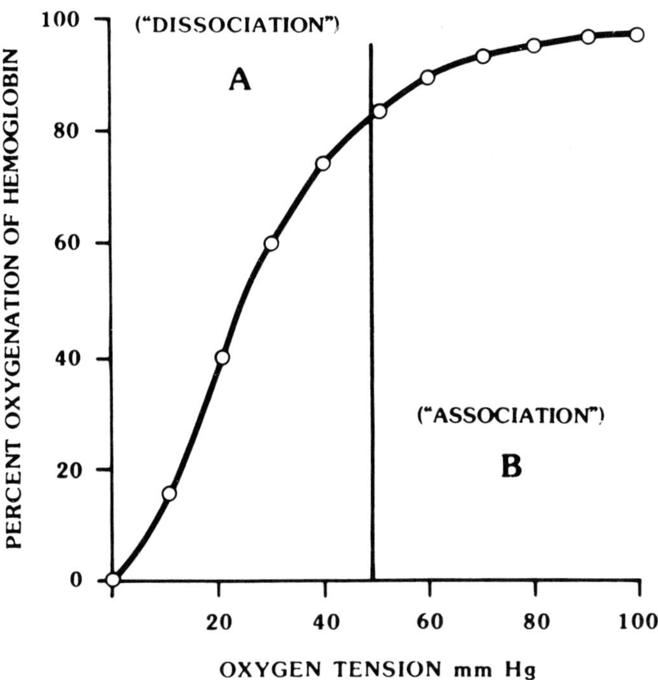

FIGURE 27.2 Oxyhemoglobin dissociation curve divided into a dissociation limb corresponding to the capillary tissue environment (A) and an association limb corresponding to the alveolar-capillary environment (B). Note that at a 90% hemoglobin saturation, the patient will be operating on the flat portion of the association limb of the curve.

Prophylactic antibiotics for the aspiration syndrome, especially in the young pregnant woman, also appear not to be efficacious. In an excellent review that was not limited to parturients, Wynne and Modell concluded that prophylactic antibiotics neither decreased infection nor increased survival. Antibiotics in this setting should be reserved for documented or clinically suspicious infections.[16]

HEPATITIS

Liver necrosis after halothane exposure was first reported in 1958. Clinically, liver involvement varies from hepatitis to fulminant and fatal necrosis, the latter occurring in 1/35,000 cases of halothane exposure.[16] Enflurane is also reported to result occasionally in hepatotoxicity.[17] At highest risk are obese, middle-aged women with repeated exposures to halothane over a short (4- to 8-week) period. Severe damage is unlikely to occur following a single exposure to halothane in the previously healthy individual. Hence, this is an unlikely postanesthetic complication in obstetrics. Treatment is essentially supportive and is directed at maintaining good nutrition and correction of any coagulopathies while permitting the liver an opportunity to regenerate.

SPINAL HEADACHE

Postpuncture spinal headache is the most common complication of conduction anesthesia in the postpartum period. The incidence of headache correlates directly with the size of the needle puncture. For instance, the use of a 16-gauge needle is associated with development of headache in 70% of the patients, whereas as few as 2% experience this complication with a 25-gauge needle.[18] Diagnosis of this condition is relatively easy; an intense headache to the point of causing nausea accompanies upright posture and is relieved by recumbency or maneuvers to increase intra-abdominal pressure. The headache is hypothesized to result from a leak of cerebrospinal fluid (CSF) into the epidural space, with resultant falls in CSF pressure and possible stretching of the dura and intracranial blood vessels.

The traditional treatment, consisting of 24 to 48 hours of strict bed rest, intravenous hydration, and sedation, is not only impractical but has recently been shown to be of limited efficacy.[19] Similarly, although reducing severe headaches from 70% to 20% following large dural punctures, infusion of 1.5 L of saline into the epidural space over 24 to 36 hours is impractical in the woman who has just given birth.[20] By contrast, epidural blood patches are over 90% effective in completely relieving spinal headaches and permit earlier ambulation.[21,22] Using the technique described by DiGiovanni and Dunbar, 10 mL of the patient's blood is injected into the epidural space.[23,24] Following this, she is placed supine for 30 minutes and hydrated with 1 L of crystalloid solution. The clot formed in the epidural space seals the leak of CSF and relieves the patient's discomfort almost immediately. Because the blood patch has a high rate of success and virtually no complications, early consultation with anesthesia personnel should be considered for all patients with significant spinal headaches.

BLADDER DYSFUNCTION

Innervation of the bladder is ablated by effective conduction anesthesia; thus, close attention to the bladder is mandatory if bladder overdistention is to be prevented. This entails visual and palpable assessment of the bladder during labor and postpartum. If distention is noted, the patient is encouraged to void; if she is unable to do so, the bladder is emptied by straight catheterization. The need to perform more than two straight catheterizations postpartum warrants indwelling catheter placement and bladder rest. Surveillance for urinary tract infections is performed by periodic urine cultures as long as catheterization is required.

If an indwelling catheter has been required as a complication of conduction anesthesia and bladder overdistention, bladder "training" is frequently necessary prior to removing the catheter. This consists of alternatively clamping and unclamping the catheter at hourly intervals to restore bladder tone. After removal of the catheter, the patient is instructed to chart the time and amount of all voided urines. After the second spontaneous voiding, she is recatheterized. If the residual is > 100 mL, the catheter is left in place; otherwise, it is removed. If the patient fails to void within 3 to 4 hours, she is instructed to void voluntarily, even if the desire or urge is absent. She is then catheterized for a postvoid residual and managed as previously outlined.

Failure to remove the catheter does not require continued hospitalization. Barring other reasons for hospitalization, these patients may be discharged with a Foley catheter and a leg bag and followed as outpatients. Bladder training by intermittent clamping of the catheter tubing is continued during waking hours, and another attempt at removal is made in 1 week. For prolonged indwelling catheterization, the woman is given prophylactic urinary tract suppression, usually with 100 mg of nitrofurantoin macrocrystals, one to three times per day.

HORNER'S SYNDROME

Horner's syndrome, consisting of ptosis, miosis, and anhydrosis, results from interruption of the cervical sympathetic ganglia and has been reported as a complication of conduction anesthesia.[25] Although one British study reported a 75% incidence of pupillary changes or other manifestations of cervical sympathetic blockage,[26] this has been rarely encountered in our patient population. Expectant management by allowing the anesthetic effects to subside usually results in prompt and complete recovery within 12 to 24 hours. During this period of recovery or in the event of persistent Horner's syndrome, tears and/or an eyepatch may be useful to prevent corneal damage.

DIRECT PHYSICAL INJURY

Injuries of the spinal cord, nerve roots, and vascular structures have been reported, but are exceedingly rare.[18,27] Nerve root or cord injury by the needle or catheter will almost always evoke sudden and severe pain, resulting in prompt removal or repositioning of the needle or catheter. Any resultant physical derangements are characteristically maximal acutely and resolve quickly. Failure to improve or deterioration of the patient's status is an indication for neurologic consultation and physical therapy.

Unless the patient has a coagulopathy, there is little risk of significant bleeding in or around the spinal cord.[28] This conclusion is supported by the frequent appearance of a few drops of blood or blood-tinged CSF in conjunction with conduction anesthesia without associated symptoms. Moreover, the use of an epidural blood patch, where up to 10 mL of autologous blood is deliberately injected into the epidural space, has not been associated with adverse consequences. Continued bleeding into the epidural or subdural space, however, can create a large hematoma capable of exerting pressure on the spinal cord to cause paraparesis and sensory loss. These findings constitute a neurosurgical emergency and require prompt neurosurgical consultation.[27] Diagnosis can be established with computed tomography (CT) scan or myelography. If paralysis is to be avoided, prompt surgical decompression of the cord is frequently necessary.

INFECTION

Epidural or subarachnoid space infections are exceedingly rare events. These infections usually result from a blood-borne infection from a different site in the body and are only rarely a consequence of direct inoculation via the catheter or anesthetic agent.[18,27–30] These infections can present either as meningitis or as an epidural abscess, and may occur either early or late in the postpartum course. Headache, fever, meningeal signs, and leukocytosis favor meningitis, whereas localizing severe back pain and overlying tenderness are more indicative of an abscess. Lumbar puncture for CSF analysis and aerobic and anaerobic cultures, as well as Gram stains, are essential parts of the evaluation. If an abscess is suspected, diagnosis can be confirmed by CT scan or myelography. Broad-spectrum antibiotic coverage should be instituted. In the setting of recent pregnancy and labor, the combination of penicillin and gentamicin is preferred because the overwhelming odds favor hematogenous seeding of the central nervous system[29]; the likely sources of infection are chorioamnionitis or metritis. Both of these are polymicrobial mixed infections in which anaerobes and the Enterobacteriacea predominate.[31] As in hematoma formation, compression exerted by the abscess can result in paralysis and sensory loss, which, if not promptly relieved, may be permanent. Accordingly, neurosurgical consultation should be obtained promptly because emergency laminectomy and decompression may be surgically necessary.

The opinions expressed in this chapter are those of the authors and not necessarily those of the United States Air Force or the Department of Defense.

REFERENCES

1. Cohen SE: The aspiration syndrome. *Clin Obstet Gynaecol* 9:235, 1982.
2. Bonica TT: Principles and practice of obstetric analgesia and anesthesia, in *Maternal Mortality*. Philadelphia, FA Davis Co, 1967, pp 748–760.
3. Phillips DC, Frazier TM, David GH, et al: The role of anesthesia in obstetric mortality: A review of 455,553 live births from 1936–1958 in the city of Baltimore. *Anesth Analg* 40:557, 1961.

4. Krantz ML, Edwards WL: The incidence of nonfatal aspiration in obstetric patients. *Anesthesiology* 39:359, 1973.
5. Department of Health and Social Security: *Report on Confidential Inquiries into Maternal Deaths in England and Wales, 1973–1975.* London, HM, Stationery Office, 1979.
6. Mendelson CL: The aspiration of stomach contents into the lungs during obstetric anaesthesia. *Am J Obstet Gynecol* 52:191, 1946.
7. Awe WB, Fletcher WS, Jacob SW: The pathophysiology of aspiration pneumonitis. *Surgery* 60:232, 1966.
8. Schwartz DJ, Wynne JW, Gibbs CP, et al: The pulmonary consequences of aspiration of gastric contents at pH values greater than 2.5. *Am Rev Respir Dis* 121:119, 1980.
9. Bond VK, Stoelting RK, Gupta CD: Pulmonary aspiration syndrome after inhalation of gastric fluid containing antacids. *Anesthesiology* 51:452, 1979.
10. Hankins GDV: Acute pulmonary injury and respiratory failure in pregnancy, in Clark SL, Phelan JP, Cotton DB (eds): *Critical Care Obstetrics.* Oradell, NJ, Medical Economics Books, 1987, pp 290–314.
11. Cameron TL, Mitchell WH, Zuidema GD: Aspiration pneumonia. Clinical outcome following documented aspiration. *Arch Surg* 106:49, 1973.
12. Cameron JL, Sebor J, Anderson RP, et al: Aspiration pneumonia. Results of treatment by positive pressure ventilation in dogs. *J Surg Res* 8:447, 1968.
13. Downs JB, Chapman RL, Modell JH, et al: An evaluation of steroid therapy in aspiration pneumonitis. *Anesthesiology* 40:129, 1974.
14. Chapman RL, Modell JR, Ruiz BC, et al: Effect of continuous positive pressure ventilation and steroids in aspiration of hydrochloric acid (pH 1.8) in dogs. *Anesth Analg* 53:556, 1974.
15. Dudley WR, Marshall BE: Steroid treatment for acid-aspiration pneumonitis. *Anesthesiology* 40:136, 1974.
16. Wynne TW, Modell TH: Respiratory aspiration of stomach contents. *Ann Intern Med* 87:466, 1977.
17. Nimmo WS, Wilson T, Prescot LF: Narcotic analgesia and delayed gastric emptying during labor. *Lancet* 1:890, 1975.
18. Subcommittee on the National Study of the Committee on Anaesthesia. National Academy of Sciences, National Research Council: Summary of the National Halothane Study. *JAMA* 197:775, 1966.
19. Eger IE, Smackler EA, Ferrell LD, et al: Is enflurane hepatotoxic? *Anesth Analg* 65:21, 1986.
20. Bromage PR: Neurologic complications of regional anesthesia, in Shnider SM, Levinson G (eds): *Anesthesia for Obstetrics.* Baltimore, Williams & Wilkins Co, 1979, pp 301–311.
21. Carbaat PAT, Van Crevel H: Lumbar puncture headache: Controlled study on preventive effects of twenty-four hours bed rest. *Lancet* 2:1133, 1981.
22. Moir DD: *Obstetric Anesthesia and Analgesia.* Baltimore, Williams & Wilkins Co, 1976, p 181.
23. DiGiovanni AT, Dunbar BS: Epidural injections of autologous blood for postlumbar-puncture headache. *Anesth Analg* 49:268, 1970.
24. DiGiovanni AT, Galbert MW, Wahle WM: Epidural injections of autologous blood for postlumbar-puncture headache II. Additional clinical experience and laboratory investigation. *Anesth Analg* 51:226, 1972.
25. Evans TM, Gauci CA, Watkins G: Horner's syndrome as a complication of lumbar epidural block. *Anaesthesia* 30:747, 1975.
26. Carrie LES, Mohan T: Horner's syndrome following obstetric epidural block. *Br J Anaesth* 48:611, 1976.

27. Graham TG: Neurological complications of pregnancy and anaesthesia. *Clin Obstet Gynaecol* 9:333, 1982.
28. Harik SI, Raichle ME, Reis DT: Spontaneous remitting spinal epidural hematoma in a patient on anticoagulants. *N Engl J Med* 284:1355, 1971.
29. Baker AS, Ojemann RG, Swartz MN, et al: Spinal epidural abscess. *N Engl J Med* 293:463, 1975.
30. Usubiaga TE: Neurological complications following epidural analgesia. *Int Anesthesia Clin* 13:19 1975.
31. Gilstrap LC III, Cunningham FG: The bacterial pathogenesis of infection following cesarean section. *Obstet Gynecol* 53:545, 1979.

Chapter 28

Thromboembolic Disorders and Anticoagulant Therapy in the Cesarean Patient

Susan E. Rutherford, MD, and
Jeffrey P. Phelan, MD

Thromboembolic disease during pregnancy is an uncommon event but remains a major cause of maternal morbidity and mortality. The greatest incidence in the puerperium is among cesarean patients. An accurate estimation of the true incidence of thromboembolic disorders related to pregnancy is difficult due to differing diagnostic and inclusion criteria. Deep venous thrombosis (DVT) of the lower extremities, however, has been reported to occur in about 0.24% of all deliveries.[1–3] The duration of pregnancy and the mode of delivery affect this incidence. For instance, the risk of DVT after cesarean delivery is three to five times greater than after vaginal delivery.[4–6] In addition to pregnancy, other risk factors include age, parity, obesity, and an inability to ambulate. In those patients with untreated DVT, 15%–24% will develop a pulmonary embolus (PE) and 12%–15% will sustain a fatal embolus. If treated appropriately, the risks of PE and death are reduced to 4.5% and 0.7%, respectively.[2,4]

Thus, it becomes immediately apparent that in the appropriate management of the cesarean patient, the clinician must consider the risks associated with the hypercoagulable state of pregnancy. With a review of hemostasis and those coagulation changes unique to pregnancy, this chapter will provide the clinician with a clearer understanding of the pathophysiology of DVT and PE. Moreover, an understanding of the underlying pathophysiology will serve as a basis for establishing the diagnosis and management of these thromboembolic disorders. Finally, a management schema will be suggested to assist with perioperative patients on anticoagulant therapy.

HEMOSTASIS

Normal blood flow requires intact, patent blood vessels. The vessel wall, platelets, coagulation cascade, and fibrinolysis work together to protect vascular integrity and assist in repair after injury. If an insult occurs, localized vasoconstriction reduces local blood flow initially, thus limiting the size of the thrombus needed to seal a defect.[5] Platelets adhere to the exposed vessel wall at the site of injury, change shape, and secrete their granule contents, leading to the accumulation of more platelets, a process termed "aggregation." Platelets also release the following: thromboxane A_2 (TxA_2),[6,7] a potent vasoconstrictor and proaggregatory agent; serotonin,[7] a vasoconstrictor; and adenosine diphosphate, which enhances aggregation. On the platelet surface, platelet factor 3 (PF_3) binds factor V and catalyzes the formation of thrombin. Then thrombin stimulates aggregation.[8]

Endothelial cells synthesize prostacyclin (PGI_2). PGI_2 acts counter to TxA_2 by aggregation and by stimulating vasodilation. The deeper an injury to a vessel wall, the greater the concentration of proaggregatory substances and the lower the amount of PGI_2 produced.

While platelets aggregate to seal the vascular defect, the coagulation cascade produces fibrin, which is polymerized as clot and becomes part of the platelet plug. Two pathways, intrinsic and extrinsic, lead to execution of the final common pathway and the production of fibrin. These pathways are initiated by components of the vessel wall, whereas circulating clotting factors are activated at the site of injury by means of proteolytic cleavage or conformational changes.

Small amounts of the early factors repetitively activate subsequent factors, resulting in progressively larger amounts of activated factors, a process termed "amplification." In the intrinsic pathway, high molecular weight kininogen and kallikrein are cofactors for the initial step, which is activation of factor XII. By catalyzing the formation of kallikrein from prekallikreins, factor XIIa also helps to initiate fibrinolysis, activate complement, and produce kinins.[5] Factor XI is activated by XIIa and then cleaves factor IX to form factor IXa.

The extrinsic pathway relies on tissue thromboplastin as a cofactor. With this pathway, tissue thromboplastin is exposed to the circulation by overlying membrane damage or proteolysis.[5] Factor VII is then activated to factor VIIa, which, with tissue thromboplastin, can activate factors IX or X.

The vitamin K–dependent factors, II, VII, IX, and X, undergo a reaction in the liver in which gamma-carboxyglutamic acid residues are attached to the protein structure. This permits them to complex with calcium ion and phospholipid receptors on the platelet or endothelial cell membrane. Subsequent steps in the clotting cascade occur at those sites.

The common pathway is initiated with the activation of factor X by either factors IXa or VIIa, together with the protein cofactor VIII:C (the antihemophilic factor) and calcium ion on the platelet surface (PF_3). Factor Xa and cofactor Va enzymatically cleave prothrombin. This process liberates thrombin into the fluid phase. Subsequently, thrombin catalyzes the formation of fibrin monomers from fibrinogen, known as "fibrinopeptides A" and "B." In a manner similar to positive feedback, thrombin also facilitates activation of factors V, VIII:C, and XIII.

The hydrophobic and electrostatic interactions of the fibrin monomer chains create a fibrin gel. A stable polymerized fibrin clot incorporating water is then formed when factor XIIIa cross-links the fibrin monomer chains with covalent bonds.

The purpose of fibrinolysis is to restore a patent vascular channel. Plasminogen and plasminogen activators are trapped within the clot. Once activated, plasmin enzymatically digests the fibrin matrix, yielding protein fragments known as "fibrin degradation products (FDP)." These fragments have anticoagulant properties that inhibit the formation and cross-linking of fibrin.[5] The measurement of FDP is an indirect measurement of fibrinolysis. Regulation of fibrinolysis is accomplished by inhibitors of plasmin or plasminogen activity that are found in serum, platelets, and within the clot, such as alpha-2 antiplasmin, which binds to fibrin and fibrinogen.[11]

Events such as exercise, emotional stress, trauma, and surgery may trigger fibrinolysis. Hypotensive shock, pharmacologic agents, activated protein C,[5,9,10] and the enzymes streptokinase and urokinase also activate plasminogen.[11]

Because antithrombin III (AT III) is a potent inhibitor of thrombin, it serves as a regulator of hemostasis. Additionally, AT III binds and inactivates factors IXa, Xa, XIa, and XIIa and acts as a substrate for these serine proteases. As a result, AT III forms stable intermediate bonds with the active portion and neutralizes the enzyme.[12] As heparin binds to AT III, its affinity for thrombin increases. The otherwise slow inactivation of thrombin by AT III is accelerated by small amounts of heparin. Once a stable thrombin–antithrombin complex is formed, heparin is released and is made available to bind with AT III again. The presence of heparan on intact endothelial cell surfaces and its binding of AT III reduce the risk of local extension of a thrombus beyond the site of vessel injury.[13] If AT III is deficient, a higher incidence of thrombosis is encountered.

Another important anticoagulant system involves proteins C and S. Their synthesis is vitamin K dependent and involves the addition of gamma-carboxyglutamic acid residues. This permits binding, via calcium ions, to cell surfaces. Binding of thrombin to thrombomodulin, a specific protein receptor for thrombin on endothelial cell surfaces, activates protein C. Protein S is bound to endothelial and platelet membranes. Complexes of protein C and protein S serve as a second mechanism to prevent extension of the thrombus beyond the area of vessel injury.[13,14] This is accomplished by proteolyzing factors VIII:Ca and Va.

HEMOSTATIC CHANGES DURING PREGNANCY AND THE IMMEDIATE POSTCESAREAN PERIOD

Pregnancy can be characterized as a hypercoagulable state. Factors V, VII, VIII, IX, X, and XII and fibrinogen levels increase during pregnancy. For instance, circulating fibrinogen increases twofold, whereas other factors, such as XI and XIII, decrease. At the same time, platelet counts remain in the normal range. Plasma fibrinolytic activity, however, decreases during pregnancy due to placental inhibitors, but usually returns to normal soon after delivery.[15] This hypercoagulable state is partially offset by a heparin-like, pregnancy-specific protein, (PAPP-A), which facilitates the neutralization of thrombin by AT III.[12]

In summary, the risk of thrombosis is increased during pregnancy because of higher levels of coagulation factors and diminished fibrinolysis. These changes reach their peak near term and in the immediate postcesarean period. In many respects, these changes serve as a protective mechanism to control blood loss after placental separation.

DIAGNOSIS OF THROMBOEMBOLIC DISEASE IN THE POSTCESAREAN PATIENT

Clinical symptoms and signs may arouse suspicion of DVT but are frequently nondiagnostic. Approximately one-half of the patients with symptoms are ultimately proven to have venous thromboses, using objective tests. The classic symptoms of DVT are unilateral pain, tenderness, and swelling of a leg. A 2-cm difference in leg circumference between the affected and normal limbs is frequently described. Clinical signs include edema, changes in limb color, and a palpable cord. In the postcesarean patient, these signs and symptoms may be masked by the swelling and edema that usually accompany pregnancy and by incisional pain. Clinical tests that are useful in ruling in or ruling out a DVT are Homan's sign and Lowenberg's test. Homan's sign is the presence of calf pain upon passive dorsiflexion of the foot. A positive Lowenberg test is the presence of pain occurring distal to a blood pressure cuff that has been rapidly inflated to 180 mm Hg. This suggests a DVT. Obstructive iliofemoral vein thrombosis may also lead to marked swelling, cyanosis, and impairment of arterial blood flow, with diminished pulses and a cold extremity. To complicate matters, postcesarean patients with a prior history of severe DVT may develop signs and symptoms consistent with DVT but in reality have postphlebitic syndrome. This condition is characterized by skin stasis, dermatitis, or ulcers.

Often the first sign of deep venous disease is the occurrence of PE. The cardinal symptoms include dyspnea (>80%), pleuritic chest pain with or without splinting (>70%), apprehension (~60%), and cough (>50%).[16,17] Tachypnea is the major sign and occurs in about 90%. Additional clinical findings include tachycardia (40%), atelectatic rales, hemoptysis, fever, diaphoresis, a friction rub, cyanosis, and changes in heart sounds (accentuated second heart sound, gallop, or murmur). Clinical evidence of pulmonary embolism is variable and often depends on the patient's preexisting health. For instance, in the postcesarean patient, atelectasis, splinting from incisional pain, and tachypnea are not unusual findings. Nevertheless, the possibility of DVT or PE exists and must be considered in any patient with persistent signs and symptoms. In cases of fatal PE, cardiac arrest usually occurs within the first hour and death within 2 hours.

Embolization is defined as massive whenever more than 50% of the pulmonary arterial circulation has been obstructed. Such patients frequently present with signs of right-sided heart failure, as evidenced by jugular venous distention, liver enlargement, left parasternal heave, and fixed splitting of the second heart sound. Not infrequently, this situation may mimic myocardial infarction with hypotension, syncope, or convulsions. Multiple small emboli may resemble a massive embolus in effect and have a range of symptoms from none at all to common pregnancy discomforts to right-sided heart failure. Pulmonary infarction may occur in less than 10% of patients.[17] When it does, pleuritic chest pain, a friction rub, or hemoptysis may develop. In postcesarean patients with conditions such as pneumonia, congestive heart failure, or cancer, PE is more difficult to diagnose.

THE DIAGNOSIS OF DVT

As a first step in confirming the presence or absence of lower extremity DVT, noninvasive testing[18] is preferable in the pregnant patient. The primary advantages are the avoidance of fetal exposure to radiation and the detection of proximal lower extremity obstruction. Although false-positive tests may occur during pregnancy or in the immediate postpartum period due to uterine compression of the inferior vena cava or postoperative edema and stasis in the pelvic veins, it is essential to exclude DVT when suspected. In addition to a baseline clotting profile, noninvasive diagnostic techniques, such as Doppler studies and impedance plethysmography, are the most widely used to confirm the diagnosis (Figure 28.1).

With normal blood flow, Doppler auscultation of the proximal leg or pelvic veins demonstrates a frequency shift due to changes in blood flow velocity with respiration. Additional manipulations such as the Valsalva maneuver, release of pressure on a distal vein, and squeezing of the muscles will produce greater shifts. Complete occlusion of a deep vein

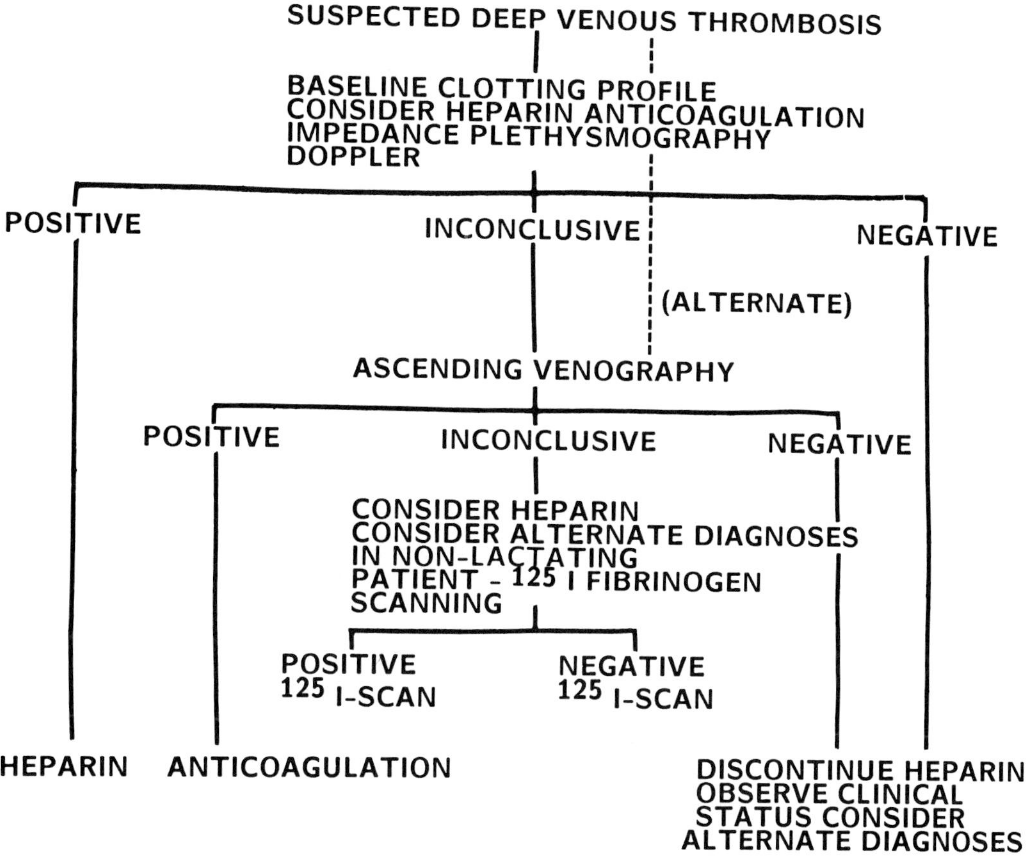

FIGURE 28.1 Proposed clinical management scheme for the postcesarean patient suspected of having DVT.

obstructs flow; consequently, there is no Doppler shift. Incomplete or partial occlusion is frequently manifested by a decreased amplitude, especially when compared with the opposite leg. However, minimal obstruction is very likely to remain undetected. The use of Doppler to detect popliteal, femoral, or iliac thromboses is effective in approximately 90% of the cases.[18] But if the calf of the leg is involved, about 50% of the thrombi will be missed[18] due to the abundance of collateral venous channels (Table 28.1)

Impedance plethysmography (IPG) is 95% sensitive (Table 28.1) in detecting thrombi in the same vessels, as is Doppler, but it is less effective than Doppler in detecting pelvic vein thrombosis.[18] This technique requires the inflation of a thigh cuff to a level between the systolic and diastolic pressures to prevent venous return. Once the cuff is inflated, a decrease in electrical resistance is observed. Sudden deflation of the thigh cuff results in an immediate outflow of blood from the leg and a sudden increase in electrical resistance. If the outflow is impaired, as with partially

TABLE 28.1 Comparison of Noninvasive Techniques with Venography for Diagnosis of DVT

Diagnostic Study	Sensitivity (%)	Specificity (%)
Doppler ultrasound		
Proximal veins	85–95	90
Calf veins	50 maximum	50 maximum
IPG		
Nonpregnant		
Proximal veins	95	98
Calf veins	<30	
Pregnant		36
^{125}I fibrinogen distal to mid-thigh		92
Thermography		75–80
Radionuclide venography proximal veins	>90	>90
^{111}In platelet imaging	90–95	95–100

Source: Rutherford SE, Phelan JP: Deep venous thrombosis and pulmonary embolism, in Clark SL, Phelan JP, Cotton DB (eds): *Critical Care Obstetrics.* Oradell, NJ, Medical Economics Books, 1987, p 133, with permission. Data collected from references 1, 18, and 19.

obstructing thrombus or vena caval occlusion, a slower increase in electrical resistance is observed.

When the results from Doppler or IPG examinations are inconclusive, ascending venography, the most useful and clinically accurate diagnostic technique (Table 28.1), should be considered (Figure 28.1). Ascending venography can also be used primarily in the nonlactating postcesarean patient when small amounts of radiation exposure are not a concern to confirm DVT, rather than using noninvasive techniques first. To perform venography, a radiopaque dye is injected into a leg vein. Gradual and complete filling of the leg veins up to the level of the mid-thigh can usually be accomplished. Above this point, incomplete filling may result in missed thrombi. Below the mid-thigh, a well-defined filling defect that is found in more than one radiographic view is diagnostic of venous thrombosis (Figure 28.2). In addition, diversion of blood flow to superficial veins or abrupt termination of filling are also suggestive of thrombosis. False-positive studies may be caused by poor technique, poor choice of injection site, tightening of leg muscles, or other leg pathology such as hematoma, popliteal cyst, cellulitis, edema, or muscle rupture. The major disadvantages of this technique include pain, swelling and tenderness, and thrombophlebitis from the procedure.

^{125}I fibrinogen scanning is contraindicated during pregnancy and lactation because unbound ^{125}I may collect in the fetal or neonatal thyroid. In nonlactating postcesarean patients, ^{125}I-labeled fibrinogen[20] may be used to identify DVT, and is preferred over ^{131}I because of its smaller radiation dose and a longer half-life. As illustrated in Figure 28.1, this

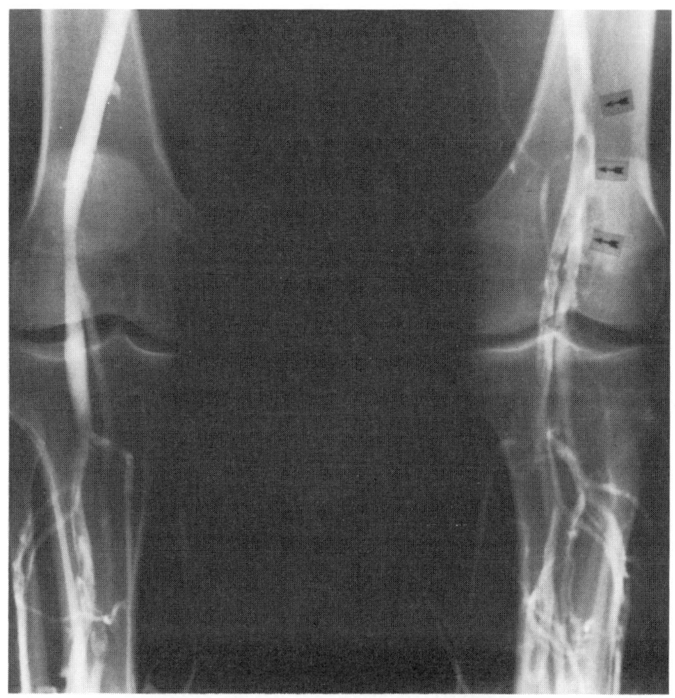

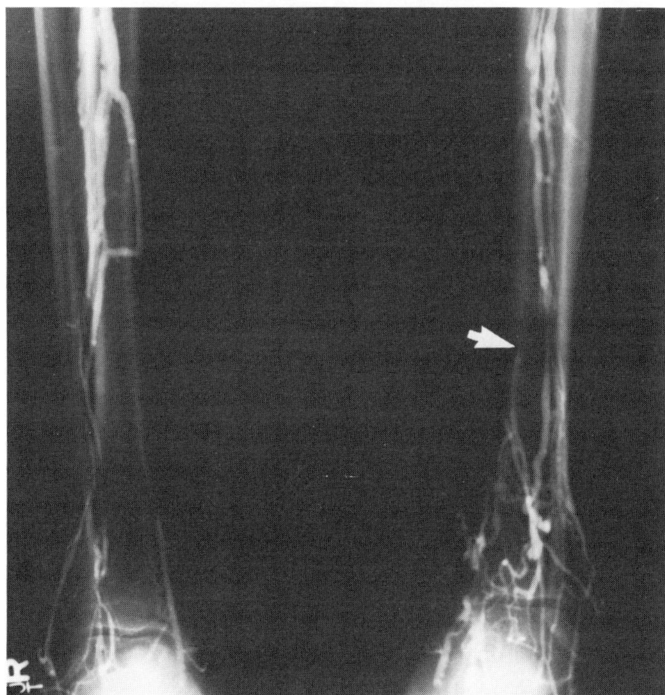

FIGURE 28.2 A contrast venogram shows a cutoff sign in the posterior tibial vein (white arrow) and filling defects in the popliteal vein in one leg (black arrows) and a normal study in the other leg. (From Clark SL, Phelan JP, Cotton DB [eds]: *Critical Care Obstetrics.* Oradel, NJ, Medical Economics Books, 1987, with permission.)

technique is useful in circumstances when venography results are inconclusive and the patient is not lactating. After intravenous injection, ^{125}I is incorporated, like normal fibrinogen, into developing thrombi. Sequential scintillation scanning is usually performed 24, 48, and 72 hours after injection. With each scan, the radioactivity is compared to background precordial values in the search for a "hot spot." Accuracy is greatest in the lower thigh and calf. Background counts in the femoral artery, the bladder, and the overlying muscle mass make detection of thrombi in the common femoral and pelvic veins more difficult. Because ^{125}I has a prolonged half-life, women who desire to breast-feed should pump their breasts and discard the milk for a minimum of 3 weeks.[21]

Finally, radionuclide venography using ^{99m}Tc particles is a relatively new technique that carries little risk to the fetus. However, this approach requires a rapid-sequence gamma camera that may not be available in many institutions. In cases of DVT above the knee,[20] the technique is more than 90% accurate.

DIAGNOSIS OF POSTCESAREAN PULMONARY EMBOLUS

In the postcesarean patient with suspected PE, baseline laboratory studies such as arterial blood gas (ABG), chest x-ray (CXR), electrocardiogram (ECG), and a clotting profile consisting of the prothrombin time (PT), partial thromboplastin time (PTT), fibrinogen and platelet counts, and oxygen therapy should be considered (Figure 28.3).

ABG, CXR, and ECG may be suggestive but are inconclusive in the diagnosis of PE. PE is unlikely with a PO_2 of >85 mm Hg on room air, but is not excluded. In one study, 14% of 43 patients with angiographically proven PE had a PO_2 of 85 mm Hg or more.[22] With a low PO_2, PE may not be the only reason, but it is frequently the most immediately life-threatening. Thus, heparin anticoagulation should be considered to reduce the risk of additional emboli.

The CXR, although frequently abnormal, may be normal in up to 30% of patients with PE.[17] The most common CXR findings consistent with PE are hemidiaphragm elevation, atelectasis, and pleural effusion.[23] Not infrequently, focal oligemia, an area of reduced vascular markings and increased radiolucency, can be seen on CXR. In cases of massive PE, changes in cardiac size or shape may be seen. Findings such as infiltrates or pleural effusion are usually later signs of parenchymal infarction. The importance of the CXR is not to confirm the presence of a PE, but to exclude other reasons for the patient's signs and symptoms and to assist in the interpretation of a lung scan.

In most patients, transient tachycardia is the most common ECG change. Classic ECG signs of acute cor pulmonale are infrequently seen and, when present, are associated with massive embolism. ECG findings

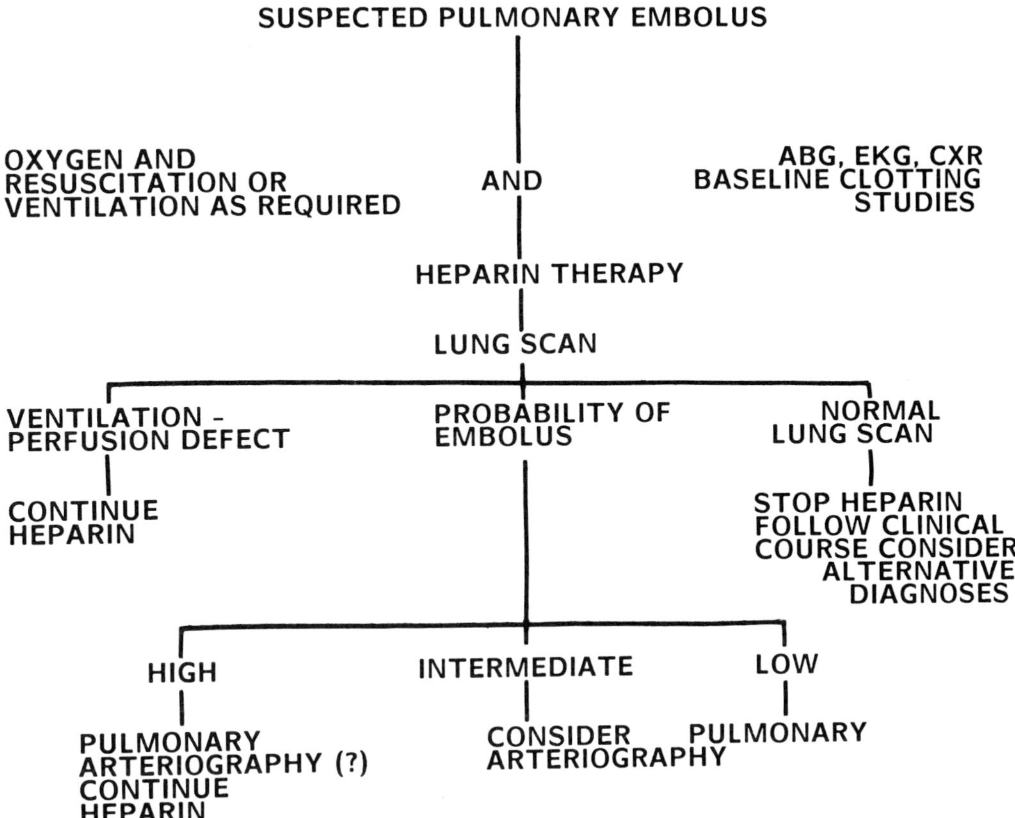

FIGURE 28.3 Proposed clinical management scheme for the postcesarean patient suspected of having PE.

consistent with cor pulmonale are right axis shift with an S_1 Q_3 T_3 pattern and nonspecific T-wave inversion.

Postcesarean patients with suspected PE should be started on heparin therapy and should undergo a perfusion lung scan. A normal scan virtually excludes the possibility of PE.[24] A perfusion lung scan is performed by intravenously injecting ^{99m}Tc-labeled albumin microspheres or macroaggregates. These particles are trapped within the pulmonary precapillary arteriolar bed, but usually not enough to affect pulmonary function.[25] The injection is performed with the patient in the supine position to increase apical perfusion. When the patient is upright, scanning is done to visualize the bases more effectively. Anterior, posterior, lateral, and posterior oblique views should be obtained. Ventilation scans with ^{133}Xe complement perfusion scans increase their specificity and may be obtained either pre- or postperfusion.

Scans are interpreted as normal or as indicating a low, intermediate, or high probability of PE. When CXR opacification corresponds to perfusion defects, the scan is considered nondiagnostic. Moreover, altered

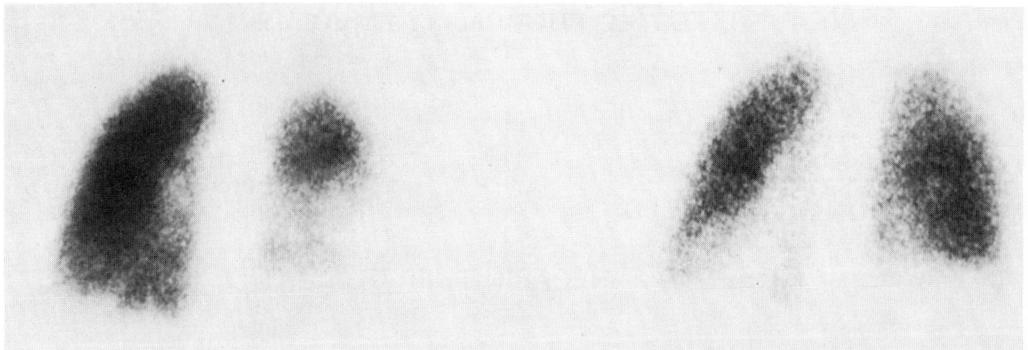

FIGURE 28.4 In these posterior views, the perfusion lung scan (left) reveals segmental defects that are not matched in the normal ventilation scan (right). This is consistent with a high probability of pulmonary embolism. (From Clark SL, Phelan JP, Cotton DB [eds]: *Critical Care Obstetrics.* Oradel, NJ, Medical Economics Books, 1987, with permission.)

pulmonary perfusion due to pneumonia, atelectasis, tumor, or effusion may produce an abnormal scan. Subsequent angiography has shown that the likelihood of PE is low with isolated subsegmental defects or matching ventilation/perfusion (V/Q) defects. In the presence of V/Q mismatching or multiple defects (Fig. 28.4), the possibility of PE is high and anticoagulation should be continued.

Although no adverse fetal effects have been reported from the performance of a lung scan during pregnancy, caution should be exercised to minimize fetal exposure to radiation. Compared with arteriography, the chance of such exposure from a lung scan is significantly less.[19] Of clinical importance, the fetal exposure to radiation from both these techniques is less than that associated with an effect in the human fetus.[26]

If the lung scan demonstrates an intermediate probability of a PE in a postcesarean patient, pulmonary arteriography is recommended to confirm the diagnosis. With the injection of contrast into lobar or segmental branches of the pulmonary artery, clear visualization of vessels larger than 2.5 mm[27] is possible. Findings consistent with a clot are a filling defect that does not obstruct flow or an abruptly terminated vessel, possibly with a trailing edge of dye where the clot incompletely fills the lumen (Figure 28.5). Morbidity and mortality with the procedure have been reported at 4%–5% and 0.2%–0.3%, respectively.[24,28] Most complications are related to catheterization and dye use.

In addition, pulmonary arteriography is recommended whenever the lung scan results do not correlate with the clinical suspicion or the risks of thrombolytic therapy (eg, streptokinase) or when surgical interruption of the vena cava necessitate a firm diagnosis prior to institution. Confirmation of DVT cannot substitute for angiographic demonstration of pulmonary embolism, as there is significant "mis-matching" of these radiographically determined diagnoses.[29]

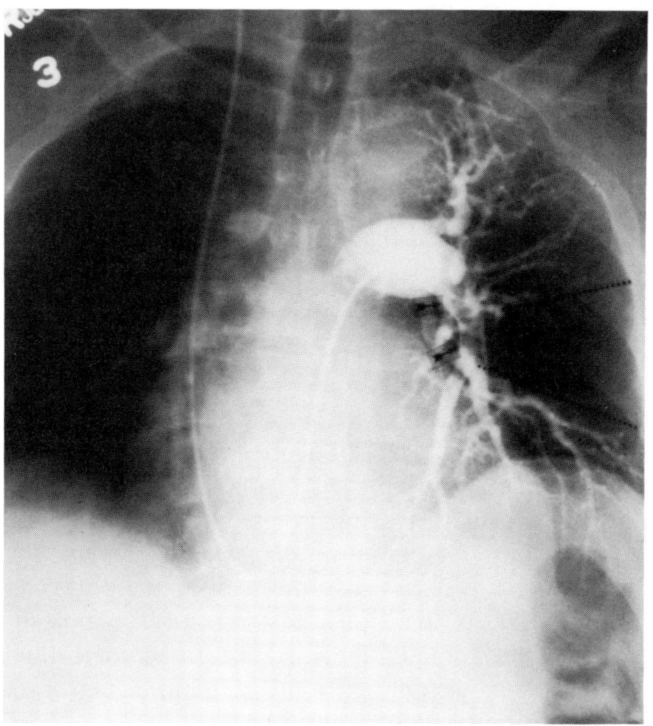

FIGURE 28.5 Arteriogram of the left pulmonary artery shows filling defects (illustrated by arrows) and an unperfused segment of lung, as indicated by the absence of contrast dye (outlined by broken line). (From Clark SL, Phelan JP, Cotton DB [eds]: *Critical Care Obstetrics*. Oradel, NJ, Medical Economics Books, 1987, with permission.)

Newer techniques to diagnose PE include digital subtraction pulmonary angiography and Indium platelet imaging. Digital subtraction pulmonary angiography is a relatively noninvasive tool that holds promise with continued technological improvement. Contrast is injected into a peripheral vein and computerized subtraction of the preinjection CXR from the postinjection film is performed to create an image of the pulmonary arterial vasculature. However, poor imaging frequently results from respiratory and cardiac motion and insufficient resolution. Additionally, it is difficult to obtain multiple projection views, and nonselective filling causes vessel overlap.

Although not yet readily available, ^{111}In platelet imaging[30] shows promise in the diagnosis and management of patients with thromboembolic disease. The patient's own platelets are extracted, labeled, and reinjected. Once injected, these ^{111}In-labeled platelets accumulate at sites of active thrombosis. Images are obtained using gamma camera scintigraphy. As long as active thrombosis is continuing, uptake of platelets can be visualized and anticoagulation monitored with this technique.

THE POSTCESAREAN PATIENT WITH A THROMBOEMBOLIC DISORDER

DVT is helped by bed rest and elevation of the affected extremity to promote venous return and decrease edema. After the initial therapy, movement and ambulation help prevent extension of thrombosis or recurrence and should be symptom limited. Acutely, oxygen is the most important adjunct in the treatment of PE (Figure 28.3). In addition, mechanical ventilation may be necessary in severe cases. Not infrequently, patients will experience pain that can be treated with narcotics in amounts small enough to prevent respiratory depression.

ANTICOAGULATION THERAPY

Heparin is the agent of choice in an acute situation in which thrombosis is suspected. Therapeutic blood levels can be rapidly achieved when it is administered intravenously. During pregnancy, heparin is the anticoagulant of choice because its high molecular weight prevents it from crossing the placenta. Actually, heparin is an acidic mucopolysaccharide that is found in commercial preparations as a mixture of molecular weights from 4,000 to 40,000. Some of the variation in biological activity is attributable to the varying weight fractions, with molecules of 4,000–5,000 daltons suggested to have higher, more uniform activity.[31]

Heparin facilitates the anticoagulant action of circulating AT III by binding to it and causing a configurational change. After AT III has irreversibly combined with thrombin or the activated factors IXa, Xa, XIa, or XIIa, the heparin is released and can interact similarly with other AT III molecules. The inactivation of small amounts of spontaneously formed factor Xa is the mechanism behind low-dose heparin prophylaxis. Much larger quantities of heparin are required to inhibit coagulation once a thrombus has been formed. With clot stabilization, as thrombin production diminishes, the heparin requirement decreases.

A disadvantage of heparin is the need for parenteral administration via intravenous or subcutaneous routes. Heparin is not absorbed via the gastrointestinal tract, and intramuscular injections have erratic absorption and involve the risk of hematoma formation. The half-life of heparin varies from less than 1 to more than 2.5 hours, and higher doses result in both a higher peak and a longer half-life.[32] Heparin levels may become abnormally elevated in patients with hepatic or renal failure.[33] Continuous intravenous infusion is clearly superior to an intermittent intravenous bolus in causing fewer hemorrhagic events. Subcutaneous administration gives adequate therapeutic levels, but slower absorption results in a 2- to 4-hour delay in achieving peak levels.

Adequate and safe anticoagulation with heparin requires careful laboratory monitoring of its bioeffect. The primary risk of heparin anticoagulation is bleeding, which is estimated to occur in 5% to 10% of patients[1,34] but may affect up to one-third.[35] Prior to initiating anticoagulation, a baseline clotting profile is reasonable to identify those patients with an underlying coagulant defect and to prevent hemorrhagic complications.

The most commonly available test used to measure the bioeffects of heparin is the activated PTT. When it is prolonged to 1.5 to 2.5[35,36] times the control value, a therapeutic heparin level has been achieved. Alternatives to the PTT include the whole blood clotting time and the thrombin time. Although no single laboratory test appears clearly superior in predicting bleeding, the heparin assay may be the most helpful.[34] Heparin levels are measured indirectly using the protamine sulfate neutralization test, in which the amount of protamine sulfate needed to reverse the effects of heparin on the thrombin clotting time is measured. Therapeutic plasma levels are in the range of 0.2–0.4 IU/mL.[1]

There are a few practical and clinical disadvantages to heparin therapy. For instance, the primary hemostatic defense in heparinized patients is platelet aggregation. Drugs that reduce platelet number or interfere with their function, such as nonsteroidal anti-inflammatory agents or dextran, may induce bleeding. For example, patients receiving aspirin may have twice the risk of bleeding of those who do not.[33] Because heparin is an acidic molecule, it is incompatible with many solutions containing medications (such as aminoglycosides). But when heparin is administered at a separate site, its activity appears to be unaffected.[37]

Other adverse effects of heparin include thrombocytopenia, hypersensitivity, and osteoporosis. Estimates of the incidence of thrombocytopenia vary from 1% to 30%.[38] The mechanism is unclear but may involve platelet clumping and sequestration, immune-mediated destruction, or consumption through low-grade disseminated intravascular coagulation. An alternative method of anticoagulation should be sought in a patient with a history of heparin-induced thrombocytopenia. Hypersensitivity is rare but may result in urticaria or anaphylaxis.

The most significant complication associated with heparin therapy is osteoporosis. Osteoporosis has been demonstrated in patients who have received at least 15,000 units/day for 6 months or more.[39] Bone demineralization specifically in pregnancy has been associated with doses of 20,000 units/day for more than 20 weeks.[40] Reversal of the osteoporosis after discontinuation of therapy may be slow[40,41] and, in some instances, incomplete.

Warfarin, a coumarin derivative, is the most commonly used oral anticoagulant. It inhibits regeneration of active vitamin K in the liver. Vitamin K is required to carboxylate the glutamic acid residues on factors II, IV, IX, and X and protein C. Otherwise, these factors would be inactive and unable to complex with calcium and phospholipid receptors.

In the postcesarean patient, warfarin use is usually limited to long-term anticoagulant therapy. During pregnancy, except in the rare situation where it is impossible to use heparin, warfarin is contraindicated because

TABLE 28.2 Examples of Drug Interactions with Coumarin Derivative Anticoagulants

Potentiate Oral Anticoagulants	May Antagonize Oral Anticoagulants
Alcohol—dose dependent	Antacids
Chlorpromazine	Antihistamines
Cimetidine	Barbiturates
Danocrine	Carbamazepine
Metronidazole	Corticosteroids
Neomycin	Oral contraceptives
Nonsteroidal anti-inflammatory drugs	Phenytoin
Salicylates—large doses	Primidone
Thyroxine	Rifampin
Trimethoprim	Vitamin K

Source: Rutherford SE, Phelan JP: Deep venous thrombosis and pulmonary embolism, in Clark SL, Phelan JP, Cotton DB (eds): *Critical Care Obstetrics.* Oradell, NJ, Medical Economics Books, 1987, p 141, with permission. Data from reference 43.

its low molecular weight of 1,000 permits it to cross the placenta easily. During pregnancy, administration in the first 9 weeks of gestation is associated with an embryopathy that includes nasal hypoplasia, depression of the bridge of the nose, and epiphyseal stippling such as that seen in Conradi-Hunermann chondrodysplasia punctata.[34] Exposure during the second two trimesters is associated with a variety of central nervous system and ophthalmologic abnormalities that may be related to fetal hemorrhage and scar tissue formation. There is also a higher risk of fetal hemorrhage with delivery due to the anticoagulant effects of the drug on the fetus.

Measurement of the PT is used to monitor the anticoagulant effect of warfarin. Therapeutic levels may be reached after 3 days and should yield a PT 1.5 to 2.5 times control values. Reversal depends on regeneration of clotting factors and is slow. Administration of parenteral vitamin K may lead to reversal in 6 to 12 hours. In an acute situation, fresh frozen plasma is given to provide clotting factors.

The major complication of warfarin use is bleeding, which occurs more often than with subcutaneous heparin.[42] Warfarin anticoagulation is also more sensitive to changes in clotting factors and plasma volume, and requires more frequent monitoring and dose adjustments. Numerous medications, such as some antibiotics, will augment or inhibit warfarin activity (Table 28.2).

MANAGEMENT OF ANTICOAGULATION

The suspicion of thromboembolism must be weighed against the risk of severe hemorrhage with anticoagulation. Except for ^{125}I fibrinogen scanning,[37] heparin does not interfere with performance or interpretation of the diagnostic procedures. Unless the patient shows evidence of active bleeding or a coagulopathy, anticoagulation with heparin should be un-

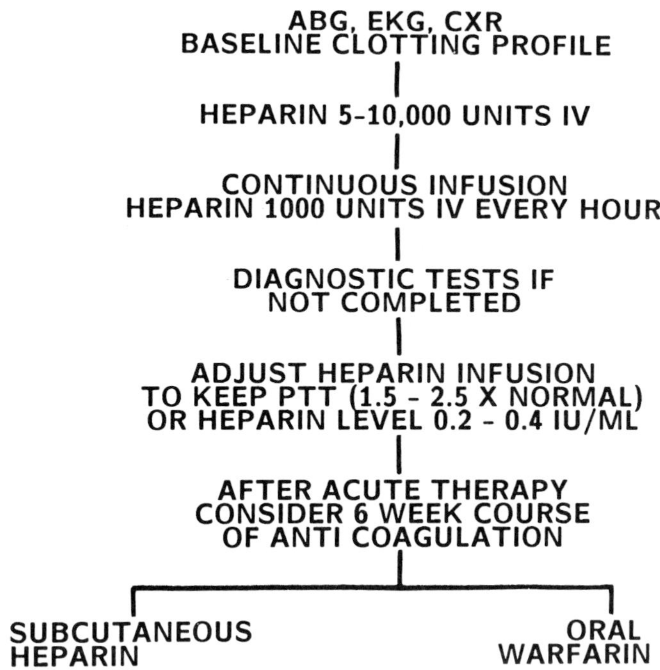

FIGURE 28.6 Proposed scheme for the initiation of anticoagulant therapy with sodium heparin in the postcesarean patient.

dertaken prior to diagnostic studies to prevent an embolic event during the interval.

After a blood sample for a baseline clotting profile is obtained, rapid anticoagulation is most easily achieved with an initial intravenous bolus of 70–100 units/kg or 5,000 to 10,000 units. For PE, as much as 15,000 units may be recommended.[44] Initial continuous infusion rates may be calculated at 15–20 units/kg/hr or 1,000 units/hr. Therapeutic doses are considered to be those that prolong the PPT 1.5–2.5 times normal or give a heparin level of around 0.2–0.4 IU/mL. Excessive doses that prolong the PTT 2.5–3.0 times normal or give levels above 0.4 IU/mL are associated with a greater likelihood of maternal bleeding.[1] It is essential that all blood samples be drawn remote from the site of heparin infusion. After initial adjustment and stabilization of the heparin dose, daily laboratory testing is adequate. The infusion dose required may change as active thrombosis is halted (Figure 28.6).

Duration of the intravenous infusion is quite variable but should be continued for a minimum of 2 days with DVT and 5 days with PE, depending on the severity of the disease. Many authors recommend intravenous therapy for a minimum of 7 to 10 days. Historically, the goal was to continue intravenous heparin until active thrombosis had stopped, thrombi were firmly attached to the vessel wall, and organization had begun.[1] An adequate therapeutic response may also be achieved, however, by the use of subcutaneous heparin.[45] The period of continuous intravenous infusion is followed in pregnancy by therapeutic subcutaneous injection for the duration of the pregnancy and anticoagulation for 6 weeks postpartum.

Subcutaneous sodium heparin may also be adjusted after measurement of the PTT or heparin level. Injections of heparin at 12-hour intervals are most commonly used, but more frequent intervals (8 hours) are also acceptable. A PTT of 1.5–2.0 times normal control values[46] or a heparin level of 0.2–0.3 units/mL 6 hours after injection have been shown to be associated with adequate anticoagulation and a low risk of bleeding. Peak levels occur approximately 2–4 hours after subcutaneous injection and the lowest levels just prior to the subsequent injection.[45] In a patient in whom management of anticoagulation is difficult, serial heparin levels may be necessary initially to monitor that patient's response to a specific heparin dose. When long-term treatment is necessary, anticoagulation may be evaluated weekly after a stable dose has been reached.

The dosage and timing is also affected by the type of heparin used. Both sodium and calcium salts are available. Sodium heparin is less expensive, achieves higher levels, has a longer duration of action, and is more generally preferred. In contrast, the use of calcium heparin necessitates higher and more frequent doses. In this report, the dosages suggested are for sodium heparin.

Careful technique in administration of subcutaneous heparin prevents erratic absorption and local bruising. The anterior flank (lateral abdominal wall) subcutaneous fat is preferable to sites in the arms and legs that are more painful and subject to rapid absorption of heparin associated with movement. An 0.5-inch or 1.5-cm needle is fully inserted vertically into a raised fold of skin and withdrawn atraumatically after injection. Further manipulation of the area (eg, massage) is avoided.

Recently reported alternatives to long-term intermittent injections in pregnancy have included continuous infusions of heparin via a Hickman catheter[47] or subcutaneous pump.[48] Six patients received continuous subcutaneous infusion to reach a therapeutic PTT of 1.5 to 2 times control values. Although there were no recurrences of thrombosis, five of the patients experienced major or minor bleeding complications.[48] Studies are needed to show a more acceptable complication rate before this technique could be recommended.

THE PREOPERATIVE CESAREAN PATIENT ON ANTICOAGULANT THERAPY

Patients on heparin and coumadin must be considered differently due to the great differences in mechanism of action, half-life, and reversal of these drugs. At the beginning of labor and delivery, a clotting profile and hematocrit should be drawn on any patient who has been receiving either therapeutic or prophylactic anticoagulants.

For the patient on heparin therapy, there are several alternatives for management. Therapeutic heparinization should be continued in high-risk patients such as those with recent PE or iliofemoral thrombosis. Additionally, patients with mechanical heart valve prostheses should also be considered for continued therapy. For this purpose, continuous intravenous infusion, aiming for a heparin level of 0.1–0.2 units/mL or a low therapeutic PTT, about 1.0–1.5 times normal, will avoid wide swings in the heparin level. Under the circumstances of continued heparin therapy, intraoperative bleeding is increased; thus, meticulous surgical technique is essential to minimize blood loss.

In the absence of an active clotting process and when minimal circulating heparin is desired, 5,000 units every 12 hours may be given perioperatively. Thoughtful consideration of individual situations is needed to guide the transition from the therapeutic dose to this low dose. A 12-hour interval prior to surgery may be sufficient.

For patients other than those at very high risk of thromboembolism, stopping heparin administration prior to cesarean and resuming it sometime afterward is recommended. This is the easiest way to manage the anticoagulated patient clinically. If continuous intravenous heparin infusion is being given, it should be stopped at least 4 hours prior to cesarean delivery and resumed without an intravenous bolus no earlier than 6 hours postoperatively. The last adjusted dose of subcutaneous heparin should be given no later than 6 to 8 prior to after the cesarean. It can be seen from the heparin half-life that with these guidelines a very small amount of heparin is still likely to be present and useful prophylactically. In contrast to a patient undergoing vaginal delivery, in whom blood loss is not much different from that of her anticoagulated state, the woman undergoing cesarean delivery has a significantly greater chance of bleeding. Thus, these guidelines are not rigid and require weighing of the risk of thromboembolism against the risk of perioperative bleeding.

When urgent cesarean delivery is necessary and heparin has been administered recently, protamine sulfate may be used to reverse heparinization. Each milligram of protamine sulfate administered intravenously will neutralize 100 units of heparin. The amount of circulating heparin may also be estimated by figuring the plasma volume at a rate of 50 mL per kilogram of body weight and multiplying the plasma volume by the heparin concentration.[9] Alternatively, the normal therapeutic level can be assumed to be 0.2–0.4 IU/mL, and a half-life of 1–1.5 hours can be used to estimate the unmetabolized heparin after a subcutaneous dose. A conservative estimate of the amount of protamine sulfate is required because excess protamine can act as an anticoagulant. The maximum allowable single dose should not exceed 50 mg. A dose that high is rarely required in these patients. If rapid laboratory services are not available, the administration of protamine may be titrated to the Lee-White clotting time. It should be given intravenously over 20 to 30 minutes to prevent hypotension. If there is sufficient time, the preferable and safest approach is to wait for the clearance of heparin.

Patients anticoagulated with warfarin who undergo cesarean delivery are at a greater risk for bleeding compared with those receiving heparin. The action of warfarin is much more difficult to reverse because its duration of action is 4 to 5 days. Parenteral vitamin K given at least 12 hours prior to cesarean may sufficiently regenerate maternal clotting factors. If it does not, 2 to 4 units of fresh frozen plasma may be given to supply the necessary clotting factors.[49] However, the fetal effects are reversed much more slowly. In utero vitamin K injections are followed approximately 48 hours later by normal neonatal PT at delivery. If warfarin is simply discontinued, up to 2 weeks is required for fetal reversal.[49] Atraumatic delivery is desirable to avoid fetal hemorrhage. Fetal anticoagulation, especially in a premature infant, may itself be an indication for cesarean delivery.

POSTCESAREAN ANTICOAGULANT THERAPY

In the postcesarean patient, tissue injury and venous stasis contribute to the overall increased risk of thromboembolism. Patients on therapeutic anticoagulation therapy prior to cesarean should be treated for 6 weeks postpartum. Therapy may consist of either adjusted-dose subcutaneous heparin injections or warfarin.

The potential disadvantages of oral anticoagulation with warfarin include a higher risk of bleeding complications and the necessity for frequent monitoring with the PT. If warfarin is selected, hospitalization and heparin should be continued until the appropriate therapeutic effect of warfarin has been achieved. This is usually 3 days after warfarin therapy has been initiated. Although warfarin therapy in lactating mothers remains somewhat controversial, investigators have not detected significant amounts of warfarin in breast milk. Thus, lactating women on warfarin therapy should be permitted to breast-feed their infants.[50]

Postcesarean thrombosis or embolism also requires therapeutic anticoagulation for a minimum of 6 weeks. If thrombosis occurs remote from delivery, the patient should be treated as a nonpregnant person, for whom longer periods of anticoagulation (eg, 3 months) are recommended.

SEPTIC PELVIC THROMBOPHLEBITIS

Because endometritis occurs most commonly in the postcesarean patient, the sequelae of septic pelvic thrombophlebitis and ovarian vein thrombophlebitis are also more likely to occur. Most often, the former condition is suspected in postcesarean patients who fail to respond to parenteral antibiotic therapy.

In general, septic thrombophlebitis of the pelvic veins is a diagnosis of exclusion. About 0.5%–2% of patients with endometritis or operative site infection develop this complication.[51] Puerperal ovarian vein thrombophlebitis occurs preponderantly on the right side and may be suspected in the presence of lateralized pain, fever, and a tender, rope-like abdominal mass extending laterally and cephalad from the uterine cornu. The tenderness and guarding found in the postoperative abdomen may make detection of unusual tenderness and palpation of a mass more difficult. Untreated ovarian vein thrombosis may extend to the inferior vena cava or, if on the left side, to the left renal vein, causing renal vein thrombosis.[52] In addition to parenteral antibiotics, treatment consists of anticoagulation with heparin. In septic pelvic thrombophlebitis, heparin is continued for 7–10 days. In ovarian vein thrombophlebitis, heparin therapy may be continued for up to 3 weeks.[50]

SURGICAL TREATMENT OF THROMBOEMBOLIC DISORDERS

Surgical intervention may be indicated in two clinical situations: embolectomy of a life-threatening, massive PE or vena caval interruption for recurrent venous emboli in spite of adequate anticoagulation. There are a variety of methods for interruption of the vena cava, including complete ligation, Teflon clips, and devices inserted transvenously such as the umbrella filter or the Greenfield filter.[53]

THROMBOEMBOLUS PROPHYLAXIS

Heparin doses used for prophylaxis do not pose as great a hazard for the patient undergoing cesarean delivery as therapeutic anticoagulation. Patients may be receiving prophylaxis for a variety of reasons: a history of PE or DVT, artificial heart valves, or primary hypercoagulable disorders such as AT III deficiency. Specific peripartum prophylaxis may benefit individuals with other risk factors such as older age, higher parity, obesity, operative delivery, and prolonged immobilization. If thromboembolism is not associated with pregnancy (eg, while taking oral contraceptives), authors vary as to the need for prophylaxis during pregnancy. All agree that prophylaxis is important during the puerperium.

Prophylaxis consists of subcutaneous heparin injections every 12 hours, and the dose varies during gestation. Increasing uteroplacental coagulation and platelet activity as pregnancy progresses lead to progressive neutralization of heparin. Doses should be adjusted to reflect these changes. This may result in an increase from 5,000 to 7,500 units and possibly 10,000 units in the third trimester.[1] A dose of 8,000 units every 12 hours is suggested for the puerperium.[54] To minimize perioperative bleeding complications, patients receiving prophylactic heparin for reasons such as obesity and immobilization are frequently given 5,000 units every 12 hours. Cautious administration is important in patients with diminished renal function, who may experience elevated heparin levels. Though less frequent, bleeding complications or osteopenia[46,54] may occur with low-dose heparin.

Antiplatelet agents such as aspirin and dipyridamole, which are most helpful in preventing thrombosis in the arterial circulation or with some prosthetic heart valves, have no known role in the prevention of pregnancy-associated thromboembolic disease.

SUMMARY

Suspicion of DVT or thromboembolism is critical to early diagnosis and treatment prior to the development of severe or life-threatening pathology. If the clinical situation is strongly suggestive, treatment with intravenous heparin can be immediately initiated, followed by definitive diagnosis. Because the consequences of treatment are long-term inconvenience and the risk of major complications, objective studies are necessary to confirm the diagnosis. Radiographic procedures such as angiography and lung scanning provide valuable information with low risk to the mother and fetus. When indicated, anticoagulation can be instituted with relative safety, providing there is careful monitoring. Heparin is unquestionably the drug of choice for treatment and prophylaxis during pregnancy. Because warfarin carries a significant risk to the fetus of anomalies and hemorrhage and is undesirable near delivery due to its poor reversibility, its use in a cesarean patient is very limited. It may be given postoperatively, even if the mother is breast-feeding, but is generally begun after the initial use of heparin. There is no practical value to other treatment modalities such as thrombolysis in the peripartal cesarean patient.

The opinions expressed in this chapter are those of the authors and not necessarily those of the United States Navy or the Department of Defense.

REFERENCES

1. Bonnar J: Venous thromboembolism and pregnancy. *Clin Obstet Gynecol* 8:455, 1981.
2. Villasanta U: Thromboembolic disease in pregnancy. *Am J Obstet Gynecol* 93:142, 1965.
3. Bergqvist A, Bergqvist D, Hallbook T: Acute deep vein thrombosis (DVT) after cesarean section. *Acta Obstet Gynecol Scand* 58:473, 1979.
4. Hirsh J, Cade JF, Gallus AS: Anticoagulants in pregnancy: A review of indications and complications. *Am Heart J* 83:301, 1972.
5. Stead RB: Regulation of hemostasis, in Goldhaber SZ (ed): *Pulmonary Embolism and Deep Venous Thrombosis*. Philadelphia, WB Saunders Co, 1985, pp 27–40.
6. Needleman P, Minkes M, Raz A: Thromboxanes: Selected biosynthesis and distinct biologic properties. *Science* 193:163, 1976.
7. Thompson AR, Harker CA: *Manual of Thrombosis and Hemostasis*. Philadelphia, FA Davis Co, 1983.
8. Holmsen H: Platelet secretion, in Colman RW, Hirsh J, Marder VJ, et al (eds): *Hemostasis and Thrombosis*. Philadelphia, JB Lippincott Co, 1982, p 392.

9. Letsky EA: Coagulation problems during pregnancy, in Lind T (ed): *Current Review in Obstetrics and Gynecology*. Edinburgh, Churchill Livingstone, 1985.
10. Comp PC, Esman CT: Generation of fibrinolytic activity by infusion of activated protein C in dogs. *J Clin Invest* 68:1221, 1981.
11. Robbins KC: The plasminogen-plasmin enzyme system, in Colman RW, Hirsh J, Marder VJ, et al (eds): *Hemostasis and Thrombosis*. Philadelphia, JB Lippincott Co, 1982.
12. Brandt JT: Current concepts of coagulation. *Clin Obstet Gynecol* 28:3, 1985.
13. Comp PD, Clouse L: Plasma proteins C and S: The function and assay of two natural anticoagulants. *Lab Management* 23:29, 1985.
14. Moake JL, Levine JD: Thrombotic disorders. *Clin Symposia* 37: 1985.
15. Bonnar J, McNichol GP, Douglas AS: Fibrinolytic enzyme system and pregnancy. *Br Med J* 3:387, 1969.
16. Laros RK, Alger LS: Thromboembolism and pregnancy. *Clin Obstet Gynecol* 22:871, 1979.
17. Rosenow EC III, Osmundson PJ, Brown ML: Pulmonary embolism. *Mayo Clin Proc* 56:161, 1981.
18. Markisz JA: Radiologic and nuclear medicine diagnosis, in Goldhaber SZ (ed): *Pulmonary Embolism and Deep Venous Thrombosis*. Philadelphia, WB Saunders Co, 1985, pp 41–72.
19. Henkin RE: Radionuclide detection of thromboembolic diseases, in Kwaan HC, Bowie EJW (eds): *Thrombosis*. Philadelphia, WB Saunders Co, 1982, pp 236–252.
20. Kakkar V: The diagnosis of deep vein thrombosis using the ^{125}I fibrinogen test. *Arch Surg* 104:152, 1972.
21. Ahlgren L, Ivarsson S, Mattson S, et al: Excretion of radionuclides in human breast milk after the administration of radiopharmaceuticals. *J Nucl Med* 26:1085, 1985.
22. Robin ED: Overdiagnosis and overtreatment of pulmonary embolism: The emperor may have no clothes. *Ann Intern Med* 87:775, 1977.
23. Sors H, Safran D, et al: An analysis of the diagnostic methods for acute pulmonary embolism. *Intensive Care Med* 10:81, 1984.
24. Kipper MS, Moser KM, Kortman KE, et al: Long-term follow-up of patients with suspected pulmonary embolism and a normal lung scan. Perfusion scans in embolic subjects. *Chest* 82:411, 1982.
25. Mills SR, Jackson DC, Older RA, et al: The incidence, etiologies, and avoidance of complications of pulmonary angiography in a large series. *Radiology* 136:295, 1980.
26. National Council on Radiation Protection and Measurements: *Medical Radiation Exposure of Pregnant and Potentially Pregnant Women*. Washington, DC, 1977.
27. Hull RD, Hirsch J, Carter CJ, et al: Pulmonary angiography, ventilation lung scanning, and venography for clinically suspected pulmonary embolism with abnormal perfusion lung scan. *Ann Intern Med* 98:891, 1983.
28. Dalen JE, Brooks HL, Johnson LW, et al: Pulmonary angiography in acute pulmonary embolism: Indications, techniques, and results in 367 patients. *Am Heart J* 81:175, 1979.
29. Goldhaber SZ: Strategies for diagnosis, in Goldhaber SZ (ed): *Pulmonary Embolism and Deep Venous Thrombosis*. Philadelphia, WB Saunders Co, 1985, pp 79–97.
30. Ezekowitz MD, Pope CF, Smith EO: Indium-111 platelet imaging, in Goldhaber SZ (ed): *Pulmonary Embolism and Deep Venous Thrombosis*. Philadelphia, WB Saunders Co, 1985, pp 261–267.
31. Bratt G, Tornebohm E, Lockner D, et al: A human pharmacological study comparing conventional heparin and a low molecular weight heparin fragment. *Thromb Haemost* 53:208, 1985.
32. DeSwart CAM, Nijmeter B, Roelofs JMM, et al: Kinetics of intravenously administered heparin in normal humans. *Blood* 60:1251, 1982.

33. Walker AM, Jick H: Predictors of bleeding during heparin therapy. *JAMA* 244:1209, 1980.
34. Holm HA, Abildgaard U, Kalvenes S: Heparin assays and bleeding complications in treatment of deep venous thrombosis with particular reference to retroperitoneal bleeding. *Thromb Haemost* 53:278, 1985.
35. Hyers TM, Hull RD, Weg JG: Antithrombotic therapy for venous thromboembolic disease. *Chest* 89:265, 1986.
36. Basu D, Gallus A, Hirsh J, et al: A prospective study of the value of monitoring heparin treatment with the activated partial thromboplastin time. *N Engl J Med* 287:324, 1972.
37. *1984 Drug Information for the Health Care Provider,* vol I. Rockville, MD, USPDI, 1983, pp 562–566.
38. Chang BH, Pitney WR, Castaldi PA: Heparin-induced thrombocytopenia: Association of thrombotic complications with heparin-dependent IgG antibody that induces thromboxane synthesis and platelet aggregation. *Lancet* 2:1246, 1982.
39. Griffith GC: Heparin osteoporosis. *JAMA* 143:85, 1965.
40. deSwiet M, Ward PD, Fidler J, et al: Prolonged heparin therapy in pregnancy causes bone demineralization. *Br J Obstet Gynecol* 90:1129, 1983.
41. Zimran A, Shilo S, Fisher D, et al: Histomorphometric evaluation of reversible heparin-induced osteoporosis in pregnancy. *Arch Intern Med* 146:386, 1986.
42. Mant MJ, O'Brien BD, Russell DB: Diagnostic leg scanning for deep venous thrombosis in the recently heparinized patient. *Arch Intern Med* 141:1757, 1986.
43. Standing Advisory Committee for Haematology of the Royal College of Pathologists: Drug interaction with coumarin derivative anticoagulants. *Br Med J* 185:274, 1982.
44. Moser KM, Fedullo PF: Venous thromboembolism: Three simple decisions (part 2). *Chest* 83:256, 1983.
45. Anderson G, Fagrell B, Holmgren K, et al: Subcutaneous administration of heparin: A randomized comparison with intravenous administration of heparin to patients with deep-vein thrombosis. *Thromb Res* 27:631, 1982.
46. Hull R, Delmore T, Carter C, et al: Adjusted subcutaneous heparin versus warfarin sodium in the long-term treatment of venous thrombosis. *N Engl J Med* 306:189, 1982.
47. Nelson DM, Stempel LE, Fabri PJ, et al: Hickman catheter use in a pregnant patient requiring therapeutic heparin anticoagulation. *Am J Obstet Gynecol* 149:461, 1984.
48. Barss VA, Schwartz PA, Greene MF, et al: Use of the subcutaneous heparin pump during pregnancy. *J Reprod Med* 30:899, 1985.
49. Knuppel RA, Petrucha RA: The anticoagulated patient in labor: An obstetric dilemma. *South Med J* 74:1084, 1981.
50. Orme ML, Lewis PJ, deSwiet M, et al: May mothers given warfarin breast-feed their infants? *Br Med J* 1:1564, 1977.
51. Duff P, Gibbs RS: Pelvic vein thrombophlebitis: Diagnostic dilemma and therapeutic challenge. *Obstet Gynecol Surv* 38:365, 1983.
52. Brown TK, Munsick RA: Puerperal ovarian vein thrombophlebitis: A syndrome. *Am J Obstet Gynecol* 109:263, 1974.
53. Hux CH, Wagner R, Rattan P, et al: Surgical treatment of thromboembolic disease in pregnancy. *Proceedings of the Society of Perinatal Obstetricians,* January 30–February 1, 1986, San Antonio, TX, p 62.
54. Howell R, Fidler J, Letsky E, et al: The risks of antenatal subcutaneous heparin prophylaxis: A controlled trial. *Br J Obstet Gynaecol* 90:1124, 1983.

Chapter 29

Diagnosis and Management of the Patient with a Fistula

Donald G. Gallup, MD, and
O. Eduardo Talledo, MD

Occurrence of fistula following cesarean delivery or cesarean hysterectomy is directly related to the technical difficulties encountered in performing the procedure and inversely related to the surgeon's experience. Failure to recognize injury to the urinary or digestive tract at the time of surgery is of major significance in the pathogenesis of such fistulas. The diagnosis, timing of repair, approach to repair, and technical guidelines for the more common obstetrically related fistulas will be reviewed.

VESICOVAGINAL FISTULA

Major injuries to the lower urinary tract reported in this country often occur during the course of gynecologically related procedures, usually hysterectomy.[1–3] The incidence of vesicovaginal fistula following cesarean delivery is about 0.04%; the incidence following cesarean hysterectomy ranges between 0.3% and 0.9%.[4] Vesicovaginal fistula may result from unrecognized bladder injury due to aggressive clamping or suture placement. Fistulas can occasionally follow forceps delivery and cerclage procedures.

Diagnosis of Unrecognized Injury

The diagnosis of a vesicovaginal fistula is often difficult. For instance, the patient's only complaint may be a variable amount of vaginal discharge. With small fistulas, the discharge, watery in character, may be episodic, related to changes in position or to bladder fullness, and normal micturation may be possible. Patients with vesicouterine fistula may be intermittently incontinent or complain only of dampness, and hematuria may be present during menses (menouria).[5] Because ureterovaginal fistulas occasionally occur with vesicovaginal fistulas, evaluation of the upper genitourinary tract is indicated. The bladder is distended with sterile milk or dilute congo red dye. Spillage into the vagina indicates a vesicovaginal fistula. If there is no spillage, the substance is left in the bladder and indigo carmine (5 mL) is given intravenously. If only dark blue dye is seen in the vagina, a ureterovaginal fistula should be suspected. If powder blue or a mixture of red and blue is noted, a combined ureterovaginal and vesicovaginal fistula should be suspected. A duck bill speculum in the vagina often aids in locating these fistulas. The three-tampon technique is also helpful in determining the location of small fistulas. After three tampons are inserted into the vagina, dilute methylene blue or indigo carmine is inserted into the bladder. The patient is ambulated. If the lower tampon is wet and blue and the others are dry, a urethral vaginal fistula is probably present. If the upper tampon is wet and blue, a vesicovaginal fistula is probable. If the upper tampon is wet only, a ureterovaginal fistula should be suspected.[6] Pyridium has also been used successfully in cases of persistent watery discharge to detect small fistulas.

Other tests include voiding cystography with a lateral view and CO_2 or air cytoscopy performed in the knee-chest position with the vagina partially filled with liquid medium. Bubbling is observed in patients with fistulas. An intravenous pyelogram (IVP) is essential for determination of the possible involvement of one or both ureters. Retrograde pyelography will confirm the location of ureteral lesions. Hysterography is helpful when vesicouterine fistula is suspected. A vesicocolonic fistula can be detected by noting the appearance of dye in the urine previously administered by an enema. If the fistula is between the small bowel and the bladder, orally administered congo red will appear in the urine.[7]

Timing of Repair

Timing of the repair of a vesicovaginal fistula must be determined on an individual basis and depends on the cause, size, and site of the fistula. The old dictum of waiting 6 months or more prior to closure is unreasonable for most patients.[8] Small, uncomplicated fistulas, which follow hysterectomies, can usually be closed after about 8 weeks using the Latzko technique. Some have reported high success rates in repairing acute fistulas transvaginally within 2–12 weeks of occurrence when preoperative steroids were given.[9,10] In general, repair can be undertaken when the bladder and vaginal sites are without inflammation and free of edema.

Large, complicated fistulas should not be repaired early. Some obstetric-related fistulas may require a delay of 4 to 6 months prior to closure after involution of the birth canal is completed.[11,12] Furthermore, spontaneous closure following catheterization with a large indwelling Foley catheter has been noted in 10% to 20% of patients.[13–15] Most fistulas

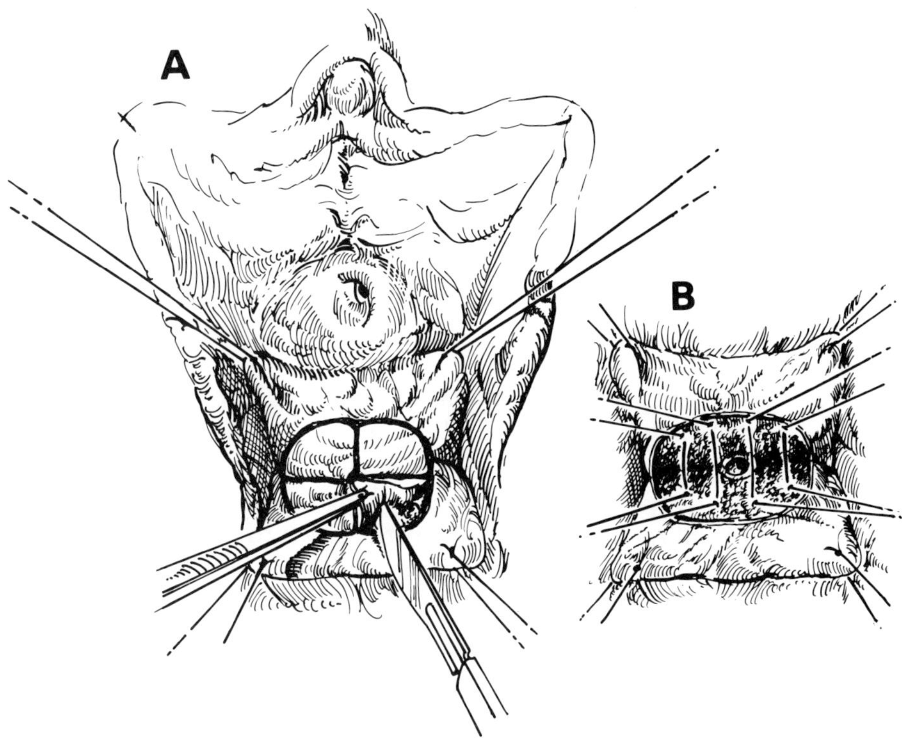

FIGURE 29.1 Latzko technique. (A) The vaginal mucosa is divided around the fistula in a four-quadrant technique. The fistula tract is left intact. (B) Interrupted sutures invert the divided vagina, covering the tract. Three layers are used.

that close spontaneously are millimeter-sized and close within 3 weeks. A conservative trial of catheter drainage is indicated for at least that period of time.

Surgical Considerations

Whether vesicovaginal fistulas are closed transabdominally or transvaginally, a ureteral catheter should be placed prior to surgery if the ureteral orifices are less than 1 cm from the tract or if the fistula is so large that the integrity of the ureter may be compromised during repair. In small fistulas, threading a small catheter through the fistula tract during cystoscopy from the bladder to the vagina may be helpful. All patients are placed on prophylactic broad-spectrum antibiotics. Although cortisone, given 1 week to 10 days preoperatively, may help decrease edema more quickly,[9,10] the possibility of impaired wound healing makes its use controversial.

There is no single approach for all fistulas. However, many gynecologists use the Latzko technique of partial colpocleisis for small- to medium-sized fistulas. Surgery is performed with the patient in the dorsal

TABLE 29.1 Indications for Abdominal Closure of Vesicovaginal Fistula

Absolute indications
Complex fistulas involving bowel or uterus
Ureteral involvement
Inaccessible location of fistula
Contracted bladder that requires patching
Excessive vaginal scarring
Relative indications
Large fistula
Multiple prior repairs
Fistulas associated with x-ray therapy

lithotomy position. Schuchardt's incision may be required in patients with small-caliber vaginas. A dilute solution of neosynephrine (1:200,000) injected into the area around the fistula will facilitate dissection and decrease blood loss. Traction sutures and a small Foley catheter inserted into the tract allow one to pull the fistula toward the operative field. The area around the fistula tract is removed in four quadrants, using a number 11 blade, the lower quadrants first (Figure 29.1). The tract is not removed or denuded, but the surrounding tissues are sufficiently mobilized. The area is closed over the fistula, using 000 PGA sutures in an inverting manner. The suprapubic approach of bladder drainage for 10 to 14 days with a No. 20 to 22 French catheter is preferable. Coitus should be avoided for a minimum of 8 weeks.

Suprapubic extraperitoneal, transvesical, and transabdominal procedures have a limited place in repairing fistula related to obstetric injuries. Moir[16] noted that the transabdominal approach was necessary in less than 5% of cases. There are few contraindications to transvaginal repair. Most of them are relative (Table 29.1). Even with large fistulas, a modified bulbocavernosus myocutaneous flap, as suggested by Hoskins et al,[17] may be successful and should be tried prior to an abdominal approach.

According to O'Conor,[18] the key to successful abdominal closure of difficult fistulas is bisection of the bladder, with wide mobilization of the bladder and vagina in separate planes. The dome of the bladder is opened, and a vertical incision is carried down to the fistula. The tract is excised, and the vagina is closed separately. Fat, peritoneum, or a pedicle of omentum is placed between the bladder and the vagina. Ureteral catheters should be inserted if the lesion is close to the trigone. Suprapubic drainage is preferred.

URETERAL FISTULA

Ureteral injuries are usually associated with pelvic surgical procedures. Their incidence varies from 0.4% to 2.5% of all gynecologic procedures.[1,19] Because only about one-third of ureteral injuries are recognized, this estimated incidence is probably low. Ureteral injuries associated with

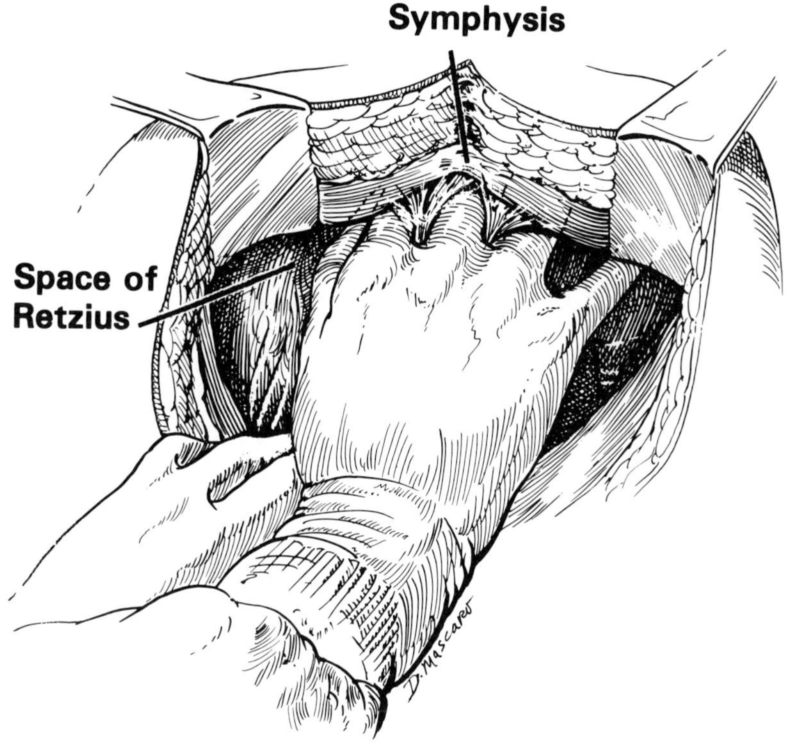

FIGURE 29.2 Developing the space of Retzius for mobilization of the bladder in order to make safe incisions in the bladder. The weight of the hand of the operator in the midline separates the bladder from its anterior attachment to the symphysis. Cephalad traction with the opposite hand of the operator on the peritoneum will aid in exposure of the space.

cesarean delivery are sporadically reported. They are usually associated with lateral extension of the uterine incision and aggressive suturing or clamping to control bleeding.[8,20,21] Following prolonged labor, ureteral fistulae cannot always be attributed to the cesarean, as pressure from the presenting part may contribute to ischemia of the distal ureter.[22] The vascular anastomotic ureteral adventitia network cannot be interrupted for more than 2 cm without the risk of necrosis. Because of dextrorotation of the pregnant uterus, the left ureter is at particular risk of injury. The ureters may be protected from injury during cesarean by adequately dissecting the bladder flap and using a broad-based bladder retractor.

Intraoperative ureteral injuries associated with cesarean hysterectomy occur in 0.3%–0.4% of cases,[23,24] whereas the frequency of postoperative ureterovaginal fistulas is about 0.7%.[25] When cesarean hysterectomy is necessary, large pedicles in the cardinal ligament area should be avoided. The use of the cautery to control bleeding is also not advisable. Furthermore, in emergency situations, eg, ruptured uteri, a supracervical hysterectomy in selected cases will not only expedite the procedure but will help avoid ureteral injury. During reperitonealization after a total hysterec-

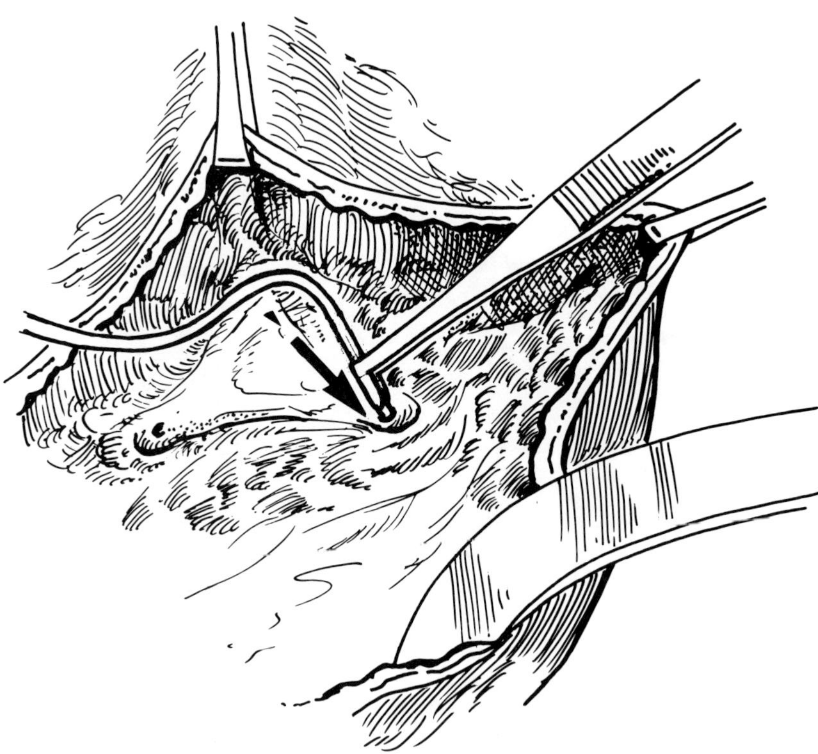

FIGURE 29.3 The bladder has been opened. A ureteral silastic catheter is threaded up the ureter through the orifice. A Campbell ureteral catheter passer aids in passage of the No. 6–8 French catheter.

tomy, a carelessly placed suture on the medial leaf can result in kinking or even ligation of the ureter.

An unrecognized injury may lead to permanent renal impairment. If an injury is suspected, indigo carmine can be injected intravenously or directly into the ureteral lumen to check for extravasation. If dye does not appear in the urine, obstruction should be suspected. If there is any doubt, the bladder should be opened. Mobilization of the bladder should first be accomplished by developing the space of Retzius (Figure 29.2). A vertical incision is carried along the dome of the bladder to expose the trigone. Indigo carmine (5 cc) is given intravenously. After 3 to 5 minutes, the ureteral orifices are observed for efflux *or* blue urine. Urinary output can be increased by giving 12.5 g of mannitol intravenously prior to injecting the dye.[19] If no urine is noted, a No. 6 to 8 French ureteral catheter is passed with the aid of a grooved Campbell's forceps (Figure 29.3). If there is difficulty in passing the catheter from below, a stab wound in the proximal ureter is made and the catheter is passed caudad.

The management of intraoperative injuries is discussed in Chapter 19. In cases of crush injuries, an indwelling silastic No. 6–8 French ureteral catheter for 10 to 14 days is often sufficient.

Postoperative Diagnosis of Ureteral Injury

Most of the techniques noted in the discussion of bladder injury apply to ureteral injuries as well. The IVP is the mainstay of postoperative diagnosis. Cystoscopy and ipsilateral retrograde pyelography are often needed to determine the exact location of the obstruction or lesion. The classic symptoms of fever, chills, flank pain, and passage of urine through the vagina, skin, or rectum should lead to initiation of these diagnostic tests. One should be aware that some patients with ureteral injuries present with abdominal distention, paralytic ileus, incontinence, or even a mass—the pseudocystic urinoma.

Timing of Repair of Unrecognized Injury

Because most of the techniques for ureteral reconstruction require a lengthy operation, the patient's general condition has an important bearing on when repairs should be attempted, although immediate repair has been suggested by some.[26–28] After 72 hours, such intervention is indicated only if pyelonephritis develops and IVP studies indicate progressive damage to the ipsilateral kidney. Repair of injuries diagnosed after 72 hours is, in general, postponed because of edema and associated local inflammation.

If a silastic catheter can be passed at the time of retrograde studies, obstruction can be circumvented in some patients. Often a percutaneous nephrostomy using a small Teflon catheter will produce immediate drainage and can sometimes be passed beyond the area of injury.[29–31] As many as 15% of ureteral fistulas will heal spontaneously if a ureteral splint can be left in place for at least 7 to 10 days.[32,33] Periodic renal sonograms every 4 weeks should be done to evaluate the upper urinary tract, because worsening of the obstructive uropathy may be an indication for earlier surgical intervention.

Surgical Considerations

If the fistula has not healed within 4 to 6 months, or if there is progressive deterioration of renal function, operative intervention is indicated. The time-honored principles of repair (hemostasis, lack of tension, watertightness) should be maintained. The type of repair to be used depends on the cause and extent of the injury, as well as its location.

Generally, lesions within 4 to 5 cm of the ureterovesical junction can be repaired using a ureteroneocystostomy. There must be *no* tension on the reimplantation site. To ensure a tension-free anastomosis, the bladder should be mobilized as noted in Figure 29.2, or the bladder can be attached to the ipsilateral psoas muscle with nonabsorbable sutures. When a long segment of distal ureter is involved, the gap can be bridged by utilizing a flap from the bladder, as described in the Boari-Okerbland method.[34] The Demel technique is a good alternative and is less prone to stricture development. The bladder is simply opened transversely and closed longitudinally.[35] The ureter is anastomosed to the bladder mucosa with interrupted 4-0 or 5-0 chromic [or polyglycolic acid (PGA)] suture. Fine, nonabsorbable sutures approximate the outside of the bladder wall and the ureteral adventitia. A silastic ureteral splint is inserted and left in place for 14 to 21 days. The retroperitoneal space is drained, using a closed system for 7 to 10 days or until drainage is minimal.

Tunneling to avoid reflux has been advocated by some investigators,[36] whereas others find this unnecessary and advocate direct, open implantation in the dome area.[37,38] Recently, Wheeless[39] reported more long-term complications in adult patients who had tunneling procedures, compared to those who had direct implantation, and suggested that tunneling was unnecessary in adults.

For injuries located above the pelvic brim, an end-to-end ureteroureterostomy is done. The damaged area must be excised. The ureter ends should be spatulated, one anteriorly and one posteriorly, to create a larger lumen. Repair is accomplished with interrupted stitching of 4-0 or 5-0 chromic or PGA sutures. A vertical ureterostomy about 2 cm in length, 5 cm cephalad to the anastomosis, is advocated.[1,19,40] A No. 6 to 8 French silastic catheter is threaded into the ureter and left in place for 2 to 3 weeks. A soft retroperitoneal closed drainage system, away from the sutured area, is also left in place for 2 to 3 weeks, or until drainage is less than 30 mL/24 hr. Mobilization of the ipsilateral kidney may be necessary to reduce tension. Many feel that the anastomotic site should be reinforced with omental fat.[19,41]

Transureteroureterostomy is a valuable option when a large segment of ureter has been injured.[19] The proximal ureter is tunneled retroperitoneally across the midline and sutured to the contralateral ureter. The prerequisite is an intact urinary drainage system on the opposite side. This procedure may be associated with stenosis, leakage, and possible damage to the intact urinary system. Other options include insertion of the ureter into an intestinal segment, which is then sutured to the bladder (ureteroileocystoplasty), and in rare cases ligation and nephrectomy.[19] The latter should be performed only after other methods have failed or if the kidney is nonfunctioning and infected.

INTESTINAL TRACT FISTULA

Intestinal injuries may result in fistula formation involving both the large and small bowels. The former are classified into those above or below the peritoneal reflection. Most of the small bowel injuries related to obstetrics and gynecology occur in the ileum. Intestinal fistulas are usually associated with endometriosis, surgical trauma, radiation therapy, pelvic infections,

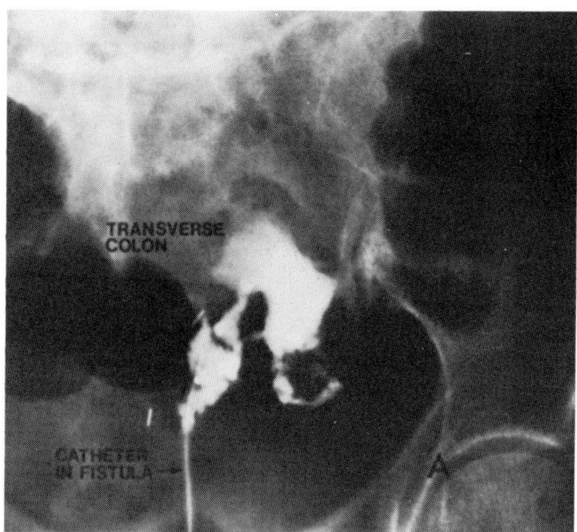

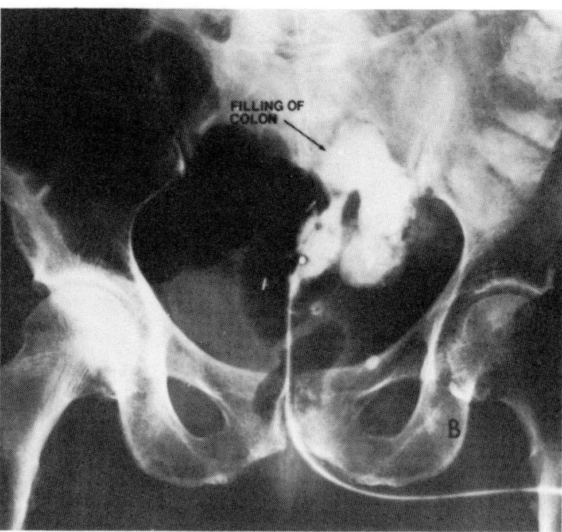

FIGURE 29.4 Fistulogram in a 60-year-old woman who has had persistent drainage thought to be caused by a stitch abscess. (A) Injection of hypoque into the catheter in the fistula. (B) Filling of the fistula and transverse and descending colons.

retained sponges, obstruction, appendicitis, granulomatous pelvic diseases, and inflammatory bowel disease. The injuries and fistulas associated with obstetrics usually occur upon entry into the abdomen; during hysterectomy; and during closure of the abdomen, when a knuckle of bowel may become incorporated into a suture. Prolonged labor, forceps delivery, and extension of episiotomies are rarely associated with bowel injuries and fistulas and are not within the scope of this chapter.

Unrecognized Bowel Injuries and Fistulas

Most enterovaginal or enterocutaneous fistulas have fairly typical signs of foul drainage, sometimes interpreted by the surgeon as a "deep stitch abscess." With persistent drainage, whether through the vagina or the skin, some simple diagnostic tests are helpful. Patients can ingest charcoal, congo red dye, carmine dye, or Povan.* Appearance of one of these materials at the drainage site confirms the diagnosis of bowel fistula. A fistulogram usually pinpoints the origin (Figure 29.4). A barium enema may be helpful in selected cases. Milk or methylene blue inserted into the rectum may help identify small rectovaginal fistulas. For complex fistulas involving the bladder or ureter, other studies may be necessary.

Timing of Fistula Repair

In the absence of acute abdominal signs, there is no need to rush to repair any gastrointestinal fistula. Obviously, high small bowel fistulas and re-

* Parke-Davis Company, Morris Plains, NJ.

TABLE 29.2 One-Day Whole Gut Lavage with Golytely[a] Solution

Two days prior to operation, give patient 1 oral biscodyl tablet to be taken at home hs.
One day prior to operation:
1. Clear liquid diet.
2. Begin chilled Golytely po at 0900 hours. The rate of ingestion should be 1.2–1.8 L/hr for a total of 3–8 hours.
3. Golytely is discontinued when clear liquid passes per rectum.
4. Neomycin sulfate, 1 g po at 1300, 1400, and 2300 hours.
5. Erythromycin base, 1 g po at 1300, 1400, and 2300 hours.
6. No enemas are needed.

Day of surgery:
1. Fleet's enema at 0630 hours.
2. Cefoxitin sodium may be given: 2 g IV push on call and 2 g IV push q6h $\times$ 3.

For patients who cannot tolerate Golytely, the solution may be infused via a nasogastric tube.

[a] Braintree Laboratories, Braintree, MA.

sulting electrolyte imbalance can result in significant morbidity and mortality. These fistulas are rarely seen in obstetric and gynecologic patients. Spontaneous closure of other small bowel and large bowel fistulas occurs in over 50% of nonirradiated patients when bowel rest and total parenteral nutrition are used.[42] Thus, the decision to repair a fistula surgically can often be delayed for 4 to 6 weeks. Bury and associates[43] have found that an elemental diet led to spontaneous closure in 54% of patients with a variety of fistulas. It is conceivable that the majority of small, obstetrically related fistulas may close if patients are placed on elemental or low-residue diets. On the other hand, as stated by Lichtman and McDonald,[44] fistulas are unlikely to close spontaneously if they are associated with foreign bodies such as permanent sutures, obstruction distal to the fistula, epithelialization of the fistula tract, or a size more than 1 cm.

Management of Intestinal Tract Fistulas

In addition to bowel preparation (Table 29.2),[45] patients are placed on an elemental diet 7 days prior to repair. Some gynecologic and general surgeons have reservations about using antibiotics for bowel sterilization and rely solely on mechanical preparation.

Some bowel fistulas are sometimes difficult to locate once celiotomy is done. Placing a Foley catheter in the fistula aids in its location. Unless the fistula is pinhole sized, resection is required. Reanastomosis can be accomplished by suture or staple techniques.[46,47]

A bypass colostomy for colonic fistulas below the peritoneal reflection is not needed. On the other hand, fistulas that occur after prior surgical attempts or in association with pelvic irradiation require a temporary diversion of the fecal stream. After colostomy, the fistula can be repaired in about 8 weeks, when edema and cellulitis have resolved. Moreover, colostomy closure should be delayed for an additional 6 weeks. When colostomies are closed, the previous colostomy site is packed open, and secondary closure is done 5 to 7 days later.

Small- to medium-sized rectovaginal or sigmoid vaginal fistulas can be repaired by the Latzko technique. Large, high, obstetrically related fistulas can be closed by the vaginal or the rectal route. Complex fistulas require a transabdominal approach. Gynecologists have successfully used the vaginal route, although a Martius flap is usually advocated. Other myocutaneous flaps, including gracilis flaps, can be used.[17] The key to operative management of fistulas is resection of the tract and surrounding scar tissue, mobilization of the vagina and rectum, hemostastis, and three-layer suturing with no tension on the suture lines.[48–50] The use of fine PGA suture material is suggested.

Colorectal surgeons suggest a transrectal approach to fistulas, with the patient in the knee-chest position. The vaginal wall and rectal wall must be mobilized for at least 4 cm. The fistula is removed along with the scar. The defect is closed in three layers. The rectal wall is advanced, brought down in an envelope fashion, and sutured to the internal sphincter for further support and to provide an additional layer.[51,52] It is advisable to use the paradoxical 5 to 6 o'clock sphincter incision, as described by Miller and Brown,[53] to decrease rectal distention by accumulation of gas in patients with midvaginal lesions.

Postoperative care is critical for successful fistula repair, particularly with large fistulas.[49] Postoperatively, patients should be placed on an elemental diet for the first week and then on a low-residue diet for an additional 3 weeks. Lescher and Pratt[49] suggest sewing a rectal tube about 1 cm in diameter at the anal margin, to decrease distension. A Foley catheter is left in place for 48 hours. Antibiotics are given as noted in Table 29.2. Stool softeners, such as Metamucil, are prescribed for at least 3 weeks. Once the patient begins to defecate, perineal toilet is done with a dilute povidone-iodine solution (1 oz added to 2 oz warm water). Sitz baths are initiated after the fourth postoperative day. Coitus is prohibited for 12 weeks. If the repair fails, a repeated attempt should not be made for at least 4 to 6 months.

REFERENCES

1. Symmonds RE: Ureteral injuries associated with gynecologic surgery: Prevention and management. *Clin Obstet Gynecol* 19:623, 1976.
2. Amirikia H, Evans TW: Ten year review of hysterectomies: Trends, indications and risks. *Am J Obstet Gynecol* 134:431, 1979.
3. Tancer ML: The post-hysterectomy (vault) vesicovaginal fistula. *J Urol* 123:839, 1980.
4. Kunz J: Lesions affecting the efferent urinary pathways during gynaecologico-obstetrically indicated operations. *Contributions Gynecol Obstet* 11:84, 1984.
5. Sammour MB: Cystouterine fistula following cesarean section with discharge of menstrual blood per urethram. *Am J Obstet Gynecol* 107:321, 1970.

6. Moir JC: Vesicovaginal fistula. *Proc R Soc Med* 59:1019, 1966.
7. Farringer JL, Hrabovsky E, Marsh J, et al: Vesicocolic fistula. *South Med J* 67:1043, 1974.
8. Goodwin WE, Scardino PT: Vesicovaginal and ureterovaginal fistulas: A summary of 25 years of experience. *J Urol* 123:370, 1980.
9. Collins CG, Pent D, Jones FB: Results of early repair of vesicovaginal fistula with preliminary cortisone treatment. *Am J Obstet Gynecol* 80:1005, 1960.
10. Collins CG, Collins JH, Harrison BR, et al: Early repair of vesicovaginal fistula. *Am J Obstet Gynecol* 111:524, 1971.
11. McCausland AM, Caillouette JC, Bennallack DA, et al: A comparative study of vesicovaginal fistulas following delivery. *Am J Obstet Gynecol* 79:1110, 1960.
12. Wein AJ, Mallory TR, Capiniello VL, et al: Repair of vesicovaginal fistula by a suprapubic transvesical approach. *Surg Gynecol Obstet* 150:57, 1980.
13. Latzko W: Postoperative vesicovaginal fistulas: Genesis and therapy. *Am J Surg* 58:211, 1942.
14. Keettel WC, Sehring FG, Prosse CA, et al: Surgical management of urethrovaginal and vesicovaginal fistulas. *Am J Obstet Gynecol* 131:425, 1978.
15. Marshall VF: Vesicovaginal fistulas on one urological service. *J Urol* 121:25, 1979.
16. Moir JC: Vesicovaginal fistula: Thoughts on the treatment of 350 cases. *Proc R Soc Med* 59:1019, 1966.
17. Hoskins WJ, Park RC, Long R, et al: Repair of urinary tract fistulas with bulbocavernosus myocutaneous flaps. *Obstet Gynecol* 63:580, 1984.
18. O'Conor VJ Jr: Review of experience with vesicovaginal fistula repair. *J Urol* 123:367, 1980.
19. Zinman LM, Libertino JA, Roth RA: Management of operative ureteral injury. *Urology* 12:290, 1978.
20. Flunter-Jones O: Cesarean section in present-day obstetrics. *Am J Obstet Gynecol* 126:52, 1976.
21. Jequier AM, Piper JV: Utero-uterine fistula after lower segment caesarean section. *J Obstet Gynecol Br Commonw* 80:276, 1973.
22. Oumachigui A, Son SB, Nayak PN: Uretero-urinary fistulas in pregnancy: Report of three cases. *Int J Gynaecol Obstet* 18:258, 1980.
23. Mickal A, Begnaud WP, Hawes TP Jr: Pitfalls and complications of cesarean hysterectomy. *Clin Obstet Gynecol* 12:660, 1969.
24. Barclay DL: Cesarean hysterectomy. A thirty years' experience. *Obstet Gynecol NY* 35:120, 1970.
25. Haynes DM, Martin BJ: Cesarean hysterectomy: A twenty-five year review. *Am J Obstet Gynecol* 134:393, 1979.
26. Hoch WH, Kursh ED, Persky L: Early aggressive management of intraoperative ureteral injuries. *J Urol* 114:530, 1975.
27. Beland G: Early treatment of ureteral injuries found after gynecologic surgery. *J Urol* 118:25, 1977.
28. Blandly JP, Anderson JD: Management of the injured ureter. *Proc R Soc Med* 70:187, 1977.
29. Ho PC, Talner LB, Parsons CL, et al: Percutaneous nephrostomy: Experience in 107 kidneys. *Urology* 16:532, 1980.
30. Lang EK, Lanasa JA, Garrett J, et al: The management of urinary fistulas and strictures with percutaneous stent catheters. *J Urol* 122:736, 1979.
31. Fisher HAG, Bennett AH, Rivard DJ, et al: Nonoperative supravesical urinary diversion in obstetrics and gynecology. *Gynecol Oncol* 14:365, 1982.
32. Hulse CA, Sawtelle WW, Naydig PW, et al: Conservative management of ureterovaginal fistula. *J Urol* 99:42, 1968.

33. Lang EK: Diagnosis and management of ureteral fistulae by percutaneous nephrostomy and antegrade stent catheter. *Radiology* 138:311, 1981.
34. Okerblad NF: Reimplantation of the ureter into the bladder by a flap method. *J Urol* 57:845, 1947.
35. Demel R: Plastic reconstruction of ureter from bladder. *Zentbl Chir* 51:2008, 1924.
36. Politano VAQ, Leadbetter WF: An operative technique for the correction of vesicoureteral reflux. *J Urol* 79:932, 1958.
37. Thompson IM, Ross G Jr: Long-term results of bladder flap repair of ureteral injuries. *J Urol* 111:483, 1974.
38. Lee RA, Symmonds RE: Ureterovaginal fistula. *Am J Obstet Gynecol* 109:1032, 1971.
39. Wheeless SCR: Ureteroneocystostomy associated with gynecologic malignancy—to tunnel or not to tunnel. Presented at the Society of Gynecologic Oncologists. Palm Springs, California, February 4, 1986 (abstract).
40. Fry DE, Milholen L, Harbrecht PJ: Iatrogenic ureteral injury. Options in management. *Arch Surg* 118:454, 1983.
41. Beland G: The abdominal surgeon and the ureter. *Can J Surg* 22:540, 1979.
42. Hew LR, Deitel M: Total parenteral nutrition in gynecology and obstetrics. *Obstet Gynecol* 55:464, 1980.
43. Bury KD, Stephens RV, Randall HT: Use of a chemically defined liquid, elemental diet for nutritional management of fistulas of the alimentary tract. *Am J Surg* 121:174, 1971.
44. Lichtman AL, McDonald JR: Fecal fistula. *Surg Gynecol Obstet* 78:449, 1944.
45. Oral electrolyte solutions for colonic lavage before colonoscopy or barium enema. *Med Lett* 27 (issue 686): 39–40, 1985.
46. Gambee LP, Garnjobst W, Hardwick CE: Ten years' experience with a single layer anastomosis in colon surgery. *Am J Surg* 92:222, 1956.
47. Wheeless CR Jr: Stapling techniques in operations for malignant disease of the female genital tract. *Surg Clin North Am* 64:591, 1984.
48. Given FT: Rectovaginal fistula. A review of 20 years' experience in a community hospital. *Am J Obstet Gynecol* 108:41, 1970.
49. Lescher TC, Pratt JH: Vaginal repair of the simple rectovaginal fistula. *Surg Gynecol Obstet* 124:1317, 1967.
50. Boronow RC: Management of radiation-induced fistulas. *Am J Obstet Gynecol* 110:1, 1971.
51. Russell TR, Gallagher DM: Low rectovaginal fistulas. Approach and treatment. *Am J Surg* 134:13, 1977.
52. Greenwald JC, Hoexter B: Repair of rectovaginal fistulas. *Surg Gynecol Obstet* 146:443, 1978.
53. Miller NF, Brown W: The surgical treatment of complete perineal tears in the female. *Am J Obstet Gynecol* 34:196, 1937.

Chapter 30

Reducing the Cesarean Delivery Rate

Richard H. Paul, MD

Currently, there is major concern regarding the incidence of cesarean birth and the continual escalation of this method of delivery in recent years. Current data document a national rate in excess of 20% and institutional rates that approach 50%.[1] This escalation has occurred in spite of concern expressed by both the lay and scientific communities, as evidenced by the consensus report issued by the National Institutes of Health.[2]

Recent data also demonstrate that suggested methods to reduce the rate of cesarean birth have resulted in minimal change in specific areas, such as permitting a trial of labor following a previous cesarean birth.[3] In addressing this problem, it is important to consider the probable reasons for the rise in cesarean birth, as well as to ennumerate the methods that may cause a plateau or a decline of cesarean birth—which is a stated goal of the scientific community and the consumer.

REASONS FOR THE INCREASED USE OF CESAREAN BIRTH

One of the laudable and easily documentable benefits of contemporary obstetrical health care has been the dramatic decline in morbidity and mortality associated with cesarean delivery. Although maternal morbidity and mortality are increased when compared to uncomplicated vaginal birth, the relative occurrence of catastrophic injury and/or mortality is infrequent. Current statistics indicate that the occurrence of maternal mortality is 20 per 100,000 births, or 1 mortality per 5,000 cesarean deliveries in the United States.[4] It is clear that one of the major reasons for the increased utilization of cesarean birth is the enhanced safety of this procedure when compared to the situation just 10–20 years ago.

In addition to the improved safety of cesarean birth, the concept held by the lay public that every fetus is destined to have an uncompromised and "perfect" outcome places great pressure on the team providing health care services. This particular demand for perfection, coupled with the presumed apparent benefits attributed to cesarean delivery from the fetal standpoint, frequently prompts this method of delivery. If one considers only the fetal aspect of obstetrical care, a strong argument can be made that the incidence of compromised outcome in a group of fetuses delivered by cesarean is less than in those exposed to the stress and potential insult imposed during labor and vaginal delivery. This same argument becomes even stronger when one deals with the very-low-birth-weight infant in whom asphyxial stress and/or minimal trauma during the delivery process seemingly give rise to subsequent newborn morbidity and mortality. Although this concept is widely held by the practitioner, little data are available that demonstrate a clear benefit of cesarean delivery over vaginal birth for even the very-low-birth-weight infant group. In spite of these factors, this concept, which is held by many lay persons and health care providers, undoubtedly leads to the election of cesarean birth rather than permitting labor and attempting vaginal delivery. Unfortunately, in addition to the concerns that affect the fetus, health care providers must concern themselves with the consequences of a major operative procedure for the mother's well-being. The increased incidence of blood loss, the trauma of a surgical procedure, and the risk of anesthetic accident are well known to all practitioners. Maternal postpartum infectious morbidity, even given the benefits of antibiotic prophylaxis, is clearly higher in women subjected to cesarean delivery. Thus, the dilemma is how to balance maternal and fetal interests appropriately without compromising either one. The problems posed by providing simultaneous care to two individuals are faced by few medical personnel other than the obstetrician or the delivering practitioner.

Complicating the picture is the ever-increasing amount of information available to the practitioner. Sophisticated ultrasonic imaging techniques reveal circumstances that would previously have remained unrecognized but that, when identified, may lead to cesarean birth in order to provide the fetus with its "best chance." In addition, continuous monitoring of the fetal heart rate provides a continuous measure of fetal status, even though these observations are, at times, imprecise or confusing to the observer. Often due to a lack of understanding or apprehension, fetal heart rate patterns that are interpretable as demonstrating less than a distress state may provoke unindicated operative intervention. Such intervention is not unreasonable to the practitioner who is faced with the patient demands for a "perfect" child. This expectation comes into conscious focus particularly when major alterations in fetal heart rate are dramatically observable and audible not only to the patient but often to other persons who are in attendance during the birth process. All of these pressures undoubtedly lead to the increased utilization of cesarean birth under the assumption that this, by itself, will meet those demands.

An additional consequence of the high rate of cesarean births is the emerging deficiencies in physician experience and acquisition of operative skills provided by obstetrical training programs. Thus, with the continual condemnation of procedures such as midforceps and/or vaginal breech delivery, the emerging generation of practitioners will necessarily lack sufficient skill to undertake such procedures. Thus, in spite of studies and reports that address the acceptability of these procedures, practitioners have become increasingly less proficient as training programs fail to teach them.

One may ask, why have we been led to the abandonment of classical operative obstetrics? Again, this situation is related partially to the unrealistic expectations ingrained in the public mind and reinforced constantly by the medicolegal climate that exists in the United States. Although most often unjustified, the continual threat of medicolegal action and the unjust assumption that compensation is due whenever an outcome is less than perfect provoke and catalyze the increased use of cesarean birth.

A final consideration that may relate to the use of cesarean birth is the indirect incentives for both the mother and the health care providers. Cesarean delivery generally requires less than 1 hour, compared to the long hours of attempted vaginal delivery. This is particularly true in the case of elective repeat sections, which are medically unnecessary in the vast majority of circumstances. Yet, in spite of supportive studies and professional pleas to undertake a trial of labor in eligible patients, recent data suggest that minimal change has occurred since the 1979 consensus report.[2] Inhibiting implementation are the factors of convenience and the use of traditional hospital services including the operating room, laboratory, ancillary support services, and professional staff, all of which benefit economically by cesarean birth compared to vaginal delivery. In addition, the third-party payments of greater fees for this operative procedure, in contrast to those for vaginal birth, provide incentives for the use of cesarean birth.

APPROACHES FOR DECREASING THE CESAREAN DELIVERY RATE

The primary area in which a dramatic decrease in cesarean delivery could be accomplished relates to the widely used concept of "once a cesarean, always a cesarean." Current data demonstrate that approximately 10% of women entering obstetrical facilities will have had a prior cesarean birth. As discussed in Chapters 31–35, when trial of labor (TOL) is offered to this group, one can anticipate that as many as 50% will achieve a successful vaginal delivery. Thus, a potential decrease of 5% in the overall section rate would be achieved by the liberal use of TOL and VBAC.[5]

In spite of the repeated demonstration of the success of TOL and VBAC, current data reveal that more than 90% of women with prior cesarean births continue to undergo repeat cesarean delivery.[3] One of the factors that may alter this disappointing situation is the more liberalized approach to the demands made upon health care providers and facilities, as presented by the American College of Obstetrics and Gynecology in 1985.[6]

Another area where cesareans could be reduced is selected vaginal breech delivery (Chapter 3). The potential decrease that might be associated with this approach is probably in the area of 1%–2%, but the general acceptability of this practice is unlikely. The decreased familiarity with attempted vaginal breech delivery and lack of practical experience also make this potential decrease impractical. The utilization of midforceps and vacuum extraction in carefully chosen cases would probably result in a similar decrease (1%–2%) in the section rate; but again, this area remains controversial and is the focus of condemnation by some prominent experts. Again, this poses a dilemma for the qualified practicing obstetrician and for physicians in training. As a result, these physicians lack confidence or experience with this method of delivery. It is unlikely, therefore, that a significant impact in this area will occur.

One promising approach being used to decrease the cesarean birth rate is version. External version may be successfully employed during late pregnancy for breech presentation and is generally effective in 60%–70% of attempts. The net effect of version on the overall cesarean delivery rate, assuming a routine cesarean delivery for the breech presentation, would be in the range of 1%–2%. Repeated studies have demonstrated the efficacy of this approach, as detailed in Chapter 36. Clearly, this is an attractive alternative when one identifies a breech presentation during the latter weeks of pregnancy.

Another area in which version, both external and internal, may play a role is in the management of multiple or twin gestation (Chapter 4). When the second twin assumes a nonvertex presentation, careful external version following the delivery of the first twin will often bring the fetus into a position where a successful vaginal delivery may be accomplished. Likewise, internal version and extraction of the second twin, when properly performed, is an acceptable approach to the delivery of the second twin. In view of the infrequent occurrence of twin gestation (less than 1%), and the even lower incidence of eligible candidates for this procedure, it is unlikely that this approach will have an appreciable effect on decreasing the cesarean rate.

A major potential method of decreasing the cesarean delivery rate would be an improved understanding of the indicators of fetal well-being, such as fetal heart rate patterns. A more definitive focus on and understanding of this indicator of fetal condition would be associated with a higher success rate of vaginal delivery. Particular emphasis should be given to emerging concepts related to acceleration patterns and concepts of fetal heart rate interpretation (Chapter 5). At times, the utilization of fetal scalp sampling, when applicable, can successfully avoid an unwarranted operative delivery. The diagnosis of fetal distress during labor, warranting operative intervention, is most probably in the range of 1%–3% of total deliveries. This number is based on observations in our facility and on the documented information in the randomized trial performed in the National Maternity Hospital in Dublin.[7]

Finally, the public, particularly the legal profession, must be educated to the fact that not all imperfect outcomes are a result of negligent care. This understanding would do much to neutralize the sometimes reflexive response to possible signs of fetal stress and inappropriate cesarean birth as a quick solution. The latter suggestion, unfortunately, is unlikely in view of all current trends, as judged by the activity of the legal profession. Thus, this lack of understanding, coupled with the continued threats posed by medicolegal action, remain major stumbling blocks to proper obstetrical care. As a result, the thoughtful and patient observations required during the normal labor process are abandoned and the expeditious "easy way out" of cesarean birth is chosen.

REFERENCES

1. Rutkow I: Obstetric and gynecologic operations in the United States, 1979 to 1984. *Obstet Gynecol* 67:755, 1986.
2. *Cesarean Childbirth: Report of a Consensus Development Conference Sponsored by the National Institute of Child Health and Human Development.* DHHS Pub No NIH 82-2067. Washington, DC, Government Printing Office, 1980.
3. Shiono PA, McNellis D, Rhoads GS: Reasons for the rising cesarean delivery rates 1978–1984. *Obstet Gynecol* 69:696, 1987.
4. Petitti DB: Maternal mortality and morbidity in cesarean section. *Clin Obstet Gynecol* 28:763, 1985.
5. Paul RH, Phelan JP, Yeh SY: Trial of labor in the patient with a prior cesarean birth. *Am J Obstet Gynecol* 151:297, 1985.
6. ACOG Newsletter: Vaginal birth after cesarean. *Focus of New Guidelines* 29: 1985.
7. MacDonald D, Grant A, Sheridan-Pereira M, et al: The Dublin randomized controlled trial of intrapartum fetal heart rate monitoring. *Am J Obstet Gynecol* 152:524, 1985.

Chapter 31 Once a Cesarean, Always a Cesarean?

Richard P. Porreco, MD

> The occurrence of pregnancy after cesarean section is not devoid of danger, as cases have been reported in which the uterine cicatrix ruptured in the latter part of the subsequent gestation. Certain authors consider it so real a danger that they have layed down the dictum "Once a cesarean, always a cesarean." This is an exaggeration.
>
> J. Whitridge Williams, 1917[1]

Several years have past since the dean of American obstetrics wrote that repeat cesarean delivery is an exaggerated response to the small risk of uterine scar dehiscence. Nevertheless, his admonition fell on deaf ears, as this dogma still clouds the management of the majority of women with previous cesarean births in the United States. The true risk of dehiscence has diminished considerably during this time period with the advent of the low transverse uterine incision, antibiotics, and blood banking. Even so, enlightened thinking regarding labor and vaginal birth in these patients has only recently gained a modicum of acceptance in this country.

The next 10 years should witness a major change in the management of these patients. Resident physicians are leaving training programs that strongly endorse vaginal birth after cesarean (VBAC). The rest of this chapter and the subsequent four chapters address the major considerations in attending patients who are laboring following previous cesarean births.

LIKELIHOOD OF VAGINAL BIRTH

The success rate in planned VBAC is dependent on selection criteria, approaches to management, and indications for primary cesarean delivery.[2] Further, it has been stated that physician and patient motivation and confidence influence the outcome in VBAC.[3] In this regard, many communities

TABLE 31.1 VBAC Success Rates

Author	Years	No. of Patients	VBAC	Percent
Lavin et al[4]	1950–1980	3,214	2,143	67
Flamm[2]	1980–1984	6,258	5,356	86
TOTAL		9,472	7,499	79

Source: After Flamm BL: Vaginal birth after cesarean section: Controversies old and new. *Clin Obstet Gynecol* 28:735, 1985, with permission.

have witnessed an expanding number of VBAC support groups and hospital-based classes centered on VBAC issues.

Table 31.1 summarizes the modern experience in the expected success rates of VBAC.

The apparent increase in the success rate in recent years undoubtedly reflects increasing physician confidence and experience, as well as more aggressive management policies. Selection criteria have been broadened over the more recent time period, and the increased success rate serves as a reminder that differences in patient "suitability" for labor after previous cesarean delivery may not be as important as was once thought (Chapter 32).

A vaginal birth prior to the cesarean(s) may increase the likelihood of a successful VBAC,[5] though it is our opinion that this is an artifact of lower overall success rates related to less aggressive management approaches. Paul et al, with an overall success rate above 80%, were unable to show a significant impact of prior vaginal birth.[6] Not surprisingly, a previous successful VBAC was associated with a higher success rate in the index labor (94%). This has been our own experience as well, with only a rare patient failing a second (or third) VBAC.

Since 1980, we have consistently noted VBAC success rates above 80%.[3,7,8] Clearly, the approach to the management of these patients is the overwhelming influence on success and will be explored in greater detail in subsequent chapters.

UTERINE SCAR DEHISCENCE

The term "uterine rupture" has catastrophic connotations and encompasses a variety of complications that are irrelevant to a discussion of VBAC. True uterine rupture can indeed be catastrophic; it is generally associated with the unscarred uterus where there has been a history of blunt trauma, obstetric manipulation (ie, internal version and extraction), or pitocin use in grand multiparous patients.[9,10] It is also associated with fundal or vertical scars of the uterus, occasionally without labor. Rarely, however, does catastrophic rupture occur in a patient with a low transverse uterine incision(s). In these instances, "occult rupture" or "occult dehiscence" is the more descriptive term.

TABLE 31.2 Maternal and Fetal Risks with Uterine Scar Dehiscence

Patient with a Previous Cesarean	Deaths from Classical Rupture			Deaths from Lower Segment Rupture		
	No.	Maternal	Fetal	No.	Maternal	Fetal
5,392	30 (0.55%)	0	17 (56.7%)	25 (0.46%)	0	3 (12%)

Source: After O'Sullivan M, Fumia F, Holsinger K, et al: Vaginal delivery after cesarean section. *Clin Perinatal* 8:131, 1981, with permission.

There have been a number of reviews of uterine rupture in the recent literature, all supporting the notion that symptomatic rupture of a low transverse scar is an exceedingly infrequent event unassociated with maternal mortality. Indeed, Eden et al have recently presented data demonstrating that the incidence of dehiscence of the uterine scar has remained relatively constant (about 1/150) over 50 years at their institution, despite changing practice patterns.[10] Clearly, one must conclude that the pathogenesis of uterine scar dehiscence relates to the nonunion of the primary uterine incision rather than to subsequent pregnancy, labor, or delivery.

Table 31.2 summarizes the real issues in uterine scar dehiscence, namely, maternal and fetal risks.

Among 5,400 patients in this summary of published American studies prior to 1980, there were no maternal deaths from rupture of even classical uterine scars. Fetal deaths were common in patients with ruptured fundal incisions, occurring in more than one-half of the cases; there were only three fetal deaths in lower segment dehiscence, all prior to the era of electronic fetal monitoring. In reviews by Lavin et al[4] and Flamm,[2] encompassing nearly 10,000 patients, no maternal mortality was reported. Of the eight fetal deaths recorded, seven were either in patients with vertical or fundal incisions or in unmonitored patients; detailed intrapartum information about the eighth fetal death is lacking. Intrapartum fetal demise secondary to the dehiscence of a low transverse uterine incision(s) while the mother was properly attended and the fetus was electronically monitored must be a rare event indeed.

The inability confidently to exclude fetal deaths in labor with ruptured vertical scars has prompted us not to encourage planned VBAC in these patients. Moreover, a brief examination of the previous scar after the expulsion of the placenta will provide insight into the natural history of pregnancy and birth in patients with known dehiscences. Repair of such dehiscences is not necessary unless bleeding unresponsive to standard oxytocic agents occurs.

Finally, with regard to perinatal morbidity and mortality, several authors have hypothetically investigated labor and conservative VBAC success rates compared to those of elective repeat cesarean delivery.[12,13] With all risks considered, these authors have concluded that morbidity and

TABLE 31.3 Incidence of Urgent Cesarean Births

	Total No.	Urgent Cesarean
Laboring patients without a scarred uterus	3,176	38 (1.2%)
Laboring patients with low transverse uterine scar(s)	146	2 (1.4%)

Source: Data from St. Luke's/Children's Perinatal Program, 1982–1983. Porreco RP, Meier PR: Repeat cesarean—most unnecessary. *Contemp Obstet Gynecol* 21:55, 1984.

mortality of the mother and infant can be reduced by anticipating labor and vaginal birth and reserving a repeat cesarean for specific indications following a trial of labor.

FACILITY

The ACOG Committee on Obstetrics: Maternal and Fetal Medicine published guidelines for vaginal delivery after a previous cesarean birth in 1985.[14] They suggest that a physician capable of performing a cesarean delivery should be "immediately available." The suggested response time for urgent cesarean birth is 30 minutes. In truth, such guidelines really apply to any inhospital birthing unit. The indications for urgent cesarean birth are numerous and varied, and include acute fetal distress, antepartum hemorrhage, footling breech presentation, and prolapsed umbilical cord. Patients with prior cesareans are not immune to these complications, but any increased risk related to symptomatic rupture is impossible to measure (Table 31.3).

Urgent cesarean deliveries were defined as those necessary within 30 minutes in the 2-year review summarized in Table 31.3. Both patients laboring in anticipation of a VBAC were found to have intact scars at surgery; indications for their repeat cesarean births were acute placental abruption and fetal distress in the second stage of labor. The majority of VBAC patients having a repeat cesarean during labor fail to progress in the first or second stage of labor, neither of which requires urgent intervention.[7]

The Canadian Consensus Conference on Cesarean Childbirth noted the probability of emergency cesarean as being 2.7% among 11,819 births. They compared this to an observed symptomatic dehiscence rate of 0.22% from four prospective studies. The panel concluded that "hospitals providing obstetric care should insure the availability of blood, operating theatre, neonatal resuscitation, nursing, anesthetic and surgical personnel such that a cesarean section can be started approximately within 30 minutes for any labouring woman, including a woman undergoing 'trial of labour.'"[15]

In summary, then, planned VBAC should occur in a setting of preparedness that would allow timely intervention if it becomes necessary. *This is the same setting applicable to all laboring patients, whose risks of urgent intervention are not measurably different from those of patients seeking a VBAC.* Minimum requirements on our service for such patients include only the establishment of intravenous access (heparin lock) and electronic fetal monitoring in the active phase of labor. These patients should not be excluded arbitrarily from inhospital birthing room settings, as the emotional support frequently associated with such facilities may be especially useful in the context of a planned VBAC.

CONFOUNDING ISSUES

A variety of complications may confuse the proper approach to patients with previous cesarean birth(s). Most commonly, patients seeking VBAC may complete 41 or 42 weeks of gestation without spontaneous labor. Some authors have recommended repeat cesarean delivery in such women.[16] It seems more prudent to approach the postdates VBAC patient as one would other patients who proceed significantly beyond their estimated date of confinement, namely, surveillance with selective induction.[17] Other patients are not advised to accept cesarean birth for postdates, and there is no information suggesting that patients with low transverse uterine scars should do so.

Other confounding complications include twin gestation, breech presentation, fetal macrosomia, and an assortment of medical illnesses. Although some authorities discourage VBAC in these circumstances, it has been our policy to counsel such patients on the merits of the specific situation, rarely if ever allowing a low transverse uterine scar(s) to influence decisions regarding management.

Finally, most obstetricians would agree that the morbidity of a simple postpartum tubal ligation cannot be compared to that of a repeat cesarean delivery. Elective sterilization is not an indication for abdominal delivery in most instances. Thirteen percent of successful VBAC patients in one study had routine postpartum tubal ligations performed without incident, and only minor prolongation of their hospital stay.[3]

PATIENT EDUCATION

Women approach pregnancy and birth with a wealth of information gathered since childhood. This undoubtedly is true of cesarean birth as well, with a variety of myths confusing attitudes and undermining a positive approach to the subsequent pregnancy and labor experience. It is the physician's responsibility to take the time necessary during the antepartum period to dispel these myths and correct misinformation. He or she must cultivate a positive attitude in the patient, as well as instill in her confidence that she will succeed in the pursuit of a VBAC. Other members of the health care team should contribute to this positivism; this is especially important for labor and delivery nurses, from whom nonverbal communication indicating lack of support for a VBAC can be exceedingly damaging.

Specific consent forms for women laboring after previous cesarean(s) should not be required and should be reserved for women in whom interventive management is planned (ie, repeat cesarean delivery). Instead, outpatient notes can be made indicating that the patient has been informed that labor following cesarean is an acceptable alternative, though there are some attendant risks.

Women frequently regret the decision to labor during the course of that labor.[3] This does not indicate a lack of resolve, but rather is a reflection of vulnerability and the understandable attempt to escape from a painful experience. This is when emotional support, anesthesia as required, and a confident, caring environment are most useful. A change of heart is not an indication for a repeat cesarean, and patients should be so counseled prior to labor.

VBAC support groups and classes can be very useful in helping to prepare the patient psychologically for her labor. Physicians and nurses should take an active role in organizing and educating these lay groups, as it is necessary that they have the correct information as a foundation on which to build their other activities. An adversarial relationship between the medical community and cesarean support groups is not in the best interest of the patient and will undermine the ultimate goal of proper education and psychological support.

IMPACT ON CESAREAN DELIVERY RATES

In 1985 the national cesarean delivery rate was 22.8% (nonfederal hospitals).[18] Although detailed data are incomplete for this most recent year, it is anticipated that the leading indication for cesarean delivery will be the same as in the last several years, namely, previous cesarean birth. Elective repeat cesarean delivery has been consistently noted as one of the leading causes of the escalating cesarean delivery rate over the last 30 years.[19]

Meier and Porreco, in an earlier study, demonstrated a reversal of the upward trend in cesarean deliveries in their hospital after inaugurating a VBAC program; a 40% reduction in elective abdominal deliveries was documented after merely offering a trial of labor to their population.[3] O'Driscoll and Foley illustrated that the difference in the U.S. and Irish cesarean birth rates is explained, in part, by the management of patients with previous cesarean delivery.[20] In comparing clinic and private services, Porreco showed that the major difference in cesarean birth rates was due to the large number of elective cesareans done among private patients.[8] Anderson and Lomas concluded that repeat cesarean delivery was responsible for more than two-thirds of the increase in cesareans between 1979 and 1982 in their community and recommended:

TABLE 31.4 Cesarean Birth Rates

Type of Cesarean Delivery	Dublin (1980)[20]	St. Luke's Clinic (1982–1985)[23]	St. Luke's Private (1982–1985)[23]	United States (1983)[22]
Primary (%)	3.7	5.1	11.6	13.2
Repeat (%)	1.1	0.9	6.2	7.1
Total (%)	4.8	6.0	17.8	20.3

> In the short term, primary advances in reducing the cesarean birth rate can be achieved only by addressing the self perpetuating contribution of previous cesarean birth.[21]

Table 31.4 outlines the impact that an aggressive policy on VBAC can have on the total cesarean birth rate. On the first two services, an aggressive approach to labor after prior cesarean birth is practiced. On the private service at St. Luke's, approximately 50% of the patients were offered a trial of labor; in the United States, only 5% of patients were offered a trial of labor in 1983.[22]

The financial impact of elective cesarean birth as a major management strategy is considerable. Assuming an elective repeat cesarean delivery rate of 6% (which may be conservative) and 3.5 million births in the United States each year, Flamm estimated that this would translate into more than one-half billion dollars in increased health care costs compared to the costs of vaginal delivery (using Southern California cost comparisons).[2] Most obstetricians would agree that this vast sum of money could be better spent in improving the welfare of mothers and infants, a goal to which elective repeat cesarean delivery clearly does not contribute.

Although it has been suggested that convenience and financial considerations support such a high elective repeat cesarean delivery rate, this may not be the case. Most physicians in this country are subject to the pressures of time; given a busy office and hospital schedule, time is a scarce commodity. Clearly, it is more time efficient to deliver a patient with a previous cesarean birth abdominally rather than to support her in a subsequent labor and possible vaginal birth.

In addition, the current medicolegal atmosphere prohibits many physicians from "risking" VBAC. Sandberg noted that "every American obstetrician has come to recognize that physicians are almost never sued for erring in the direction of cesarean section or for performing an unnecessary abdominal delivery. Allegations of such are seldom taken seriously by the court, especially if the infant is normal and alive."[24] Haynes de Regt et al concluded that the currently observed high rates of cesarean birth, supported in large part by elective repeat procedures, may be another result of the current malpractice crisis in obstetrics.[25] Neilson, in a review of cesarean births, stated that "any further increase of the incidence of cesarean section should be followed by documented improvement in neonatal outcome."[26] Certainly the procedure of elective repeat cesarean delivery does not meet the criterion of improved newborn outcome; indeed, it may be counterproductive in that regard.[27]

CONCLUSION

"Once a cesarean, always a cesarean is an outmoded dictum. Mortality fears for mother and infant resulting from uterine rupture in a trial of labor are not borne out by existing data."[28] Most enlightened obstetricians would agree with this conclusion by a recent president of the American College of Obstetricians and Gynecologists. It has already been stated that the specific approach to management is important in order to achieve a successful outcome in patients laboring after previous cesareans. Appreciation of the prognosis for a successful VBAC as it relates to the indication for the primary cesarean delivery is necessary in counseling these patients. The use of oxytocics (Chapter 33) and conduction anesthesia (Chapter 35) in planning and supporting labor are two specific issues of which the attending physician must have a clear understanding in order to achieve success rates of 80%–90%. Finally, the data available on patients with multiple uterine scars (Chapter 34) need to be assessed carefully before such patients are arbitrarily excluded from labor in a subsequent pregnancy. These considerations are of overwhelming importance in the modern approach to VBAC. Perhaps future generations of obstetricians will view elective repeat cesarean delivery, along with the craniotome and Willett forceps, as being of historical interest only.

REFERENCES

1. Williams JW: *Obstetrics,* ed. 4 New York, D. Appleton and Co, 1917, p 488.
2. Flamm BL: Vaginal birth after cesarean section: Controversies old and new. *Clin Obstet Gynecol* 28:735, 1985.
3. Meier P, Porreco R: Trial of labor following cesarean section: A two year experience. *Am J Obstet Gynecol* 144:671, 1982.
4. Lavin JP, Stephens RJ, Miodovnik M, et al: Vaginal delivery in patients with a prior cesarean section. *Obstet Gynecol* 59:135, 1982.
5. Riva H, Teich J: Vaginal delivery following cesarean section. *Am J Obstet Gynecol* 81:501, 1964.
6. Paul RH, Phelan JP, Yeh S: Trial of labor in the patient with a prior cesarean birth. *Am J Obstet Gynecol* 151:297, 1985.
7. Porreco RP, Meier PR: Repeat cesarean—most unnecessary. *Contemp Obstet Gynecol* 21:55,1984.
8. Porreco RP: High cesarean section rate: A new perspective. *Obstet Gynecol* 65:307, 1985.
9. Plauche WC, Von Almen W, Muller R: Catastrophic uterine rupture. *Obstet Gynecol* 64:792, 1984.
10. Eden RD, Parker RT, Gall SA: Rupture of the pregnant uterus: A 53 year review. *Obstet Gynecol* 68:671, 1986.

11. Gibbs CE: Planned vaginal delivery following cesarean section. *Clin Obstet Gynecol* 23:507, 1980.
12. O'Sullivan M, Fumia F, Holsinger K, et al: Vaginal delivery after cesarean section. *Clin Perinatal* 8:131, 1981.
13. Pauerstein CJ: Labor after cesarean section: From precept to practice. *J Reprod Med* 26:409, 1981.
14. Shy KK, LoGerfo JP, Karp LE: Evaluation of elective repeat cesarean section as a standard of care: An application of decision analysis. *Am J Obstet Gynecol* 139:123, 1981.
15. Guidelines for vaginal delivery after a previous cesarean birth. *ACOG Newsletter*. February, 1985, p 8.
16. Hannah W: Final statement of the panel from the National Consensus Conference on Aspects of Cesarean Birth, Hamilton, Ontario, Canada, 1986.
17. Yeh SY, Huang XH, Phelan JP: Post-term pregnancy after previous cesarean section. *J Reprod Med* 29:41, 1984.
18. *Advance Data, Vital and Health Statistics*. No. 127. Department of Health and Human Services Pub. (PHS) 86-1250. Washington, DC, September 1986.
19. Bottoms SF, Rosen MG, Sokol RJ: The increase in the cesarean birth rate. *N Engl J Med* 302:559, 1980.
20. O'Driscoll K, Foley M: Correlation of decrease in perinatal mortality and increase in cesarean section rates. *Obstet Gynecol* 61:1, 1983.
21. Anderson GM, Lomas J: Determinants of the increasing cesarean birth rate. *N Engl J Med* 311:887, 1984.
22. Taffel SM, Placek PJ, Moien M: One-fifth of 1983 US births by cesarean section. *Am J Public Health* 75:190, 1985.
23. Burke MS, Porreco RP: High cesarean section rates unnecessary for good perinatal outcome. *Fam Pract Recert* (in press), 1987.
24. Sandberg EC: Trial labor following cesarean section (comment). *Am J Obstet Gynecol* 149:41, 1984.
25. Haynes de Regt R, Minkoff HL, Feldman J, et al: Relation of private or clinic care to the cesarean birth rate. *N Engl J Med* 315:619, 1986.
26. Nielson TF: Cesarean section: A controversial feature of modern obstetric practice. *Gynecol Obstet Invest* 21:57, 1986.
27. Cohen M, Carson BS: Respiratory morbidity benefit of awaiting onset of labor after elective cesarean section. *Obstet Gynecol* 65:818, 1985.
28. Klein L: Cesarean birth and trial of labor. *Female Patient* 9:106, 1984.

Chapter 32

Effect of Previous Indications for Cesarean on Subsequent Outcome

Gary S. Eglinton, MD

"Once a cesarean, always a cesarean"[1] is a dictum that will die slowly. As discussed previously in Chapter 31, evidence is mounting in favor of a trial of labor (TOL) after a prior cesarean. Extensive scholarly reviews of TOL after prior cesarean have appeared recently,[2,3] documenting the wisdom of this approach for most women with a history of a single prior low transverse uterine incision. In 1980, a National Institutes of Health Consensus Development Conference convened in Dallas to consider the provocative rise in the cesarean rate in the United States.[4] The conferees found that the diagnoses of dystocia and elective repeat cesarean had contributed most to the recent rise. The published recommendations of the conference included methods to decrease the influence of both of these diagnoses on the cesarean rate.

Our struggle in the United States with these concepts has stimulated a response from the other side of the Atlantic in the form of a gentle prod from the staff of the National Maternity Hospital, Dublin.[5] Of course, there are practical differences other than simple geography that contribute to disparate cesarean rates on opposite sides of the Atlantic.[6] But the Dallas respondents to our Irish critics acknowledged that a falling rate of elective repeat cesarean could have a dramatic impact on our total cesarean rate.

The reasons for the persistent high elective repeat cesarean rate in the United States cannot be divorced from the indications for the primary cesarean. The high rate of primary cesarean for dystocia complicates the issue tremendously. A great prejudice against TOL by women with prior cesareans for dystocia remains in the minds of many U.S. obstetricians and their patients. In this chapter, we will review the data that suggest the abandoning of that prejudice.

TABLE 32.1 Outcome of Trial of Labor by Indication for Prior Cesarean: Recurring Causes

Prior Indication	No. of Patients	Success	Percentage of Success	Author	Year
CPD/FTP	83	49	59	Riva	1961
	28	14	50	Pauerstein	1969
	24	14	58	McGarry	1969
	49	29	59	Morewood	1973
	90	25	28	Saldana	1979
	33	13	39	Demianczuk	1982
	58	40	69	Seitchik	1982
	83	65	78	Meier	1982
	62	22	35	Wadhawan	1983
	89	55	62	Graham	1984
	61	39	64	Clark	1984
	78	42	54	Jarrell	1985
	319	245	77	Paul	1985
	822	622	77	Phelan	1987
Totals	1879	1274	68		
Labor arrest	8	6	75	Saldana	1979
	17	12	71	Wadhawan	1983
Totals	25	18	72		
Prolonged labor	97	65	67	McGarry	1969
	57	42	74	Morewood	1973
Totals	154	107	70		
Failed induction	25	11	44	McGarry	1969
	23	8	35	Morewood	1973
Totals	48	19	40		

THE INFLUENCE OF PRIOR INDICATION ON SUCCESSFUL TOL

In 1982, Lavin et al published a detailed review of the English language literature on TOL through 1980.[3] With this work, we have brought that review up to present day. Some groups have not permitted a planned TOL for patients with a prior cesarean for cephalopelvic disproportion/failure to progress (CPD/FTP).[7,8] Other groups apparently have permitted TOL for these patients, but their reports did not permit stratification of the patients by indication for the index cesarean.[9–11] The papers of others listed patients by indication for prior cesarean, and reported success in 12%–30% with prior CPD/FTP, but the proportion of patients with this diagnosis permitted a TOL is obscure.[12–15]

Table 32.1 lists reports of TOL after prior cesarean, grouped by indication for prior cesarean, for several diagnoses of interest. In some instances, we interpreted the authors' data differently than did Lavin et al. The greatest discrepancy is for those patients listed under CPD/FTP. Lawrence displayed "What results may be expected if previously-sectioned patients are allowed to go into labour."[16] Because his group did not necessarily permit a TOL, but merely onset of labor, their published success rate was only 121/449 (27%) after a prior low segment incision. Because it is not clear what proportion of these patients had a TOL, or what the indications for repeat cesarean in labor were, we omitted the Lawrence series. For the series by Pauerstein et al, we included both nulliparous and parous patients.[17] To avoid the semantic difficulties raised by McGarry, we cited CPD, as the author did, and accepted his separate category of prolonged labor.[18] In each of the other referenced series, we also recorded the data directly from the authors' own results, including separate categories for labor arrest and prolonged labor.[19–28]

Several of the referenced works warrant special comment. The report by Meier and Porreco from the Kaiser Permanente Hospital in San Diego noted that some attending physicians were initially reluctant to support a TOL policy, especially after prior CPD/FTP.[23] And yet, the Kaiser success rate was the highest in this group. The first Los Angeles County/University of Southern California Medical Center (LAC/USC) series was gathered retrospectively[26] and revealed a lower success rate than the second and subsequent prospective series from that facility.[28,29] The differences could have arisen from bias of ascertainment on a busy service or from increasing security of the staff with the TOL policy over the years of the studies.

Perhaps most interesting in this group is the report by Seitchik and Rao.[22] Through a retrospective computer search, they identified 58 patients who had cesareans for CPD/FTP for their first deliveries and then returned to the same hospital to be managed by the same staff for a later delivery. Each patient had entered her first labor spontaneously and had received oxytocin augmentation prior to the diagnosis of FTP in labor. Although the patients were managed on the same service for both the index failed labor and the subsequent TOL, the success rate for TOL was 69%. The authors were unable to identify any significant prognostic factor that could be applied to predict the outcome of an individual TOL. They concluded that most women who had a prior cesarean for "failure to progress" or "relative cephalopelvic disproportion" deserved a TOL in a subsequent pregnancy.

The LAC/USC authors did not have the advantage of a uniform population of patients who had all had their primary cesareans at the same facility.[26,28,29] But most of their patients had primary cesareans in the same facility or in Latin America, where the cesarean rate is lower than it is in the United States, and we must presume an adequate trial of labor prior to the decision for cesarean in most cases. The implication of these studies is that even when the patient failed to progress despite an adequate trial in a prior labor, there is a high probability that a TOL in the current pregnancy will be successful. Although there are no recent data, studies by McGarry and Morewood et al suggested that prior failure of induction leading to cesarean may indicate a lower anticipated successful TOL rate.[18,19] These authors also provided data on patients attempting TOL after primary cesarean for "prolonged labor." Neither this term nor the

TABLE 32.2 Outcome of Trial of Labor by Indication for Prior Cesarean: Nonrecurring Causes

Prior Indication	No. of Patients	Success	Percentage of Success	Author	Year
Breech	19	16	84	McGarry	1969
	3	3	100	Saldana	1979
	68	62	91	Meier	1982
	90	67	74	Graham	1984
	94	81	86	Clark	1984
	72	54	75	Jarrell	1985
	135	123	90	Paul	1985
	332	294	89	Phelan	1987
Totals	813	700	86		
Fetal distress	45	36	80	McGarry	1969
	56	44	79	Morewood	1973
	16	10	65	Saldana	1979
	27	25	93	Meier	1982
	20	15	75	Wadhawan	1983
	25	13	52	Graham	1984
	38	31	82	Clark	1984
	67	56	84	Paul	1985
	168	140	83	Phelan	1987
Totals	462	370	80		
Placental[a]	54	45	83	McGarry	1969
	27	23	85	Morewood	1973
	5	3	60	Saldana	1979
	8	7	88	Meier	1982
	34	27	79	Wadhawan	1983
	17	14	82	Clark	1984
Totals	145	119	82		

[a] Placental = previa, abruptio, or hemorrhage.

term "labor arrest" cited by both Saldana et al and Wadhawan and Narone was specifically defined by the authors.[20,24] But certainly all these diagnoses might be considered together as "mechanical" or "recurring" causes for failed labor. Comparing these cases to those in Table 32.2, for which the indication for the index cesarean was a "nonrecurring" cause, there is a clear difference. Yet, the success rate is far too high for those series listed in Table 32.1 to support prohibition of TOL for patients with a history of prior cesarean for "recurring" causes.

Some authors have demonstrated a different prognosis for successful TOL dependent upon prior vaginal deliveries (Table 32.3). In the retrospective report by Eglinton et al, the success rate was 81% for those who had one or more vaginal deliveries prior to primary cesarean, compared to 77% for those who had no vaginal deliveries prior to primary cesarean.[30] The contrast was slightly greater (87% versus 75%) for those who had vaginal deliveries after the prior cesarean compared to those with no intervening vaginal deliveries. From the same series, Clark et al reported an even greater contrast in the subgroup whose primary cesarean had been for CPD/FTP. The success rate was 86% for those with any prior vaginal

TABLE 32.3 Outcome of Trial of Labor by Prior Deliveries

	Number of Prior Vaginal Deliveries					
	None			One or More		
Author	Patients	Success	Percentage of Success	Patients	Success	Percentage of Success
Eglinton						
Before CS	221	170	77	80	65	81
After CS	226	170	75	75	65	87
Clark						
CS for CPD			51			86
Pauerstein						
Before or after CS	30	16	53	13	10	77
Riva						
Before CS	130	85	65	84	74	88
Paul						
Before CS	552	443	80	169	144	85
After CS	600	473	79	119	112	94

CS = cesarean section.

delivery, compared to 51% for those with only one prior delivery, that being by cesarean for CPD/FTP.[26] The data of Pauerstein et al were similar to those of Clark et al, although the former authors did not restrict the outcome reference to patients with prior cesarean for CPD/FTP.[17]

Riva and Teich permitted TOL for patients with a history of more than one prior cesarean and for patients with prior classical cesareans.[31] In fact, 32.3% of their patients had prior classical cesareans and another 11% had unknown incisions, but the uterine scars were "classical in type." Even for patients with two prior deliveries, both by cesarean, the success rate was 65%. In a more contemporary prospective series, Paul et al demonstrated success rates as high as 94% for patients with a history of vaginal delivery after prior cesarean.[28]

THE INFLUENCE OF PRIOR INDICATION ON COMPLICATIONS

Table 32.4 presents morbidity data stratified by type of current delivery from the prospective data of Phelan et al.[29] These data are similar to the prior retrospective[30] and prospective[28] data from LAC/USC. In these studies, "dehiscence" was used to describe the scar separation that did not penetrate the uterine serosa, did not cause hemorrhage, and appeared clinically unimportant. Patients who attempted TOL were at no higher risk for dehiscence than those who had elective repeat cesareans, either antepartum or early intrapartum. A restratification of patients by indication for prior cesarean did not reveal any statistically significant differences in dehiscence rates.[28] In the study by Tahilramaney et al, the rate was 1.6% for those with a history of prior cesarean for any other indi-

TABLE 32.4 Morbidity Measures and Hospital Stay Comparisons for Study Groups

	Trial of Labor (*N* = 1796)				**No Trial of Labor (*N* = 847)**					
	Successful Vaginal Delivery (*N* = 1465)		Failure Cesarean (*N* = 331)		Vaginal Delivery (*N* = 69)		Elective Cesarean (*N* = 314)		Other Cesarean (*N* = 464)	
	N	%	*N*	%	*N*	%	*N*	%	*N*	%
Dehiscence	22	1.5	17	5.1	3	4.3	7	2.2	10	2.2
Febrile morbidity	53	3.6	106	32	4	5.8	56	18	103	22
Hospital stay (days)	2.2		4.2		2.3		4.2		4.3	

Elective repeat cesarean was performed in 12% of the total population with a prior cesarean.
Source: Phelan JP, Clark SC, Diaz F, et al: Vaginal birth after cesarean. *Am J Obstet Gynecol* 157:1510, 1987, with permission from the CV Mosby Co.

cation.[32] Further, among the patients with prior cesarean for CPD/FTP, 1/46 (2.2%) delivered vaginally, compared to 3/149 (2.0%) delivered by repeat cesarean in labor, had a dehiscence. This difference was not significant.

Other authors have also compared dehiscence or rupture rates among patients with prior cesarean for differing indications. Salzmann calculated rates of symptomatic true complete or nearly complete rupture of a low segment scar to be highest at 2% or 3% after prior cesarean for placenta previa or abruptio placentae, intermediate for other diagnoses, and zero for those with a history of CPD/FTP.[33] Pedowitz and Schwartz published higher rates of rupture of 13%–23% for patients with prior cesarean for abruptio, previa, or fetal distress, compared to 6.3% for those with prior cesarean for CPD during labor.[34] On the basis of all these series, one might argue that it is safer to permit labor after prior cesarean for a recurring condition (CPD/FTP) than after prior cesarean for a nonrecurring condition. Salzmann's explanation for this paradox is that cesarean performed after adequate thinning of the lower segment avoids the muscular upper segment, resulting in a lower risk of separation in a subsequent pregnancy.

The risk of fetal distress in labor is no higher for patients attempting TOL than for those delivering by elective repeat cesarean. Paul et al found the risk of fetal distress to be 2% among 1209 patients with prior cesarean, 2.4% for those attempting TOL, compared to 1.5% for those scheduled for repeat cesarean.[28] For patients with a history of prior cesarean for fetal distress, the risk for recurrence of fetal distress during TOL was 2/67 (3%), no higher than the 16/684 (2.3%) risk among patients with a history of prior cesarean for any other indication.

CONCLUSIONS

Many physicians believe that prior cesarean for CPD or FTP contraindicates a subsequent TOL. An abundance of evidence gathered both retrospectively and prospectively contradicts that belief. CPD is too difficult to define, and FTP is too all-encompassing. We do not yet have data on the probabilities of successful TOL after cesarean for specific labor arrest disorders (secondary arrest of dilatation, prolonged deceleration phase, failure of descent, arrest of descent)[35] occurring singly or in combination with other labor aberrations. The most pessimistic estimate available from contemporary data suggests a probability of success of 50% for a patient attempting TOL after cesarean for failure to progress in her only prior labor. If the parturient has had a prior vaginal delivery, her chance of successful TOL rises to 86%, despite a history of prior cesarean for FTP.[26] This success rate is in the range we might quote for a patient with a history of prior cesarean for any other indication. If the patient has a history of prior cesarean for a nonrecurring condition and subsequent vaginal delivery, her probability of successful TOL might be as high as 94%,[28] which is higher than that for a low-risk primigravida in uncomplicated labor in many U.S. hospitals. Because the risk of complications in a TOL is very low, and probably is essentially independent of the indication for the prior cesarean, there is no justification for a bias against the patient with a history of prior cesarean for CPD or FTP.

The opinions expressed in this chapter are those of the author and not necessarily those of the United States Air Force or the Department of Defense.

REFERENCES

1. Cragin EB: Conservatism in obstetrics. *NY State J Med* 104:1, 1916.
2. Shy KK, LoGerfo JP, Karp LE: Evaluation of elective repeat cesarean section as a standard of care: An application of decision analysis. *Am J Obstet Gynecol* 139:123, 1981.
3. Lavin JP, Stephens RJ, Miodovnik M, et al: Vaginal delivery in patients with a prior cesarean section. *Obstet Gynecol* 59:135, 1982.
4. *Cesarean Childbirth.* NIH Pub. No. 82-2067. Bethesda, Md, 1981.
5. O'Driscoll K, Foley M: Correlation of decrease in perinatal mortality and increase in cesarean section rates. *Obstet Gynecol* 61:1, 1983.
6. Leveno KJ, Cunningham FG, Pritchard JA: Cesarean section: An answer to the House of Horne. *Am J Obstet Gynecol* 153:838, 1985.
7. Harris JR: Vaginal delivery following cesarean section. *Am J Obstet Gynecol* 66:1191, 1953.
8. O'Connell W: Vaginal delivery following cesarean section. *Pac Med Surg* 74:343, 1966.
9. Allahbadia N: Vaginal delivery following cesarean section. *Am J Obstet Gynecol* 85:241, 1963.
10. Meehan FP, Moolgaoker AS, Stallworthy J: Vaginal delivery under caudal analgesia after caesarean section and other major uterine surgery. *Br Med J* 2:740, 1972.
11. Gibbs CE: Planned vaginal delivery following cesarean section. *Clin Obstet Gynecol* 23:507, 1980.
12. Cosgrove RA: Management of pregnancy and delivery following cesarean section. *JAMA* 145:884, 1951.

13. Birnbaum SJ: Postcesarean obstetrics: Management of subsequent pregnancy. *Obstet Gynecol* 7:611, 1956.
14. Wilson A: Labor and delivery after cesarean section. *Am J Obstet Gynecol* 62:1225, 1951.
15. Browne ADH, McGrath J: Vaginal delivery after previous caesarean section: A survey of 800 cases at the Rotunda Hospital, Dublin. *J Obstet Gynaecol Br Commonw* 72:557, 1965.
16. Lawrence RF: Vaginal delivery after caesarean section. *J Obstet Gynaecol Br Emp* 60:237, 1953.
17. Pauerstein CJ, Karp L, Muher S: Trial of labor after low segment cesarean section. *South Med J* 62:925, 1969.
18. McGarry JA: The management of patients previously delivered by caesarean section. *J Obstet Gynaecol Br Commonw* 76:137, 1969.
19. Morewood GA, O'Sullivan MJ, McConney J: Vaginal delivery after cesarean section. *Obstet Gynecol* 42:589, 1973.
20. Saldana LR, Schulman H, Reuss L: Management of pregnancy after cesarean section. *Am J Obstet Gynecol* 135:555, 1979.
21. Demianczuk NN, Hunter DJS, Taylor DW: Trial of labor after previous cesarean section: Prognostic indicators of outcome. *Am J Obstet Gynecol* 142:640, 1982.
22. Seitchik J, Rao VRR: Cesarean delivery in nulliparous women for failed oxytocin-augmented labor: Route of delivery in subsequent pregnancy. *Am J Obstet Gynecol* 143:393, 1982.
23. Meier PR, Porreco RP: Trial of labor following cesarean section: A two-year experience. *Am J Obstet Gynecol* 144:671, 1982.
24. Wadhawan S, Narone JN: Outcome of labor following previous cesarean section. *Int J Gynaecol Obstet* 21:7, 1983.
25. Graham AR: Trial labor following previous cesarean section. *Am J Obstet Gynecol* 149:35, 1984.
26. Clark CL, Eglinton GS, Beall M, et al: Effect of indication for previous cesarean section on subsequent delivery outcome in patients undergoing a trial of labor. *J Reprod Med* 29:33, 1984.
27. Jarrel MA, Ashmead GG, Mann LI: Vaginal delivery after cesarean section: A five-year study. *Obstet Gynecol* 65:628, 1985.
28. Paul RH, Phelan JP, Yeh S: Trial of labor in the patient with a prior cesarean birth. *Am J Obstet Gynecol* 151:297, 1985.
29. Phelan JP, Clark SL, Diaz F, et al: Vaginal birth after cesarean. *Am J Obstet Gynecol* 157:1510, 1987.
30. Eglinton GS, Phelan JP, Yeh S, et al: Outcome of a trial of labor after prior cesarean delivery. *J Reprod Med* 29:3, 1984.
31. Riva HL, Teich JC: Vaginal delivery after cesarean section. *Am J Obstet Gynecol* 81:501, 1961.
32. Tahilramaney MP, Boucher M, Eglinton GS, et al: Previous cesarean section and trial of labor. Factors related to uterine dehiscence. *J Reprod Med* 29:17, 1984.
33. Salzmann B: Rupture of low-segment cesarean section scars. *Obstet Gynecol* 23:460, 1964.
34. Pedowitz P, Schwartz RM: The true incidence of silent rupture of cesarean section scars: A prospective analysis of 403 cases. *Am J Obstet Gynecol* 74:1701, 1957.
35. Friedman EA: *Labor: Clinical Evaluation and Management.* New York, Appleton-Century-Crofts, 1967.

Chapter 33

Vaginal Birth after Cesarean

The Role of Oxytocin

Janet Horenstein, MD, and
Jeffrey P. Phelan, MD

Cesarean delivery has now become the number one hospital-based operative procedure in the United States and accounts for approximately 25% of all live births.[1] Since 1978, the cesarean rate has risen 44%; 47% of the rise has been due to the performance of an elective repeat cesarean.[2] During the same period, vaginal birth after cesarean has been shown to be an acceptable alternative to this traditional approach[3–8] (Chapter 31). However, clinicians practicing obstetrics today have been reluctant to adopt attempted vaginal delivery as an alternative in their prior cesarean patients.[2] This is due, in large part, to the fear that the uterus would rupture during a trial of labor. However, this fear has not been realized.[8] Moreover, the use of oxytocin in these patients has been a considerable point of controversy. The major concern is that the intrapartum administration of oxytocin would be associated with an increased risk of uterine rupture. As a consequence, this would expose the mother and fetus to a greater risk of morbidity and mortality. As with the trial of labor without oxytocin, these fears have not been realized. In fact, the use of oxytocin during a trial of labor has increased dramatically in this decade[1,9–11] and has not been associated with an increased risk of morbidity or mortality.

In light of the rapid increase in oxytocin usage in recent times, the purpose of this chapter is to review the overall experience of oxytocin usage in patients with a prior cesarean who have undergone a trial of labor. Finally, a management scheme for these patients when oxytocin in considered medically necessary will be suggested.

OXYTOCIN USAGE

At the Los Angeles County/University of Southern California Medical Center, the incidence of oxytocin use has increased 140% over a 4-year

TABLE 33.1 Trend in Oxytocin Usage for Prior Cesarean Patients Who Underwent a Trial of Labor

	1980[9]	1982–1983[10]	1983–1984[11]
Trial of labor	292	751	1045
Oxytocin	58 (20%)	289 (38%)	504 (48%)
Vaginal delivery	31 (53%)	200 (69%)	357 (71%)

period (Table 33.1). During this time, the vaginal delivery rate has remained fairly constant. The greater use of oxytocin is partly due to a greater familiarity with its usage in prior cesarean patients. It also reflects the fact that patients with two or more prior cesareans were permitted a trial of labor and a similar percentage received oxytocin.[11]

As demonstrated by Table 33.2, of 3,211 reported prior cesarean patients, 1,111 (35%) received oxytocin during a trial of labor.[3,9–17] The incidence of oxytocin use ranged from 2% to 48%. Those studies reporting little or no use of oxytocin were made during periods where oxytocin was considered unsafe. Subsequent studies that permitted oxytocin usage in prior cesarean patients who underwent a trial of labor have contributed to a greater incidence of usage and a clearer understanding of its effects.

VAGINAL DELIVERY RATES

Although the overall reported incidence of oxytocin usage during a trial of labor in prior cesarean patients is 35%, the experience in patients receiving oxytocin for *induction* of labor is limited. For instance, in those series with detailed information on the administration of oxytocin, 11% of patients received it for induction of labor (Table 33.3). Nonetheless, the vaginal delivery rates do not appear to be significantly affected by whether oxytocin is used for induction or augmentation of labor.[9–11,13,14,17,18] For instance (Table 33.3), the overall rates of successful vaginal delivery with induction (60%) and augmentation (68%) of labor are similar.

Of interest is that prostaglandin gels have also been used to ripen the cervix in prior cesarean patients who desired a trial of labor.[19] This was followed by oxytocin induction or augmentation of labor. In the series

TABLE 33.2 Incidence of Oxytocin Usage and the Rate of Uterine Dehiscence for Prior Cesarean Patients Who Received Oxytocin during a Trial of Labor

Trial of labor	3211
Oxytocin usage	1111 (35%)
Dehiscence	43 (3.9%)

TABLE 33.3 Vaginal Delivery Rates for Prior Cesarean Patients Who Received Oxytocin for Induction or Augmentation of Labor

	Number	Vaginal Delivery
Induction	123	774 (60%)
Augmentation	968	662 (68%)

by Mackenzie et al,[19] the repeat cesarean delivery rate was 24%. The usual indications for cesarean delivery were encountered, and the rate of fetal distress was 4%. Moreover, there were no uterine dehiscences or ruptures in the study population.

The vaginal delivery rates for prior cesarean paticnts who underwent a trial of labor with or without oxytocin[5,9–13,16,17] are contrasted in Table 33.4. Successful vaginal delivery was significantly higher in the nonoxytocin group. Of the 2916 prior cesarean patients who underwent a trial of labor where oxytocin use was known (Table 33.4), 1,096 (38%) received oxytocin. The repeat cesarean delivery rate was 14% versus 32% in the nonoxytocin and oxytocin groups, respectively. The incidence of repeat cesarean delivery in the oxytocin group was 2.3 times higher than in the population who did not receive oxytocin.

The most common indications for repeat cesarean delivery for patients who underwent a trial of labor with or without oxytocin[11] are presented in Table 33.5. Three-fourths of the patients who received oxytocin underwent cesarean delivery for cephalopelvic disproportion (CPD) or failure to progress (FTP). When the oxytocin group was contrasted with the nonoxytocin group, the incidence of fetal distress by indication was significantly higher in the nonoxytocin group. However, the overall rates of repeat cesarean delivery for fetal distress in the oxytocin and nonoxytocin groups were 3.0% and 2.6%,[11] respectively. These results were not significantly different. Finally, the delivery outcome, as measured by hemorrhage, transfusions, uterine atony, and hysterectomy, was unaffected by the administration of oxytocin during a trial of labor.[10]

TABLE 33.4 Vaginal Delivery Rates for Prior Cesarean Patients Who Underwent a Trial of Labor with or without Oxytocin

	Number	Vaginal Delivery
Oxytocin	1096	747 (68%)
No oxytocin	1820	1572 (86%)

TABLE 33.5 Indications for Repeat Cesarean in Prior Cesarean Patients Who Underwent a Trial of Labor with or without Oxytocin

Indication for Repeat Cesarean	Oxytocin (*N* = 236)	No Oxytocin (*N* = 95)
CPD/FTP	183 (78%)	57 (60%)
Fetal distress	24 (10%)	26 (28%)
Breech	4 (2%)	6 (6%)
Other	25 (10%)	6 (6%)

Source: After Horenstein J, Phelan JP: Previous cesarean section: The risks and benefits of oxytocin usage in a trial of labor. *Am J Obstet Gynecol* 151:564, 1985.

UTERINE SCAR SEPARATION RATE WITH OXYTOCIN USAGE

As previously noted, clinicians were frequently concerned about the administration of oxytocin during a trial of labor. Their fear was that its administration would expose the mother to a greater probability of uterine scar separation and its sequelae. The overall rate of uterine scar separation for the published reports listed in Table 33.2 was 3.9%. In the series by Phelan and associates,[11] the incidence of dehiscence was similar whether or not oxytocin was administered. The rates in their series were 3% and 2%, respectively. These results were not significantly different. Moreover, in those patients undergoing a repeat cesarean delivery during a trial of labor, the overall incidence of scar separation was less in the oxytocin group (4.7%) than in the nonoxytocin (5.3%) group. The higher incidence of dehiscence in the repeat cesarean patient is due to the fact that the scar can be visualized at cesarean delivery. Finally, as demonstrated by Tahilramaney and associates,[8] "neither the administration of oxytocin nor the duration of its administration had an impact on the rate of uterine dehiscence."

PREDICTORS OF VAGINAL DELIVERY

When oxytocin is considered for the induction or augmentation of labor in the prior cesarean patient, several factors can serve as predictors of subsequent vaginal delivery. One important factor is the prior indication for cesarean delivery. As demonstrated by Table 33.6, those patients whose primary indications for cesarean delivery were CPD/FTP and fetal distress had the lowest probability of delivering vaginally if oxytocin was required. While the increased rate of cesarean delivery following primary cesarean for CPD/FTP is understandable, the reasons for the higher rate in patients whose primary cesarean was for fetal distress are less clear. As noted by Horenstein and Phelan,[10] the indication for repeat cesarean delivery in these patients was not recurrent fetal distress but CPD/FTP.

TABLE 33.6 Prior Indication for Cesarean Delivery and a Subsequent Trial of Labor with or without Oxytocin

	Oxytocin		No Oxytocin	
Prior Indication	Number	Vaginal Delivery	Number	Vaginal Delivery
CPD/FTP	416	272 (65%)	404	352 (87%)
Breech	122	93 (76%)	210	200 (95%)
Fetal Distress	78	54 (69%)	94	87 (93%)
Other	177	138 (78%)	276	250 (91%)

Source: After Horenstein J, Phelan JP: Previous cesarean section: The risks and benefits of oxytocin usage in a trial of labor. *Am J Obstet Gynecol* 151:564, 1985.

One of the best single predictors of successful vaginal delivery in patients with prior cesarean who require oxytocin is a history of prior vaginal delivery.[10,18] Whether the patient had a vaginal delivery before or after the cesarean, her chances of subsequent vaginal delivery were found to be 85%.

Lastly, as demonstrated by Silver and Gibbs,[18] the prior birth weight of the patient's last baby in comparison to that of the current fetus is also a reliable predictor of subsequent vaginal delivery when oxytocin is medically necessary. As demonstrated by these investigators, if the past birth weight was greater than the present birth weight, the patient had an 84% chance of delivering vaginally. In contrast, if the present birth weight was larger than the past birth weight, the chances of successful vaginal delivery were less than 50%. This concern over birth weight is borne out by the work of Phelan and associates.[20] Birth weights that were equal to or exceeded 4,000 g indicated a significantly lower probability of vaginal delivery and a higher rate of repeat cesarean delivery. For instance, the repeat cesarean delivery rate in mothers whose infants weighed 4,000 g or more was 42% in the oxytocin group versus 25% in the nonoxytocin group.[20]

Finally, once oxytocin administration has been initiated, an early response to the drug is a positive predictor of whether the patient will deliver vaginally or not. In the series by Silver and Gibbs,[18] if cervical dilatation occurred within 2 hours of oxytocin administration, vaginal delivery was more likely to occur.

In summary, the use of oxytocin is associated with a two- to threefold greater probability of repeat cesarean delivery. In those patients whose prior cesarean deliveries were for fetal distress or CPD/FTP, the probability of vaginal delivery is reduced, but more than 60% of the patients still achieve a vaginal delivery. In addition, patients whose present estimated birth weight is greater than the past birth weight, and those in whom the estimated fetal weight is 4,000 g or more have a greater probability of requiring a repeat cesarean delivery. In contrast, patients who have had a prior vaginal delivery or who demonstrate an early response to oxytocin have the greatest probability of successful vaginal delivery.

MANAGEMENT IN LIGHT OF THE CURRENT LITERATURE

In light of the recent literature, the use of oxytocin in prior cesarean patients who undergo a trial of labor appears to be reasonable. The indications for oxytocin administration should be the same as those for patients with an unscarred uterus. When oxytocin is administered for induction or augmentation of labor, it should be in a dilute solution and by controlled infusion in accordance with the ACOG Technical bulletin No. 49.[21] Other alternatives include an approved protocol for such administration in each obstetrician's hospital setting or the one suggested by Seitchik et al.[22] This would be in keeping with current American College of Obstetricians and Gynecologists guidelines on vaginal birth after cesarean.[23]

During a trial of labor in the patient with a prior cesarean birth who requires oxytocin, the mother and the fetus should be closely monitored, as outlined in Chapter 2. An early response to oxytocin is frequently associated with a greater probability of vaginal delivery.[18] However, if the patient has an adequate response but fails to dilate sufficiently within a reasonable period of time, cesarean delivery should be considered.

In conclusion, it appears that the use of oxytocin, when carefully monitored, is a safe and reasonable consideration in the prior cesarean patient who desires a trial of labor. Although its use is associated with a greater probability of cesarean delivery, approximately 65% to 70% of patients who receive oxytocin will ultimately deliver vaginally. This increased rate of vaginal delivery does not appear to be associated with an increased risk of maternal or fetal morbidity or mortality.

REFERENCES

1. Rutkow IM: Obstetric and gynecologic operations in the United States, 1979 to 1984. *Obstet Gynecol* 67:755, 1986.
2. Shiono PH, McNellis D, Rhoads GG: Reasons for the rising cesarean delivery rates: 1978–1984. *Obstet Gynecol* 69:696, 1987.
3. Riva H, Teich J: Vaginal delivery after cesarean section. *Am J Obstet Gynecol* 81:501, 1961.
4. Gibbs C: Planned vaginal delivery following cesarean section. *Obstet Gynecol* 23:507, 1980.
5. Meier PR, Porreco RP: Trial of labor following cesarean section: A two-year experience. *Am J Obstet Gynecol* 144:671, 1982.
6. Eglinton GS, Phelan JP, Yeh SY, et al: Outcome of a trial of labor after prior cesarean delivery. *J Reprod Med* 29:3, 1984.
7. Paul RH, Phelan JP, Yeh SY: Trial of labor in the patient with a prior cesarean birth. *Am J Obstet Gynecol* 151:297, 1985.
8. Tahilramaney MP, Boucher M, Eglinton GS, et al: Previous cesarean section and trial of labor. Factors related to uterine dehiscence. *J Reprod Med* 29:17, 1984.
9. Horenstein J, Eglinton G, Tahilramaney M, et al: Oxytocin use during a trial of labor in patients with previous cesarean section. *J Reprod Med* 29:26, 1984.

10. Horenstein JP, Phelan JP: Previous cesarean section: The risks and benefits of oxytocin usage in a trial of labor. *Am J Obstet Gynecol* 151:564, 1985.
11. Phelan JP, Clark SL, Diaz F, et al: Vaginal birth after cesarean. *Am J Obstet Gynecol* 157:1510, 1987.
12. Saldana L, Schulman H, Reuss L: Management of pregnancy after cesarean section. *Obstet Gynecol* 135:555, 1979.
13. Flamm BL, Dunnett C, Fischerman E, et al: Vaginal delivery following cesarean section: Use of oxytocin augmentation and epidural anesthesia with internal tocodynamic and internal fetal monitoring. *Am J Obstet Gynecol* 148:759, 1984.
14. Martin JN, Harris BA, Huddleston JF, et al: Vaginal delivery following previous cesarean birth. *Am J Obstet Gynecol* 146:255, 1983.
15. Meehan FP, Moolgaoker AS, Stallworthy J: Vaginal delivery under caudal anesthesia after cesarean section and other major uterine surgery. *Br Med J* 2:740, 1972.
16. McGarry J: The management of patients previously delivered by cesarean section. *J Obstet Gynecol Br Commonw* 76:137, 1969.
17. Demianczuk NN, Hunter DJS, Taylor DW: Trial of labor after previous cesarean section: Prognostic indicators of outcome. *Am J Obstet Gynecol* 142:640, 1982.
18. Silver RK, Gibbs RS: Prediction of vaginal delivery in patients with a previous cesarean section who require oxytocin. *Am J Obstet Gynecol* 156:57, 1987.
19. Mackenzie IZ, Bradley S, Embrey MP: Vaginal prostaglandins and labor induction for patients previously delivered by cesarean section. *Br J Obstet Gynecol* 91:7, 1984.
20. Phelan JP, Eglinton GS, Horenstein JM, et al: Previous cesarean birth: Trial of labor in women with macrosomic infants. *J Reprod Med* 29:36, 1984.
21. Induction of Labor. American College of Obstetricians and Gynecologists Technical Bulletin No. 49, May 1978.
22. Seitchik J, Amico J, Castillo M: Oxytocin augmentation of dysfunctional labor. V. An alternative oxytocin regimen. *Am J Obstet Gynecol* 151:757, 1985.
23. Practice perspectives: Guidelines for vaginal delivery after previous cesarean birth. *ACOG Newsletter*, February, 1985, p 8.

Chapter 34

Vaginal Birth after Multiple Prior Cesareans

Jeffrey P. Phelan, MD

Vaginal birth after one prior cesarean is becoming an acceptable alternative to routine elective repeat cesarean delivery.[1–9] Experience to date indicates that these patients have an 80%–85% chance of achieving a vaginal delivery. These data further suggest that a trial of labor appears to be the safest option for both mother and fetus.[10] But physicians often ask, "What are the possibilities for a trial of labor in patients with two or more prior cesareans?" Current ACOG guidelines for vaginal birth after cesarean do not specify the number of prior cesareans a patient can have for attempted vaginal delivery. Regardless, recent evidence suggests that a trial of labor in the patient with two or more prior cesareans[5–9,11] is a reasonable consideration. Moreover, a trial of labor appears to offer no greater risk of harm to the pregnant woman and her fetus than that incurred by undertaking a trial of labor in a patient with one prior cesarean.

In light of the accumulating evidence regarding the safety of trial labor in the patient with multiple prior cesarean births, the purpose of this chapter is to review current reports on these patients. Lastly, this chapter will address the role of oxytocin and conduction anesthesia in those patients who have undergone a trial of labor after two or more prior cesarean births.

VAGINAL BIRTH AFTER TWO OR MORE CESAREANS

In the published reports to date,[5–9,11] the incidence of trial of labor has not been routinely described. However, three reports[5,8,9] do provide detailed information. Of the 892 patients with two or more prior incisions, 209 (23%) decided in favor of attempted vaginal delivery. This incidence varied with the series and ranged from 10% to 32%. In contrast to patients with one prior cesarean delivery, where the incidence approximates 60%–

TABLE 34.1 Trial of Labor Incidence and Vaginal Delivery Rates for Patients with Two or More Prior Cesareans

Study	Patients	Trial of Labor	Vaginal Delivery
Phelan et al[5]	608	159 (26%)	116 (73%)
Riva and Teich[6]	—	76 —	50 (66%)
Saldana et al[7]	—	38 —	17 (81%)
Wadhawan and Narone[9]	96	31 (32%)	22 (71%)
Porreco and Meier[12]	—	21 —	17 (81%)
Martin et al[8]	192	19 (10%)	12 (63%)

65%,[5] this incidence is markedly reduced. One reason for this relatively low incidence is the lack of clinical familiarity in handling these patients. With greater experience, the incidence of trial of labor should approximate that of patients with one prior cesarean.

Overall, 344 patients with two or more prior uterine incisions have undergone a trial of labor (Table 34.1). Of these, 239 (70%), with a range from 58% to 81%,[5–9,11] have delivered vaginally. If the patients with two (Table 34.2) or three or more (Table 34.3) prior uterine incisions are contrasted, the experience with patients with three or more incisions is quite limited and the vaginal delivery rates are decidedly reduced. For instance, of the 248 patients with two prior uterine incisions, 179 (72%) achieved vaginal delivery,[5,6,8,9] whereas of 37 patients with three or more prior uterine incisions,[5,6,8] 21 (57%) achieved a vaginal delivery.

In those patients who failed to achieve vaginal delivery, the usual indications for cesarean delivery were encountered, such as cephalopelvic disproportion and fetal distress. These incidences were comparable to those encountered in patients with one prior uterine incision.

OXYTOCIN AND EPIDURAL USAGE DURING TRIAL OF LABOR

With the increase in the number of patients undergoing a trial of labor after prior cesarean delivery, oxytocin usage has increased dramatically (Chapter 33). Although the data have been gathered primarily in patients

TABLE 34.2 Vaginal Delivery Rate for Patients with Two Prior Cesareans Who Underwent a Trial of Labor

	Trial of Labor (*N*)	Vaginal Delivery
Phelan et al[5]	149	107 (72%)
Riva and Teich[6]	55	41 (75%)
Wadhawan and Narone[9]	31	22 (71%)
Martin et al[8]	13	9 (69%)

TABLE 34.3 Vaginal Delivery Rates for Patients with Three or More Prior Cesareans Who Underwent a Trial of Labor

	Trial of Labor (*N*)	Vaginal Delivery
Riva and Teich[6]	21	9 (43%)
Phelan et al[5]	10	9 (90%)
Martin et al[8]	6	3 (50%)

with one prior incision, oxytocin usage in patients with multiple prior cesarean deliveries has also shown an increase. For instance, during a 1-year period (Table 34.4), there was a 140% increase in the number of patients with two or more prior uterine incisions who received oxytocin during a trial of labor.[5] Of note is that by the second year of the report by Phelan and associates,[5] the incidence of oxytocin use had risen to 48%. This is considerably higher than the 33% incidence described by Porreco and Meier.[11] These data suggest that with greater experience comes a higher incidence of use that is not associated with a greater risk of uterine dehiscence or rupture[5] (Chapter 33).

If the patients with two or more prior cesareans who did and did not receive oxytocin are contrasted, the patients who received oxytocin were less likely to achieve a vaginal delivery. For instance, in the 69 patients with two or more incisions who received oxytocin, 42 (61%) delivered vaginally. In contrast, in the nonoxytocin group, 74 of 90 patients (82%) achieved a vaginal delivery. Thus, the administration of oxytocin to a patient with two or more prior cesareans was associated with a twofold increase in the incidence of cesarean delivery. The most common indication for repeat cesarean delivery was cephalopelvic disproportion/failure to progress. Of note is that the incidences of fetal distress and uterine dehiscence were comparable to those of patients with one prior incision and no oxytocin usage. Though the experience is limited, the use of oxytocin, when administered for the usual and customary indications and in a judicious manner, appears to be a reasonable consideration in the patient with two or more prior cesareans.

The experience with epidural anesthesia in these patients is limited to two reports.[5,11] For these combined series, the overall oxytocin use was in 22 of 134 patients (16.4%). In those patients receiving a combination

TABLE 34.4 Incidence of Oxytocin Usage and Vaginal Delivery in Patients Undergoing a Trial of Labor with Two or More Prior Uterine Incisions

	1982–1983	1983–1984
Trial of labor	25	134
Oxytocin	5 (20%)	64 (48%)
Vaginal delivery	3 (60%)	39 (61%)

TABLE 34.5 Incidence of Uterine Scar Separations Based on the Number of Prior Uterine Incisions

Study	Year	Number of Prior Uterine Incisions		
		1	2	3
Pedowitz and Schwartz[13]	1957	29/327 (8.9%)	8/47 (17%)	1/2 (50%)
Case et al[14]	1971	17/491 (3.5%)	5/228 (2.2%)	3/37 (8.1%)
Tahilramaney et al[15]	1980	17/643 (2.6%)	4/133 (3.0%)	3/40 (7.5%)

of epidural anesthesia and oxytocin, the probability of vaginal delivery was 47%.[5] In contrast, in those patients who received conduction anesthesia without oxytocin, 100% achieved a vaginal delivery. Of note is that the use of epidural anesthesia alone or in combination with oxytocin was not associated with a greater risk of maternal or fetal morbidity.

UTERINE DEHISCENCE

For purposes of this chapter, a uterine dehiscence was defined as a palpable and/or visualized uterine defect that did not require operative intervention. A uterine rupture was defined as a uterine defect that did require operative intervention.[2]

Previous reports (Table 34.5) have shown an increasing rate of uterine dehiscence rupture as the number of prior uterine incisions increased.[12–14] The overall incidence of uterine dehiscence in these reports was 1%–4.3%, 2%–4.2%, and 3%–8.9%. In these reports, the patients reported by Pedowitz and Schwartz[12] and Case et al[13] underwent an elective repeat cesarean delivery and were not permitted a trial of labor. But in the report by Tahilramaney and associates,[14] 37% of the patients underwent a trial of labor. The uterine scar separation rate for the trial and nontrial groups was 1.6% and 3.8%, respectively. Moreover, recent experience indicates that there is not a greater incidence of dehiscence in patients with two or more prior cesareans. For example, of 268 patients who underwent a trial of labor (Table 34.6), 6 (2.6%) with two or more prior incisions were found to have a uterine defect. Finally, the overall incidence of uterine dehiscence for patients with two and three or more prior cesareans was

TABLE 34.6 Maternal Morbidity in Relation to a Trial of Labor in Patients with Two or More Prior Incisions (N = 268)

Maternal Morbidity	Number	Percent
Dehiscence	6	(2.6%)
Hysterectomy	0	(0.0%)
Maternal mortality	0	(0.0%)

3.1% and 3.3%, respectively. Thus, in contrast to prior reports,[12–14] the incidence of uterine scar separation does not appear to increase with the number of prior uterine incisions.

Furthermore, as demonstrated by Table 34.6, the incidence of hysterectomy and maternal mortality was not increased for patients with two or more prior incisions who underwent a trial of labor.

SUMMARY

Based on the aforementioned data, patients with two prior uterine incisions should be permitted a trial of labor and managed similarly to patients with one prior uterine incision. Although the data do suggest that a trial of labor is a reasonable consideration in patients with three or more prior uterine incisions, the experience to date is too limited and more experience is necessary. Thus, patients with two prior incisions should be offered the option of a trial of labor. If accepted, these patients should be managed as patients with one prior incision. During labor, epidural anesthesia would seem reasonable, depending upon the individual circumstances. Similarly, if oxytocin administration is considered medically necessary to either augment or induce labor, it appears to be a reasonable consideration.

During the trial of labor, the guidelines suggested by the American College of Obstetricians and Gynecologists should be followed.[15] Continuous electronic fetal monitoring should be employed throughout the course of labor to detect any evidence of intrapartum fetal distress. A physician capable of performing a cesarean delivery should be immediately available in the event of an acute emergency. The use of oxytocin and epidural anesthesia would appear reasonable so long as a contraindication does not exist. When oxytocin is to be administered to patients with two prior uterine incisions, the guidelines set forth in ACOG Technical Bulletin No. 49 should be followed.[16] Finally, circumstances in the individual practitioner's hospital may be such that a trial of labor in patients with two prior uterine incisions may be unreasonable. If not, guidelines should be established to allow attempted vaginal delivery in patients with two or more prior cesarean births.

With an increasing number of patients with one prior cesarean birth achieving a vaginal delivery, fewer patients with two or more prior incisions will be encountered in the future. It is anticipated, therefore, that chapters such as this will be of historical interest only.

REFERENCES

1. Eglinton GS, Phelan JP, Yeh SY, et al: Outcome after prior cesarean delivery. *J Reprod Med* 29:3, 1984.

2. Paul RH, Phelan JP, Yeh SY: Trial of labor in the patient with a prior cesarean birth. *Am J Obstet Gynecol* 151:297, 1985.
3. Meier PR, Porreco RP: Trial of labor following cesarean section: A two-year experience. *Am J Obstet Gynecol* 144:671, 1982.
4. Gibbs CE: Planned vaginal delivery following cesarean section. *Clin Obstet Gynecol* 23:507, 1980.
5. Phelan JP, Clark SL, Diaz F, et al: Vaginal birth after cesarean. *Am J Obstet Gynecol* 157:1510, 1987.
6. Riva HL, Teich JC: Vaginal delivery after cesarean section. *Am J Obstet Gynecol* 81:501, 1961.
7. Saldana LR, Schulman H, Reuss L: Management of pregnancy after cesarean section. *Am J Obstet Gynecol* 135:555, 1979.
8. Martin JN, Harris BA, Huddleston JF, et al: Vaginal delivery following previous cesarean birth. *Am J Obstet Gynecol* 146:255, 1983.
9. Wadhawan S, Narone JN: Outcome of labor following previous cesarean section. *Int J Gynecol Obstet* 21:7, 1983.
10. Boucher M, Tahilramaney M, Eglinton GS, et al: Maternal morbidity related to trial of labor after previous cesarean delivery: A quantitative analysis. *J Reprod Med* 29:12, 1984.
11. Porreco RP, Meier PR: Trial of labor in patients with multiple previous cesarean sections. *J Reprod Med* 28:770, 1983.
12. Pedowitz P, Schwartz RM: The true incidence of silent rupture of cesarean section scars. A prospective analysis of 403 cases. *Am J Obstet Gynecol* 74:1071, 1957.
13. Case BD, Corcoran R, Jeffcoate N, et al: Cesarean section and its place in modern obstetric practice. *J Obstet Gynecol Br Commonw* 78:203, 1971.
14. Tahilramaney MP, Boucher M, Eglinton GS, et al: Previous cesarean section and trial of labor. Factors related to uterine dehiscence. *J Reprod Med* 29:17, 1984.
15. Practice perspectives: Guidelines for vaginal delivery after previous cesarean birth. *ACOG Newsletter*, February, 1985, p 8.
16. *Induction of Labor*. ACOG Technical Bulletin 49. Washington, DC, American College of Obstetricians and Gynecologists, 1978.

Chapter 35

Epidural Anesthesia in Patients Undergoing Trial of Labor after a Previous Cesarean Birth

Janet Horenstein, MD, and
Steven L. Clark, MD

In many areas of the United States, epidural anesthesia for pain relief of labor has become standard practice. The advantages of such regional techniques over intravenous medication include more effective pain relief and fewer potential fetal effects.[1,2] Under many circumstances, epidural anesthesia is also the anesthetic method of choice for cesarean delivery.[3,4] Here again, epidural block offers superb pain relief and avoids potential maternal and fetal side effects associated with either spinal or general anesthesia. With the increasingly common practice of allowing a trial of labor following a previous cesarean delivery, controversy has arisen over the safety of epidural anesthesia for labor in patients with a scarred uterus.[5–10]

Traditionally, epidural anesthesia was viewed as being relatively contraindicated in patients laboring with a uterine scar. Concerns regarding the safety of epidural anesthesia under these circumstances centered principally on the theoretical possibility of masking the pain associated with uterine scar separation.[7,11] Under such circumstances, it was felt that epidural anesthesia would obviate this early warning sign of scar separation and thus delay timely intervention, with possible serious consequences for the mother and fetus. Recent experience from a number of centers has refuted this concept. In 1980, Carlson et al reported two patients with rupture of a uterine scar.[12] In both cases, the patients were aware of uterine pain and tenderness despite epidural analgesia, confirming earlier observations by Crawford.[13] Golan et al reviewed 93 cases of uterine rupture.[14] In this population, uterine or scar tenderness was an infrequent presenting sign of uterine rupture and occurred with equal frequency (approximately 25%) among patients with spontaneous uterine rupture and those suffering from scar separation. In a similar manner, Uppington examined six patients who developed uterine rupture in labor following a previous cesarean, and concluded that epidural anesthesia did not obliterate the signs and symptoms of uterine separation at the site of a previous low transverse uterine scar.[10] Both of these studies indicated that other presenting signs, such as fetal distress and alterations in uterine contraction pattern, were more common than was acute pain. Alterations in the uterine contraction pattern may occur in the forms of increased intensity and increased frequency of contractions, or if monitored with an internal pressure catheter system, may present with loss of intrauterine pressure.

It is also important to note that, if properly managed, such uterine scar separations are not nearly as catastrophic as those associated with spontaneous uterine rupture, and usually result in a good outcome for both the mother and fetus. In a review of world literature, Flamm et al uncovered only a single case of scar separation resulting in fetal death in a *monitored* patient.[9] Thus, it appears highly unlikely that restriction of epidural anesthesia in patients undergoing a trial of labor would have any appreciable effect on maternal or fetal morbidity in patients with a previous cesarean delivery.

Further, there are several reports of patients undergoing emergency cesarean for uterine tenderness (presumably heralding uterine scar separation) in which no separation was found.[15,16] In one study of 20 patients undergoing repeat cesarean delivery due to uterine pain and tenderness, actual scar separation was found in only 1 (5%).[15] This observation further supports the contention that uterine pain is neither a sensitive nor a specific symptom of uterine rupture.

In patients laboring with an epidural catheter, the usual precautions regarding laboring patients with a uterine scar remain important. Careful fetal monitoring including, when technically feasible, application of an internal scalp electrode is essential. An intrauterine pressure catheter is also a consideration in order to monitor carefully the uterine pressure generated. A sudden increase in baseline tonus or a sudden absence of uterine pressure, either alone or coupled with evidence of acute fetal distress, should lead to consideration of expeditious abdominal delivery.

Thus, despite theoretical concerns, the available clinical experience conclusively supports the belief that the administration of epidural anesthesia is appropriate in patients undergoing a trial of labor with a low transverse uterine incision.[8–10,12,13,17–21] The decision to use epidural anesthesia in such a patient should be made after consideration of the usual obstetric indications and contraindications; it appears that the presence of a uterine scar should not influence this decision. With this principle correctly applied, it is hoped that lack of adequate pain relief for labor will no longer be a deterrent for patients desiring a trial of labor.

REFERENCES

1. Ralston DH, Shnider SM: The fetal and neonatal effects of regional anesthesia in obstetrics. *Anesthesiology* 48:34, 1978.

2. Faure EAM, Bart AJ, Koht A: A comparison of continuous infusion epidural analgesia vs. intermittent injection techniques for obstetrical pain relief. *Anesthesiology* 53S:294, 1980.
3. Jumes FM, Crawford JS, Hopkinson R, et al: A comparison of general anesthesia and lumbar epidural analgesia for elective cesarean section. *Anesth Analg* 56:228, 1977.
4. Abboud TK, Nagappala S, Murakawa K, et al: A comparison of the effects of general and regional anesthesia for cesarean section on neonatal neurologic and adoptive capacity scores. *Anesth Analg* 64:996, 1985.
5. Albright GA: *Anesthesia in Obstetrics: Maternal, Fetal and Neonatal Aspects.* Reading, Mass, Addison-Wesley Pub Co, 1978, p 198.
6. Bromage PR: *Epidural Analgesia.* Philadelphia, WB Saunders Co, 1978, p 582.
7. Brundenell M, Chakravarti S: Uterine rupture in labour. *Br Med J* 2:122, 1975.
8. Rudick V, Niv D, Hetman-Perim, et al: Epidural analgesia for planned vaginal delivery following previous cesarean section. *Obstet Gynecol* 64:621, 1984.
9. Flamm BL, Dunnett C, Fischermann E, et al: Vaginal delivery following cesarean section: Use of oxytocin augmentation and epidural anesthesia with internal tocodynamic and internal fetal monitoring. *Am J Obstet Gynecol* 148:759, 1984.
10. Uppington J: Epidural analgesia and previous caesarean section. *Anaesthesia* 38:336, 1983.
11. O'Driscoll K: An obstetrician's view of pain. *Br J Anaesth* 47:1053, 1975.
12. Carlson C, Lybell-Lindahl G, Ingemarsson I: Extradural block in patients who have previously undergone cesarean section. *Br J Anaesth* 52:827, 1980.
13. Crawford JS: The epidural sieve and MBC (minimal blocking concentration): A hypothesis. *Anaesthesia* 31:1278, 1976.
14. Golan A, Sandbank O, Rubin A: Rupture of the pregnant uterus. *Obstet Gynecol* 56:349, 1980.
15. Case B, Corcoran R, Jeffcoate N: Cesarean section and its place in modern obstetric practice. *J Obstet Gynecol Br Commonw* 78:203, 1971.
16. Cosgrove RA: Management of pregnancy and delivery following cesarean section. *JAMA* 145:884, 1951.
17. Meehan FP, Moolgaoker AS, Stallworthy J: Vaginal delivery under caudal analgesia after cesarean section and other major uterine surgery. *Br Med J* 2:740, 1972.
18. Wilson AL: Labor and delivery after cesarean section. *Am J Obstet Gynecol* 62:1225, 1951.
19. Rudick V, Niv D, Golan A, et al: Epidural analgesia in 1200 monitored parturients. *Isr J Med Sci* 1:20, 1983.
20. Editorial comments. *Ob Gyn Survey* 39:204, 1984.
21. Horenstein JM, Clark SL, Phelan JP: Prior cesarean birth: Trial of labor with epidural anesthesia. Las Vegas, Nevada, Society of Perinatal Obstetricians, 1985, p 264.

Chapter 36

The Role of External Version in Modern Obstetrics

Gary S. Eglinton, MD

Breech presentation complicates about 3% of all term pregnancies. Yet, this single complication has been the third greatest contributor to the recent rise in the rate of cesarean delivery in the United States.[1] Although the cesarean rate for all deliveries increased from 5.5% to 15.2% from 1970 to 1978, the rate for breech deliveries increased from 11.6% to 60.1% over the same period, accounting for 10%–15% of the increase in the overall rate. Since these data were published, the rates of cesarean delivery have continued to increase for both breech and nonbreech indications.

Why has the rate of cesarean for breech presentation increased so dramatically? There is a large body of retrospectively gathered data implicating the breech presentation in higher neonatal and perinatal morbidity and mortality rates[2–6] and later neurologic abnormalities[4,5,7–9] when compared to the vertex presentation. The difference is most pronounced for vaginally delivered breech infants. Proponents of abdominal delivery for breech fetuses cite data from these sources implying the neonatal performance of the abdominally delivered breech approaches that of the vaginally delivered vertex.

Congenital anomalies and prematurity explain much of the increase in morbidity and mortality for breech infants. But even after correction for these confounding variables, Brenner et al found the perinatal mortality rate for fetuses at 32 weeks gestational age or greater to be 3.2% for those delivered vaginally, compared to zero for those delivered by cesarean.[3] Similarly, Todd and Steer studied only term breech deliveries at the Sloane Hospital for Women from 1949 through 1959 and found a corrected perinatal mortality of 1.1% attributable solely to the breech presentation.[10] This rate was four times higher than the rate for fetuses presenting as a term vertex after the same corrections. The private service had a 31%

cesarean rate and a corrected perinatal mortality rate of 0.3%. Although the patient populations may not have been identical in this retrospective chart review, the question of the role of operator experience in contributing to the vaginal breech outcome was raised. After a review of each of the cases, the authors concluded that an increase in the cesarean rate from 23% to approximately 30% by adherence to a rigid protocol that included x-ray pelvimetry and cesarean for any labor aberration could have decreased the corrected perinatal mortality to 1 in 1,006 cases.

In 1980, Gimovsky et al reported a retrospective study of the application of this protocol at the Sloane Hospital for Women from 1972 to 1977.[11] These investigators concluded that the breech presentations managed by protocol had a significantly lower perinatal morbidity than those managed off protocol (15.4% versus 3%, $P < 0.001$).

Following a strict protocol, Collea et al published the results of a randomized trial of labor versus elective cesarean for term fetuses in frank breech presentation.[12] Qualifying patients were at 36 or more gestational weeks, with estimated fetal weights of 2500–3800 g. The authors found that neonatal morbidity was significantly higher in the intentionally labored neonates than in the planned cesarean neonates ($P < 0.01$). Although there were no maternal deaths, maternal morbidity was significantly more frequent in cesarean delivery patients ($P < 0.01$). Subsequently, Gimovsky et al reported the results of the randomized management of the nonfrank breech presentation at term.[13,14] Unlike the previous frank breech study by Collea et al, [12] neonatal morbidity, despite five cord prolapses and one perinatal death, was similar among all study groups. There was no maternal mortality, but as in the study of Collea et al, maternal morbidity was markedly higher among the cesarean delivered mothers.

In 1985, Westgren et al published the results of a prospective study to determine the frequency of breech presentation at 32 weeks gestation and at delivery.[15] With a universal ultrasound screening program at 32 weeks, they identified 310 of 4600 (6.7%) fetuses in breech presentation. They then followed the patients with breech presentations weekly and chronicled the spontaneous cephalic version (SCV) rates compared to the persistent breech rates with increasing gestational age. They noted that 43% of the fetuses persisted in the breech presentation until delivery. The persistent breech fetuses had more preterm deliveries, lower mean gestational age at delivery, and lower birth weight at delivery at each gestational week from 37 to 42 weeks. Also, 80% of the persistent breech group had legs extended at the knees at 32 weeks (frank breech) compared to only 48% of the SCV group. At lower gestational ages, there appeared to be a marked difference in the probability of spontaneous conversion to vertex presentation based on parity and prior breech history. The highest spontaneous conversion rate was among parous women without a history of prior breech delivery, followed by nulliparas and then by parous women with a history of prior breech delivery. By the completion of 37 weeks gestation, the spontaneous conversion rate for parous women without a breech history was about 20% and was negligible for the other two groups. By 38 weeks, all women had less than a 10% probability of spontaneous conversion.

In summary, the route of delivery and management of the pregnant woman with a breech presentation requires the balancing of risks between the mother and her fetus. If cesarean delivery is routinely performed for the breech presentation, the risks to the fetus are reduced but the risks to the mother are significantly increased.[12,13] Conversely, attempted vaginal breech delivery exposes the fetus to a greater risk of morbidity and mortality[12,13,15]; but if the fetus is delivered vaginally, maternal morbidity and mortality are significantly reduced. With either approach, however, a high cesarean delivery rate results.

A SOLUTION TO THE BREECH DILEMMA—EXTERNAL CEPHALIC VERSION

Although obstetricians have expressed consternation over management of the breech delivery and have advocated either vaginal or cesarean approaches, neither of these strategies addresses the primary issue: persistence of the breech presentation at term. A potential solution to the problem has existed for centuries: external cephalic version (ECV). Recently, Jordan adopted an anthropological cross-cultural approach in tracing the history and breadth of experience with the application of this simple technique.[16] She offered the opinion that

> in obstetric communities where ECV is accepted and routinely practiced—and that was as true for the earlier American period as it is in present-day Europe—advocates of ECV maintain that it is associated with little risk and should constitute the conservative method of first choice. They argue logically and from their clinical experience that version is superior to either breech delivery or section. Where it is not accepted, on the other hand, practitioners believe with equal conviction that the risks associated with ECV are too high and justify abandoning it in favor of, usually, surgical delivery.

Jordan discusses three approaches to ECV: the traditional approach, as practiced in primitive societies; the conventional approach, as practiced with some medical technological application, such as stethoscopes and anesthesia; and the tocolytic approach, as introduced by Saling et al in 1975.[17] Subsequently, there have been four published, randomized, prospectively controlled studies assessing the efficacy of ECV in decreasing the rate of breech presentation at term and in decreasing the rate of cesarean delivery.[18–21] To understand the role of ECV in the modern management of the breech presentation, a review of ECV is necessary.

TABLE 36.1 Initial Reports of External Cephalic Version under Tocolysis

	Saling and Muller-Holve[17]	Berg and Kunze[28]	Fall and Nilsson[29]
Number	57	10	53
Agent	Fenoterol	Fenoterol	Terbutaline
Success	43 (75%)	7 (70%)	37 (70%)
Cesarean delivery rate	NA	1 (10%)	NA

NA = not available.

EXTERNAL CEPHALIC VERSION—THE INTRODUCTION OF TOCOLYSIS

Although tocolysis is not required to facilitate ECV prior to term, the traditional and conventional approaches to ECV, especially remote from term, probably play minor roles in modern obstetrics. After a review of the available version literature, several conclusions become evident: first, the spontaneous conversion rates and the postversion reversion rates are too high to warrant attempted ECV prior to term; second, the success of version at term without tocolysis or general anesthesia generally has been unsatisfactory; third, the addition of general anesthesia to facilitate version in later pregnancy has resulted in complication rates of 1%–4%, including perinatal death rates of over 1%.[22–27]

Saling and Muller-Holve (Table 36.1) attempted ECV at term after a continuous intravenous infusion of fenoterol.[17] Version was attempted after 37 weeks gestation for several reasons. Prior to term, the spontaneous conversion rate is high. Because the spontaneous conversion rate is low at term, it seemed unlikely that a fetus would revert spontaneously after successful ECV at term. If a complication occurred during a version, necessitating emergency delivery, a term baby should be at limited neonatal risk.

Saling and Muller-Holve preferentially attempted a new technique: a back flip, in which the operator began the procedure by first applying pressure through the maternal abdominal wall on the fetus's forehead to initiate rotation, before adding pressure with the other hand to elevate and rotate the breech. They also added light penthrane or nitrous oxide anesthesia by mask during the procedure. They were successful in 43 of 57 (75%) patients after a total of 67 attempts. Their data also indicated success in six of nine attempts at 32–36 weeks. During the study period, the number of singleton breech fetuses weighing more than 2,500 g decreased to 1.6% of all deliveries. During the immediately preceding 16 months, the rate had been 3.8%. At the time of their report, 54 study patients had delivered, 40 with a vertex presentation. The reversion rate was 26%.

The authors emphasized the importance of pre- and postversion external fetal heart rate (FHR) monitoring and ultrasonographic confirmation of the presentation. Of the 57 patients studied, 9 had evidence of FHR abnormalities. Of these, there were five cases of fetal bradycardia, two cases of fetal tachycardia, and two cases of fetal deceleration. In the latter two instances, the FHR pattern led to the delivery of infants small for gestational age.

In 1977, Berg and Kunze (Table 36.1) reported their experience with the application of a regimen similar to that of Saling and Muller-Holve.[28] They succeeded in 7 of 10 attempted versions under tocolysis but had abnormal perinatal outcomes in 2 neonates. After a successful version, one fetus had an abnormal FHR pattern but remained in utero for another 5 weeks. Intrapartum, the fetus again had abnormal FHR but had Apgar scores of 9 and 10 and an umbilical artery pH of 7.31. The infant had spastic cerebral palsy. Another fetus had abnormal FHR patterns both before and after an unsuccessful version and died in utero 7 hours after the procedure.

In 1977, Fall and Nilsson (Table 36.1) asked for referral of all breech patients in the county of Uppsala, Sweden, in their 36th or 37th gestational week.[29] Essentially all deliveries in the county occurred in their hospital. After a group of patients was excluded from consideration for ECV because of contraindications, ECV was successful in 37 of 53 (70%) attempts by a single operator, using continuous terbutaline infusion at a rate of 2.5–5.0 μg/min. One patient experienced a spontaneous conversion after a failed version attempt. The subsequent cesarean rate among the vertex patients was 3%. Among the 15 failed version patients and the 26 other patients who either were not referred, had contraindications, or were not evaluated until labor, the cesarean rate was 56%. Unlike the Saling–Muller–Holve and Berg–Kunze groups, these investigators did not use anesthesia or sedation. But, as in these groups, version was attempted by a single operator. No serious maternal or fetal/neonatal complications of the ECV attempts were encountered.

These reports[17,28,29] established that ECV under tocolysis is a reasonable consideration in the breech presentation at term and, more importantly, can be safely done with minimal risk to the mother and fetus. However, these reports failed to address some critical questions about ECV. For instance, did ECV, in fact, reduce the incidence of breech presentation at term? Was there a reduction in the cesarean delivery rate? These questions could only be answered by prospective, randomized clinical studies of ECV.

RANDOMIZED CONTROL TRIALS OF ECV UNDER TOCOLYSIS

In 1979–1980, Van Dorsten et al enrolled 51 low-risk patients at 37–39 weeks gestation in a prospective, randomized study to assess the efficacy of ECV under tocolysis in decreasing the rate of breech presentation at delivery and in decreasing the rate of cesarean delivery for breech pre-

TABLE 36.2 Results of Four Randomized, Prospectively Controlled Studies That Assessed the Value of External Cephalic Version

	Van Dorsten et al[18]	Hofmeyr[19]	Brocks et al[20]	Kasule et al[21]
Number	48 (ECV—25; C—23)	60 (ECV—30; C—30)	65 (ECV—31; C—34)	640 (ECV—310; C—330)
Version successful	17 (68%)	29 (97%)	13 (41%)	250 (80%)
Spontaneous conversion rate (controls)	4 (17%)	10 (33%)	5 (15%)	156 (47%)
Cesarean rate				
ECV	7 (28%)	6 (20%)	7 (23%)	51 (17%)
C	17 (74%)	13 (43%)	12 (35%)	52 (16%)

ECV = external cephalic version group; C = control group.

sentation at the time of referral (Table 36.2).[18] After confirmation of the presentation, eligible patients were randomized either to a control or a study group. Careful ultrasonographic and external FHR monitor screening determined comparable low-risk groups. Patients received no anesthesia or sedation. Using a continuous infusion of terbutaline or ritodrine, and adding a second operator for the last several patients in the study, the success rate for version was 68%. All 17 fetuses remained vertex until labor, for an intrapartum vertex presentation rate of 68%. There were 4 spontaneous conversions among the 23 control patients, for an intrapartum vertex rate of only 17% ($P < 0.01$). None of the failed version patients had a spontaneous conversion. The cesarean rate was 28% in the study group and 74% ($P < 0.01$) in the control group. All the cesareans in the control group and all but one in the failed version group were related to the abnormal presentation intrapartum. The indication for the one cesarean in the successful version group and for the other cesarean in the failed version group was secondary arrest of dilatation. There were no clinically significant maternal or fetal/neonatal complications of the procedure. Although the rate of nuchal cords was higher in the successful version group than in either the failed version group or the control group, the differences were not statistically significant. This study clearly demonstrated the efficacy of ECV under tocolysis. Within the limitations of a small sample size, the procedure also appeared safe.

After completion of the initial randomized study, the control arm was terminated; ECV was offered to all eligible patients referred for consideration for version.[30,31] Of the 212 patients considered for ECV from 1979 to 1983, 148 were considered candidates. Of these, version was successful in 108 (73%). The spontaneous reversion rate to breech was 7%. No fetus spontaneously converted to vertex after a failed attempted version. Cesarean rates were 24% in the successful version group and 85% in the unsuccessful version group. Among the successful version patients, the most common indication for cesarean was failure to progress. Among the failed version patients, the most common indication for cesarean was breech related.

There were few complications during the study period. Six of 145 (4.1%) patients had evidence of fetal-maternal bleeding on Kleihauer-Betke (KB) testing. Two patients (1.4%) required transfer to the labor and delivery area for intensive fetal monitoring for prolonged bradycardia after successful version. Upon arrival, the FHR patterns were normal and the KB tests were negative. Subsequently, both patients delivered vaginally and had infants with Apgar scores greater than 7 at 1 and 5 minutes. In the series, one fetal death occurred 3 weeks after a successful version. At delivery, there was no evidence of abruption or a nuchal cord. Autopsy failed to reveal the cause of death.

Adequate FHR monitor strips were available for a retrospective study by Phelan and associates[32] of 137 of 148 (92%) attempted version patients. All patients had reactive nonstress tests (NST) prior to version, but 16 of the 137 (11.7%) had diminished variability. During the tocolytic infusion and the version attempt, 30.7% had some abnormality of the FHR, primarily deceleration or bradycardia (28.5%). Patients with non-anterior placentas were more likely to have FHR deceleration than were those with anterior placentas (38.5% versus 18.5%, $P < 0.01$). Neither success or failure of the version, number of attempts, duration of attempt, tocolytic agent used, duration of infusion, nor subsequent neonatal outcome correlated with intraversion FHR pattern changes. The incidence of positive postversion KB tests was higher in the group with normal patterns during the version, but not statistically so (5.3% versus 2.4%). After the version, 27 (19%) had abnormal patterns, primarily bradycardia and deceleration, and 50 (36%) had diminished variability. A positive KB test was more common among those with postversion FHR abnormalities (14.8% versus 1.8%, $P < 0.01$). There were no other significant differences between the groups with and without postversion FHR changes after comparison for the factors listed above.

Hofmeyr reported a prospective, randomized, controlled study of ECV among African women (Table 36.2) at 36 weeks gestation.[19] He described a new technique, with the patient lying on her side and the operator seated facing her abdomen. Of 30 patients who underwent version, 29 (97%) were successful. Of note, only seven (23%) patients required tocolysis. But the spontaneous conversion rate was 33% in the control group. Clearly, this population was different from that reported by Stine and associates.[31] Hofmeyr also demonstrated a higher rate of vertex presentation in labor in the study group than in the control group (97% versus 33%, $P < 0.001$). Because the spontaneous conversion rate was so high in the control group, the cesarean rates were not significantly different.

In Denmark, Brocks et al evaluated for ECV 153 patients (Table 36.2) with breech presentations at 37 weeks gestation.[20] They considered 130 low-risk patients candidates, but only 65 consented to randomization (31 study, 34 control). Although the spontaneous conversion rate in the control group was similar to that of Van Dorsten et al, [18] the success rate was only 41%. Moreover, the cesarean rate was not significantly different.

Kasule et al (Table 36.2) reported another prospective, randomized, controlled trial of ECV from Africa.[21] Without the use of analgesia, sedation, or tocolysis, 310 patients were randomized to attempted version after 33 weeks. Although there was an 80% success rate, only 132 (43%) fetuses remained vertex at delivery. The reversion rate among nulliparas was significantly lower than among multiparas (16% versus 43%, $P < 0.05$), but the vertex rate at delivery was the same for nulliparas in both groups (46% versus 45%). The spontaneous conversion rate after failed version was 23%. Cesarean delivery rates were 17% and 16% for the study and control groups, respectively. Perinatal mortality, however, was 10 times higher than among their U.S. counterparts. In their study, three perinatal deaths were attributed to the attempted version. Kasule and associates concluded that in their population attempted version prior to term without tocolysis had a greater risk than benefit.

In summary, the randomized, controlled trials of ECV under tocolysis demonstrated generally a reduction in the incidence of breech presentation at term and in the cesarean delivery rate. Moreover, as demonstrated by Van Dorsten et al,[18] Hofmeyr, [19] and Brocks et al,[20] the risks of ECV to the mother and fetus are minimized with the use of ultrasonographic screening, FHR monitoring, and tocolysis. In the absence of these safeguards, the risks to the fetus from ECV exceed the benefits.[21]

THE EXPANDING ROLE OF ECV

Since these initial reports, the role of ECV under tocolysis has grown considerably. For instance, Eglinton demonstrated that the procedure could be transported from the major university research-oriented medical center to a smaller residency teaching hospital.[33] To save the 10–20 minutes required for the preversion infusion of intravenous tocolytic, an intravenous bolus of 0.125–0.25 mg of terbutaline sulfate was administered over 1 minute, with occasional additional small boluses administered up to a maximum of 0.45 mg. In contrast to prior experiences, all versions were performed by residents with little or no prior version experience under the supervision of a single experienced operator. During 30 months' experience in 1982–1985, the success rate was 74%, including two successes with magnesium sulfate tocolysis (a severe preeclamptic and a class F diabetic), who both had normal spontaneous vaginal deliveries after induction postversion. The cesarean rate was 20% in the successful ECV group and 94% in the failed ECV group. There was one reversion after successful version, and one fetus sustained a prolapsed cord 4 days after attempted version and died before a cesarean could be accomplished.

TABLE 36.3 Intrapartum External Version for the Second Twin (N = 25) without Tocolysis

	Second Twin	
	Transverse Lie	Breech
Number	14	11
Version successful	12 (86%)	8 (73%)
Cesarean birth	4 (29%)	1 (9%)

Source: Adapted from Chervenak FA, Johnson RE, Berkowitz RL, et al: Intrapartum external version of the second twin. *Obstet Gynecol* 62:160, 1983.

During Labor

Using the same inclusion/exclusion criteria and techniques as for antepartum ECV, version has been attempted in the breech presentation in active labor.[33,34] Under these circumstances, version was attempted on the labor and delivery floor. Each patient received a bolus of terbutaline to relax the uterus. In this limited study population, the success rate was 5/9 (56%). More recently, Ferguson and Dyson reported a larger experience with intrapartum ECV.[35] They used a continuous ritodrine infusion and were successful in 11 of 15 (73%) attempts with intact membranes. They noted universal failure in an unstated number of attempts with ruptured membranes. Cesarean occurred after only 1 of 11 successes but after all 4 failures. With more patients, the overall success rate will probably decline. However, this approach illustrates quite clearly that version remains an alternative whenever a patient in early labor has a breech presentation and intact membranes.

The Second Twin

In recent years, multiple gestation has also increased in prominence as an indication for cesarean, especially if the presenting fetus is not vertex. But some also consider a nonvertex second twin an indication for cesarean.[36–38] Chervenak et al (Table 36.3) reported attempted intrapartum external version of the nonvertex second twin without tocolysis.[39] The successful version rates were 86% for the transverse lie and 73% for the breech second twin. The overall vaginal delivery rate was 80%. Although the authors thought the procedure useful, they admitted that their findings were based on selected retrospective data and offered several precautions for the application of a similar technique. In addition to standard safeguards for all versions, they suggested amniotomy and possible oxytocin administration after successful version, and cautioned against attempted version for vaginal delivery if the second twin is significantly larger than the first. If version is unsuccessful, or if the second twin evidences fetal distress during the attempt, breech extraction or cesarean may be nec-

TABLE 36.4 Results of Intrapartum External Cephalic Version for the Transverse Lie in Labor with Intact Membranes

	Transverse Lie
Number	12
Version successful	10 (83%)
Cesarean delivery	6 (50%)

essary. There is no clear impression of a lower limit of fetal weight for which this approach might be safe.

The Transverse Lie

Transverse lie is an unusual intrapartum presentation, occurring in only 69 of 16,674 (0.4%) patients delivered during 1 year at the LAC/USC Medical Center. Phelan et al (Table 36.4) considered 27 of these patients candidates for attempted ECV and offered ECV to 13, of whom 12 consented.[40] Using a continuous ritodrine infusion, they converted 9 of 12 to vertex presentations, and 6 of 9 delivered vaginally. All three cesareans were for labor arrests. They converted one to a breech presentation, but elected cesarean for suspected macrosomia and delivered a 4720-g neonate without incident. The two patients for whom they failed to convert the fetus to a longitudinal lie underwent cesarean delivery, without evidence of maternal or fetal/neonatal harm from the attempted version. Although six patients (50%) still had cesarean deliveries, the four who had been converted to longitudinal lies avoided vertical uterine incisions, and were thus candidates for trial of labor in their subsequent pregnancies.

Recent Reports

Two large series on antepartum ECV under tocolysis have recently been reported by Dyson et al[41] and Morrison and associates.[42] As demonstrated by these reports (Figure 36.1), the overall success rate for version was

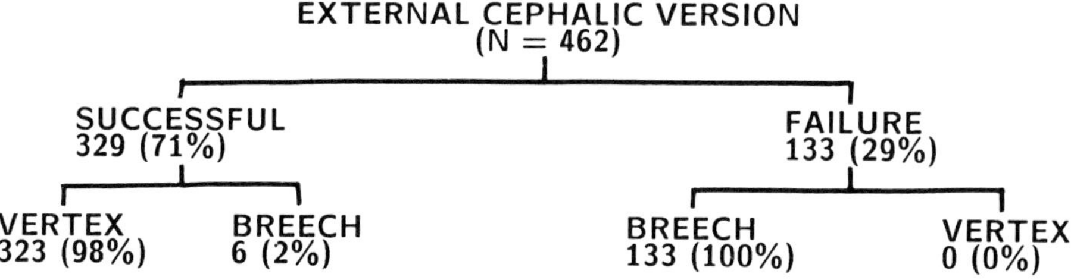

FIGURE 36.1 Outcome of attempted external cephalic version in 462 patients with a breech presentation.[41,42]

71%. Of the 329 patients converted to a cephalic lie, 98% remained vertex. In the 133 (29%) patients who failed attempted version, all of the fetuses remained breech.

During the version process, FHR abnormalities such as tachycardia, change in baseline, and variable deceleration or bradycardia occurred in 18% of the patients in the series of Morrison et al. None of the patients from either series required emergency delivery. Of note, no fetal or neonatal deaths were recorded.

Overall, cesarean delivery was indicated in 135 (29%) patients. The cesarean delivery rates for the successful and failed version groups were 13% and 70%, respectively. These results were significantly different.

In conclusion, these reports illustrate quite clearly that antepartum ECV can reduce the frequency of breech presentation at term. But, most of all, a program such as the one described by these investigators can reduce the cesarean delivery rate for the breech presentation by as much as 60%.

PERFORMANCE OF ECV

Indications

Indications for ECV include persistent breech presentation antepartum near term,[17–31] persistent breech presentation intrapartum,[33–35] second twin nonvertex during delivery of the first twin,[39] and persistent transverse lie at term[43] and intrapartum.[40] Westgren et al suggested that an appropriate time to consider version is 37–38 weeks in paras and 36–37 weeks in nulliparas because of the relative probabilities of spontaneous conversion in each population.[15] The probability of spontaneous conversion this late in gestation is especially remote for the frank breech.

Contraindications

Contraindications to ECV include maternal reluctance to undergo the procedure, contraindications to vaginal delivery, multiple gestation antepartum, placenta previa, ruptured membranes or oligohydramnios (amniotic fluid index <5.1 cm),[44] undiagnosed vaginal bleeding, significant fetal anomaly on ultrasound, FHR deceleration on NST, and fetal breech fixed in the maternal pelvis that requires vaginal manipulation to gain any mobility. Previous low transverse cesarean birth currently is a relative contraindication, but this may change as experience with this group grows.

Preversion Evaluation

An essential component of the version process is the preversion evaluation (Table 36.5) of the pregnant woman and her breech fetus. As demon-

TABLE 36.5 Evaluation and Management of the Patient Who Presents with a Breech or Transverse Lie for Attempted External Cephalic Version

History
Examination
Ultrasound evaluation
Nonstress test
Informed consent
Tocolytic agent
External cephalic version
Postversion nonstress test
RH immune globin

strated by Stine and associates,[31] approximately 22% of patients are not considered candidates for the procedure. First, the maternal history is taken, with a focus on the indications and contraindications for version. In addition, a maternal history of preexistent myocardial disease or diabetes mellitus would indicate the use of magnesium sulfate for tocolysis rather than a beta-mimetic. Second, an abdominal exam is warranted to assess the mobility of the breech and to determine whether or not the breech is engaged. An engaged breech is more difficult to turn and is associated with a lower success rate.

An ultrasound evaluation is then conducted to confirm the breech presentation, to rule out any significant fetal anomalies, placenta previa, or intrauterine growth retardation; to determine the fetal gestational age; and to assess the amniotic fluid volume. If the ultrasound evaluation is normal, an NST is done to assure fetal well-being. An NST with variable decelerations should alert the physician to the possibility of an abnormal cord position such as a nuchal cord.[45] Ultrasound may be helpful in identifying a fetus with one or more nuchal cords (Figure 36.2). If the evaluation discloses the patient to be a candidate for version, informed consent should be provided.

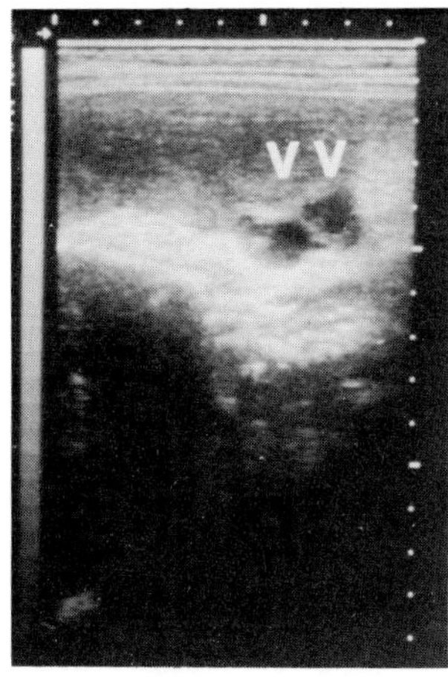

FIGURE 36.2 An ultrasound evaluation of the fetal neck in a breech fetus demonstrates a double nuchal cord at the arrows.

TABLE 36.6 Tocolytic Agents, Dosages, and Mode of Administration Found to Be Effective for External Cephalic Version

Terbutaline	5 μg/min IV by infusion pump, 0.125–0.25 mg IV slowly
Ritodrine	100 μg/min IV by infusion pump
Magnesium sulfate	4.0 g IV over 15–20 minutes, followed by 2.0 g/hr by infusion pump

ECV should be performed in a hospital setting with ready access to a delivery room for emergency cesarean delivery. The patient is not necessarily fasting but has eaten only lightly, is dressed in a hospital gown, has an intravenous line in place, and has signed consent forms for ECV. The patient assumes a semirecumbent posture with left lateral tilt for the preoperative NST, and has the head of the bed lowered to a level position only during the procedure.

Many tocolytic regimens have been successful (Table 36.6). The most common regimens have been continuous intravenous infusion for a period of 10–15 minutes before manipulation or longer, if necessary, to abolish spontaneous uterine activity. In the United States, infusions have consisted of 5–10 μg/min of terbutaline or 50–100 μg/min of ritodrine. Reinfusion after failed version or with continued elevation of uterine tone or contractile activity may require higher infusion rates. The manufacturers of terbutaline do not support the intravenous use of terbutaline, but a body of English-language literature does.[46–50] The use of an intravenous bolus of a beta-mimetic for acute uterine relaxation is not new,[46,49,51] and the metabolic,[52] acid-base,[53] and cardiovascular effects[33,54] have been studied. An isolated report of a possible severe complication of administration in this fashion exists, but it is not certain that the terbutaline was responsible for uterine tetany in this case.[55] At least two groups have found the terbutaline bolus technique satisfactory for ECV with tocolysis.[33,41] After a dose of 0.25 mg by slow IV push, the maternal pulse generally peaks at 100–110 beats per minute within 1 to 2 minutes, and the uterus is relaxed enough to begin manipulation at that time. Monitoring of maternal vital signs is required immediately before and frequently after administration of the bolus. When beta-mimetics are contraindicated, magnesium sulfate, as outlined in Table 36.6, can also be used with similar monitoring precautions.

The fetal monitors must be removed during the manipulation, but leaving the monitor turned on provides a convenient time flow sheet for recording vital signs, administration of tocolytics, etc. The ultrasound imager should remain at the bedside, to be used to monitor the FHR continuously or intermittently during the manipulation of the fetus. Generous application of ultrasound couplant to the maternal abdomen facilitates the "pushing" motion on the fetus necessary for successful ECV.

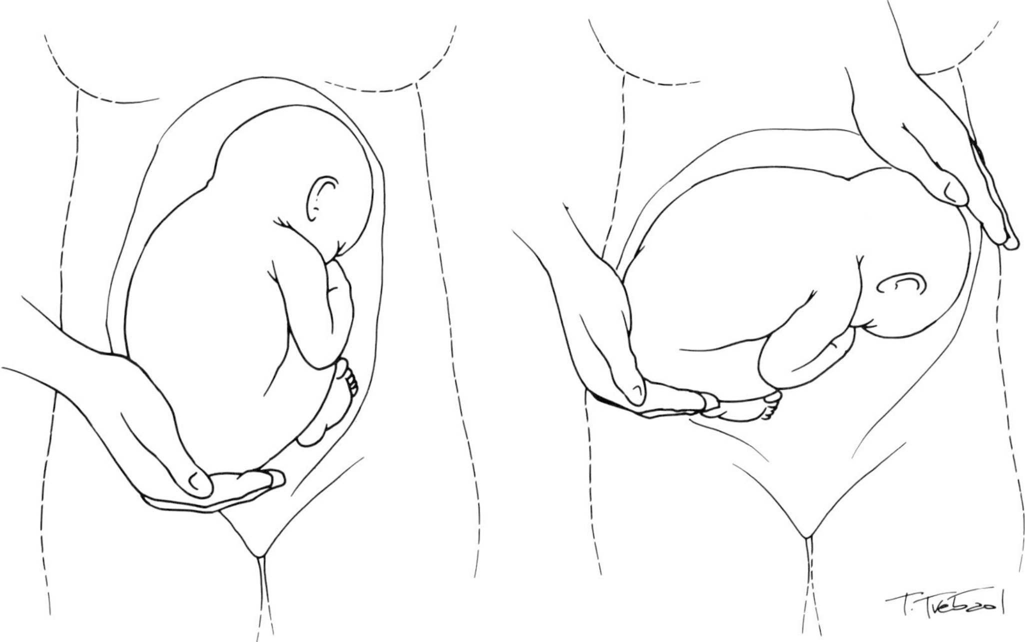

FIGURE 36.3 The buttocks of the breech are elevated with the right hand. The fetus is rotated clockwise, and the left hand guides the fetal vertex.

After the tocolytic has been administered, version is usually begun by first elevating the breech (Figure 36.3). Whether a "front flip" (Figures 36.3, 36.4) or "back flip" is used will depend upon whether the fetal spine crosses the maternal midline.

If the fetal spine crosses the maternal abdominal midline, a front flip is attempted first (Figure 36.3). However, a back flip is attempted first if the fetal head and spine are on the same side of the maternal abdominal midline. If we fail in one direction, we generally make the next attempt in the opposite direction. Attempting to maintain the fetal spine flexed may be important. If a back flip is attempted, the fetal breech should be elevated first, then moved laterally, before applying pressure to the fetal head to bring it down toward a transverse lie. If a front flip is attempted, the fetal head might be brought down laterally before manipulating the breech up and laterally to approach the transverse position. Regardless of the number of operators and which direction is tried first, gentle, slow, deliberate manipulation is mandatory. Often an alternating or simultaneous "rocking" motion on the fetal poles is helpful. Sometimes it is necessary to "hold" in or near the transverse position because of maternal discomfort or fetal bradycardia; the fetus may begin to move and may seem to complete the version without further assistance. If fetal bradycardia persists, it may be necessary to reverse the procedure and return the fetus to the original position. Some patients will be more comfortable

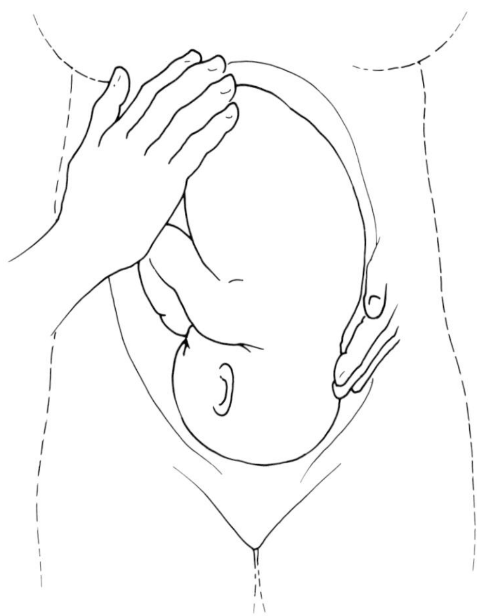

FIGURE 36.4 Once the fetus has been rotated, the vertex is guided into the maternal pelvis.

and better able to cooperate if they flex their thighs slightly. In more difficult cases, maternal position changes may improve maternal comfort and may provide some aid from gravity in completing the version.

Maternal participation as a team member is paramount. Her degree of discomfort and ability to cooperate control the manipulation. Although most successful versions are completed in only several minutes, there is no need for a sense of urgency. Several reinfusions and reattempts to complete a version successfully may be necessary. Key is the understanding that reattempt does not mean "push harder." Continued observation with ultrasound may dictate a different approach, such as moving the other fetal pole first, changing maternal position, placing a hand behind the maternal flank to aid in control of the fetal head, etc. Flexibility and gentle persistence are frequently rewarded with success.

A technique for twin delivery when the twins are relatively concordant with the presenting twin vertex has been to attempt version for the nonvertex second twin for a short time, during the period immediately after delivery of the first twin, when uterine activity noticeably diminishes. In the rare circumstance when version has failed, breech extraction has been successful. An equally acceptable alternative, if the breech can be settled into the pelvis, is to await the return of spontaneous labor, or to augment with oxytocin, and monitor closely for anticipated assisted breech delivery. The keys to success with this technique are the avoidance of haste or undue force, the full understanding and cooperation of the mother, and the willingness to remain flexible and change the plan as necessary. At the same time, it is wise to avoid excessive delay in attempting ECV because the cervix may return to a state of less than complete dilatation, eliminating breech extraction as an option.[56] Generally, version of the second twin should be completed within 5 minutes of the birth of the first. If this does not happen, the physician should abandon the effort and begin careful, atraumatic manipulation for total breech extraction or movement of the breech down deeply into the maternal pelvis. Chervenak et al recommended epidural analgesia as an aid[39] for successful version. Attendance of the anesthesia and pediatric services and prior preparation for cesarean for all planned twin deliveries ensure a smooth transition to cesarean should the mother or the fetus evidence intolerance of the pursuit for vaginal delivery.

Precautions

Careful maternal and fetal evaluation is required before and during manipulation. Avoid iatrogenic complications of tocolytics, excessive force, and preterm delivery. Obtain the patient's consent for ECV. Prepare the patient and staff for possible cesarean. Require normal antepartum FHR and ultrasound evaluation prior to and after an attempt, successful or unsuccessful, and weekly until delivery. Postversion, administer 300 μg of Rh immune globulin to Rh-negative, unsensitized women after the procedure, unless immediate delivery (48 hours) is planned.[57] If version fails, spontaneous conversion is extremely unlikely. Therefore, protect the fetus from the consequences of prolapsed cord at term and as suggested in Chapter 3.

Risk/Benefit Considerations

The observed risks of ECV under tocolysis have been minimal. If ECV doubles any important spontaneous risks, such as increasing the risk of abruptio placentae from 1% to 2%, it would take 400 randomized cases to demonstrate a statistically significant difference at $P < 0.05$ and nearly 800 cases at $P < 0.01$.[16] Although only a few hundred cases of ECV under tocolysis have been published, thousands of cases of version have been presented, combining the conventional and the tocolytic approaches. Considering the total experience, it seems unlikely that ECV doubles any important risks. Application of ECV with tocolysis as described above should permit at least a 10%–15% reduction in overall cesarean rates without increased morbidity or mortality.

The opinions expressed in this chapter are those of the author and not necessarily those of the United States Air Force or the Department of Defense.

REFERENCES

1. *Cesarean Childbirth*. Pub. No. 82-2067. Bethesda, Md, National Institutes of Health, 1981.

2. Bowes WA, Taylor ES, O'Brien M, et al: Breech delivery: Evaluation of the method of delivery on perinatal results and maternal morbidity. *Am J Obstet Gynecol* 135:965, 1979.
3. Brenner WE, Bruce RD, Hendricks CH: The characteristics and perils of breech presentation. *Am J Obstet Gynecol* 118:700, 1974.
4. Franu S: Fetal mortality and morbidity following breech delivery. *Acta Obstet Gynecol* 56(suppl):1, 1976.
5. Kauppila O: The perinatal mortality of breech deliveries and observations on affecting factors. *Acta Obstet Gynecol Scand* 39(suppl):1, 1975.
6. Rovinsky JJ, Miller JA, Kaplan S: Management of breech presentation at term. *Am J Obstet Gynecol* 115:497, 1973.
7. Alexopoulos KA: The importance of breech delivery in the pathogenesis of brain damage: End result of a long-term followup. *Clin Pediatr* 12:248, 1973.
8. Fianu S, Jackson I: Minimal brain dysfunction in children born in breech presentation. *Acta Obstet Gynecol Scand* 58:295, 1979.
9. Ingemarsson I, Westgren M, Svenningsen WW: Long-term followup of preterm infants in breech presentation delivered by cesarean section: A prospective study. *Lancet* 2:172, 1978.
10. Todd WD, Steer CM: Term breech: Review of 1006 term breech deliveries. *Am J Obstet Gynecol* 22:583, 1963.
11. Gimovsky ML, Petrie RH, Todd WD: Neonatal performance of the selected term vaginal breech delivery. *Obstet Gynecol* 56:687, 1980.
12. Collea JV, Rabin SC, Weghorst GR, et al: The randomized management of term frank breech presentation: Vaginal delivery vs. cesarean section. *Am J Obstet Gynecol* 131:186, 1978.
13. Gimovsky ML, Wallace RL, Schifrin BS, et al: Randomized management of the nonfrank breech presentation at term: A preliminary report. *Am J Obstet Gynecol* 146:34, 1983.
14. Taylor ES: Randomized management of the nonfrank breech presentation at term: A preliminary report. *Obstet Gynecol Surv* 38:608, 1983.
15. Westgren M, Edvall H, Nordstrom L, et al: Spontaneous cephalic version of breech presentation in the last trimester. *Br J Obstet Gynaecol* 92:19, 1985.
16. Jordan B: External cephalic version as an alternative to breech delivery and cesarean section. *Soc Sci Med* 18:637, 1984.
17. Saling E, Muller-Holve W: External cephalic version under tocolysis. *J Perinat Med* 3:115, 1975.
18. Van Dorsten JP, Schifrin BS, Wallace RL: Randomized control trial of external cephalic version with tocolysis in late pregnancy. *Am J Obstet Gynecol* 141:417, 1981.
19. Hofmeyr GJ: Effect of external cephalic version in late pregnancy on breech presentation and cesarean section rate: A controlled trial. *Br J Obstet Gynaecol* 90:392, 1983.
20. Brocks V, Philipsen T, Secher NJ: A randomized trial of external cephalic version with tocolysis in late pregnancy. *Br J Obstet Gynaecol* 91:653, 1984.
21. Kasule J, Chimbira THK Brown IMcL: Controlled trial of external cephalic version. *Br J Obstet Gynaecol* 92:14, 1985.
22. Bonnar J, Howie PW, MacLennan H: External cephalic version with anesthesia. *JAMA* 205:87, 1968.
23. Bradley-Watson PJ: The decreasing value of external cephalic version in modern obstetric practice. *Am J Obstet Gynecol* 123:237, 1975.
24. Brosset A: The value of prophylactic external version in cases of breech presentation. *Acta Obstet Gynecol Scand* 35:555, 1956.
25. Ellis R: External cephalic version under anaesthesia. *J Obstet Gynaecol Br Commonw* 75:865, 1968.

26. Friedlander D: External cephalic version in the management of breech presentation. *Am J Obstet Gynecol* 95:906, 1966.
27. Ranney B: The gentle art of external cephalic version. *Am J Obstet Gynecol* 116:239, 1973.
28. Berg D, Kunze U: Critical remarks on external cephalic version under tycolysis. Report on a case of antepartum fetal death. *J Perinat Med* 5:32, 1977.
29. Fall O, Nilsson BA: External cephalic version in breech presentation under tocolysis. *Obstet Gynecol* 53:712, 1979.
30. Wallace RL, Van Dorsten JP, Eglinton GS, et al: External cephalic version with tocolysis. Observations and continuing experience at the Los Angeles County/University of Southern California Medical Center. *J Reprod Med* 29:745, 1984.
31. Stine LE, Phelan JP, Wallace RL, et al: Update on external cephalic version performed at term. *Obstet Gynecol* 65:642, 1985.
32. Phelan JP, Stine LE, Mueller E, et al: Observations of fetal heart rate characteristics related to external cephalic version and tocolysis. *Am J Obstet Gynecol* 149:658, 1984.
33. Eglinton GS: External cephalic version at term update on the travis experience. Abstract 98. Presented at the 31st annual meeting of the Armed Forces District (AFD) of the American College of Obstetricians and Gynecologists (ACOG), San Diego, California, 1986.
34. Roukema JE, Eglinton GS: Bolus terbutaline tocolysis for external cephalic version in advanced labor. Abstract 138. Presented at the 29th annual meeting of the Armed Forces District (AFD) of the American College of Obstetricians and Gynecologists (ACOG), Atlanta, Georgia, 1984.
35. Ferguson JE II, Dyson DC: Intrapartum external cephalic version. *Am J Obstet Gynecol* 152:297, 1985.
36. Cetrulo CL, Ingardia CJ, Sbarra AJ: Management of multiple gestation. *Clin Obstet Gynecol* 23:533, 1980.
37. Keith L, Newton WP: Twin gestation, in Dilts PV, Gergie AB, Sciarra JJ (eds): *Gynecology and Obstetrics,* ed 2, vol 2. New York, Harper & Row, 1985, pp 8–9.
38. Taylor ES: Editorial. *Obstet Gynecol Surv* 31:535, 1976.
39. Chervenak FA, Johnson RE, Berkowitz RL, et al: Intrapartum external version of the second twin. *Obstet Gynecol* 62:160, 1983.
40. Phelan JP, Stine LE, Edwards NB, et al: The role of external version in the intrapartum management of the transverse lie presentation. *Am J Obstet Gynecol* 151:724, 1985.
41. Dyson DC, Ferguson JE II, Hensleigh P: Antepartum external cephalic version under tocolysis. *Obstet Gynecol* 67:63, 1986.
42. Morrison JC, Myatt RE, Martin JN, et al: External cephalic version of the breech presentation under tocolysis. *Am J Obstet Gynecol* 154:900, 1986.
43. Phelan JP, Boucher M, Mueller E, et al: The nonlaboring transverse lie: A management dilemma. *J Reprod Med* 31:184, 1985.
44. Phelan JP, Smith CV, Broussard P, et al: Amniotic fluid volume assessment using the four quadrant technique in the pregnancy between 36 and 42 weeks gestation. *J Reprod Med* 32:540, 1987.
45. Phelan JP, Lewis P: Fetal heart rate decelerations during a nonstress test. *Obstet Gynecol* 57:228, 1981.
46. Andersson KE, Bengtsson LP, Gustafson I, et al: The relaxing effect of terbutaline on the human uterus during term labor. *Am J Obstet Gynecol* 121:602, 1975.
47. Ingemarsson I: Effect of terbutaline on premature labor. *Am J Obstet Gynecol* 125:520, 1976.
48. Wallace RL, Caldwell DL, Ansbacher R, et al: Inhibition of premature labor by terbutaline. *Obstet Gynecol* 51:387, 1978.

49. Arias F: Intrauterine resuscitation with terbutaline: A method for the management of acute intrapartum fetal distress. *Am J Obstet Gynecol* 131:39, 1978.
50. Ingemarsson I, Bengtsson B: A five-year experience with terbutaline for preterm labor: Low rate of severe side effects. *Obstet Gynecol* 66:176, 1985.
51. Lipschitz J: Use of a beta(2)-sympathomimetic drug as a temporizing measure in the treatment of acute fetal distress. *Am J Obstet Gynecol* 129:31, 1977.
52. Ingemarsson I, Westgren M, Lindberg C, et al: Single injection of terbutaline in term labor: Placental transfer and effects on maternal and fetal carbohydrate metabolism. *Am J Obstet Gynecol* 139:697, 1981.
53. Ingemarsson I, Arulkumaran S, Ratnam SS: Single injection of terbutaline in term labor. I. Effect on fetal pH in cases with prolonged bradycardia. *Am J Obstet Gynecol* 153:859, 1985.
54. Ingemarsson I, Arulkumaran S, Ratnam SS: Single injection of terbutaline in term labor. II. Effect on uterine activity. *Am J Obstet Gynecol* 153:865, 1985.
55. Bhat N, Seifer D, Hensleigh P: Paradoxical response to intravenous terbutaline. *Am J Obstet Gynecol* 153:310, 1985.
56. Pritchard JA, MacDonald PC, Gant NF: *Williams Obstetrics,* ed 17. New York, Appleton-Century-Crofts, 1985, pp 520–522.
57. *Management of Isoimmunization in Pregnancy*. Technical Bull. 90. Washington, DC, American College of Obstetricians and Gynecologists, 1986.

Additional Cesarean Considerations

Chapter 37

Cesarean Delivery in Developing Countries

Thomas E. Elkins, MD, MAR,
Charles Drescher, MD,
J. O. Martey, MD, and
Richard Anane, MD

In 1981, the World Health Organization (WHO) highlighted a program entitled "Health Care for All By the Year 2000." A goal of this program was to improve maternal and child health care in the developing countries of the world. Statistics produced by that organization in 1980 underline the importance of this goal for the significant improvement in overall world health.[1] They found three-fourths of the world's population of 4.4 billion living in developing countries. Of the 122 million children born worldwide each year, more than 80% are born in these same areas. Additionally, more than 90% of the low-birth-weight infants delivered each year are born in developing countries. Their perinatal mortality is approximately 20-fold that of their counterparts born in the Western world. Maternal mortality in developing countries commonly ranges from 500 to 1,000 maternal deaths per 100,000 live births, whereas rates of 10–20 per 100,000 live births occur in developed countries. Such a high mortality rate indicates the importance of better understanding of the birthing processes that occur in these areas. The focus of this chapter will be on the role of cesarean delivery in developing countries. Although a general discussion of this topic is limited because of unique problems found in specific areas, several valid generalizations can still be made.

The delivery of obstetric care and the performance of a cesarean in developing countries are complicated by problems no longer seen in most developed areas. Poor communication and transportation systems make the absence of antenatal care the rule rather than the exception. Mail systems, telephone, and radio are usually unavailable or inefficient. A scarcity of maintained roads makes travel of any distance in most tropical areas during the rainy season nearly impossible. Compound these problems with a severe personnel shortage and the result is less than 30% of deliveries being performed by trained staff.[2] Consequently, significantly fewer cesareans are being performed than the estimated need.[3] Equally important are the limited supplies of medicines, surgical equipment, and transfusable blood. In some rural areas, operations are still delayed or not performed because of lack of water or electricity.[4] The patients who present to these poorly supplied areas, in addition to bearing the normal stresses of pregnancy, are often malnourished, anemic, and suffer from chronic parasitic infections. Finally, physicians who elect to work in these areas are usually singlehandedly responsible for obstetric, pediatric, and anesthetic care.

INDICATIONS FOR CESAREAN

The reported incidence of cesarean delivery in developing countries ranges from 3% to 29%,[5–7] with most larger series indicating an incidence of around 10% of deliveries. As pointed out in the series from the Korle Bu teaching hospital in Accra, Ghana, cesarean birth rates from centers will most likely be inflated because of the large referral services that these institutions support. When those authors recalculated their rates for the true population base served, the cesarean rate decreased from 10.9% to 7%. A large series from Khartoum, Sudan, reported a cesarean rate of 12.0%. Cesarean delivery rates reported from developing areas may be somewhat unreliable because of the limited time and facilities for record keeping. Lawson and Steward[8] emphasized the importance of developing an accurate record system so that trends may be observed. Although large longitudinal series that would allow reliable estimates in changes of cesarean rates over time are lacking, there is currently no evidence to indicate an increase in the overall cesarean rate in developing countries similar to that observed in many industrialized areas. For instance, the cesarean delivery rate at Komfo Anokye Teaching Hospital, Kumasi, Ghana, in 1985 was 7.7%, which is not significantly different from the 7.0% reported from nearby Accra, Ghana, in 1971.

In all reported series, the most common indication for cesarean delivery was cephalopelvic disproportion (CPD), which accounted for 20.8%–53% of all cesarean births. A major reason for this is the very high incidence of android pelvis configurations found in Africa and other Third World regions, as well as rickets and other bony anomalies of the pelvis and spine. Although CPD is frequently the most common indication for cesarean delivery in developed countries, the presentation in developing countries is much different. Ross[9] described a series of 341 patients who presented in Nigeria with obstructed labor. Most patients had been in labor for at least 24 hours and, not uncommonly, for 2–5 days. Mothers were dehydrated, ketotic, exhausted, and frequently infected. They presented with all the clinical findings of ignored labor, including obvious contraction rings and gross vulvar edema. Usually the fetal head was out of the pelvis, but occasionally the presenting part was at the mid-pelvis

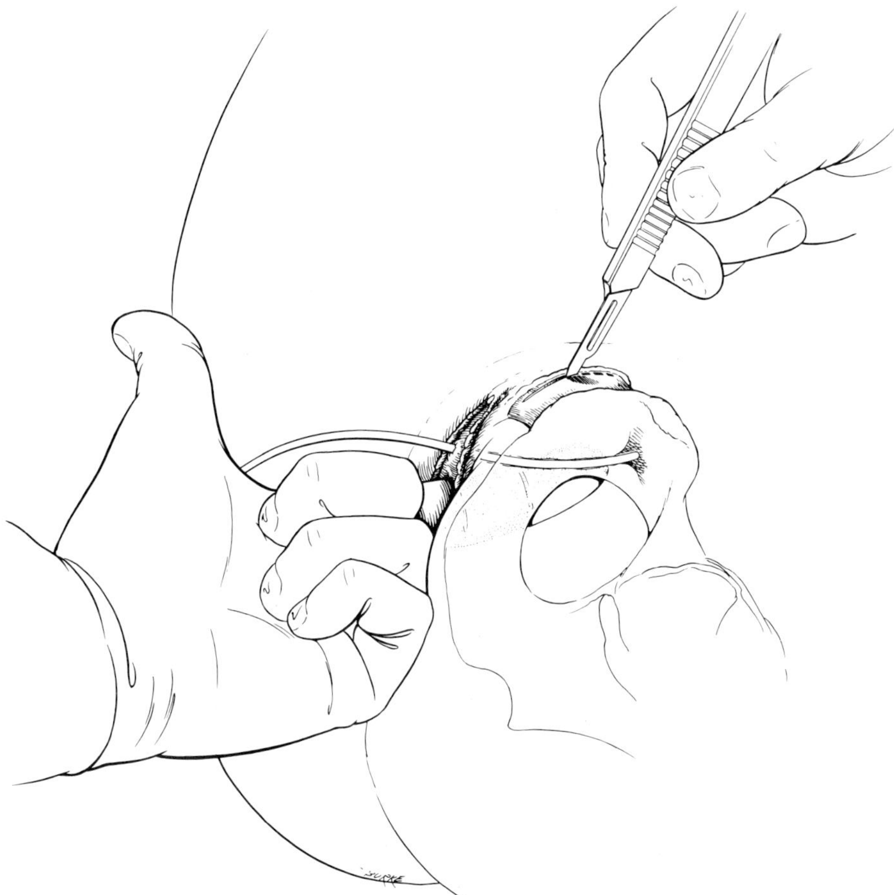

FIGURE 37.1 The technique of symphysiotomy. The midline cartilage is carefully incised while the urethra is pushed laterally.

or even the perineum because of molding. Of these patients, 11.1% presented with a ruptured uterus. Not infrequently, the fetus was dead or moribund, with the fetal heart rate being auscultated at admission in only 35.5%. Only 71.8% of those infants presenting with audible fetal heart tones survived. The maternal mortality in this population was 11.6%. Other complications included fever (69.4%), vesicovaginal fistula (7.7%), rectovaginal fistula (0.6%), and peripheral nerve palsies (1.0%).

Cesarean delivery for CPD in this setting is much different and often technically more difficult than when performed for similar indications in Western countries. Because of the potential high morbidity and mortality associated with cesarean delivery under these circumstances, many authors[10–12] have suggested symphysiotomy (Figure 37.1) or destructive procedures, as alternatives, particularly when the fetus is already dead. Of 210 patients who presented with CPD, 105 underwent a cesarean delivery, and 105 were treated with symphysiotomy, with and without forceps or vacuum extraction.[10] Indications for symphysiotomy were moderate to severe CPD and the absence of deformities of the back, leg, or pelvis. There were three maternal deaths, two in the cesarean group and one in the symphysiotomy group. The causes of death in the two groups were sepsis and eclampsia, respectively. Perinatal deaths totaled 17 in the symphysiotomy group and 7 in the cesarean group. The authors felt that this difference was primarily related to poor patient selection in the symphysiotomy group during the earlier part of the study. Both groups suffered from approximately equal numbers of immediate complications; however, the types of complications were different. Patients undergoing symphysiotomy more frequently suffered from walking difficulties, stress urinary incontinence, local hematoma, and vesicovaginal fistula. The incidence of vesicovaginal fistula may again have been affected by patient selection. Cesarean patients more frequently required blood transfusion, had pneumonia, or suffered wound breakdown. Follow-up at 6 weeks showed similar results for the two groups, with 65% and 70% of the patients being free of symptoms.

The technique for performing a symphysiotomy is shown in Figure 37.1. Local anesthesia is infiltrated through the mons pubis into the pubic bone periosteum and midline cartilage. Local or pudendal anesthesia should also be used to anesthetize the perineum. A Foley catheter is inserted to drain the bladder and to allow lateral displacement of the urethra with digital pressure. Using sterile technique, a 2-cm incision is made in the mons pubis. This incision is carried downward with a pushing motion of the fingers until the midline cartilage of the pubic bone is entered. The knife blade should separate the pubic bone by pushing through the cartilage. Great care should be taken to avoid entering other structures. Pushing the blade too deeply may result in vaginal infection, hemorrhage of the periurethral vessels, or urethral fistula formation.

Following incision of the pubic symphysis, a widening of the pelvic bony structure is readily noticed. A vacuum extractor is then applied to the fetal vertex to assist in vaginal delivery.

Postpartum management of patients following symphysiotomy includes prophylactic antibiotics and heparinization, pelvic support with a tight girdle or binder, urethral catheterization, and immobilization for 7–10 days. Most patients begin ambulating without difficulty after this initial period of rest.*

The outcome of future pregnancies was essentially the same, except for a higher incidence of cesareans in the group of women treated primarily by cesarean. In 5 of 68 subsequent pregnancies, repeat symphysiotomy

---

* The authors are indebted to Dr. Fran Greenway, Nalerigu, Ghana, for sharing this technique and protocol.

was performed. There was one ruptured uterus in each group. Greisen[13] followed eight patients for 2–5 years after symphysiotomy and found no long-term complications. Currently, there is general agreement regarding the indications and contraindications for symphysiotomy. Current indications include moderate CPD and the fetal head at least $^{3}/_{5}$ into the pelvis. Contraindications include (1) greater than moderate CPD; (2) true conjugate less than 8.0 cm; (3) fetal weight greater than 4,000 g; (4) cervix dilated less than 6 cm; (5) breech, brow, mentum posterior, or transverse presentation; (6) extreme obesity; (7) existing hip or pelvic disorder; and (8) prior cesarean.

When one is confronted with CPD and a dead fetus, destructive procedures such as cleidotomy, craniotomy, and decapitation should be considered in the Third World, where cesarean delivery for fetal demise carries a high risk of maternal mortality.

Craniotomy can be performed with Smellie scissors or a Simpson perforator, and decapitation may be accomplished with either a blunt hook or sickle knife. Cleidotomy involves the surgical division of the clavicle to facilitate delivery of the shoulders through the birth canal. It can be accomplished with any instrument capable of cutting bone but may be most easily performed with the Dubois scissors. Evisceration with and without spondylotomy may be used for management of an undeliverable transverse presentation. Any instrument that can cut through the fetal abdominal and thoracic cavities may be used.

When performing a fetal destructive procedure, care must be used to avoid injury to maternal tissues. Cluat[14] reported the following complications among 62 patients undergoing craniotomy: maternal death—2 patients, ruptured uterus—2 patients, and significant lacerations—10 patients. Contraindications to fetal destructive procedures include (1) a living fetus, (2) a markedly contracted pelvis, (3) cervical dilatation less than 7 cm, and (4) obstructing pelvic tumors.[15]

Previous cesarean birth is the second most common indication for cesarean delivery in many of the series reported. At Khartoum, 11.1% of 341 cesarean deliveries were performed solely because of prior cesarean.[6] The two series from Ghana reported repeat cesarean delivery rates of 24.5% and 8.2%.[5,7] The percentage of repeat cesareans performed electively prior to the onset of labor varies widely. The Khartoum series had an exceptionally high rate, with 37 of 38 repeat sections being performed electively. The series from Ghana reported elective cesarean rates of 1.2% and 1.7%. When one considers the great difficulties with communication, transportation, lack of antenatal care, and subsequent inadequate gestational dating, it is likely that most repeat cesareans are performed after the onset of labor. This has been our experience. Although the authors of the Khartoum series did not address the incidence of prematurity with such a high elective repeat rate, they did indicate that there were 2 neonatal deaths within the first week of life among the 38 infants managed this way.[6] Additionally, because of the great concern regarding subsequent pregnancies after cesarean delivery and the inability to achieve timely repeat cesarean delivery, classical uterine incisions are rarely performed in developing countries. These incisions usually account for less than 1% of cesarean scars. When a classical cesarean is performed, simultaneous sterilization is usually done.

In the United States, many patients with a prior cesarean are permitted a trial of labor (Chapter 31). Although many recent reports in developed countries document the advantages of this approach in carefully monitored situations, there is little information regarding this practice from these parts of the world. There are theoretical concerns regarding the adequacy of healing of the uterine incision, including the high incidence of postoperative infection, anemia, and malnutrition associated with cesareans performed on patients from these areas. However, Klufio et al, in Accra, Ghana,[16] noted a favorable outcome for attempted vaginal birth after cesarean. In their report, 572 patients with one or more previous cesarean deliveries presented to their institution in active labor, and 294 (52%) delivered vaginally. Of the 294 vaginal deliveries, 225 were spontaneous vertex, 10 were breech, and 59 required either vacuum or forceps. The likelihood of successful vaginal delivery was inversely related to the number of prior cesarean deliveries. The successful vaginal delivery rate by the number of prior cesareans was one (60.6%), two (21.7%), and three (9.5%). The most common indications for a repeat cesarean birth were previous cesarean (42.6%), CPD (34.1%), and fetal distress (7.8%). There were 16 cases (2.8%) of ruptured uterus, and all fetuses were delivered abdominally. There was one maternal mortality in a patient with a ruptured uterus.

Other less common indications for cesarean in large studies include fetal distress, malpresentation, antepartum hemorrhage, hypertensive disorders of pregnancy, cord prolapse, and failed induction. The percentage of cesareans performed for these indications varies but ranges from 1% to 10%. Perhaps fetal distress is the least well-defined of the above-mentioned indications because of variations in fetal monitoring techniques. Electronic fetal monitoring is rarely, if ever, performed. Fetal well-being is assessed by auscultation with the fetoscope or the unaided ear if a fetoscope is unavailable. The interval and duration of monitoring are not standardized and are often dependent upon the discretion of the labor attendant. With these monitoring techniques, many cases of fetal distress go undetected. Cesarean delivery for antepartum hemorrhage due to placenta previa or abruptio placenta is often associated with high morbidity because of the limited blood banking facilities. However, if a cesarean is clinically indicated, the procedure is performed despite these conditions.

COMPLICATIONS ASSOCIATED WITH CESAREAN DELIVERY

Cesarean delivery in developing countries carries a much greater risk of complications than similar operations performed in the Western world.

Hemorrhage, infection, uterine rupture, and anesthetic complications occur frequently. The potential for serious complications, including maternal death, must be carefully considered before a cesarean is undertaken.

Chattopadhyay et al[17] reviewed maternal mortality associated with cesarean delivery in Riyadh, Saudi Arabia, and found an incidence of 0.3 maternal deaths per 100 cesarean births. This was six times higher than the overall maternal mortality rate in the same area. Causes of death included hemorrhage, infection, pulmonary embolus, and anesthesia. The maternal death rate associated with cesarean delivery in Kumasi, Ghana, in 1985 was 1.3%, which is consistent with data reported from other studies in West Africa.[7]

Infectious complications are a serious problem in these countries. Inadequate hygiene, poor sterilization techniques, limited antibiotics, anemia, malnutrition, neglected labor with prolonged rupture of the membranes, and intravaginal application of native medicines all contribute to this problem. Maternal mortality following cesarean delivery, though infrequent in the United States (0.15 deaths in 10,000 live births), is one of the leading causes of death in these countries. Gogoi[18] reported on infectious complications following cesarean delivery in 103 high-risk patients in Assam, India. The overall maternal mortality rate was 12.6%, but it was 50% in those who underwent a classical cesarean. Other complications included postoperative shock (17%), peritonitis (66%), fever (98%), and wound infection (25%). In that series, ominous clinical findings included vomiting, abdominal distention, and diarrhea.

Antibiotics are employed whenever available. Specific regimens vary from region to region, but intravenous penicillin or ampicillin and streptomycin is a commonly used combination. Tetracycline compounds are also frequently employed. Metronidazole is used when coverage of anaerobic infections is deemed important. Extraperitoneal cesarean seems to be used infrequently.

Uterine rupture remains a major problem in developing areas, and many series have demonstrated a strong association between prior cesarean and uterine rupture.[19–21] Lawson and Ajabor[19] reported on 57 cases of uterine rupture following cesarean from the University of Ibadan, Nigeria. They called attention to the tendency for classical incisions, but not lower segment incisions, to rupture prior to the onset of labor. Pain was the most consistent clinical finding noted in rupture prior to onset of labor, whereas vaginal bleeding occurred more frequently with rupture during labor. Other findings included a change in the shape of the lower pole of the uterus, suprapubic tenderness, fetal distress, hematuria, and progressive abdominal distention. With prompt diagnosis and intervention, the maternal mortality was relatively low (5%), but perinatal mortality was 31%. Elkins et al[21] reviewed 45 cases of uterine rupture and found maternal death to be associated with sepsis, birth of a macerated infant, vulvar edema, prolonged labor, abnormal presentation, and performance of a hysterectomy. Repair of the defect with tubal ligation if the defect is in the upper segment is the treatment of choice in developing countries. Hysterectomy is reserved for those cases in which the uterus has been extensively damaged. Simultaneous rupture of the urinary bladder was observed in both series and probably accounts for the complications of urinary incontinence and vesicovaginal fistula noted after uterine rupture.

Anemia is a frequent finding among people living in developing countries. Common etiologies include generalized malnutrition, vitamin deficiencies, parasitic infections, hereditary hemoglobinopathies, and anemia secondary to chronic illness. Compound these factors with the physiologic anemia associated with pregnancy and it is easy to understand why many pregnant patients in these countries suffer from profound anemia. A generalized lack of adequate blood banking facilities makes cesarean delivery a high-risk procedure. Disasters are often averted by arranging blood donations from family members, hospital workers, or previously identified members of the local town or village. Unfortunately, suitable donors cannot always be found, and this system is particularly inefficient when emergency procedures are performed.

The above problems can be avoided by using the technique of autotransfusion of blood lost at the time of surgery. This can be easily accomplished using a simple system consisting of a blood-collecting device, an in-line filter system, and a container for anticoagulation, usually with citrate phosphate dextrose. The usefulness of this technique has been repeatedly demonstrated in the battlefield hospitals worldwide and in hospitals in developed countries prior to the advent of safe blood banking techniques.[22] The recent trend toward performance of surgical procedures that require large quantities of blood, the reduction in the supply of blood products, and the increasing risks associated with transfusion of donor products have created renewed interest in this technique in the Western world. Although not used uniformly in developing countries, this technique certainly can be of great value in those areas. The authors have personally seen an autotransfusion system in use at the Komfo Anokye Teaching Hospital in Kumasi, Ghana. Although there are no data currently available, the staff physicians at the hospital felt that this technique resulted in a significant decrease in maternal mortality and morbidity.

In this rural setting, the surgeon is frequently the only medical professional present at the time of cesarean. As a result, the surgeon must be prepared to administer anesthesia for the delivery. Most surgeons operating under these conditions have little or no formal training in anesthesia and anesthetic techniques; as a result, anesthetic options are limited.

General inhalation anesthesia is used infrequently for cesarean in developing countries because it is labor intensive, requires continuous cardiopulmonary monitoring, and is associated with significant neonatal depression. Additionally, delivery systems are expensive and difficult to maintain, and inhalation agents are often unavailable. Regional techniques such as lumbar block or local infiltration are used more commonly. Intravenous administration of anesthetic agents such as ketamine or pethidine and Pentothal is also used. Ketamine may be particularly advantageous because of its high therapeutic index and lack of maternal circulatory or fetal neurologic depression. It may, however, be associated with maternal hallucinations or suboptimal analgesia.[23]

CONCLUSIONS

Many cesarean deliveries are being performed in areas of the world where there is inadequate medical care. A lack of skilled personnel, patient education, sanitation, transportation, communication, and medical supplies all contribute to the problem. That patients receive necessary operations at all is a credit to the physicians who elect to work under these conditions. Unfortunately, operative procedures, such as cesarean delivery performed in these settings, are often associated with high complication rates.

With improvement in overall health care delivery systems, cesarean birth statistics for the Third World will probably show a similar improvement. Future studies will be necessary to assess ongoing needs and evaluate further progress.

REFERENCES

1. Petros-Barvazian A: World priorities and targets in maternal and child health for the year 2000. *Int J Gynaecol Obstet* 22:439, 1984.
2. Ogunbode O: Problems of obstetric care in Nigeria. *Int J Gynaecol Obstet* 22:475, 1984.
3. Nordbert EM: Incidence and estimated need for cesarean section, inguinal hernia repair, and operation for strangulated hernia in rural Africa. *Br Med J* 289:92, 1984.
4. Aggarwal VP: Obstetric emergency referrals to Kenyatta National Hospital. *East Afr Med J* 57:144, 1980.
5. Klufio CA, Ardayfio SAW, Nartey IN, et al: A retrospective survey of cesarean sections at Korle Bu Teaching Hospital, Accra: 1971—a review of 1077 cases. *Ghana Med J* 14:142, 1973.
6. Verzin JA: The role of caesarean section in communities with large families. *East Afr Med J* 41:276, 1964.
7. Anane R, Martey JO: Komfo Anokye Teaching Hospital—Department of Obstetrics and Gynecology Statistics—1985. Unpublished data.
8. Lawson JB, Steward D (eds): *Obstetrics and Gynecology in the Tropics and Developing Countries.* London, Edward Arnold, 1977.
9. Ross SM: Obstructed labour. *Niger Med J* 5:344, 1966.
10. Hartfield VJ: A comparison of the early and late effects of subcutaneous symphysiotomy and of lower segment cesarean section. *J Obstet Gynaecol Br Commonw* 80:508, 1973.
11. Bird GC, Bal JS: Subcutaneous symphysiotomy in association with the vacuum extractor. *J Obstet Gynaecol Br Commonw* 74:266, 1967.
12. Gebbie D: Symphysiotomy. *Clin Obstet Gynaecol* 9:663, 1982.
13. Greisen G: Three-year follow-up of eight patients delivered by symphysiotomy. *J Gynaecol Obstet* 23:203, 1985.

14. Cluat B: Destructive operations on the dead fetus. *Am J Obstet Gynecol* 87:258, 1963.
15. Quilligan EJ, Zuspan FP: *Operative Obstetrics,* ed 4. Appleton-Century-Crofts, 1982, pp 673–696.
16. Klufio CA, Arkutu ARA, Bentsi-Enchill KK: The outcome of pregnancy and labour following previous cesarean section at the Korle Bu Teaching Hospital. *Ghana Med J* 14:250, 1973.
17. Chattopadhyay SK, Sengupta BS, Chattopadhyay C, et al: Maternal mortality in Riyadh, Saudi Arabia. *Br J Obstet Gynaecol* 90:809, 1983.
18. Gogoi MP: Maternal mortality from cesarean section in infected cases. *J Obstet Gynaecol Br Commonw* 78:373, 1971.
19. Lawson JB, Ajabor LN: Ruptured cesarean section scar. *J Obstet Gynaecol Br Commonw* 75:1296, 1968.
20. Megafu U: Factors influencing maternal survival in ruptured uterus. *Int J Gynaecol Obstet* 23:475, 1985.
21. Elkins T, Onwuka E, Stovall T, et al: Uterine rupture in Nigeria. *J Reprod Med* 30:195, 1985.
22. Jacobs LM, Hsieh JW: A clinical review of autotransfusion and its role in trauma. *JAMA* 251:3283, 1984.
23. Mankowitz E, Downing JW, Brock-Utne JG, et al: Total intravenous anaesthesia using low-dose ketamine infusion for caesarean section. *S Afr Med J* 65:246, 1984.

Chapter 38

Ethical Considerations in Cesarean Birth

Thomas E. Elkins, MD, MAR

Despite the existence of codes of behavior that have long served as general guidelines for physicians, biomedical ethics is a relatively new area of concern in obstetric and gynecologic literature. This chapter presents some of the general concerns about cesarean births that are becoming prominent in an era of rapidly increasing obstetric technology[1] and to present some of the specific ethical concerns about cesarean birth when its use represents the whole topic of maternal–fetal conflict.[2] This discussion will demonstrate both the similarity of ethical concerns that cesarean delivery shares with any surgical procedure and the uniqueness of ethical concerns about cesarean birth because of the impact such a procedure may have when more than one patient (ie, mother and fetus) is affected. Cesarean birth shares the ethical concerns about truth telling and a covenant relationship between doctor and patient that allows informed consent in any surgical procedure. However, when the recommendation for cesarean delivery runs counter to maternal desires, ethical concerns unique to obstetrics are also involved.

GENERAL ETHICAL ISSUES IN CONTEMPORARY CESAREAN BIRTHS

Few procedures in our society are ever performed with as much emotion and uncertainty as cesarean deliveries. The birth of a child is one of life's most natural and rewarding processes, and the decision to interrupt this process with surgery naturally stirs ethical and legal concerns. To have a clearer understanding of the ethical concerns, the fundamental principles of biomedical ethics are emphasized and are related to cesarean births and the doctor–patient relationship.

Truth Telling: Physician Responsibility and Fallibility

Popular novelists, opposed to contemporary obstetric practice, have painted a picture of the paternalistic obstetrician who strides into a laboring patient's room, glances at a wavering fetal heart rate on a monitor strip, and announces that a cesarean birth must be done for the safety of both mother and fetus. The dips and squiggles of the tracing are shown to the parents, who listen with awe and appreciation. One author has even presented the following negative description of contemporary obstetric practice:

> Picture this not very rare scenario: The patient is admitted at 7:00 A.M. The doctor stimulates her labor while at the same time scheduling her for a cesarean delivery at 5:30 P.M. If the patient is lucky and has all the various factors (size of pelvis, size of baby, efficiency of labor) aligned just perfectly, she will deliver before the schedule time for the operation. If, however, she is among the group who commonly take much longer than that to complete their labor, she most likely will be subjected to a cesarean delivery that evening—for the doctor's convenience! Except for previously scheduled cesarean sections . . . by far the greatest number are done immediately after office hours.[1]

The physician's honesty, competence, and integrity were once never questioned. For instance, parents did not question the truthfulness of the counseling given to them, yet were overjoyed by the unnecessary cesarean delivery of a normal, healthy child. In reality, such a time has passed, and honesty in counseling has now become a central issue in cesarean births. This has occurred for at least two reasons: (1) a rapidly changing technology and (2) the public's recent emphasis on physician accountability. Many in society appear convinced that the decision to perform a cesarean is always a straightforward "right or wrong" decision. Nothing could be further from the truth. Often the urgency of decision making in obstetrical emergencies leaves little time for lengthy patient–physician interaction. In this chapter, the assumption is that there is sufficient time for an informed, consenting decision.

A review of "The Principle of Honesty" by Robert Veatch supports truthfulness as "a fundamental moral claim on human interaction."[2] Immanuel Kant saw dishonesty as a formal wrongdoing and concluded that "to be truthful in all declarations is therefore a sacred unconditional command of reason, and not to be limited by any expediency."[3] Such thinking had been challenged in the past by utilitarians like Henry Sidgwick who claimed that "where deception is designed to benefit the person deceived, common sense seems to concede that it may sometimes be right."[4] As Veatch notes, contemporary medicine has shifted away from the utilitarian view of Sidgwick to the more formalist thinking of Kant in terms of truth telling. In fact, the most recent AMA code of ethics included for the first time the exhortation to physicians "to deal honestly with patients and colleagues."[5]

Two major problems now face the obstetrician who recommends cesarean delivery. First, rapidly advancing technology often makes the "truth" concerning the necessity of cesarean delivery a highly debatable subject. For instance, should all women with a breech presentation or a prior cesarean undergo a cesarean? Studies revealing the true maternal risks of vaginal delivery after cesarean birth(s) have made the dictum "once a cesarean, always a cesarean" obsolete. The responsibility of the practicing physician to keep well informed about current information in a rapidly changing field like obstetrics is especially vital because of the contemporary demand for honesty in counseling and patient involvement in decision making. However, in a rapidly evolving technological environment, providing truthful information is made increasingly difficult even for the physician who remains current. Even the most honest counseling may therefore appear retrospectively to be inadequate and inaccurate.

Second, the current malpractice climate has brought an increased awareness of the fallibility of physicians. In claims involving medical malpractice, the truthfulness of medical facts may be viewed completely differently by competing experts. Thus, physicians are fallible in their ability both to recognize the truth and to present its consequences honestly to patients.

In such times, truthfulness in counseling includes a recognition that technology (and the physician's understanding of it) is constantly evolving, and the potential for technological or human fallibility is equally constant. The principle of honesty in patient counseling has become the contemporary obstetrician's responsibility and a burden of conscience that underscores every recommendation for a cesarean delivery.

Motivational Ethics: Contemporary Influence and Physician Promise Keeping

In teaching biomedical ethics to residents, it becomes obvious that concern for the moral rightness of any medical procedure is motivational for the majority of physicians. May notes that the task of ethics in a professional setting is "corrective vision."[6] Both May and Veatch emphasize the ethical image of the physician–patient relationship as a form of covenant response. Intertwined in that response are the concepts of gifts (provided by physicians *and* by patients), of promise keeping, and of mutual responsibility. The health and well-being of the patient become the overriding concern for a physician viewing his or her responsibilities as part of a covenant response. However, the rising rate of cesarean births in our country has fostered many societal concerns about the covenant response of physicians and their vulnerability to many nonmedically related influences in contemporary decision making.

The rising rate of cesarean births in the United States has caused great concern about the underlying motives for such a rise. In 1970, the cesarean rate was about 5.5% of all deliveries, but by 1978 it had risen to 15.2%.[7] Today it is not uncommon for hospitals to report a 30% incidence of cesarean delivery. Danforth has noted the following "new" indications for cesarean section as being responsible for the rising rate: (1) an awareness of the hazards of vaginal breech and midforceps delivery, (2) the implication that cesarean birth is much less traumatic for the tiny fetus and in some cases of multiple pregnancy, and (3) the early recognition of present or anticipated fetal distress by fetal monitoring. He also states that cephalopelvic disproportion and failure to progress in labor are also increasingly common indications for cesarean births.[8] In the United States, the increase in cesarean rates has been accompanied by a dramatic fall in perinatal mortality rates.[8] But, as Danforth notes, similar decreases in the perinatal mortality rate have been noted in other countries despite a stable cesarean rate of 4%–5%.[9] Indeed, even after a national consensus development conference on cesarean childbirth in 1980, cesarean rates continued to rise in the United States rather than declining, while perinatal mortality rates have stabilized.[10]

Furthermore, the high cesarean rates do not necessarily reflect the distribution of high-risk populations, in whom a higher rate would be expected.[11] In fact, some studies have noted a direct correlation between the availability of private third-party insurance payments and the cesarean delivery rate. For instance, nonpaying patients have lower rates of cesarean birth.[12] Some authors contend that it is more cost effective to perform a cesarean than for a physician to be in attendance throughout a lengthy, oxytocin-augmented labor and vaginal delivery. This "convenience factor" has also been mentioned as a potential factor in the rising rate but is difficult to document.[13] Finally, fear of litigation has compelled physicians to practice defensive medicine. In many respects, this is perhaps one of the most important factors responsible for the current increase in cesarean births in the United States. Publicity surrounding the aforementioned concerns often leads American consumers to question the motivation of physicians who recommend cesarean deliveries even when the procedure is medically indicated.

Thus, contemporary obstetricians may feel compelled to perform more cesarean deliveries in response to consumer demands for the "perfect baby," while at the same time feeling pressured to avoid contributing to the cesarean rate. Neither extreme opinion provides an acceptable basis for medical decision making. Seitchik has recently commented on the fallibility of allowing societal opinion to be the basis for the formulation of ethical reasoning in medical decision making.[14] Such relativism has long been a concern of developers of moral theory.[15] Without a renewed emphasis on the merits of objective medical decision making, physicians will once again be faced with increasing criticism for the rising use of cesarean delivery in this country. This suggests that it is time for the decision to perform a cesarean delivery to undergo review, not only for the medical indications but for the ethical ones as well. Ultimately, this will ensure a higher quality of care to our patients.

THE COURT-ORDERED CESAREAN BIRTH: PHYSICIAN RESPONSIBILITY IN MATERNAL–FETAL CONFLICTS

Consideration of a specific case may be helpful in illustrating ethical concerns about cesarean births.

> A 19-year-old unmarried, indigent female G1P0 was admitted at 34 weeks gestation in early labor with ruptured membranes and severe preeclampsia. The cervix was 2 cm dilated, 75% effaced, and the presenting vertex at −2 station. Heavy meconium fluid was noted, and the fundal height measured 28 cm. Ultrasound evaluation demonstrated oligohydramnios and intrauterine growth retardation. The fetal heart rate tracings revealed diminished beat-to-beat variability, a baseline tachycardia, and severe atypical variable fetal heart rate decelerations. The fetal heart rate pattern persisted despite maternal oxygen administration, position change, and intravenous hydration. Her clotting profile was within an acceptable range for surgery, and her liver enzymes were elevated. A cesarean for severe preeclampsia and fetal distress was recommended; however, the mother refused the surgery. When told that her refusal could result in death or severe brain damage to her infant, she remained unconcerned and stated that she never wanted this pregnancy.

It is important for practicing obstetricians to understand the ethical concerns of those who would support the mother's decision in the above instance and of those who would seek legal means to intervene by cesarean delivery on behalf of the fetus. Both opinions, depending on the focus of values, could be seen as representing one of medicine's first ethical principles, "Primum non nocere," or "First, do no harm."

Those who would support the mother in refusing cesarean delivery usually site the principle of autonomy as the ethical basis for such a decision. Autonomy is a form of liberty of action whereby the individual determines his or her own course of action in accordance with a personally chosen plan.[16] It is a cherished right of persons within a constitutional democracy and has become a prominent part of biomedical ethics theory since the 1960s. The concept of informed consent is the most obvious manifestation of autonomy in medical practice today. When the guidelines for informed consent are met and the patient is a competent adult, our society has supported an individual's right to make personal decisions in most situations. This right is supported by two traditional principles of our legal system.[17] One is the right of privacy. This has included the protection of parental autonomy, which allows parents to make decisions on behalf of their children [*Meyer v Nebraska,* 262 US 390 (1923)]. The second is the right of bodily integrity, which means that persons have the qualified right to be free of unwarranted and unreasonable bodily intrusions [*Terry v Ohio,* 392 US 1, 8–9 (1968)]. However, these legal rights are not absolute, and the state has the power to overrule parental decisions when those decisions place a child's health or life in jeopardy [*Prince v Massachusetts,* 321 US 158 (1944)]. Reasonable bodily intrusions have included compulsory vaccinations [*Jacobson v Massachusetts,* 197 US 11, 31 (1905)] and evidence gathering [*Rivas v United States,* 368 F2d 703 (6th Cir 1966)]. Although these legal rights are based upon individual autonomy and yet are limited, the principle of autonomy itself is now being challenged as an absolute in medical literature.[18] Regardless of one's view of autonomy, a physician's decision to intervene against the wishes of a competent adult, either medically or surgically, sets a dangerous precedent that may have grave consequences. Moreover, a charge of assault and battery is a real possibility for physicians [*Mohr v Williams,* 95 Minn 261 (1905)], especially if court-ordered approval for intervention is not obtained prior to the intervention. The ethical implications of denying persons their basic liberty and self-determination allow visions of a "slippery slope" that could become terrifying for pregnant women. As Angela Holder has noted, such denials of individual autonomy in an effort to control maternal behavior (and thus protect or benefit the fetus) could result in legal regulation of drug usage, smoking, working, and other behaviors for the woman who elects to become pregnant.[19] To some, such extreme possibilities make medical intervention on behalf of the fetus, but against the mother's will, unreasonable under any circumstances.

On the other hand, others would defend the physician's obligation to intervene on behalf of the fetus in the above case. A similar situation that led to a court-ordered intervention has been discussed in the obstetric literature.[20] Such actions are generally based upon the beneficent concern of the obstetrician for fetal as well as maternal well-being.[21] The principle of beneficence means "wishing the good for another." It is one of the most time-honored principles of medicine and is marked by a compassionate approach to patient care. Among the ancient philosophers, the term "philanthrophy" was used to describe Galen's "love for mankind . . . and concern for its future." Scribonius claimed that a physician has two essential characteristics: competence and compassion/humaneness. Early Christian writers explained beneficence in terms of the word *agape:* the God-like love that is unlimited, freely given, sacrificial, and not dependent on the character of its object.[22] It remains today a central motivating theme in health care, and is emphasized by the physician's desire to protect the well-being of the third-trimester fetus, even in the face of maternal refusal to permit medically necessary care for the fetus. However, two factors have recently enhanced the concern of the obstetrician and of society for fetal well-being: (1) the consideration of the fetus as a patient and (2) the increased concern over fetal value resulting from the abortion controversy.

Medical therapy, given to the mother but aimed at enhancing fetal well-being, has been accepted for many years. Interventions as simple as dietary restrictions and additional insulin injections for diabetic mothers are examples of such approaches. Some medical interventions involve significant but usually acceptable medical risks for mothers who choose to support fetal well-being. An example would be ritodrine (or other tocolytic) therapy for premature labor. In April 1981, surgical correction of in utero fetal anomalies was first attempted, though the operation posed risks for the mother.[23] Although the value of such surgical attempts in some situations remains controversial, the availability of these techniques and the willingness of physicians to treat conditions that threaten fetal well-being greatly enhance the image of the fetus as a patient.[24] Such advances in technology make beneficent concerns about fetal well-being seem reasonable.

The current abortion controversy has also led to an expanded literature concerned with fetal value and the ethical/legal status of the fetus. As an example, the American College of Obstetricians and Gynecologists has issued a statement of policy entitled "Further Ethical Considerations in Induced Abortion" (1977) that includes the following:

> Since the status of the fetus involves widely divergent theological and philosophical opinions in a pluralistic society, unanimity should not be expected. However, there appears to be a greater agreement on this matter than some positional statements suggest.
>
> This agreement is to be found in a general consensus in at least two main areas: 1) without going at length into the basis of the difference, the fetus has a qualitatively different nature and value from that of other human tissue or organs, and 2) this value derives, at least in part, from its potential for developing into an obvious member of the human family.
>
> The value of the fetus is thus related to that placed on all human beings. It is therefore not possible fully to dissociate fetal life from human life so as to disvalue the one without posing some measure of threat, however subtle, to the value of the other. There are circumstances where individual judgement may suggest that an abortion expresses and even deepens the concern for humanness, as in instances where the fetal presence threatens to diminish the human quality of the maternal life. But in no case should its destruction be treated as a casual matter without regard for the ethical issues involved; for it is human value that is jeopardized by attitudes which devalue the fetus. Our society will probably never be able to agree on the precise worth to be assigned to a fetus, but its value certainly should be afforded whatever level of concern is required to maintain our sensitivity to that larger human value with which it is, at least symbolically, associated.[25]

Another recent article reviewing the instances in which third trimester abortion could be justified ethically included the following comment:

> [For anomalies other than anencephaly] . . . the obligation to care for the fetus carries more weight than the mother's desire for third trimester termination.[26]

In the case of *Roe v Wade* [410 US 113, 93 Ct 705, 35 L Ed2d 147 (1973)] the court's decision reflected society's concern for the potentially viable fetus and afforded it some protection.

Engelhardt has recently reviewed the gradually increasing tendency of the court system to recognize fetal rights.[27] Wrongful-life suits have upheld the right of the fetus to sue as a damaged person when its right to be born with a sound mind and body has been abridged. The fetus thus possesses rights as "a place-holder for a future person."[27] In 1981, a Georgia court ruled that "[when we] weighed the right of the mother to practice her religion and to refuse surgery on herself, against her unborn child's right to live, we found in favor of her child's right to live."[28] Lieberman et al reviewed the varying inheritance laws that also emphasize the rights of the viable fetus.[29] His claim, that refusal by the mother to undergo surgery for the benefit of the fetus would constitute a felony, was contradicted by an accompanying discussion.[30] All of these legal discussions have revealed society's concern for the safety and well-being of the potentially viable fetus, and therefore enhance the obstetrician's dilemma when a mother refuses a medically necessary cesarean delivery. The need to assess the ethical basis for solving such dilemmas is more urgent now than ever before.

Some authors have offered partial solutions to the question of forced cesarean deliveries against the mother's will. Myron Gordon, reflecting concerns for the personal autonomy of the mother, included only gross cephalopelvic disproportion or placenta previa as valid indications for forced cesarean delivery; under these circumstances, the risk of maternal death is substantial.[31] Others have considered the possibility of delivering a severely damaged infant to be an indication for forced cesarean delivery, while denying that prevention of fetal demise would be a similar indication. This would imply that severe fetal distress, if death in utero could be reliably predicted, would not be an indication for cesarean birth, and that a breech presentation with a hyperextended vertex (associated with a high percentage of neonatal spinal cord injuries when delivered vaginally) would constitute a reasonable indication for cesarean. Both of these theories place diminished value on fetal survival when compared to the wishes of the mother and the small risk of morbidity or mortality to her. Other authors have concluded that when the risk of fetal death or damage is significant, this justifies seeking court approval against the wishes of the mother, in an effort to provide beneficent health care that shows reasonable respect for human life.[20,21] As Engelhardt states, policies will need to be developed to determine what level of risk can justify certain levels of interference.[27] However, the risks of cesarean birth, although still significant for the mother, now appear to be small enough to honor a woman's decision to choose cesarean birth electively.[32,33] This serves as an impetus to physicians to encourage this form of delivery when it is medically necessary for the mother and/or the fetus.

MEDICAL DECISION MAKING IN AN ERA OF CONTROVERSY REGARDING THE USE OF CESAREAN DELIVERY

An awareness of ethical issues is an important component in the medical decision making that accompanies cesarean births. The principle of distributive justice in providing care for the indigent; the principle of "Primum non nocere" in performing cesareans for the very-low-birth-weight fetus; and the principle of informed consent when it appears to be medically indicated to perform a cesarean section for a mentally handicapped minor with no guardian are all examples of ethical concerns that must be understood in order to formulate appropriate medical decisions. However, an understanding of these principles will not provide the physician with a clear-cut decision on every question concerning cesarean births. But such vast concerns expressed throughout history by all of society should make any physician pause before making a hasty decision. It is that agonizing pause that ethics ensures. During that time, the physician must consider whether all the issues have been addressed and whether adequate consultation has occurred (including peer review, contacts with social services, legal counsel, ethics committees, and/or the court system) in order to avoid poor medical decisions. The physician must also question if enough sensitive, patient, and educational counseling has been provided to the mother. The practicality of an understanding of ethics, as it relates to cesarean birth, "lies not in aiding one to follow a road map to a right answer, but in providing an adequate framework for reflection that will insure thoughtful, reasonable medical decisions, even in the face of controversial issues."[34]

REFERENCES

1. Keyser HH: in Barrett S (ed): *Women Under the Knife.* New York, Warner Books, 1984, pp 74–75.
2. Veatch RM: The principle of honesty, in *A Theory of Medical Ethics.* New York, Basic Books, 1981, pp 214–226.
3. Kant I: On the supposed right to tell lies from benevolent motives, Trans by TK Abbott, in Kant I: *Critique of Practical Reason and Other Works on the Theory of Ethics.* London, Longmans, 1909, p 363.
4. Sidgwick H: *The Methods of Ethics.* New York, Down Publications, 1966, p 316.
5. American Medical Association: Text of the American Medical Association's new principles of medical ethics. *Am Med News* August 1–8:9, 1980.
6. May WF: *The Physician's Covenant: Images of the Healer in Medical Ethics.* Philadelphia, Westminster Press, 1983, p 13.

7. Placek PJ, Taffel SM: The frequency of complications in cesarean and noncesarean deliveries, 1970 and 1978. *Public Health Rep* 98:396, 1983.
8. Danforth DM: Cesarean section. *JAMA* 253:811, 1985.
9. O'Driscoll K, Foley M: Correlation of decrease in perinatal mortality and increase in cesarean section rates. *Obstet Gynecol* 61:1, 1983.
10. Gleicher N: Cesarean section rates in the United States. *JAMA* 252:3273, 1984.
11. Williams RL, Chen PM: Controlling the rise in cesarean section rates by the dissemination of information from vital records. *Am J Public Health* 73:863, 1983.
12. Placek PJ, Taffel S, Moren M: Cesarean section delivery rates: United States, 1981. *Am J Public Health* 73:861, 1983.
13. Evans MI, Richardson DA, Sholl JS, et al: Cesarean section: Assessment of the convenience factor. *J Reprod Med* 29:670, 1984.
14. Seitchik J: Words, thoughts, and things. *Am J Obstet Gynecol* 154:699, 1986.
15. Niehbur R: *Moral Man and Immoral Society.* New York, Charles Scribner's Sons, 1932.
16. Beauchamp TL, Childress JF: *Principles of Biomedical Ethics.* New York, Oxford University Press, 1979, p 56.
17. Hallisey PL: The fetal patient and the unwilling mother: A standard for judicial intervention. *Pacific Law J* 14:1065, 1984.
18. Clements CD, Sider RC: Medical ethics' assault upon medical values. *JAMA* 250:2011, 1983.
19. Holden AR: Maternal–fetal conflicts and the law. *Female Patient* 10:80, 1985.
20. Bowes WA, Selgestad B: Fetal versus maternal rights: Medical and legal perspectives. *Obstet Gynecol* 58:209, 1981.
21. Chervanek FA, McCullough LB: Perinatal ethics: A practical method of analysis of obligations to mother and fetus. *Obstet Gynecol* 66:440, 1985.
22. Amundsen DW, Ferngren GB: Philanthropy in medicine: Some historical perspectives, in Shelp EE (ed): *Beneficence in Health Care.* Philosophy and Medicine Series, vol II. Boston: D Reidel Publishing Co, 1982, pp 1–32.
23. Ruddick W, Wilcox W: Operating on the fetus. *Hastings Center Rep* 12:10, 1982.
24. Lenow JL: The fetus as a patient: Emerging rights as a person? *Am J Law Med* 9:1, 1983.
25. American College of Obstetricians and Gynecologists. Further ethical considerations in induced abortion. ACOG Policy Statement. Washington, DC, ACOG, 1977.
26. Chervanek FA: Anencephaly said to justify late abortion. *OB-Gyn News* 20:6, 1985.
27. Engelhardt HT: Current controversies in obstetrics: Wrongful life and forced fetal surgical procedures. *Am J Obstet Gynecol* 151:313, 1985.
28. *Jefferson v. Griffin Spalding County Hospital Authority,* 274 SE 2d 457 (Ga 1981).
29. Lieberman JR, Mazor M, Chaim W, et al: The fetal right to live. *Obstet Gynecol* 53:515, 1979.
30. Shriner TL: Maternal versus fetal rights—a clinical dilemma. *Obstet Gynecol* 53:518, 1979.
31. Gordon M: Maternal v. fetal rights. *At Issue* 1:5, 1986.
32. Johnson SR, Elkins TE, Strong C, et al: Obstetric decision-making: Responses to patients who request cesarean delivery. *Obstet Gynecol* 67:847, 1986.
33. Dugowson CE: Elective cesarean more likely in MD. *Ob-Gyn News* 20:3, 1985.
34. Elkins TE: in Ryan G (ed): *Biomedical Ethics in Maternal and Child Health.*

Chapter 39

Medical–Legal Considerations of Cesarean Delivery

Jeffrey P. Phelan, MD

Since the NIH consensus conference on cesarean birth in 1980,[1] the cesarean delivery rate has continued to rise. In fact, by 1983, cesarean delivery had become the number one hospital-based operative procedure in the United States.[2] Explanations for this rise have focused primarily on the indications for cesarean. As demonstrated by Shiono and associates, the primary reasons for the rise in cesarean births have been attributed to the performance of elective repeat cesareans and cesareans for fetal distress and dystocia.[3]

But could the rise in cesarean births be due to other factors that do not lend themselves to statistical analysis? For instance, the rise in cesarean births has paralleled the rise in malpractice claims. The average number of claims per 100 physicians has risen threefold in the last 5 years.[4] In fact, it is estimated that more than 70% of the fellows of the American College of Obstetricians and Gynecologists (ACOG) have been sued at least once.[5] Of greater concern to the practicing obstetrician is the fact that the rise in malpractice claims has been accompanied by a 2300% increase in the number of awards in excess of $1 million.[4] By 1984, the midpoint birth injury jury award was close to $1.5 million.[4]

In obstetrics, the problem is complicated by parental expectations of a "perfect child" and the belief that cesarean delivery can provide that child. But, as demonstrated throughout this book, cesarean delivery does not lend itself to simple categorization. In actuality, cesarean birth is a complex issue that cuts across all aspects of our society. Notwithstanding, and unlike other medical specialists, the obstetrical health care provider must simultaneously balance the interests of two and sometimes more individuals. When it comes to cesarean delivery, the balancing continues. Should a cesarean delivery be performed and thus expose the mother to a greater risk of morbidity and mortality? Or should vaginal delivery be

TABLE 39.1 The Four Elements of Negligence

Duty
Breach
Causation
Injury

allowed because it reduces these maternal risks, yet exposes the fetus to a greater one?[6] It may be that the circumstances of the case make cesarean delivery the only apparent option. Under different circumstances, vaginal rather than cesarean delivery would have been the best choice.

It is these complexities that have frequently contributed to the rise in malpractice claims and lawsuits. For completeness, this chapter is devoted to the medical-legal issues associated with cesarean birth and will review the basic concepts of negligence, the duty to refer, and the doctrine of informed consent.[7] Additionally, the concept of timely cesarcan delivery,[8] foreign objects left in the abdomen,[9] instruments that break during a cesarean,[10] failure to perform a proper cesarean and subsequent liability for prenatal injuries,[11] and the "captain of the ship" doctrine[12] will be discussed.

A detailed analysis of each of these issues is not within the scope of this chapter. First, the laws vary from state to state. Second, the individual circumstances of each case vary. Third, a purpose of this chapter is to provide the reader with an overview of the medical–legal issues that could arise from the performance of a cesarean. If a more detailed analysis with applicable state law is desired, the reader is referred to an attorney in the reader's state or jurisdiction. Finally, this chapter is intended to be used for educational purposes and is not designed to provide legal advice.

NEGLIGENCE

Negligence is "conduct which falls below the standard established by law for the protection of others against an unreasonable risk of harm."[13] It is important to note that the focus in negligence is on conduct and not on the health care provider's state of mind. In general, it is no different from getting a ticket for running a red light or for causing a motor vehicle accident when running a stop sign. In other words, the focus is on the act that caused someone's injuries. With respect to cesarean delivery, negligence could be construed from a physician's performance of an unindicated cesarean[7] or for the failure to perform one in a timely manner.[8]

To establish that a person is negligent in a medical malpractice action, the four elements in Table 39.1 need to be satisfied by a preponderance of the evidence. The first element, the duty of a physician and surgeon, is contained in the following jury instruction. Jury instructions are "given by the judge to the jury prior to their deliberation that informs the jury of the law applicable to the facts of the case before them."[14]

The California jury instruction given below is in the *Book of Approved Jury Instructions (BAJI). BAJI* 6.00[15] expresses the duty or obligation of a practicing physician or surgeon in California.

> In performing professional services for a patient, a physician or surgeon has the duty to have that degree of learning and skill ordinarily possessed by reputable physicians and surgeons practicing in the same or a similar locality and under similar circumstances.
>
> It is his further duty to use the care and skill ordinarily exercised in like cases by reputable members of his profession practicing in the same or a similar locality under similar circumstances, and to use reasonable diligence and his best judgment in the exercise of his skill and the application of his learning, in an effort to accomplish the purpose for which he is employed.
>
> A failure to perform any such duty is negligence.

Analysis of the instruction suggests that three elements make up a physician's duty or obligation to a patient. First, the physician has an obligation "to have that degree of learning and skill ordinarily possessed by physicians practicing in the same or similar locality under similar circumstances."[15] For instance, board certified obstetricians undergo the same or similar training and certification process. In addition, evidence in support of the maintenance of that learning and skill could be continuing medical education credits and the journals or textbooks a physician may read.

A physician also appears to have a second obligation: to use that care and skill ordinarily exercised by other physicians practicing in the same or similar locality under similar circumstances. Here physicians have frequently established their own standards. For example, standard of care guidelines can be found in current ACOG standards and guidelines[16] or in the policy and procedure manuals of each physician's hospital. In most states, local rules may no longer apply. As a result, a national standard is frequently applied in medical malpractice actions.

A third obligation of the physician is "to use reasonable diligence and his best judgment in the exercise of his skill and the application of his learning, in an effort to accomplish the purpose for which he is employed."[15] In essence, the physician is required to use that knowledge and skill to protect the pregnant woman and her child against an unreasonable risk of harm. The failure to perform any of these duties would be considered negligence. But the failure to perform these duties also needs to be linked or causally related to the injuries the patient sustained (Table 39.1).

REFERRAL TO A SPECIALIST

The technological advances and the information explosion of the last 20 years have made it harder for the practicing physician to keep pace with the changes in medicine. Subspecialization has been a necessary outgrowth of these advances. This has been especially true in obstetrics and gynecology. For example, consider what has happened during the past 15 years in obstetrics alone. Fetal monitoring and ultrasonography have been introduced and are currently used on a regular basis. In many respects, the three subspecialty areas—gynecologic oncology, reproductive endocrinology, and maternal–fetal medicine—were created as a result of the technological and information explosion of the 1970s and 1980s. Although most communities desire these clinical subspecialists, these physicians have largely limited their practices to university hospitals. However, it is estimated that, in the future, a greater number of subspecialists will be practicing in nonuniversity hospitals.

Nevertheless, a nonspecialist appears to have a duty to refer a patient to a specialist or to request the assistance of a specialist whenever circumstances warrant it. For example, with the increased availability of maternal–fetal medicine subspecialists, an increasing number of high-risk patients could be referred to these physicians, not necessarily for primary prenatal care but for consultation. If a physician fails to refer such a patient to a specialist, the physician could be held to the standard of the specialist in the same field [*Seneris v Haas,* 45 Cal 2d 811, 291 P2d 915 (1955)]. This could mean that a higher standard of care could be applied.

For example, suppose a bladder laceration occurs during the performance of a cesarean delivery. Under most circumstances, a fully trained specialist in obstetrics and gynecology can repair this laceration without calling in a consultant. But a more extensive laceration of the bladder or bowel, or a laceration of the ureter, might, depending upon the learning and skill of the physician involved and the circumstances of the case, require a physician more highly skilled in the repair of these complications. This could include, but is not limited to, a urologist, a gynecologic oncologist, or a general surgeon. If the repair is undertaken, however, by a nonspecialist and the patient sustains a causally related injury, the nonspecialist could be held to the standard of one of these specialists. Thus, the underlying rationale for this principle appears to be frequent consultation. More frequent consultation provides a direct benefit to the patient and an indirect one to her primary physician.

INFORMED CONSENT

As patients have sought greater control of their health care, informed consent has assumed a prominent role in the practice of medicine today. One concern among practitioners is not whether informed consent was given but whether the information provided was adequate to allow the patient to make an informed choice.[17] In fields other than obstetrics, the physician provides the information to the patient or, in the case of a minor, to the parent or guardian. In obstetrics, the adequacy of informed consent becomes complicated by the pain of labor, analgesics that can affect the patient's mental state, and the expanding rights of the fetus.[18] It is these complexities that make each patient dependent on her physician to provide sufficient information before undertaking the proposed operation, such as a cesarean, or treatment.

What constitutes adequate patient informed consent can also vary from state to state and according to the circumstances of the case.[7] But there appears to be a common thread. For example, the doctrine of informed consent focuses on the characteristics of the physician–patient relationship.[19] First, knowledge of medicine between the physician and the patient is not the same. Second, a competent adult has the right to decide whether to agree to lawful medical treatment. Third, before submitting to the treatment, the patient has the right to be informed. Fourth, the patient is unlearned in the medical sciences and, as a result, is dependent on her physician to provide her with sufficient information to make an informed choice.

The underlying rationale for the doctrine of informed consent is illustrated in *Cobbs v Grant,* 8 Cal 3d 229, 104 Cal Rptr 505, 502 P2d 1 (1972). In that case, the patient agreed to undergo surgery for a duodenal ulcer. However, the inherent risks associated with the surgical procedure were not discussed with the patient. Following the surgery, the patient sustained internal bleeding and required a splenectomy. A month after the second surgery, the patient was readmitted for a gastric ulcer and underwent a partial gastrectomy. Subsequently, the patient was readmitted for abdominal bleeding due to an abdominal suture dissolving prematurely. At issue in this case was whether the patient had been adequately informed of the risks of surgery.

What must be disclosed? In many respects, the information to be disclosed is that which you or I would want to know if we were considering a proposed medical treatment or surgical procedure. This would include material information so that the patient could make an informed decision. Frequently, the difficult part is deciding what is considered material. Often this decision relates to patient-oriented or professional standards.[20] In a patient-oriented standard, the health care provider would have to consider what a reasonable patient would consider significant. In contrast, the professional standard is directed at what a reasonable health care provider would disclose under the same or similar circumstances.

Under a patient-oriented standard,[20] as illustrated in the California Jury Instruction, *BAJI* 6.11,[21] the patient is entitled to know about any known risk of death or serious illness. At the same time, the disclosure or explanation to the patient should be given in lay terms or at the patient's level of understanding. What if there are lesser risks associated with a proposed procedure or treatment? Under these circumstances, disclosure of lesser risks may depend on whether physicians practicing under the same or similar circumstances would be required to disclose those risks.

But where the procedure is simple and the danger is remote and commonly appreciated to be remote, such as drawing blood or the patient's request not to be informed, there may be no duty to disclose the risks of that procedure.

With respect to cesarean delivery, the patient is generally entitled to be informed of the reason for the cesarean, the risks and potential complications of the procedure, alternative treatment approaches such as external cephalic version or vaginal birth after cesarean, and the consequences if the procedure is not performed and problems of recuperation occur. Equally important is the fact that the performance of a cesarean without the patient's consent [*Mohr v Williams,* 95 Minn 261, 104 NW 2d 523 (1905)] or where the consent is deemed invalid[22] could be considered battery.

Even though informed consent appears to be an infrequently litigated issue today,[7] it is important to understand how these cases might be approached. As noted in Table 39.1, the basic elements of negligence are also involved. But once a duty relationship is established between the physician and the patient, the question becomes whether the physician breached his duty by failing to give sufficient information so that a proposed treatment could be chosen intelligently. This again will depend on the applicable standards—patient oriented or professional.[20] This will frequently focus on whether the physician informed the patient of alternative treatments, the reasonably forseeable risks of each alternative, and the consequences of no treatment. Additionally, if the maternal risk of an alternative treatment had been disclosed, the patient or plaintiff, it seems, would have chosen either no treatment or a different one. Finally, the plaintiff would have to show that she was injured as a result of submitting to treatment. What consequences will follow if the patient has consented to a proposed treatment or operation and the physician has failed to inform the patient adequately? The failure to obtain "such consent is negligence and renders the physician or surgeon subject to liability for any injury [proximately, legally] resulting from the [treatment or operation] if a reasonably prudent person in the patient's position would not have consented to the [treatment or operation] if he had been adequately informed of all the significant perils."[21]

The issue of informed consent is illustrated in the case of *Truman v Thomas.*[17] In that case, Mrs. Truman saw her physician on several occasions between 1964 and 1969. Her physician, however, never obtained a Pap smear, nor did he specifically inform her of the risks involved in a failure to perform this test. He said "You should have a Pap smear," but this was not supported by the medical records. Subsequently, she was diagnosed as having inoperable carcinoma of the cervix and died at age 30. Suit was brought by her dependent children. The finding of the court was that the patient should have been given adequate information regarding the effects of refusing to undergo diagnostic treatment.

The failure to inform the patient of alternative treatment approaches may serve as a basis for medical malpractice claims. For instance, with the resurgence of vaginal birth after cesarean where it has been shown that maternal morbidity and mortality can be significantly reduced,[23] the performance of an elective repeat cesarean delivery without disclosing to the patient the trial of labor alternative would be one example. The same principle might also apply to external cephalic version (Chapter 36) or vaginal breech delivery (Chapter 3). Notwithstanding, the converse, elective cesarean delivery, would also be in keeping with this principle.

The issue of informed consent can also present in a different way. In a California case,[24] a 38-year-old G 3 P 2002 presented to her physician's office at 38 weeks gestation following an uncomplicated prenatal course. At that visit, the physician advised her that she might have a breech. The records contained the following notation: "Breech?" According to the mother, no discussion regarding the risks of a breech presentation or studies to confirm it occurred. Soon after the last visit, her membranes ruptured and she went immediately to the hospital. There the umbilical cord prolapsed, a cesarean delivery was done, and a child with significant neurologic damage was delivered. The informed consent issues focused on the physician's failure to inform the patient of the foreseeable risks and potential complications of a breech presentation in umbilical cord prolapse and its attendant sequelae. At trial, the defense experts maintained that it was a standard of care to wait for labor or spontaneous conversion to vertex. This defense would be considered valid were it not for the fact that the umbilical cord did prolapse before labor started.[24] In keeping with the informed consent doctrine, the patient has a right to be informed of material risks and to make a choice regarding alternative treatment.

FAILURE TO PERFORM A CESAREAN IN A TIMELY MANNER

"Cases frequently are generated by the failure of physicians or staff to recognize and manage immediate or imminent emergencies. Failure to properly assess and react is fertile ground for a negligence claim."[25] But when is it a failure to perform a cesarean in a timely manner? According to the most recent guidelines of the ACOG, any facility that provides obstetrical care should have, as a minimum, a "cesarean delivery capability within 30 minutes."[26] This would imply, therefore, that a decision–incision interval in excess of 30 minutes could constitute a breach in the standard of care. If the decision–incision interval does exceed 30 minutes and the infant is born with a neurologic handicap, should the physician be held liable for those injuries? For this reason, there may be a "fertile ground for a negligence claim,"[25] but it does not necessarily follow that the health care provider proximately caused the injuries. Circumstances may be such that cesarean delivery may not have been technically feasible within the "allotted time."

Moreover, there is a popular misconception that neonatal brain damage is proximately related to the events of labor and is due not to the natural course of events of pregnancy but to the negligent conduct of the attendant physician, nursing staff, or hospital. As suggested by Perkins,[27] "the number of infants injured before labor is highly underestimated [and those infants injured] during labor is highly overestimated." In support of Perkins' assertion, Paul and associates[28] have demonstrated that fetal injuries such as intracranial hemorrhage, myocardial infarction, and meconium aspiration can and do occur prior to the onset of labor. Then what is the role of electronic fetal monitoring? Although "fetal heart rate changes can provide an indicator of hypoxia that precedes neurologic damage,"[29] the fetal heart rate pattern at the onset of labor may be indicative of fetal prelabor injury. As suggested by the 10-year experience with electronic fetal monitoring at Los Angeles County/University of Southern California Medical Center, a major benefit of monitoring is the identification of the fetus at risk of death during labor.[30] This suggests, therefore, that "intrapartum asphyxia may be the result rather than the cause of neurologic abnormality."[31] Moreover, neonatal compromise may represent a continuum rather than a single isolated event that "is not . . . influenced markedly by the circumstances of labor and delivery."[27] This is not to say that an adverse fetal outcome cannot be related to the events of labor or to the conduct of the health care provider, but rather that fetal monitoring is imprecise and cannot reliably predict an adverse fetal outcome[32] and that the failure to perform a cesarean within a specified period of time is not necessarily the cause of the neonatal injuries.

Nevertheless, the physician should make reasonable efforts either to evaluate a patient [*Thomas v Ellis,* 329 Mass 93, 106 NE 2d 687 (1952)] or to begin a cesarean in a timely manner.[8] For example, in *Thomas v Ellis,* the pregnant woman's husband first notified her physician around 11:30 P.M. that she was bleeding heavily from her vagina. At that time, the husband was advised to keep her at home and observe her for approximately 1 hour. About a half hour later, the husband called the physician because there was "more blood all over the blanket, a lot of blood" and the patient had pain. The physician told the husband that it sounded like an abruption. He advised them to go directly to the hospital and stated that he would meet them there. The couple arrived at around 12:30 A.M. The record was unclear as to when the physician arrived, but a cesarean was done about 11:00 A.M. At the time of delivery, an abruption was confirmed and the fetus was dead.

This case illustrates the importance of a timely evaluation and delivery. An earlier evaluation and delivery might have provided a more favorable outcome for the fetus. But because that evalution and delivery were not undertaken earlier, we will never know whether it would have made a difference in this case. However, a timely evaluation is the first step in minimizing the risk of harm.

In the event of acute fetal distress such as an acute, prolonged fetal heart rate deceleration, the timeliness of the cesarean may protect the fetus from neurologic injury or death. With inhouse anesthesia, cesarean delivery can frequently be rapidly achieved. But inhouse anesthesia is not always encountered where obstetrical services are provided. Under these circumstances, cesarean delivery would be necessarily delayed while waiting for anesthesia personnel to come to the hospital.

If anesthesia personnel are not in the hospital, several options are available. One possibility is to attempt to arrest uterine activity with a beta-mimetic such as terbutaline.[33] This would allow intrauterine resuscitation of the fetus and provide additional time for anesthesia support personnel to arrive. If the beta-mimetic is contraindicated, technically not feasible, or unsuccessful, cesarean delivery under local anesthesia, as outlined in Chapter 10, is another option.

In summary, reasonable efforts to evaluate a patient or to perform a cesarean in a timely manner would appear prudent. Whether this will have an effect on the incidence of neonatal injury or death remains to be proven. It should, however, make the ground for a negligence claim less fertile.

FAILURE TO PERFORM A CESAREAN PROPERLY

The failure to perform a procedure, such as the administration of rhogam to an Rh-negative gravida, may give rise to a claim against the physician for maternal or neonatal injuries in a subsequent pregnancy.[34] This concept has been extended to include a host of cases where physicians have been held liable for a child's injuries that resulted from negligence toward the child's mother in a prior pregnancy.[11] This includes the failure to perform a cesarean properly during an earlier pregnancy. In *Bergstreser v Mitchell,* 577 F2d22 (CA8 MO, 1978), the plaintiff had undergone a cesarean in a previous pregnancy. The prior incision, however, was not described in the legal summary. At approximately 30 weeks gestation in a subsequent pregnancy, she sustained a uterine rupture that resulted in an exploratory laparotomy and delivery of the infant. The child suffered brain damage. The plaintiff alleged that the injuries sustained by the infant were due to the negligent performance of the prior cesarean and the failure to inform her of the prior uterine incision.

As outlined in Chapter 14, the various types of uterine incisions and their indications were reviewed. Furthermore, in this era, when vaginal birth after cesarean is becoming an acceptable alternative,[35] it is important to inform the patient of the type of incision performed and its consequences. In addition, reasonable efforts to avoid a cesarean birth or to reduce the necessity for an upper-segment uterine incision with external cephalic version (Chapter 36) would appear prudent. If this is done, the likelihood of liability for a subsequent pregnancy might be lessened.

TABLE 39.2 Considerations When an Instrument Breaks during a Cesarean

Actions prior to breaking of the instrument
Defective instrument
Improper or inappropriate instrument
Actions during breaking of the instrument
Subsequent actions
Removal of fragment
Disclosure

INSTRUMENTS THAT BREAK DURING A CESAREAN

During a cesarean delivery, instruments may break, requiring removal of the fragments, if possible, without injuring the patient. For example, part of a fetal scalp electrode[36] or a portion of the blade for fetal scalp blood sampling[37] may have broken off in the fetal scalp. Similar events can also occur during surgery. During surgery, needles, gloves, catheters, or instruments may break, giving rise to the question of whether the surgeon is liable.[10]

As demonstrated in Table 39.2, several factors are involved in the determination of liability. The attention required goes beyond the mere breaking of the instrument. At a minimum, and as pointed out earlier in this chapter, the patient must suffer some type of injury as a result of the break. The legal procedure, as pointed out by Zitter,[10] will be to determine, if possible, the party responsible for the breaking of the instrument and the injury. This could include a lawsuit against the manufacturer, hospital, or surgeon.

Therefore, whenever an instrument breaks during a cesarean, for example, the focus will be first on the actions prior to the use of the instrument. For example, the broken instrument may have had a design defect or become defective during the manufacturing process. In addition, the instrument may not have been defective during manufacture but may have been altered by the hospital in some way, or the hospital may have supplied it in a defective condition by not replacing it when it showed signs of wear and tear.

The selection of an improper or inappropriate instrument that breaks can also be an important part of the situation. For example, the instrument that broke may not have been the proper one under the circumstances of the case.

For physicians performing cesareans, the critical issues are their conduct during the breaking of the instrument and subsequently. In the former case, attention will center on how the instrument selected was used. For instance, if a scalpel is used and it can be shown that there is no evidence of metal fatigue or defect in the blade, the focus will be on how the surgeon used the blade and whether its use was consistent with the practice of other surgeons in similar locations under similar circumstances. The same

TABLE 39.3 Potential Areas for Medical Malpractice Action When a Foreign Body Is Left in an Abdomen Following a Cesarean

Sponge and instrument count
Disclosure
Consent for removal of foreign body

analysis could also be applied to the insertion of pulmonary artery catheter if the tip breaks off or the suturing a wound if the needle breaks off.

The conduct of the physician and hospital also comes into question after the instrument breaks. The most frequently asked questions are the following: What was done to retrieve the fragment? What was disclosed to the patient? In the former, attention will focus on whether the efforts to retrieve the fragment were reasonable under the circumstances. In most instances, the broken fragment can be safely removed without exposing the patient to an unreasonable risk of harm. But what happens if the fragment cannot be safely removed? Do you leave it alone? That will also depend on the circumstances of the case and the skill of the surgeon. What seems clear is that the patient is entitled to know whether a broken piece of an instrument could not be removed.

In summary, instruments may break during the performance of a cesarean. Once an instrument breaks, the broken fragments should be safely removed. If the fragments cannot be safely removed, full disclosure to the patient is important. Finally, as part of the usual course of practice, these events should be carefully documented in the medical record.

FOREIGN BODIES LEFT IN THE PATIENT FOLLOWING A CESAREAN

Throughout surgical history, numerous objects have been left in the abdomen following surgery. These have included beetles, needles, drains, sponges, surgical instruments, forceps, and a cloth sac.[9] At the time of cesarean, this could also include the fetal scalp electrode. Although foreign bodies may be more frequently left behind during extensive surgery, a needle, sponge, and instrument count is designed to protect against this event. The failure to follow such a procedure could be evidence of negligence [*Bowers v Olch,* 120 Cal App 2d 108, 260 P2d 997 (1953)].

Prior to the performance of a cesarean, a needle and sponge count is done by the surgical scrub nurse and the circulating nurse. Once completed, the results of the count are given audibly. Before the end of the cesarean, none of the sponges, needles, or instruments should leave the operating room. Prior to and after the closure of the peritoneum, the count is done again and the results are given audibly to the surgeons and scrub nurse. The numbers must match.

If the count indicates a missing sponge, needle, or instrument, a search for the missing item is appropriate. The failure to search for a missing item could be evidence of negligence [*Smedra v Stanek,* 187, F2d 892 (CA 10 COLO 1951)]. Fortunately, most items are radiopaque or, in the case of sponges, contain a radiopaque tape. Thus, if manual and visual exploration is unsuccessful, an abdominal x-ray may help locate the missing item.

Reliance on the needle and sponge count alone may not support the claim that a physician exercised due care.[9] For example, in the case of *Key v Caldwell* [39 Cal App 2d 698, 104 P2d 87 (1940)], a laparotomy sponge was left in a patient's abdomen following a cesarean delivery. The needle and sponge count was done and was said to be correct. Testimony demonstrated that the surgeon in this case had the practice of placing a laparotomy sponge in the same location in the abdominal cavity at each cesarean. Although the physician attempted to rebut the allegations, the sponge had nevertheless not been removed.

The *Key* case suggests that the surgeon has an independent duty to determine whether a sponge, for example, has been left behind. Thus, in addition to an accurate needle, sponge, and instrument count, manual and visual exploration of the abdomen would also appear prudent.

As noted before, when an instrument had been broken[10] during a cesarean, reasonable efforts to locate the missing object would also be appropriate. These efforts may be sufficient if the item is not located [*Roark v Peters,* 162 La 111, 110 So 106 (1926)], but the patient is entitled to be informed of the missing object unless there are medical reasons for not informing her.[9]

If an item is discovered to be missing after a cesarean, is consent required to remove it? According to Jones,[9] the operating surgeon can perform a second operative procedure for the purpose of removing a foreign body immediately following the primary procedure without the consent of the patient. If, however, a sponge is found to be missing some time after the cesarean, full disclosure and consent would be appropriate[9] [*Delahunt v Fenton,* 244 Mich 226, 221 NW 168 (1928)].

In summary, needle, sponge, and instrument counts are an important part of a cesarean delivery. In addition, a manual and visual exploration of the abdomen before closure would appear prudent. Moreover, these findings should be documented in the medical records. If it is subsequently determined that an item is missing, the physician should tell the patient and obtain her consent to remove it.

CAPTAIN OF THE SHIP DOCTRINE

The "captain of the ship" doctrine was first stated in the case of *McConnell v Williams* [361 Pa 355, 65 A2d 243 (1949)]. In that case, Mrs. McConnell underwent a cesarean. The cesarean was performed by Dr. Williams, assisted by an intern requested by him. After delivery, the infant was given to the intern to tie the cord and apply silver nitrate to the baby's eyes. According to the facts, the intern applied the appropriate strength silver nitrate once in the left eye and twice in the right eye. Subsequently, it was noted that the right eye was burned and had to be removed. One issue of the case was whether the intern was a temporary employee or agent of the surgeon or an employee of the hospital.

The court considered these questions and found the following, which is excerpted from the opinion[38]:

> And indeed it can readily be understood that in the course of an operation in the operating room of a hospital, and until the surgeon leaves that room at the conclusion of the operation (the "operation" in the present case including the tying of the cord and the insertion of the silver nitrate solution in the infant's eyes) he is in the same complete charge of those who are present and assisting him as is the captain of a ship over all on board, and that such supreme control is indeed essential in view of the high degree of protection to which an anaesthetized, unconscious patient is entitled—a protection which Mrs. McConnell could justly claim in this case by reason of her trust and confidence in, and necessary reliance upon, the surgeon she employed to take care of her and her child when born.
>
> If, then, it be true that defendant had supervisory control and the right to give orders to the intern in regard to the very act in the performance of which the latter was negligent, it would follow, according to the classical test of agency herein before stated, that a jury would be justified in concluding that the temporary relationship between defendant and the intern was that of master and servant, and that consequently defendant was legally liable for the harm caused by any negligence on the part of the intern.

This case illustrates that a physician who exercises control and authority over an intern, as in this case, could be held liable for the negligence of the intern. In a more recent case [*Schultz v Mutch,* 211 Cal Rptr 445 (1985)], the captain of the ship doctrine has been evaluated again, but with nursing personnel.

In that case, Mrs. Schultz presented to the hospital in labor. Shortly after her admission, her membranes ruptured and, due to some question of presentation, she was sent to the x-ray department. In the interim, the defendant physician became involved as primary surgeon in a cesarean delivery of another patient. During this cesarean, the physician exercised control over the nurses in the room and made no inquiries about Mrs. Schultz. Subsequently, fetal distress was diagnosed and Mrs. Schultz underwent a cesarean. A baby boy was delivered severely asphyxiated and, due to the asphyxia, was retarded and quadriplegic.

The court concluded that the captain of the ship doctrine should be followed in this case. The California jury instruction[39] that deals with the liability of surgeons for the negligence of assistants and nurses is as follows:

> Regardless of who employs or pays [a nurse or an assisting surgeon] who takes part in the performance of surgery or services incidental to such surgery, if, while engaged in any such service, [the assisting surgeon or nurse] is under the direction of a certain surgeon in charge, so as to be his temporary servant or agent, any negligence on the part of any such assisting person, occurring while the latter is under the surgeon's direction, is deemed in law to be the negligence of such surgeon.

In summary, when a physician exercises control over a nurse or assistant surgeon during the performance of a cesarean, for example, the physician could be held liable for their negligent conduct.

REFERENCES

1. Cesarean Childbirth (DHHS Pub. No. 82-2067). Report of a Consensus Development. Conference sponsored by the National Institute of Child Health and Human Development, Washington DC, 1980.
2. Rutkow I: Obstetric and gynecologic operations in the United States, 1979 to 1984. *Obstet Gynecol* 67:755, 1986.
3. Shiono PA, McNellis D, Rhoads GS: Reasons for using cesarean 1978–1984. *Obstet Gynecol* 69:696, 1987.
4. Stavish S: Malpractice costs: The pressure for relief mounts. *Med World News* July 25: 1985.
5. Church GJ: Sorry, your policy is cancelled. *Time Magazine*, March 24, 1986.
6. Petitti DB: Maternal mortality and morbidity in cesarean section. *Clin Obstet* 28:763, 1985.
7. Appelbaum PS, Lidz CW, Meisel A: *Informed Consent: Legal Theory and Clinical Practice.* New York, Oxford University Press, 1987.
8. Gee DR: Physician's failure to perform timely cesarean. 19 POF 2d 285 (1979).
9. Jones JL: Malpractice: Liability of physician, surgeon, anesthetist, or dentist for injury resulting from foreign object left in patient. 10 ALR 3d 9 (1966).
10. Zitter JM: Medical malpractice: Instruments breaking in course of surgery or treatment. 20 ALR 45h 1179 (1986).
11. Liability for child's personal injuries or death resulting from tort committed against child's mother before child was conceived. 91 ALR 3d 316 (1979).
12. *McConnell v Williams,* 361 Pa 355, 65 A2d 243 (1949).
13. *Barron's Law Dictionary,* ed 2. 1984, p 309.
14. *Barron's Law Dictionary,* ed 2. 1984, p 237.
15. *Book of Approved Jury Instructions,* ed 7. St Paul, MN, West Publishing Co, 1986.
16. *Standards for Obstetric-Gynecologic Services,* ed 6. Washington, DC, American College of Obstetricians and Gynecologists, 1985.
17. *Truman v Thomas,* 27 Cal 3d 285, 165 Cal Rptr 308, 611 P2d 902 (1980).
18. Kolder VEB, Gallagher J, Parsons MT: Court-ordered obstetrical interventions. *N Engl J Med* 316:1192, 1987.
19. *Cobbs v Grant,* 8 Cal 3d 229, 104 Cal Rptr 505, 502 P2d 1 (1972).
20. Appelbaum PS, Lidz CW, Meisel A: The legal requirements for disclosure and consent: History and current status, in *Informed Consent: Legal Theory and Clinical Practice.* New York, Oxford University Press, 1987, pp 35–65.
21. *Book of Approved Jury Instructions,* St Paul, MN, West Publishing Co, 1986.
22. *Rainer v Community Memorial Hosp,* 18 CA 3d 240, 95 Cal Rptr 901 (1971).
23. Boucher M, Tahilramaney M, Eglinton GS, et al: Maternal morbidity as related to

a trial of labor after previous cesarean delivery: A quantitative analysis. *J Reprod Med* 29:12, 1984.
24. Rubsamen DS: A greater burden for the obstetrician in managing breech deliveries? *13th Professional Liability Newsletter* 11 (October): 1982.
25. Olender JH: Obstetric negligence. *Trial* May: 52, 1984.
26. *Standards for Obstetric-Gynecologic Services,* ed 6. Washington, DC, American College of Obstetricians and Gynecologists, 1985, p 29.
27. Perkins RP: Perspective on perinatal brain damage. *Obstet Gynecol* 69:807, 1987.
28. Paul RH, Yonekura ML, Cantrell CJ, et al: Fetal injury prior to labor: Does it happen? *Am J Obstet Gynecol* 154:1187, 1986.
29. Adamson SK, Myers RE: Late decelerations and brain tolerance of the fetal monkey to asphyxia. *Am J Obstet Gynecol* 128:893, 1977.
30. Yeh SY, Diaz F, Paul RH: Ten year experience of intrapartum fetal monitoring in Los Angeles County/University of Southern California Medical Center. *Am J Obstet Gynecol* 143:496, 1982.
31. Niswander K: Asphyxia in the fetus and cerebral palsy, in Pitkin RM, Zlatnik FJ (eds): *1983 Year Book of Obstetrics and Gynecology.* Chicago, Year Book Medical Publishers, 1983, pp 107–125.
32. Schifrin BS, Dame L: Fetal heart rate patterns—predictor of Apgar score. *JAMA* 219:1322, 1972.
33. Patriarco MS, Viechnicki BM, Hutchinson TA, et al: A study on intrauterine fetal resuscitation with terbutaline. *Am J Obstet Gynecol* 157:384, 1987.
34. *Renslow v Mennonite Hospital,* 67 Ill 2d 348, 10 Ill Dec 484, 367 NE 2d 1250 (1977).
35. Phelan JP, Clark SL, Diaz F, et al: Vaginal birth after cesarean. *Am J Obstet Gynecol* 157:1510, 1987.
36. Thoulon JM, Gonnet C: les accidents de l'electrocardiographie Foetale directe (a propos d'une de l'electrode de scalp). *J Gynecol Obstet Biol Reprod* 7:1257, 1978.
37. Nieburg P, Gross SJ: Breakage of a fetal scalp blade with retention of fragments in the infant's scalp. *Am J Obstet Gynecol* 157:441, 1987.
38. *McConnell v Williams,* 361 Pa 355, 359, 65 A2d 243, 246 (1949).
39. *Book of Approved Jury Instructions,* ed 7. St Paul, MN, West Publishing Co, 1986.

Index

C

D

E